A COMPANION TO SPECIALIST SURGICAL PRACTICE: CORE TOPICS IN GENERAL AND EMERGENCY SURGERY — FOURTH EDITION

A COMPANION TO SPECIALIST SURGICAL PRACTICE: OESOPHAGOGASTRIC SURGERY — FOURTH EDITION

A COMPANION TO SPECIALIST SURGICAL PRACTICE: COLORECTAL SURGERY — FOURTH EDITION

A COMPANION TO SPECIALIST SURGICAL PRACTICE: BREAST SURGERY — FOURTH EDITION
Edited by J. Michael Dixon

A COMPANION TO SPECIALIST SURGICAL PRACTICE

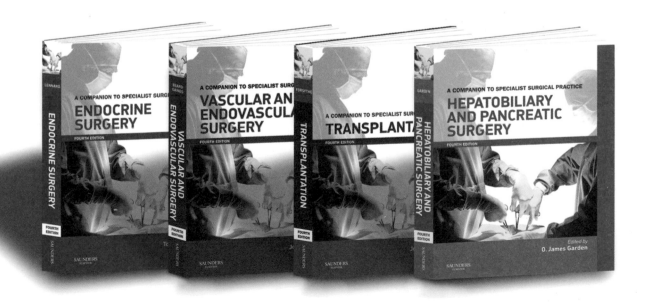

A COMPANION TO SPECIALIST SURGICAL PRACTICE: ENDOCRINE SURGERY — FOURTH EDITION

A COMPANION TO SPECIALIST SURGICAL PRACTICE: VASCULAR AND ENDOVASCULAR SURGERY — FOURTH EDITION

A COMPANION TO SPECIALIST SURGICAL PRACTICE: TRANSPLANTATION — FOURTH EDITION

A COMPANION TO SPECIALIST SURGICAL PRACTICE: HEPATOBILIARY AND PANCREATIC SURGERY — FOURTH EDITION
Edited by O. James Garden

CORE TOPICS IN GENERAL AND EMERGENCY SURGERY

A Companion to Specialist Surgical Practice

Series Editors

O. James Garden
Simon Paterson-Brown

CORE TOPICS IN GENERAL AND EMERGENCY SURGERY

FOURTH EDITION

Edited by

Simon Paterson-Brown

MB BS MPhil MS FRCS(Ed) FRCS(Engl)

Honorary Senior Lecturer
Clinical and Surgical Sciences (Surgery)
University of Edinburgh;
Consultant General and Upper Gastrointestinal Surgeon
Royal Infirmary of Edinburgh
Edinburgh, UK

SAUNDERS

ELSEVIER

Edinburgh   London   New York   Oxford   Philadelphia   St Louis   Sydney   Toronto   2009

SAUNDERS
ELSEVIER

First edition 1997
Second edition 2001
Third edition 2005
Fourth edition 2009

ISBN 9780702030178

British Library Cataloguing in Publication Data
A catalogue record for this book is available from the British Library

Library of Congress Cataloging in Publication Data
A catalog record for this book is available from the Library of Congress

Notice
Knowledge and best practice in this field are constantly changing. As new research and experience broaden our knowledge, changes in practice, treatment and drug therapy may become necessary or appropriate. Readers are advised to check the most current information provided (i) on procedures featured or (ii) by the manufacturer of each product to be administered, to verify the recommended dose or formula, the method and duration of administration, and contraindications. It is the responsibility of the practitioner, relying on their own experience and knowledge of the patient, to make diagnoses, to determine dosages and the best treatment for each individual patient, and to take all appropriate safety precautions. To the fullest extent of the law, neither the Publisher nor the Editors assumes any liability for any injury and/or damage to persons or property arising out of or related to any use of the material contained in this book.

The Publisher

ELSEVIER your source for books, journals and multimedia in the health sciences
www.elsevierhealth.com

Working together to grow libraries in developing countries
www.elsevier.com | www.bookaid.org | www.sabre.org
ELSEVIER   BOOK AID International   Sabre Foundation

The Publisher's policy is to use **paper manufactured from sustainable forests**

Printed in China

Commissioning Editor: Laurence Hunter
Development Editor: Elisabeth Lawrence
Project Manager: Andrew Palfreyman
Text design: Charlotte Murray
Cover Design: Kirsteen Wright
Illustration Manager: Gillian Richards
Illustrators: Martin Woodward and Richard Prime

Contents

Contents

Contributors

Iain D Anderson, BSc, MD, FRCS
Consultant Surgeon
Intestinal Fistula Unit
Salford Royal Hospital NHS Foundation Trust
Manchester, UK

Paul Baskerville, MD, FRCS
Consultant Surgeon and Director of Surgical Practice
King's College Hospital
London, UK

David E. Beck, MD
Chairman, Department of Colon and Rectal Surgery
Ochsner Clinic Foundation
New Orleans, LA, USA

Andrew C. de Beaux, MB, ChB, MD, FRCS
Consultant General and Upper Gastrointestinal
Surgeon
Department of Surgery Royal Infirmary of Edinburgh
Edinburgh, UK

**Kenneth D. Boffard, BSc, MB, BCh, FRCS(Gen Surg),
FRCS(Ed), FRCPS(Glasg), FCS(SA), FACS**
Professor and Clinical Head
Department of Surgery Johannesburg Hospital and
University of the Witwatersrand
Johannesburg, South Africa

Peter Chong, MB, ChB, BSc (Hons), FRCS
Consultant Colorectal Surgeon
Department of Surgery
Western Infirmary
Glasgow, UK

Dafydd A. Davies, MD
Fellow, Paediatric Trauma and Paediatric Surgery
Division of General Surgery
Hospital for Sick Children
Toronto, Ontario, Canada

Euan J. Dickson, MD, FRCS(Glasg)
Consultant Surgeon
West of Scotland Pancreatico-Biliary Unit
Glasgow Royal Infirmary
Glasgow, UK

**Michael Grounds, MD, MB, BS, LRCP,
MRCS, FRCA, DA**
Reader in Intensive Care Medicine
St George's Hospital Medical School;
Consultant in Anaesthesia and Intensive Care
Medicine
St George's Hospital
London, UK

**Steven D. Heys BmedBiol, MD, PhD, FRCS,
FRCS(Ed), FRCS(Glasg)**
Professor of Surgical Oncology
University of Aberdeen;
Honorary Consultant Surgeon
Grampian University Hospitals Trust
Aberdeen, UK

Jacob C. Langer, MD
Professor of Surgery, University of Toronto
Robert M. Filler Chair and Chief, Paediatric General
Surgery
Hospital for Sick Children
Toronto, Ontario, Canada

James Lau, MD
Professor of Surgery
Department of Surgery
Prince of Wales Hospital
Shatin, Hong Kong

Rhona M. Maclean, MB, ChB, FRCP, FRCPath
Consultant Haematologist
Royal Hallamshire Hospital
Sheffield, UK

Colin J. McKay, MB, BS, FRCA
Consultant Surgeon
Regional Upper Gastrointestinal Surgical Unit
Glasgow Royal Infirmary
Glasgow, UK

**B. James Mander, BSc, MS, MB, BS, FRCS,
FRCS(Gen Surg)**
Consultant Colorectal Surgeon
Edinburgh Colorectal Unit
Western General Hospital
Edinburgh, UK

Contributors

Jonathan A. Michaels, MChir, FRCS
Professor of Vascular Surgery
Academic Vascular Unit
Northern General Hospital
Sheffield, UK

Enders Ng, MD
Chief, Upper GI Division
The Chinese University of Hong Kong
Department of Surgery
Prince of Wales Hospital
Shatin, Hong Kong

Rowan W. Parks, MD, FRCSI, FRCS(Ed)
Senior Lecturer in Surgery
University of Edinburgh;
Honorary Consultant Surgeon
Royal Infirmary of Edinburgh
Edinburgh, UK

Hugh M. Paterson, MD, FRCS(Gen Surg)
Clinical Senior Lecturer in Coloproctology
Western General Hospital
Edinburgh, UK

**Simon Paterson-Brown, MB, BS, MPhil, MS,
FRCS(Ed), FRCS(Engl)**
Honorary Senior Lecturer
Clinical and Surgical Sciences (Surgery)
University of Edinburgh;
Consultant General and Upper Gastrointestinal
Surgeon
Royal Infirmary of Edinburgh
Edinburgh, UK

Andrew Rhodes, MB, BS, FRCA, FRCP
Consultant in Anaesthesia and Intensive Care Medicine
Department of Intensive Care Medicine
St George's Hospital
London, UK

Kathryn A. Rigby, MSc, MB, ChB, FRCS
Specialist Registrar in General Surgery
Sheffield Vascular Institute
Northern General Hospital
Sheffield, UK

William G. Simpson, MB, ChB, MRCPath
Consultant in Clinical Biochemistry
and Nutrition Support
Department of Clinical Biochemistry
Grampian University Hospitals Trust
Aberdeen, UK

Charles B. Whitlow, MD
Program Director and Staff Surgeon
Ochsner Clinic Foundation
New Orleans, LA, USA

Series preface

Since the publication of the first edition in 1997, the *Companion to Specialist Surgical Practice* series has aspired to meet the needs of surgeons in higher training and practising consultants who wish contemporary, evidence-based information on the subspecialist areas relevant to their general surgical practice. We have accepted that the series will not necessarily be as comprehensive as some of the larger reference surgical textbooks which, by their very size, may not always be completely up to date at the time of publication. This Fourth Edition aims to bring relevant state-of-the-art specialist information that we and the individual volume editors consider important for the practising subspecialist general surgeon. Where possible, all contributors have attempted to identify evidence-based references to support key recommendations within each chapter.

We remain grateful to the volume editors and all the contributors of this Fourth Edition. Their enthusiasm, commitment and hard work has ensured that a short turnover has been maintained between each of the editions, thereby ensuring as accurate and up-to-date content as possible. We remain grateful for the support and encouragement of Laurence Hunter and Elisabeth Lawrence at Elsevier Ltd. We trust that our aim of providing up-to-date and affordable surgical texts has been met and that all readers, whether in training or in consultant practice, will find this fourth edition an invaluable resource.

O. James Garden MB, ChB, MD, FRCS(Glas), FRCS(Ed), FRCP(Ed), FRACS(Hon), FRCSC(Hon)

Regius Professor of Clinical Surgery, Clinical and Surgical Sciences (Surgery), University of Edinburgh, and Honorary Consultant Surgeon, Royal Infirmary of Edinburgh

Simon Paterson-Brown MB, BS, MPhil, MS, FRCS(Ed), FRCS(Engl)

Honorary Senior Lecturer, Clinical and Surgical Sciences (Surgery), University of Edinburgh, and Consultant General and Upper Gastrointestinal Surgeon, Royal Infirmary of Edinburgh

Editor's preface

Although surgical subspecialisation within the specialty of 'general surgery' has progressed rapidly over the last decade, most general surgeons on call, irrespective as to their subspecialty interest, require a core knowledge in both elective and emergency surgery in order to be able to see and treat undifferentiated referrals and conditions outwith their normal everyday elective 'specialist' practice. This volume of the *Companion to Specialist Surgical Practice* provides the background information on these key areas of 'general surgery' for all practising general surgeons in both the elective and emergency situations. It is the only volume of this series which provides detailed descriptions of evidence-based medicine and how surgical outcomes can be measured, in addition to other important areas common to all of 'general surgical practice'. These include an overview of day case surgery, abdominal hernias, thromboembolic prophylaxis, the management of sepsis and the intensive care patient, the use of scoring systems in patient assessment, and surgical nutrition. This volume should be considered complementary to the other more specialist volumes in the series by including all the emergency areas which remain within the remit of the general surgeon on call. As in everyday practice, there remain emergency patients who, having been resuscitated and a diagnosis made, might be better served by being referred to a colleague or unit with the relevant subspecialist interest. This volume discusses those conditions which the general surgeon might be expected to deal with and, where appropriate, identifies those which might be better managed by a 'specialist'. In these cases the reader will be referred to the relevant specialist volume of this series.

Acknowledgements

I remain grateful to my long-suffering wife and family for their ongoing support and understanding in completing another edition of this volume of *Core Topics in General and Emergency Surgery*. I am also extremely grateful to Elsevier Science for their help and all the other chapter authors for once again (or for the first time) submitting, on time, such high-standard material. The additional workload required in the writing of concise, well-referenced and up-to-date chapters for a book such as this, by busy practising surgeons, should never be underestimated. Once again I would like to acknowledge the help, enthusiasm and friendship of my co-editor of the *Companion to Specialist Surgical Practice* series, James Garden, not only for helping to get this project off the ground in 1995, but for his ongoing support and commitment during these four editions.

Simon Paterson-Brown
Edinburgh

Evidence-based practice in surgery

Critical appraisal for developing evidence-based practice can be obtained from a number of sources, the most reliable being randomised controlled clinical trials, systematic literature reviews, meta-analyses and observational studies. For practical purposes three grades of evidence can be used, analogous to the levels of 'proof' required in a court of law:

1. **Beyond all reasonable doubt.** Such evidence is likely to have arisen from high-quality randomised controlled trials, systematic reviews or high-quality synthesised evidence such as decision analysis, cost-effectiveness analysis or large observational datasets. The studies need to be directly applicable to the population of concern and have clear results. The grade is analogous to burden of proof within a criminal court and may be thought of as corresponding to the usual standard of 'proof' within the medical literature (i.e. $P < 0.05$).

2. **On the balance of probabilities.** In many cases a high-quality review of literature may fail to reach firm conclusions due to conflicting or inconclusive results, trials of poor methodological quality or the lack of evidence in the population to which the guidelines apply. In such cases it may still be possible to make a statement as to the best treatment on the 'balance of probabilities'. This is analogous to the decision in a civil court where all the available evidence will be weighed up and the verdict will depend upon the balance of probabilities.

3. **Not proven.** Insufficient evidence upon which to base a decision, or contradictory evidence.

Depending on the information available, three grades of recommendation can be used:

a. Strong recommendation, which should be followed unless there are compelling reasons to act otherwise.
b. A recommendation based on evidence of effectiveness, but where there may be other factors to take into account in decision-making, for example the user of the guidelines may be expected to take into account patient preferences, local facilities, local audit results or available resources.

c. A recommendation made where there is no adequate evidence as to the most effective practice, although there may be reasons for making a recommendation in order to minimise cost or reduce the chance of error through a locally agreed protocol.

Strong recommendation

Evidence where a conclusion can be reached 'beyond all reasonable doubt' and therefore where a **strong recommendation** can be given.

This will normally be based on evidence levels:

- Ia. Meta-analysis of randomised controlled trials
- Ib. Evidence from at least one randomised controlled trial
- IIa. Evidence from at least one controlled study without randomisation
- IIb. Evidence from at least one other type of quasi-experimental study.

Expert opinion

Evidence where a conclusion might be reached 'on the balance of probabilities' and where there may be other factors involved which influence the recommendation given. This will normally be based on less conclusive evidence than that represented by scalpel icons:

- III. Evidence from non-experimental descriptive studies, such as comparative studies and case–control studies
- IV. Evidence from expert committee reports or opinions or clinical experience of respected authorities, or both.

Evidence in each chapter of this volume which is associated with either a strong recommendation or expert opinion is annotated in the text by either a **scalpel** or **pen-nib** icon as shown above. References associated with **scalpel** evidence will be highlighted in the reference lists, along with a short summary of the paper's conclusions where applicable.

1

Evidence-based practice in surgery

Kathryn A. Rigby
Jonathan A. Michaels

Introduction

Evidence-based medicine is the conscientious, explicit and judicious use of current best evidence in making decisions about the care of individual patients. The practice of evidence-based medicine means integrating individual clinical expertise with the best external clinical evidence from systematic research.[1]

The concept of evidence-based medicine (EBM) was introduced in the 19th century but has only flourished in the last few decades. Historically, its application to surgical practice can be traced back to the likes of John Hunter and the American Ernest Amory Codman, who both recognised the need for research into surgical outcomes in an attempt to improve patient care.

In mid-19th century Paris, Pierre-Charles-Alexander Louis used statistics to measure the effectiveness of bloodletting, the results of which helped put an end to the practice of leeching. Ernest A. Codman began work as a surgeon in 1895 in Massachusetts. His main area of interest was the shoulder and he became a leading expert in this topic as well as being instrumental in the founding of the American College of Surgeons. He developed his 'End Result Idea', a notion that all hospitals should follow up every patient it treats 'long enough to determine whether or not its treatment is successful and if not, why not?' in order to prevent similar failures in the future.[2] Codman also developed the first registry of bone sarcomas.

In the UK, one of the most important advocates of EBM was Archie Cochrane. His experiences in the prisoner of war camps, where he conducted trials in the use of yeast supplements to treat nutritional oedema, influenced his belief in reliable and scientifically proven medical treatment. In 1972 he published his book *Effectiveness and Efficiency*. Cochrane advocated the use of the randomised controlled trial (RCT) as the gold standard in the research of all medical treatment and, where possible, systematic reviews of these trials. One of the first systematic reviews of RCTs was of the use of corticosteroid therapy to improve lung function in threatened premature birth. Although RCTs had been conducted in this area, the message of the results was not clear from the individual studies, until the review overwhelmingly showed that corticosteroids reduced both neonatal morbidity and mortality. Had a systematic review been conducted earlier, then the lives of many babies could have been saved, as the review clearly showed that this inexpensive treatment reduced the chance of these babies dying from complications of immaturity by 30–50%.[3] In 1992, as part of the UK National Health Service (NHS) Research and Development (R&D) Programme, the Cochrane Collaboration was founded.

Subsequently, in 1995, the first centre for EBM in the UK was established at the Nuffield Department of Clinical Medicine, University of Oxford. The driving force behind this was the American David Sackett, who had moved to a new Chair in Clinical Epidemiology in 1994 from McMaster University in Canada, where he had pioneered self-directed teaching for medical students.

From these roots, the interest in EBM has exploded. The Cochrane Collaboration is rapidly expanding, with review groups in many fields of medicine and surgery. EBM is not limited only to hospital-based medicine but is increasingly seen in nursing, general practice and dentistry, and there are many new evidence-based journals appearing.

While clinical experience is invaluable, the rapidly changing world of medicine means that clinicians must keep abreast of new advances and, where appropriate, integrate research findings into everyday clinical practice. Neither research nor clinical experience alone is enough to ensure high-quality patient care; the two must complement each other. Sackett et al. identified five steps that should become part of day-to-day practice and in which a competent practitioner should be proficient:[4]

1. to convert information needs into answerable questions;
2. to be able to track down efficiently the best evidence with which to answer them (be it evidence from clinical examination, the diagnostic laboratory, research evidence or other sources);
3. to be able to appraise that evidence critically for its validity and usefulness;
4. to apply the results of this appraisal in clinical practice;
5. to evaluate performance.

This chapter discusses the steps that are necessary to identify, critically appraise and combine evidence, to incorporate the findings into clinical guidance, and to implement and audit any necessary changes in order to move towards EBM in surgery. Many of the organisations and information sources that are relevant to EBM are specific to a particular setting. Therefore, the emphasis in this chapter is on the health services within the UK, although there are comparable arrangements and bodies in many other countries. Links to a number of these are given in the Internet resources described at the end of the chapter.

The need for evidence-based medicine

In 1991, there was still a widely held belief that only a small proportion of medical interventions were supported by solid scientific evidence.[5] Jonathan Ellis and colleagues, on behalf of the Nuffield Department of Clinical Medicine, conducted a review of treatments given to 109 patients on a medical ward.[6] The treatments were then examined to assess the degree of evidence supporting their use. The authors concluded that 82% of these treatments were in fact evidence based. However, they did

suggest that similar studies should be conducted in other specialties. The importance of evidence-based health care in the NHS was formally acknowledged in two government papers, *The new NHS*[7] and *A first class service*.[8] These led to the development of the National Service Frameworks and the National Institute of Clinical Excellence (NICE).

In surgery there is a limited body of evidence from high-quality RCTs. For an RCT to be ethical there needs to be a clinical equipoise. That is to say, there needs to be a sufficient level of uncertainty about an intervention before a trial can be considered. For example, it would be unethical to conduct an RCT in the use of burr holes for extradural haematomas, because the observational data alone are so overwhelming as to the high degree of effectiveness that it would be unethical to deny someone a burr hole to prove the point.

Many surgeons feel unhappy with having to explain to a patient that there is clinical uncertainty about a treatment, as patients have historically put their trust in surgeons' hands. This reluctance to perform RCTs and the belief that they would be difficult to carry out has led to practices that are poorly supported by high-quality evidence. For example, there is widespread use of radical prostatectomy to treat localised prostatic carcinoma in the USA, despite a distinct lack of evidence to support this procedure.[9]

New technologies in surgery may be driven into widespread use by market forces, patients' expectations and clinicians' desire to improve treatment options. For example, with laparoscopic surgery, many assumed that it must be 'better' because it made smaller holes, there was less pain involved and therefore patients left hospital sooner. It was only after many hospitals had instituted its use that concerns were raised about its real benefits and the adequacy of training in the new technology. In 1996, a group of surgeons from Sheffield published a randomised, prospective, single-blind study that compared small-incision open cholecystectomy with laparoscopic cholecystectomy.[10] They demonstrated that in their hands the laparosopic technique offered no real benefit over a mini-cholecystectomy in terms of the postoperative recovery period, hospital stay and time off work, but it took longer to perform and was more expensive.[10] There were, however, other factors which may have influenced the results from this study, including surgeon experience, and mini-cholecystectomy has not been widely adopted.

The MRC Laparoscopic Groin and Hernia Trial Group undertook a large multicentre randomised comparison between laparoscopic and open repair of groin hernias.[11] The results demonstrated that the laparoscopic procedure was associated with an earlier return to activities and less groin pain 1 year after surgery but it was also associated with more serious surgical complications, an increased recurrence rate and a higher cost to the health service. They suggested that laparoscopic hernia surgery should be confined to specialist surgical centres. NICE have since published guidelines which suggest that it is patients with bilateral or recurrent hernias who benefit most from laparoscopic repair.

Some would argue that surgery, unlike drug trials, is operator dependent and that operating experience and skill can affect the outcome of an RCT and cite this as a reason for not undertaking surgical trials. Although operator factors can introduce bias into a trial, the North American Symptomatic Carotid Endarterectomy Trial has shown that such problems can largely be overcome through appropriate trial design.[12] Only surgeons who had been fully trained in the procedure, and who already had a proven low complication rate, were accepted as participants in the trial.

These examples illustrate a clear need for high-quality research to be undertaken into any new technology to assess both its efficacy and its cost-effectiveness before it is introduced into the healthcare system.

However, concerns have been raised about EBM. Sceptics have suggested that it may undermine clinical experience and instinct and replace it with 'cookbook medicine' or that it may ignore the elements of basic medical training such as history-taking, physical examination, laboratory investigations and a sound grounding in pathophysiology. Another fear is that purchasers and managers will use it as a means to cut costs and manage budgets.

Nevertheless, EBM can formalise our everyday procedures and highlight problems. It can provide answers by ensuring that the best use is made of existing evidence or it can identify areas in which new research is needed. Although it has a role in assessing the cost-effectiveness of an intervention, it is not a substitute for rationing and often results in practice that, despite being more cost-effective, has greater overall cost.[13]

The process of evidence-based medicine

EBM requires a structured approach to ensure that clinical interventions are based upon best available evidence. The first stage is always to pose a clinically relevant question for which an answer is required. Such a question should be clear, specific, important and answerable. One way of formulating questions is to think of them as having three key elements:

- the population to whom the question applies;
- the intervention of interest (and any other interventions with which it is to be compared);
- the outcome of interest.

Therefore the question 'What is the best treatment for cholecystitis?' needs to be much more clearly formulated if an adequate, evidence-based approach is to be used. A much better question would be 'For adult patients admitted to hospital with acute cholecystitis (the **population**), does early open cholecystectomy, laparoscopic cholecystectomy or best medical management (the **interventions**) produce the lowest mortality, morbidity and total length of stay in hospital (the **outcomes**)?' Even this may require more refinement to define further the exact interventions and outcomes of interest.

Once such a question has been clearly defined, a number of further stages of the process can follow:

1. Relevant sources of information must be searched to identify all available literature that will help in answering the question.
2. Published trials must be critically appraised to assess whether they possess internal and external validity in answering the question posed (**internal validity** is where the effects within the study are free from bias and confounding; **external validity** is where the effects within the study apply outside the study and the results are therefore generalisable to the population in question).
3. Where relevant, a systematic review and meta-analysis may be required to provide a clear answer from a number of disparate sources.
4. The answers to the question need to be incorporated into clinical practice through the use of guidelines or through other methods of implementation.
5. Adherence to 'best practice' needs to be monitored through audit, and the process needs to be kept under review in order to take account of new evidence or clinical developments.

Sources of evidence

Once a question has been formulated, the next step in undertaking EBM is the identification of all the relevant evidence. The first line for most practitioners is the use of journals. Many clinicians will subscribe to specific journals in their own specialist area and have access to many others through local libraries. However, the vast increase in the number of such publications makes it impossible for an individual to access or read all the relevant papers, even in a highly specialised area.

There has been a huge expansion in the resources that are available for identifying relevant material from other publications, including indexing and abstracting services such as MEDLINE (computerised database compiled by the US National Library of Medicine) and EMBASE. The rapid technological developments of the past few years have made these widely available through Internet services, electronic publications and online databases.

There is also a rapidly expanding set of journals and other services that provide access to selected, appraised and combined results from primary information sources.

As a result, the information sources that provide the evidence to support EBM are vast and include the following:

- Media – journals, online databases, CD-ROMs and the Internet.
- Independent organisations – research bodies and the pharmaceutical industry.
- Health services – purchasers and providers at local, regional and national levels.
- Academic units.

Some of these are described in more detail below and the Appendix to this chapter provides a list of contact details for further information.

Journals

The following are a selection of journals that act as secondary sources, identifying and reviewing other research that is felt to be of key importance to evidence-based practice.

Evidence-based Medicine

First launched in October 1995, *Evidence-based Medicine* is a collaboration between the American College of Physicians (ACP) and the *British Medical Journal* (BMJ) Publishing Group. The ACP Journal Club, begun in 1991, has a large editorial team who survey a vast array of journals, identifying clinically relevant research articles and summarising the essential information. This consequently allows the reader to keep up with the latest advances in clinical practice. *Evidence-based Medicine* is the UK version of the journal and covers a wide range of specialties, and also contains extracts from the American journal, systematic reviews from the Cochrane Collaboration and reports from the York Centre for Reviews and Dissemination.

Evidence-based Nursing

Evidence-based Nursing follows similar lines to *Evidence-based Medicine*, but contains articles more relevant to the nursing field. It is edited by the Royal College of Nursing and the BMJ Publishing Group.

Evidence-based Health Care

Evidence-based Health Care and Public Health is published by Elsevier (Harcourt). It also contains abstracts and articles about evidence-based issues and results of systematic reviews, etc.

Evidence-based Mental Health

The BMJ Publishing Group publishes *Evidence-based Mental Health* in collaboration with the Health Information Research Unit, Department of Clinical Epidemiology and Biostatistics, McMaster University and the NHS R&D programme. It is a quarterly publication that identifies and appraises clinically relevant research.

Internet resources

The Internet is becoming an increasingly useful source of medical information and evidence. Details of Internet addresses for many of the sources referred to below are given in the Appendix to this chapter, although this is a rapidly progressing and changing area. There are many journals and databases that are available either free or through subscription. For example, MEDLINE can be searched free of charge through the National Library of Medicine, PubMed service; the *British Medical Journal* and the *Journal of the American Medical Association* (*JAMA*) are freely available in an electronic form. This medium also provides a number of advantages over printed material, including ease of searching, hyperlinks to other sources, access to additional supporting materials or raw data and the provision of discussion groups. There are, however, potential problems with the Internet in that there is no quality control and much of the available material is of dubious quality or published by those with particular commercial or other interests.

The OMNI (Organising Medical Networked Information) Project is a useful Internet-based resource that provides UK and worldwide coverage of resources in medicine, biosciences and health management. It has now been incorporated into the INTUTE health and life sciences group. It has been created by a network of UK universities and partners such as the Wellcome Trust.

Academic units

Cochrane Collaboration

As described above, the British epidemiologist who inspired this collaboration realised that in order to make informed decisions about healthcare, reliable evidence must be accessible and kept up to date with any new evidence. It was felt that failure to achieve this might result in important developments in healthcare being overlooked. This was to be a key aspect in providing the best healthcare possible for patients. It was also hoped that by making clear the result of an intervention then work would not be duplicated.

The Cochrane library is the electronic publication of the Cochrane Collaboration and it includes several databases:

- The Cochrane Database of Systematic Reviews contains systematic reviews and protocols of reviews in preparation. These are regularly updated and there are facilities for comments and criticisms along with authors' responses.
- The Cochrane Controlled Trials Register is the largest database of RCTs. Information about trials is obtained from several sources including searches of other databases and hand searching of medical journals. It includes many RCTs not currently listed in databases such as MEDLINE or EMBASE.
- The Database of Abstracts of Reviews of Effectiveness (DARE) contains abstracts of reviews that have been critically appraised by peer reviewers at the NHS Centre for Reviews and Dissemination (CRD) and by others.
- The Cochrane Review Methodology Database is a bibliography of articles on the science of research synthesis.
- The Reviewers' Handbook includes information on the science of reviewing research and details of the review groups. It is also available in hard copy.[14]

The Cochrane library is regularly updated and amended as new evidence is acquired. It is distributed on disk, CD-ROM and the Internet.[3] To allow the results of the reviews to be widely used no one contributor has exclusive copyright of the review.

Centre for Evidence-based Medicine

The Centre for Evidence-based Medicine is a collaboration between the Health Authority, the NHS R&D programme, medical academia and the hospitals of Oxford. Its chief remit is to promote EBM and the practice of it in healthcare. It runs workshops and courses in both the practice and teaching of EBM. The members are also involved in RCTs and work closely with the Cochrane Collaboration Methods Working Group.

Review Body for Interventional Procedures (ReBIP)

This is a joint venture between the Health Services Research Unit at Sheffield University and Aberdeen University. It works under the auspices of NICE's Interventional Procedures Programme (IPP). When there is doubt about the safety and efficacy of any procedure they will be commissioned to provide a systematic review or gather additional data.

NHS agencies

NHS Centre for Reviews and Dissemination (CRD)

The CRD was established in January 1994 at the University of York; it is funded by the NHS Executive and the health departments of Scotland, Wales and Northern Ireland but is independent of the government. Its sister organisation is the UK Cochrane Centre and they were both set up to support the NHS R&D programme. The CRD concentrates specifically on areas of priority to the NHS. It is designed to raise the standards of reviews within the NHS and to encourage research, by working with healthcare professionals. There are two databases that it maintains:

- the NHS Economic Evaluation Database contains mainly abstracts of economic evaluations of healthcare interventions and assesses the quality of the studies, stating any practical implications to the NHS;
- DARE (see above).

NHS Health Technology Assessment programme

The Health Technology Assessment (HTA) is the NHS-funded research programme that commissions research into high-priority areas. This includes many systematic reviews and primary research in key areas. The programme publishes details of ongoing HTA projects and monographs of completed research.

Critical appraisal

 This is the process by which we assess the evidence presented to us in a paper. We need to be critical of it in terms of its validity and clinical applicability.

From reading the literature, it is evident that there may be many trials on the same subject, which may all draw different conclusions. Which one should be believed and allowed to influence clinical practice? We owe a duty to our patients to be able to assess accurately all the available information and judge each paper on its own merits before changing our clinical practice accordingly.

Randomised control trials

The RCT is a comparative evaluation in which the interventions being compared are allocated to the units being studied purely by chance. It is the 'gold standard' method of comparing the effectiveness of different interventions.[15] Randomisation is the only way to allow valid inferences of cause and effect,[16] and no other study design can potentially protect as well against bias.

Unfortunately, not all clinical trials are done well, and even fewer are well reported. Their results may therefore be confusing and misleading, and it is necessary to consider several elements of a trial's design, conduct and conclusions before accepting the results. The first requirement is that there must be sufficient detail available to make such an assessment.

It has become clear that there is a need for the presentation of clinical trials to be standardised. Two groups published proposals for standardisation in 1994 and the subsequent joint publication became known as the CONSORT statement (Table 1.1).[17,18]

 The CONSORT statement listed items that should be included in any trial report, along with a flow chart identifying the patient's progress through the trial.[17,18]

Table 1.1 • CONSORT statement regarding the standardisation of presentation of randomised controlled clinical trials.

Sections	Content
Title	Identify the study as a randomised trial
Abstract	Use a structured format
Introduction	State prospectively defined hypothesis, clinical objectives and planned subgroup or covariant analyses
Methods	
Protocol	Planned study population described together with inclusion and exclusion criteria
	Planned interventions and their timing
	Primary and secondary outcome measure(s), the minimum important difference(s) and indicate how the target sample size was projected
	Rationale and methods of statistical analyses
	Prospectively defined stopping rules
Assignment	Unit of randomisation
	Method used to generate the allocation schedule
	Method of allocation concealment
	Method to separate the generator from the executor of the assignment
Masking (blinding)	Mechanism for masking (e.g. capsules, tablets)
	Similarity of treatment characteristics
	Allocation schedule control
	Evidence for successful blinding among participants, person doing intervention, outcome assessors and data analysts
Results	
Participant flow	Provide a trial profile, showing patient flow, numbers and follow-up, timing of randomisation assignments, interventions and measurements for each randomised group
Analysis	State estimated effect of intervention on primary and secondary outcome measures including a point estimate and confidence interval
	State absolute numbers when feasible
	Present summary data and appropriate statistics in sufficient detail to permit alternative analyses and replication
	Describe prognostic variables by treatment group and attempt to adjust for them
	Describe protocol deviations and the reasons why
Discussion	State specific interpretation of study findings, sources of bias and imprecision and discuss internal and external validity
	State general interpretation of the data in light of the totality of available evidence

Many journals now encourage authors to submit a copy of the CONSORT statement relating to their paper (e.g. *British Medical Journal, Journal of the American Medical Association, Lancet*).[18] A similar checklist has been proposed for the reporting of observational studies (cohort, case–control and cross-sectional). This is called the Strengthening the Reporting of Observational Studies in Epidemiology (STROBE) statement.[19] The QUORUM statement is a similar checklist that has been developed to improve the quality of reporting relating to systematic reviews of RCTs.[20]

The STROBE statement provides a recommended checklist for the reporting of observational studies[19] and the QUORUM statement provides similar recommendations for systemic reviews of RCTs.[20]

The Critical Appraisal Skills Programme (CASP) is a UK-based project designed to develop appraisal skills about effectiveness. It provides half-day workshops and has developed appraisal frameworks based on 10 or 11 questions for RCTs, qualitative research and systematic reviews.

Assuming that the relevant information is available, critical appraisal is required to ensure that the methodology of the trial is such that it will minimise effects on outcome other than true treatment effects, i.e. those owing to **chance, bias** and **confounding**:

- Chance – random variation, leading to imprecision.
- Bias – systematic variation leading to inaccuracy.
- Confounding – systematic variation resulting from the existence of extraneous factors that affect the outcome and have distributions that are not taken into account, leading to bias and invalid inferences.

All good study designs will reduce the effects of chance, eliminate bias and take confounding into account. This requires consideration of many aspects of trial design, including methods of randomisation, blinding and masking, analysis methods and sample size. It also requires the reviewer to consider aspects such as sponsorship and vested interests that may introduce sources of bias. Discussion of methodology for the critical appraisal of RCTs and other forms of study is readily available elsewhere.[21]

Systematic literature reviews

A systematic review is an overview of primary studies carried out to an exhaustive, defined and repeatable protocol.

There has been an explosion in the published medical literature, with over two million articles a year published in 20 000 journals. The task of keeping up with new advances in medical research has become quite overwhelming. We have also seen that the results of trials in the same subject may be contradictory, and that the underlying message can be masked. Systematic reviews are designed to search out meticulously all relevant studies on a subject, evaluate the quality of each study and assimilate the information to produce a balanced and unbiased conclusion.[22]

One advantage of a systematic review with a meta-analysis over a traditional subjective narrative review is that by synthesising the results of many smaller studies, the original lack of statistical power of each study may be overcome by cumulative size, and any treatment effect is more clearly demonstrated. This, in turn, can lead to a reduction in delay between research advances and clinical implementation. For example, it has been demonstrated that if the original studies done on the use of anticoagulants after myocardial infarction had been reviewed, their benefits would have been apparent much earlier.[23,24] It is obviously essential that both the benefit or any harm caused by an intervention becomes apparent as soon as possible.

Unfortunately, as in reported trials, not all reviews are as rigorously researched and synthesised as one would hope and are open to similar pitfalls as RCTs. The Cochrane Collaboration has sought to rectify this and has worked upon refining the methods used for systematic reviews. It has consequently produced some of the most reliable and useful reviews and its methods have been widely adopted by other reviewers. The Cochrane Collaboration advises that each review must be based on an explicit protocol, which sets out the objectives and methods so that a second party could reproduce the review at a later date if required.

Because of the increasing importance of systematic reviews as a method of providing the evidence base for a variety of clinical activities, the methods are discussed in some detail below. There are several key elements in producing a systematic review.

1. Develop a protocol for a clearly defined question

Within a protocol:

- the objectives of the review of the RCTs must be stated;
- eligibility criteria must be included (e.g. relevant patient groups, types of intervention and trial design);
- appropriate outcome measures should be defined.

In the Cochrane Collaboration, each systematic review is preceded by a published protocol that is subjected to a process of peer review. This helps to ensure high quality, avoids duplication of effort and is designed to reduce bias by setting standards for inclusion criteria before the results from identified studies have been assessed.

2. Literature search

All published and unpublished material should be sought. This includes examining studies in non-English journals, grey literature, conference reports, company reports (drug companies can hold a lot of vital information from their own research) and any personal contacts, for personal studies or information. The details of the search methodology and search terms used should be specified in order to make the review reproducible and allow readers to repeat the search to identify further relevant information published after the review. The most frequently used initial source of information is MEDLINE but this does have limitations. It only indexes about one-third of all medical articles that exist in libraries (over 10 million in total),[25] and an average search by a regular user would only yield about one-fifth of the trials that can be identified by more rigorous techniques for literature searching.[26] It also has a bias towards articles published in English. Other electronic and indexed databases should also be searched, but often the only way to ensure that the maximum number of relevant trials are found, wherever published and in whatever language, is to hand search the journals. This is one of the tasks of the Cochrane Collaboration through a database maintained at the Baltimore Cochrane Centre.

One must also be aware, however, that there is a potential for 'publication bias': trials that are more likely to get published are those with a positive result rather than a negative or no-effect result,[27] and these are more likely to be cited in other articles.[28]

3. Evaluating the studies

Each trial should be assessed to see if it meets the inclusion criteria set out in the protocol (eligibility). If it meets the required standards, then the trial is subjected to a critical appraisal, ideally by two independent reviewers to ascertain its validity, relevance and reliability. Any exclusions should be reported and justified; if there is missing information from the published article, it may be necessary to attempt to contact the author of the primary research. Reviewers should also, if possible, be 'blinded' to the authors and journals of publication, etc. in order to minimise any personal bias.

The Cochrane reviewers are assisted in all these tasks by instructions in the Cochrane Handbook[14] and through workshops at the Cochrane Centres.[29]

4. Synthesis of the results

Once the studies have been graded according to quality and relevance, their results may be combined in an interpretative or a statistical fashion. It must be decided if it is appropriate to combine some studies and which comparisons to make. Subgroup or sensitivity analyses may also be appropriate. The statistical analysis is called a meta-analysis and is discussed below.

5. Discussion

The review should be summarised. The aims, methods and reported results should be discussed and the following issues considered:

- quality of the studies;
- possible sources of heterogeneity (reasons for inconsistency between studies, e.g. patient selection, methods of randomisation, duration of follow-up or differences in statistical analysis);
- bias;
- chance;
- applicability of the findings.

As with any study, a review can be done badly, and the reader must critically appraise a review to assess its quality. Systematic errors may be introduced by omitting some relevant studies, by selection bias (such as excluding foreign language journals) or by including inappropriate studies (such as those considering different patient groups or irrelevant outcomes). Despite all precautions, the findings of a systematic review may differ from those of a large-scale, high-quality RCT. This will be discussed below in relation to meta-analysis.

Meta-analysis

A meta-analysis is a specific statistical strategy for assembling the results of several studies into a single estimate, which may be incorporated into a systematic literature review.[30]

Here we must make the distinction that the term 'meta-analysis' refers to the statistical techniques used to combine the results of several studies and is not synonymous with systematic review, as it is sometimes used.

A common problem in clinical trials is that the results are not clear-cut, either because of size or because of the design of the trial. The systematic review is designed to eliminate some of these problems and give appropriate weightings to the best- and worst-quality studies, regardless of size. Meta-analysis is the statistical tool used to combine the results and give 'power' to the estimates of effect.

Meta-analyses use a variety of statistical techniques according to the type of data being analysed (dichotomous, continuous or individual patient data),[14] and there are two main models used to analyse the results: the fixed-effect model (logistic regression, Mantel–Haenszel test and Peto's method) and the random-effect model. The major concern with fixed-effect methods is that they assume no clinical heterogeneity between the individual trials, and this may be unrealistic.[31] The random-effect method takes into consideration random variation and clinical heterogeneity between trials. In the presentation of meta-analysis, a consistent scale should be chosen for measuring treatment effects and to cope with the possible large scale of difference in proportions, risk ratios or odds ratios that can be used.

Heterogeneity

Trials can have many different components[21] and therefore a meta-analysis is only valid if the trials that it seeks to summarise are homogeneous: you cannot add apples and oranges.[32] If trials are not

comparable and any heterogeneity is ignored, the analysis can produce misleading results.

Figure 1.1 shows an example of this from a meta-analysis of 19 RCTs investigating the use of endoscopic sclerotherapy to reduce mortality from oesophageal varices in the primary treatment of cirrhotic patients.[33] Each trial is represented by a 'point estimate' of the difference between the groups, and a horizontal line showing the 95% confidence interval (CI). If the line does not cross the line of no effect, then there is a 95% chance that there is a real difference between the groups. It can be seen that in this case the trials are not homogeneous as some of the lower limits of the CIs are above the highest limits of CIs in other trials. Such a lack of homogeneity may have a variety of causes, relating to clinical heterogeneity (differences in patient mix, setting, etc.) or differences in methods. The degree of statistical heterogeneity can be measured to see if it is greater than is compatible with the play of chance.[34] Such a statistical tool may lack statistical power;

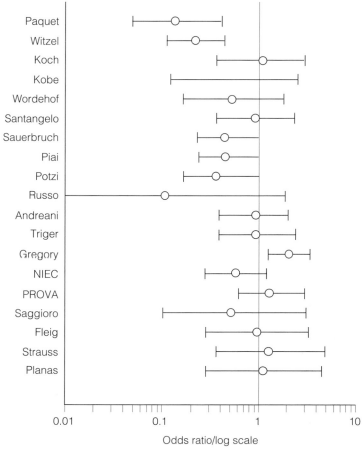

Figure 1.1 • An example of a meta-analysis of 19 randomised controlled trials investigating the use of endoscopic sclerotherapy to reduce mortality from oesophageal varices in the primary treatment of cirrhotic patients. Reproduced from Chalmer I, Altman DG. Systematic reviews. London: BMJ Publishing, 1995; p. 119. With permission from Blackwell Publishing Ltd.

consequently results that do not show significant heterogeneity do not necessarily mean that the trials are truly homogeneous and one must look beyond them to assess the degree of heterogeneity.

'Meta-analysis is on the strongest ground when the methods employed in the primary studies are sufficiently similar that any differences in their results are due to the play of chance.'[30]

Views on the usefulness of meta-analyses are divided. On the one hand, they may provide conclusions that could not be reached from other trials because of the small numbers involved. However, on the other hand, they have some limitations and cannot produce a single simple answer to all complex clinical problems. They may give misleading results if used inappropriately where there is a biased body of literature or clinical or methodological heterogeneity. If used with caution, however, they may be a useful tool in providing information to help in decision-making.

Figure 1.2 shows a funnel plot of a meta-analysis relating to the use of magnesium following myocardial infarction.[35] The result of each study in the analysis is represented by a circle plotting the odds ratio (with the vertical line being at 1, the 'line of no effect') against the trial size. The diamond represents the overall results of the meta-analysis with its pooled data from all the smaller studies shown. This study[36] was published in 1993 and showed that it was beneficial and safe to give intravenous magnesium in patients with acute myocardial infarction. The majority of the studies involved show a positive effect of the treatment, as does the meta-analysis. However, the results from this study were contradicted in 1995 by ISIS-4, a very large RCT involving 58 050 patients.[37] It had three arms, in one of which intravenous magnesium was given to patients suspected of an acute myocardial infarction. The results are marked on the funnel plot and show that there is no clear benefit for this treatment, contrary to the results of the earlier meta-analysis.

Some would say that this is one of the major problems with using statistical synthesis. An alternative viewpoint is that it is an example of the importance of ensuring that the material fed into a meta-analysis from a systematic review is researched and critically appraised to the highest possible standard. Explanations for the contradictory findings in this review have been given as:[32,35]

- publication bias, since only trials with positive results were included (see funnel plot);

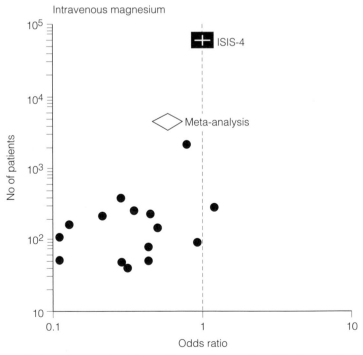

Figure 1.2 • A funnel plot of a meta-analysis relating to the use of magnesium following myocardial infarction. Points indicate values from small and medium-sized trials; the diamond is the combined odds ratio with 95% confidence interval from the meta-analysis of these trials and the square is that for a mega trial. Reproduced from Egger M, Smith GD. Misleading meta-analysis. Br Med J 1995; 310:752–4. With permission from the BMJ Publishing Group Ltd.

- methodological weakness in the small trials;
- clinical heterogeneity.

Clinical guidelines

 Clinical guidelines are systematically developed statements to assist practitioner and patient decisions about appropriate healthcare for specific clinical circumstances.[38]

EBM is increasingly advocated in healthcare, and evidence-based guidelines are being developed in many areas of primary healthcare such as asthma,[39] stable angina[40] and vascular disease.[41] Over 2000 guidelines or protocols have been developed from audit programmes in the UK alone. An observational study in general practice has also shown that recommendations which are evidence based are more widely adopted than those which are not.[42] The UK Department of Health has also endorsed the policy of using evidence-based guidelines.[43]

Guidelines may have a number of different purposes:

- to provide an answer to a specific clinical question using evidence-based methods;
- to aid a clinician in decision-making;
- to standardise aspects of care throughout the country, providing improved equality of access to services and enabling easier comparisons to be made for audit and professional assessment (a reduction in medical practice variation);
- to help to make the most cost-effective use of limited resources;
- to facilitate education of patients and healthcare professionals.

For clinical policies to be evidence-based and clinically useful, there must be a balance between the strengths and limitations of relevant research and the practical realities of the healthcare and clinical settings.[44]

There are, however, commonly expressed concerns about the use of guidelines:

- There is a worry that the evidence used may be spurious or not relevant, especially in areas where there is a paucity of published evidence.
- Guidelines may not be applicable to every patient and are therefore only useful in treating diseases and not patients.
- Clinicians may feel that they take away their autonomy in decision-making.

- A standardised clinical approach may risk suffocating any clinical flair and innovation.
- There may be geographic or demographic limitations to the applicability of guidelines; for instance, a policy developed for use in a city district may not be transferable to a rural area.

The effectiveness of a guideline depends on three areas, as identified by Grimshaw and Russell:[45]

1. How and where the guidelines are produced (development strategy) – at a local, regional or national level or by a group internal or external to the area.
2. How the guidelines have been disseminated, e.g. a specific education package, group work, publication in a journal or a mailed leaflet.
3. How the guidelines are implemented (put into use).

In the UK, there are a number of bodies that produce guidelines and summaries of evidence-based advice.

The National Institute for Clinical Excellence (NICE)

NICE is a special health authority formed on 1 April 1999 by the UK government. The board comprises executive and non-executive members. It is designed to work with the NHS in appraising healthcare interventions and offering guidance on the best treatment methods for patients. It assesses all the evidence on the clinical benefit of an intervention, including quality of life, mortality and cost-effectiveness. It will then decide using this information if the intervention should be recommended to the NHS.

Scottish Intercollegiate Guidelines Network (SIGN)

The SIGN was formed in 1993. Its objective is to improve the effectiveness and efficiency of clinical care for patients in Scotland by developing, publishing and disseminating guidelines that identify and promote good clinical practice. SIGN is a network of clinicians and healthcare professionals including representatives from all the UK Royal Medical Colleges as well as from nursing, pharmacy, dentistry and professions allied to medicine. Patients' views are represented on SIGN through the Scottish Association of Health Councils. SIGN works closely with other national groups and government agencies working in the NHS in Scotland. The SIGN Secretariat is based at the Royal College of Physicians of Edinburgh and to date they have produced over 80 guidelines.

Royal colleges

The Royal College of Surgeons of England has produced guidelines on topics such as:

- management of head injuries;
- management of groin hernias in adults;
- management of gastroscopy;
- management of ankle fractures.

Effective healthcare bulletins

Effective healthcare bulletins have been commissioned by the UK Department of Health to provide an overall summary of the clinical and cost-effectiveness of healthcare interventions.

Effective Practice and Organisation of Care (EPOC)

EPOC is a subgroup of the Cochrane Collaboration that reviews and summarises research about the use of guidelines.

Guidelines also need to be critically appraised and a framework has been developed by Cluzeau et al. to do this.[46] It uses 37 questions to appraise three different areas of a clinical guideline:

1. rigour of development;
2. content and context;
3. application.

Integrated care pathways (ICPs)

ICPs are known by a number of names, including integrated care plans, collaborative care plans, critical care pathways and clinical algorithms. ICPs are a development of clinical practice guidelines and have emerged over recent years as a strategy for delivering consistent high-quality care for a range of diagnostic groups or procedures. They are usually multidisciplinary, patient-focused pathways of care that provide a framework for the management of a clinical condition or procedure and are based upon best available evidence.

The advantage of ICPs over most conventional guidelines is that they provide a complete package of protocols relating to the likely events for all healthcare personnel involved with the patient during a single episode of care. By covering each possible contingency with advice based upon best evidence, they provide a means of both identifying and implementing optimum practice.

Grading the evidence

There is a traditional hierarchy of evidence, which lists the primary studies in order of perceived scientific merit. This allows one to give an appropriate level of significance to each type of study and is useful when weighing up the evidence in order to make a clinical decision. One version of the hierarchy is given in Box 1.1.[21] It must be remembered, however, that this is only a rough guide and that one needs to assess each study on its own merits. Although a meta-analysis comes above an RCT in the hierarchy, a good-quality RCT is far better than a poorly performed meta-analysis. Similarly, a seriously flawed RCT may not merit the same degree of importance as a well-designed cohort study. Checklists have been published that may assist in assessing the methodological quality of each type of study.[21]

Similar checklists are available for systematic reviews.[21,47,48] As already discussed, the preparation of a systematic review is a complex process involving a number of steps, each of which is open to bias and inaccuracies that can distort the results. Such lists can be used as a guide when preparing a review as well as in assessing one. One checklist used to assess the validity of a review does so by identifying potential sources of bias in each step (Table 1.2).[49]

It is hoped that the results of a systematic review will be precise, valid and statistically powerful in order to provide the highest quality information on which to base clinical decisions or to produce clinical guidelines. The strength of the evidence provided by a study also needs to be assessed before making any clinical recommendations. A grading system is required to specify the levels of evidence, and several have previously been reported (e.g. those of the Antithrombotic Therapy Consensus Conference[50] or that shown in Table 1.3.

The grading of evidence and recommendations within textbooks, clinical guidelines or ICPs should allow users easily to identify those elements of

Box 1.1 • Hierarchy of evidence

1. Systematic reviews and meta-analyses
2. Randomised controlled trials with definitive results (the results are clinically significant)
3. Randomised controlled trials with non-definitive results (the results have a point estimate that suggests a clinically significant effect)
4. Cohort studies
5. Case–control studies
6. Cross-sectional studies
7. Case reports

From Greenhalgh T. How to read a paper: the basics of evidence based medicine. London: BMJ Publications, 1997; Vol. xvii, p. 196. With permission from the BMJ Publishing Group Ltd.

Table 1.2 • Checklist for assessing sources of bias and methods of protecting against bias

Source	Check
Problem formulation	Is the question clearly focused?
Study identification	Is the search for relevant studies thorough?
Study selection	Are the inclusion criteria appropriate?
Appraisal of the studies	Is the validity of the studies included adequately assessed?
Data collection	Is missing information obtained from investigators?
Data synthesis	How sensitive are the results to changes in the way the review is done?
Interpretation of results	Do the conclusions flow from the evidence that is reviewed? Are recommendations linked to the strength of the evidence?
	Are judgements about preferences (values) explicit?
	If there is 'no evidence of effect', is care taken not to interpret this as 'evidence of no effect'?
	Are subgroup analyses interpreted cautiously?

From Oxman A. Checklists for review articles. Br Med J 1994; 309:648–51. With permission from the BMJ Publishing Group Ltd.

Table 1.3 • Agency for Health Care Policy and Research grading system for evidence and recommendations

Category	Description
Evidence	
Ia	Evidence from meta-analysis of randomised controlled trials
Ib	Evidence from at least one randomised controlled trial
IIa	Evidence from at least one controlled study without randomisation
IIb	Evidence from at least one other type of quasi-experimental study
III	Evidence from non-experimental descriptive studies, such as comparative studies and case–control studies
IV	Evidence from expert committee reports or opinions or clinical experience of respected authorities, or both
Recommendation strength	
A	Directly based on category I evidence
B	Directly based on category II evidence or extrapolated recommendation from category I evidence
C	Directly based on category III evidence or extrapolated recommendation from category I or II evidence
D	Directly based on category IV evidence or extrapolated recommendation from category I, II or III evidence

From Hadorn DC, Baker D, Hodges JS et al. Rating the quality of evidence for clinical practice guidelines. J Clin Epidemiol 1996; 49:749–54. With permission from Elsevier.

evidence that may be subject to interpretation or modification in the light of new published data or local information. It should identify those aspects of recommendations that are less securely based upon evidence and therefore may appropriately be modified in the light of patient preferences or local circumstances. This raises different issues to the grading of evidence for critical appraisal and for systematic reviews.

In 1979, the Canadian Task Force on the Periodic Health Examination was one of the first groups to propose grading the strength of recommendations.[51] Since then there have been several published systems for rating the quality of evidence, although most were not designed specifically to be translated into guideline development. The Agency for Health Care Policy and Research has published such a system, although this body considered that its level of classification may be too complex to allow clinical practice guideline development.[52] Nevertheless, the Agency advocated evidence-linked guideline development, requiring the explicit linkage of recommendations to the quality of the supporting evidence. The Centre for Evidence-based Medicine has developed a more comprehensive grading system, which incorporates dimensions such as prognosis, diagnosis and economic analysis.[53]

These systems are complex; for textbooks, care pathways and guidelines, such grading systems need to be clear and easily understood by the relevant audience as well as taking into account all the different forms of evidence that may be appropriate to such documents.

Determining strength of evidence

There are three main factors that need to be taken into account in determining the strength of evidence:

- the type and quality of the reported study;
- the robustness of the findings;
- the applicability of the study to the population or subgroup to which the guidelines are directed.

Type and quality of study

Meta-analyses, systematic reviews and RCTs are generally considered to be the highest quality evidence that is available. However, in some situations these may not be appropriate or feasible. Recommendations may depend upon evidence from other kinds of study, such as observational studies of epidemiology or natural history, or synthesised evidence, such as decision analyses and cost-effectiveness modelling.

For each type of evidence, there are sets of criteria as to the methodological quality, and descriptions of techniques for critical appraisal are widely available.[21] Inevitably, there is some degree of subjectivity in determining whether particular flaws or a lack of suitable information invalidates an individual study.

Robustness of findings

The strength of evidence from a published study would depend not only upon the type and quality of a particular study but also upon the magnitude of any differences and the homogeneity of results. High-quality research may report findings with wide confidence intervals, conflicting results or contradictory findings for different outcome measures or patient subgroups. Conversely, sensitivity analysis within a cost-effectiveness or decision analysis may indicate that uncertainty regarding the exact value of a particular parameter does not detract from the strength of the conclusion.

Applicability

Strong evidence in a set of guidelines must be wholly applicable to the situation in which the guidelines are to be used. For example, a finding from high-quality research based upon a hospital population may provide good evidence for guidelines intended for a similar setting but a lower quality of evidence for guidelines intended for primary care.

Grading system for evidence

The following is a simple pragmatic grading system for the strength of a statement of evidence, which will be used to grade the evidence in this book (and the others in the Companion series). Details of the definitions are given in Table 1.4. For practical purposes, only the following three grades are required, which are analogous to the levels of proof required in a court of law:

I. **'Beyond reasonable doubt'**. Analogous to the burden of proof required in a criminal court case and may be thought of as corresponding to the usual standard of 'proof' within the medical literature (i.e. $P < 0.05$).

II. **'On the balance of probabilities'**. In many cases, a high-quality review of literature may fail to reach firm conclusions because of conflicting evidence or inconclusive results, trials of poor methodological quality or the lack of evidence in the population to which the guidelines apply. Where such strong evidence does not exist, it may still be possible to make a statement as to the 'best' treatment on the 'balance of probabilities'. This is analogous to the decision in a civil court where all the available evidence will be weighed up and a verdict will depend upon the balance of probabilities.

III. **'Unproven'**. Where the above levels of proof do not exist.

All evidence-based guidelines require regular review because of the constant stream of new information that becomes available. In some areas, there is more rapid development and the emergence of new evidence; in these instances, relevant reference will be made to ongoing trials or systematic reviews in progress.

Grading of recommendations

Although recommendations should be based upon the evidence presented, it is necessary to grade the strength of recommendation separately from the evidence. For example, the lack of evidence regarding an expensive new technology may lead to a strong recommendation that it should only be undertaken as part of an adequately regulated clinical trial. Conversely, strong evidence for the effectiveness of a treatment may not lead to a strong recommendation for use if the magnitude of the benefit is small and the treatment very costly.

Table 1.4 • Grading of evidence and recommendations

Category	Description
Evidence	
I	'Beyond reasonable doubt'. Evidence from high-quality randomised controlled trials, systematic reviews, high-quality synthesised evidence, such as decision analyses, cost-effectiveness analyses or large observational datasets, which is directly applicable to the population of concern and has clear results
II	'On the balance of probabilities'. Evidence of 'best practice' from a high-quality review of literature, which fails to reach the highest standard of 'proof' because of heterogeneity, questionable trial methodology or lack of evidence in a relevant population
III	'Unproven'. Insufficient evidence upon which to base a decision or contradictory evidence
Recommendations	
A	A strong recommendation, which should be followed unless there are compelling reasons against to act otherwise
B	Recommendations based on evidence of effectiveness that may need interpretation in the light of other factors (e.g. patient preferences, local facilities, local audit results or available resources)
C	Recommendation where there is inadequate evidence on effectiveness but pragmatic or financial reasons to institute an agreed policy
Other considerations	
	The evidence should be presented as clear and brief points, with reference to original source material
	Individual evidence requiring early review should be identified with reference to known sources of work in progress

The following grades of recommendations are suggested and details of the definition are given in Table 1.4:

A. A strong recommendation, which should be followed.
B. A recommendation using evidence of effectiveness, but where there may be other factors to take into account in the decision-making process.
C. A recommendation where evidence as to the most effective practice is not adequate, but there may be reasons for making the recommendations in order to minimise cost or reduce the chance of error through a locally agreed protocol.

Implementation of evidence-based medicine

Healthcare professionals have always sought evidence on which to base their clinical practice. Unfortunately, the evidence has not always been available, reliable or explicit, and when it was available it has not been implemented immediately. James Lancaster in 1601 showed that lemon juice was effective in the treatment of scurvy, and in 1747 James Lind repeated the experiment. The British Navy did not utilise this information until 1795 and the Merchant Navy not until 1865. When implementation of research findings are delayed, ultimately the people who suffer are the patients.

A number of different groups of people may need to be committed to the changes before they can take place with a degree of success. These include:

• healthcare professionals (doctors, nurses, etc.);
• healthcare providers and purchasers;
• researchers;
• patients and the public;
• government (local, regional and national).

Each of these groups has a different set of priorities. To ensure that their own requirements are met by the proposal, negotiation is required, which takes time. There are many potential barriers to the implementation of recommendations, and clinicians may become so embroiled in tradition and dogma that they are resistant to change. They may lack knowledge of new developments or the time and resources to keep up to date with the published literature. Lack of training in a new technology, such as laparoscopic surgery or interventional radiology, may thwart their use, even when shown to be effective. Researchers may become detached from the practicalities of clinical practice and the needs of the health service and concentrate on inappropriate questions or produce impractical guidelines. Managers are subject to changes in the political climate and can easily be driven by policies and budgets. The resources available to them may be limited and not allow for the purchase of new technology, and even potentially cost-saving developments may not be introduced because of the difficulties in releasing the savings from elsewhere in the service.

Patients and the general public can also influence the development of the healthcare offered. They are susceptible to the persuasion of the mass media and may demand the implementation of 'miracle cures' or fashionable investigations or treatments. Such interventions may not be practical or of any proven benefit. They can also determine the success or failure of a particular treatment. For instance, a treatment may be physically or morally unacceptable, or there may be poor compliance, especially with preventative measures such as diets, smoking cessation or exercise. All these aspects can lead to a delay in the implementation of research findings.

Potential ways of improving this situation include the following:

- Provision of easy and convenient access to summaries of the best evidence, electronic databases, systematic reviews and journals in a clinical setting.
- Development of better disease management systems through mechanisms such as clinical guidelines, ICPs and electronic reminders.
- Implementation of computerised decision-support systems.
- Improvement of educational programmes – practitioners must be regularly and actively appraised of new evidence rather than relying on the practitioner seeking it out; passive dissemination of evidence is ineffective.
- More effective systems to encourage patients to adhere to treatment and general healthcare advice; the information must be clear, concise, correct and actively distributed.

There is a gap between research and practice, and there is a need for evidence about the effectiveness of different methods of implementing changes in clinical practice. The NHS Central R&D Committee set up an advisory group to look into this problem and identified 20 priorities for evaluation, as shown in Box 1.2.[54]

An EPOC review has examined the different methods of implementing evidence-based healthcare and classified them into three broad groups:[55]

- consistently effective – educational visits and interactive meetings;
- sometimes effective – audit and feedback;
- little or no effect – printed guideline distribution.

Box 1.2 • Priority areas for evaluation in the methods of implementation of the findings of research: recommendations of the advisory group to the NHS Central Research and Development Committee

1. Influence of source and presentation of evidence on its uptake by healthcare professionals and others
2. Principal sources of information on healthcare effectiveness used by clinicians
3. Management of uncertainty and communications of risk by clinicians
4. Roles for health service users in implementing research findings
5. Why some clinicians but not others change their practice in response to research findings
6. Role of commissioning in securing change in clinical practice
7. Professional, managerial, organisational and commercial factors associated with securing change in clinical practice, with particular focus on trusts and primary care providers
8. Interventions directed at clinical and medical directors and directors of nursing trusts to promote evidence-based care
9. Local research implementation and development projects
10. Effectiveness and cost-effectiveness of audit and feedback to promote implementation of research findings
11. Educational strategies for continuing professional development to promote the implementation of research findings
12. Effectiveness and cost-effectiveness of teaching critical appraisal skills to clinicians, patients/users, purchasers and providers to promote uptake of research findings
13. Role of undergraduate training in promoting the uptake of research findings
14. Impact of clinical practice guidelines in disciplines other than medicine
15. Effectiveness and cost-effectiveness of reminder and decision support systems to implement research findings
16. Role of the media in promoting uptake of research findings
17. Impact of professional and managerial change agents (including educational outreach visits and local opinion leaders) in implementing research findings
18. Effect of evidence-based practice on general health policy measures
19. Impact of national guidelines to promote clinical effectiveness
20. Use of research-based evidence by policy-makers

From NHS Central Research and Development Committee. Methods to promote the implementation of research findings in the NHS: priorities for evaluation: report to the NHS Central Research and Development Committee. London: Department of Health, 1995. © Crown copyright 2008. Reproduced under the terms of the Click-Use Licence.

Several groups have looked at implementing evidence-based practice, such as grommet use in glue ear and steroids in preterm delivery:

- PACE (Promoting Action on Clinical Effectiveness);[56]
- PLIP (Purchaser Led Implementation Projects);[57]
- GriPP (Getting Research into Practice and Purchasing).[58]

Successful implementation of research findings into practice appears to be due to a multipronged approach and the UK National Association of Health Authorities and Trusts (NAHAT) has produced an action checklist in order to facilitate this process.[59]

It must be remembered, however, that EBM is not the sole preserve of experts or clinicians. The research, dissemination and implementation of clinical and economic evaluations have wide-reaching repercussions for the health service. Managers are under increasing pressure to be effective both clinically and for costs and are accountable at local, regional and national levels. They need to be actively involved and understand the process. As with all interactions between elements in the health service, there must be collaboration, the ultimate goal being an improvement in patient care.

Audit

Audit is the systematic critical analysis of the quality of medical care, including the procedures used for diagnosis and treatment, the use of resources, and the resulting outcome and quality of life for the patient.[60]

The Department of Health has set out policy documents that outline the development and role of audit in today's healthcare system.[60,61] Everyone involved in the healthcare process has a responsibility to conduct audit and to assess the quality of care that they provide. In 1996, Donabedian categorised three important elements in the delivery of healthcare:[62]

- Structure – this relates to physical resources available, e.g. the number of theatres, hospital beds and nurses, etc.

- Process – this refers to the management of the patient, e.g. procedures carried out, drugs used, care delivered, etc.
- Outcome – this refers to the result of the intervention, e.g. the amount of time off work, incidence of complications, morbidity and length of stay.

Audit is a dynamic cyclical process (an audit loop) in which standards are defined and data are collected against these standards (**Fig. 1.3**). The results are then analysed and if there are any variances, proposals for change are developed to address the needs. These changes are then implemented and the quality of care reassessed. This closes the audit loop and the procedure begins again. The key to effective audit is that the loop must begin with the development of evidence-based standards. Any success in changing care to meet proposed standards is unlikely to produce more effective clinical care if such standards are set in an arbitrary way. The Royal College of Surgeons of England has published its own guidelines on clinical audit in surgical practice.[63]

One result of the drive to implement audit in the UK was the development in 1993 of a National Confidential Enquiry into Perioperative Deaths (NCEPOD). This is an ongoing national audit and has produced a series of reports and recommendations based upon a peer review process. The process has a high rate of participation and reports and recommendations have resulted in a number of changes in practice. For example, there has been a dramatic reduction in out-of-hours operating following recommendations suggesting that much of this was unsafe and unnecessary.

Figure 1.3 • The audit loop.

Key points

- The formulation of clear and answerable questions is a key element of EBM in surgery.
- Identification of all the relevant evidence is required.
- Critical appraisal of the evidence is necessary.
- Synthesis of information from multiple sources needs to provide a clear message through systematic review and/or meta-analysis.
- Findings should be implemented through mechanisms such as the use of clinical guidelines and ICPs.
- Monitoring through audit is necessary to ensure continuing adherence to best practice.
- Regular review to incorporate new evidence or take account of clinical developments should be carried out.
- Throughout this book and the other volumes in this series, an attempt will be made to take an evidence-based approach. This will include the identification of high-quality evidence from RCTs and systematic reviews, underlining key statements and recommendations relating to clinical practice. All clinicians have a duty to ensure that they act in accordance with current 'best evidence' in order to give patients the highest chance of favourable outcomes and make the best use of limited healthcare resources.

References

1. Sackett D, Rosenberg WMC, Muirgray JA et al. Evidence based medicine: what it is and what it isn't. Br Med J 1996; 312:71–2.

2. Kaska S, Weinstein JN. Historical perspective. Ernest Amory Codman, 1869–1940. A pioneer of evidence-based medicine: the end result idea. Spine 1998; 23:629–33.

3. Cochrane Collaboration. The Cochrane Collaboration: preparing, maintaining and disseminating systematic reviews of the effects of health care. Oxford: Cochrane Centre, 1999.

4. Sackett D, Richardson WS, Rosenberg W. Evidence-based medicine: how to practice and teach EBM. New York: Churchill Livingstone, 1997.

5. Smith R. Where is the wisdom? Br Med J 1991; 303:798–9.

6. Ellis J, Mulligan I, Rowe J et al. Inpatient general medicine is evidence based. Lancet 1995; 346:407–10.

7. Department of Health. The new NHS: modern, dependable. London: Department of Health, 1997.

8. Department of Health. A first class service. London: Department of Health, 1998.

9. Wilt T, Brawer MK. The Prostate Cancer Intervention Versus Observation Trial: a randomized trial comparing radical prostatectomy versus expectant management for the treatment of clinically localized prostate cancer. J Urol 1994; 152:1910–14.

10. Majeed A, Troy G, Nicholl JP et al. Randomised, prospective, single-blind comparison of laparoscopic versus small-incision cholecystectomy. Lancet 1996; 347:989–94.

11. Anon. Laparoscopic versus open repair of groin hernia: a randomised comparison. The MRC Laparoscopic Groin Hernia Trial Group. Lancet 1999; 354:185–90.

12. Anon. Beneficial effect of carotid endarterectomy in symptomatic patients with high-grade carotid stenosis. North American Symptomatic Carotid Endarterectomy Trial Collaborators. N Engl J Med 1991; 325:445–53.

13. Hunter D. Rationing and evidence-based medicine. J Eval Clin Pract 1996; 2:5–8.

14. Clarke M, Oxman AD (eds). Cochrane reviewers handbook 4.1.1 (updated December 2000). Oxford: Cochrane Library, 2000; Issue 4.

15. Guyatt G, Sackett DL, Sinclair JC et al. for the Evidence-Based Medicine Working Group. Users' guides to the medical literature. IX. A method for grading health care recommendations. JAMA 1995; 274:1800–4.

16. Altman D. Randomisation. Br Med J 1991; 302:1481–2.

17. Begg C, Cho M, Eastwood S et al. Improving the quality of reports on randomized controlled trials. Recommendations of the CONSORT Study Group [not in English]. Rev Esp Salvd Publa 1998; 72:5–11.

18. Altman D. Better reporting of randomised controlled trials: the CONSORT statement. Br Med J 1996; 313:570–1.

19. Elm E, Altman DG, Egger M et al. Strengthening the reporting of observational studies in epidemiology (STROBE) statement: guidelines for reporting observational studies. Br Med J 2007; 335:806–8.

20. Mober D, Cook DJ, Eastwood S et al. for the QUORUM Group. Improving the quality of reports of meta-analyses of randomized controlled trials: the QUORUM statement. Lancet 1999; 354:1896–900.

21. Greenhalgh T. How to read a paper: the basics of evidence based medicine. London: British Medical Journal Publications, 1997; Vol. xvii, p. 196.

22. Mulrow C. Rationale for systematic reviews. Br Med J 1994; 309:597–9.

23. Lau J, Schmid CH, Chalmers TC. Cumulative meta-analysis of clinical trials builds evidence for exemplary medical care. J Clin Epidemiol 1995; 48:45–57; discussion 59–60.

24. Antman E, Lau J, Kupelnick B et al. A comparison of results of meta-analyses of randomized control trials and recommendations of clinical experts. Treatments for myocardial infarction. JAMA 1992; 268:240–8.

25. Greenhalgh T. How to read a paper. The MEDLINE database. Br Med J 1997; 315:180–3.

26. Adams C, Power A, Fredrick K et al. An investigation of the adequacy of MEDLINE searches for randomized controlled trials (RCTs) of the effects of mental health care. Psychol Med 1994; 24:741–8.

27. Easterbrook P, Berlin JA, Gopalan R et al. Publication bias in clinical research. Lancet 1991; 337:867–72.

28. Gotzsche P. Reference bias in reports of drug trials. Br Med J (Clin Res) 1987; 295:654–6.

29. Fullerton-Smith I. How members of the Cochrane Collaboration prepare and maintain systematic reviews of the effects of health care. Evidence-Based Med 1995; 1:7–8.

30. Sackett D. Clinical epidemiology: a basic science for clinical medicine, 2nd edn. Boston: Little Brown, 1991; Vol. xviii, p. 441.

31. Thompson S, Pocock, S. Can meta-analysis be trusted. Lancet 1991; 338:1127–30.

32. Anon. Magnesium, myocardial infarction, meta-analysis and mega-trials. Drug Ther Bull 1995; 33:25–7.

33. Chalmers I, Altman DG. Systematic reviews. London: BMJ Publications, 1995; p. 50.

34. DerSimonian R, Laird N. Meta-analysis in clinical trials. Controlled Clin Trials 1986; 7:177–88.

35. Egger M, Smith GD. Misleading meta analysis. Br Med J 1995; 310:752–4.

36. Yusuf S, Teo K, Woods K. Intravenous magnesium in acute myocardial infarction. An effective, safe, simple, and inexpensive intervention. Circulation 1993; 87:2043–6.

37. Anon. ISIS-4: a randomised factorial trial assessing early oral captopril, oral mononitrate, and intravenous magnesium sulphate in 58050 patients with suspected acute myocardial infarction. ISIS-4 (Fourth International Study of Infarct Survival) Collaborative Group. Lancet 1995; 345:669–85.

38. Field MJ, Lohr KN. Clinical practice guidelines: directions for a new program. Washington, DC: National Academy Press, 1990; p. 160.

39. Anon. North of England evidence based guidelines development project: summary version of evidence based guideline for the primary care management in adults. North of England Asthma Guideline Development Group. Br Med J 1996; 312:762–6.

40. Anon. North of England evidence based guidelines development project: summary version of evidence based guideline for the primary care management angina. North of England Stable Angina Guideline Development Group. Br Med J 1996; 312:827–32.

41. Eccles M, Freemantle N, Mason J. North of England evidence based guideline development project: guideline on the use of aspirin as secondary prophylaxis for vascular disease in primary care. North of England Aspirin Guideline Development Group. Br Med J 1998; 316:1303–9.

42. Grol R, Dalhuijsen J, Thomas S. Attributes of clinical guidelines that influence use of guidelines in general practice: observational study. Br Med J 1998; 317:858–61.

43. NHS Executive. Clinical guidelines: using clinical guidelines to improve patient care within the NHS. Leeds: NHS Executive, 1996.

44. Gray J, Haynes RD, Sackett DL et al. Transferring evidence from health care research into medical practice. 3. Developing evidence-based clinical policy. Evid-Based Med 1997; 2:36–8.

45. Grimshaw J, Russell IT. Effect of clinical guidelines on medical practice: a systematic review of rigorous evaluations. Lancet 1993; 342:1317–22.

46. Cluzeau F, Littlejohns P, Grimshaw J et al. Appraisal instrument for clinical guidelines. London: St George's Hospital Medical School, 1997.

47. Oxman A, Guyatt GH. Guidelines for reading literature reviews. Can Med Assoc J 1988; 138:697–703.

48. Oxman A, Cook DJ, Guyatt GH. Users' guides to the medical literature. VI. How to use an overview. Evidence-Based Medicine Working Group. JAMA 1994; 272:1367–71.

49. Oxman A. Checklists for review articles. Br Med J 1994; 309:648–51.

50. Cook D, Guyatt GH, Laupacis A et al. Rules of evidence and clinical recommendations on the use of antithrombotic agents. Chest 1992; 102:3055–115.

51. Canadian Task Force on the Periodic Health Examination. The periodic health examination. Can Med Assoc J 1979; 121:1193–254.

52. Hadorn DC, Baker D, Hodges JS et al. Rating the quality of evidence for clinical practice guidelines. J Clin Epidemiol 1996; 49:749–54.

53. Centre for Evidence-based Medicine. Levels of evidence and grades of recommendations. Oxford: Centre for Evidence-based Medicine, 1999; http://cebmjr2.ox.ac.uk/docs/levels.html

54. NHS Central Research and Development Committee. Methods to promote the implementation of research findings in the NHS: priorities for evaluation: report to the NHS Central Research and Development Committee. London: Department of Health, 1995.

55. Bero L, Grilli R, Grimshaw J et al. Closing the gap between research and practice. In: Haines A, Donald A (eds) Getting research findings into practice. London: BMJ Publications, 1998; pp. 27–35.

56. Dunning M, Abi-aad G, Gilbert G et al. Turning evidence into everyday practice. London: King's Fund, 1999.

57. Evans D, Haines A. Implementing evidence based changes in healthcare. Oxford: Radcliffe Medical Press, 2000.

58. Dunning M, McQuay H, Milne R. Getting a GRiPP. Health Serv J 1994; 104:18–20.

59. Appleby JWK, Ham C. Acting on the evidence: a review of clinical effectiveness: sources of information, dissemination, and implementation. Birmingham: National Association of Health Authorities and Trusts, 1995.

60. Department of Health. Clinical audit: meeting and improving standards in health care. London: Department of Health, 1998; p. 14.

61. Department of Health. The evolution of clinical audit. Heywood: Health Publications Unit, 1994.

62. Donabedian A. Evaluating the quality of care. Millbank Memorial Federation of Quality 1996; 3:166–203.

63. Royal College of Surgeons of England. Clinical audit in surgical practice. London: Royal College of Surgeons of England, 1995.

Appendix

Possible sources of further information, useful Internet sites and contact addresses

The details below provide references to a number of sources of information, particularly those accessible through the Internet. It must be remembered that there are rapid changes in the material available online and Internet addresses are liable to change. Several of these sources provide extensive links to other sites. In particular, the ScHARR site 'Netting the Evidence' (see below) provides an extensive and regularly updated list of other useful sites.

Organisations specialising in evidence-based practice, systematic reviews, etc

Aggressive Research Intelligence Facility (ARIF)
http://www.arif.bham.ac.uk

CASP (Critical Appraisal Skills Programme)
http://www.phru.nhs.uk/Pages/PHD/CASP.htm

Centre for Evidence-based Child Health
http://www.ich.ucl.ac.uk/ich/academicunits/Centre_for_evidence_based_child_health/Homepage

Centre for Evidence-based Medicine, Department of Primary Care, Old Road Campus, Headington, Oxford OX3 7LF; Tel. 01865 289337
http://www.cebm.net

Centre for Evidence-based Mental Health
http://www.pyschiatry.ox.ac.uk/cebmh

Centre for Evidence-based Nursing
http://www.york.ac.uk/healthsciences/centres/evidence/cebn.htm

Department of Health R&D Strategy Home Page
http://www.dh.gov.uk/Policyandguidance/Researchanddevelopment/index.htm

McMaster University
http://www.mcmaster.ca

NIHR Health Technology Assessment Programme
http://www.hta.nhsweb.nhs.uk/

NHS Centre for Reviews and Dissemination University of York, Heslington, York YO1 5DD; Tel. 01904 321040
email: crd@york.ac.uk
http://www.york.ac.uk/inst/crd/

National Institute for Clinical Excellence (NICE)
http://www.nice.org.uk/
Intute: Health and Life Sciences formerly known as OMNI (Organising Medical Networked Information) Project
http://www.intute.ac.uk/healthandlifesciences/medicine

Resources for Evidence-based Surgery
A site created for all surgeons and the related medical community, hosted by the Royal College of Surgeons of England
http://www.rcseng.ac.uk//library/healthinformatics/evidence-based-practice

Sheffield Centre for Health and Related Research (ScHARR)
An introduction to evidence-based practice is available on the Internet called 'Netting the Evidence', produced by Andrew Booth from Sheffield University. This is a comprehensive guide to a range of sources and tools on the web in EBM
Regent Court, 30 Regent Street, Sheffield S1 4DA; Tel. 0114 2768555; email: mailto:a.boothsheffield.ac.uk; http://www.shef.ac.uk/scharr/ir/netting/

Evidence Network an initiative of the ESRC UK Centre for Evidence-Based Policy and Practice
http://evidencenetwork.org/index.html

UK Cochrane Centre
Summertown Pavilion, Middle Way, Oxford OX2 7LG; Tel. 01865 516300; email: crouse@cochrane.co.uk

Internet access to the Cochrane library and databases: http://www cochrane.org/index.htm

Controlled Trials Register, listings of ongoing MRC and NRR clinical trials: http://www.controlled-trials.com/

Sources of reviews and abstracts relating to evidence-based practice

ACP Journal Club
http://www.acpjc.org

Bandolier (topics in EBM reviewed for the NHS R&D Directorate)
http://www.jr2.ox.ac.uk:/bandolier/

BMJ Clinical Evidence – a compendium of evidence for effective health care
http://clinicalevidence.bmj.com/ceweb/index.jsp

Cochrane Systematic Reviews (abstracts only)
http://www.cochrane.org/reviews/index.htm

Effective Health Care Bulletins
http://www.york.ac.uk/inst/crd/ehcb.htm

Evidence-based Health Care
http://www.harcourt-international.com/journals/ebhc

Evidence-based Medicine
http://www.ebm.bmj.com/

Evidence-based Purchasing
http://www.pasa.nhs.uk/PASAWeb/NHS procurement/CEP

Journals available on the internet

eBMJ (electronic version of the *British Medical Journal*)
http://www.bmj.com

Journal of the American Medical Association (JAMA)
http://jama.ama-assn.org/

Canadian Medical Association Journal (CMAJ)
http://www.cmaj.ca/

Databases, bibliographies and catalogues

University of Hertfordshire Library
Contains up-to-date information on journals and other publications on EBM with access to many EBM internet resources

Library and Media Services, College Lane, Hatfield, Hertfordshire AL10 9AD; Tel. 01707 284678; email: c.cox@herts.ac.uk; http://www.studynet1. herts.ac.uk/lis.nsf

PUBMED (the free version of MEDLINE)
http://www.ncbi.nlm.nih.gov/PubMed/

BestBets – best evidence topics
http://www.bestbets.org

Trip database – turning research into practice
http://www.tripdatabase.com/index.html

BMJ Best Treatments
http://besttreatments.bmj.com/btuk/home.jsp

BMJ Clinical Evidence
http://clinicalevidence.bmj.com/ceweb/index.jsp

Leicester University database
http://www.le.ac.uk/li/clinical/digital/evidence/databases.html

Sources of guidelines and integrated care pathways

AHRQ (Agency for Healthcare Research and Quality)
Provides practical healthcare information, research findings and data to help consumers
http://www.ahcpr.gov/
Evidence Based Practice Centres
Develop evidence reports and technology assessments in conjunction with the AHRQ
http://www.ahcpr.gov/clinic/epc/

Cedars – Sinai Medical Center, Health Services Research
Home page: http://www.csmc.edu/

HealthCare: Clinical Information Index Page
Clinical information on evidence-based practice, clinical guidelines, medical effectiveness, pharmaceutical therapy, new technology and screening
http://www.ahcpr.gov/clinic/

Leicester GH guidelines
http://www.le.ac.uk/li/clinical/digital/evidence/governance.html

National Guideline Clearinghouse
Resource for evidence-based clinical practice guidelines and related documents. The site provides guidelines in multiple medical fields
http://www.guideline.gov/

National Library for Health
http://www.library.nhs.uk/guidelinesfinder/

National Pathways Association
http://www.the-npa.org.uk/

Scottish Intercollegiate Guidelines Network (SIGN)
http://www.sign.ac.uk

Useful texts

Cochrane Collaboration Handbook
http://www.cochrane.org/resources/handbook/index.htm

2

Outcomes and health economic issues in surgery

Jonathan A. Michaels

Introduction

Evidence-based medicine demands that all those making decisions regarding clinical management, either on an individual patient basis or at a policy level, consider existing evidence in order to maximise the chance of favourable outcomes and optimise the use of available resources. However, such evidence is rarely clear-cut and there may be conflicting advice because of differences in the way that outcomes are measured, the way in which costs are assessed or the perspective from which an economic evaluation is carried out.

This chapter deals with some of the issues around the measurement of outcomes, the calculation of costs and the methods of economic evaluation. The available outcome measures are considered, drawing the distinctions between disease-specific and generic measures and explaining concepts such as health-related quality of life, quality-adjusted life-years (QALYs) and utilities. The differences between costs, charges and resource use are highlighted, followed by a discussion of issues such as discounting, sensitivity analysis and marginal costing. Finally, a section on economic evaluation describes the different techniques available – cost minimisation, cost-effectiveness, cost–utility and cost–benefit analysis – and discusses the use of cost-effectiveness league tables. The intention is not to provide a full reference work on these subjects but to raise awareness of some of the important issues to be considered when evaluating evidence on specific interventions that may rely on differing outcome measurements or methods of economic evaluation.

Outcome measures

Clinicians tend routinely to consider health outcomes in terms of clinical or biomedical measures such as blood pressure levels, blood sugar levels or bone mineral density. Process-based outcomes such as readmission rates, reintervention or complications are readily considered alternatives. Data such as these are seen as readily available, easily measured, objective and comparable between differing settings. However, the present environment in medical services makes it necessary for the healthcare professional to consider more than just the treatment of the condition. A greater emphasis is now placed upon the consideration by the clinician of the actual status of the patient's quality of life. Now, considerations extend beyond assessing the value of an intervention and the effectiveness, or otherwise, of drug regimens. There should also be an assessment of the patient's physical, mental and social well-being. In line with such interests, there has been considerable research and a greater emphasis upon applying subjective non-biomedical measures and the development of such tools (or 'instruments') has been substantial since the early 1980s.

When considering which instrument of assessment to choose from the plethora now available, the user should carefully consider what parameter is to be measured before making a final selection of an outcome measure. Before applying this measure to a patient population, particular consideration needs to be given to deciding whether it will measure what we are interested in measuring and whether it will answer the questions that we wish to be answered.

All too often assessment tools may be applied to patients in the wrong circumstances or used when there is no realistic opportunity to measure what we wish to measure. These are important considerations because the administration and analysis of these measures can be costly, as well as taking up valuable time for both patients and clinicians. In addition, the use of unsuitable measures applied in the wrong context might yield results that are perhaps plausible but wrong, thus leading to erroneous conclusions. The implications of such findings for patients or the health service can be substantial.

Attention must also be given to the psychometric properties of the instruments chosen to measure health, with particular attention given to reliability and validity. **Reliability** refers to whether the instrument will be reproducible, such that if applied in different settings or circumstances to the same unchanged population then the same results should be achieved. This has particular implications for studies using instruments to derive longitudinal data on a particular sample of patients. In such circumstances, we need to be confident that observed changes over a given time period reflect actual change. Test–retest reliability is an important consideration and is assessed by making repeated assessments under the same circumstances at differing points in time and comparing the results using correlations or differences. Similarly, for instruments that require administration by interviewers, there needs to be a high level of agreement between different raters assessing the same patients but at different periods in time. For example, Collin et al. found a high level of agreement between the patients, a trained nurse and two skilled observers during applications of the Barthel Index to the same group of patients.[1]

Another psychometric criterion for consideration is that of **validity**, which means that instruments measure precisely what they set out to do. It should be borne in mind that measures can be reliable without being valid, but they cannot be valid without being reliable. Three types of validity are described. First, **content validity**, which relates to the choice, appropriateness and representativeness of the content of the instrument. Judging content validity involves an assessment of whether all of the relevant concepts are represented. For example, a representative sample of asthmatic patients could be used to develop an asthma questionnaire in order to ensure that it captures all the domains of interest for such a patient population. Second, there is a requirement to consider **criterion validity**, which is the degree to which the measure obtains results that are comparable to some kind of 'gold standard'. While this is theoretically a simple concept, there are very few such gold standards for comparison. Finally, there is **construct validity**. This relates to observation of

when expected patterns of given relationships are observed. For example, if a method of valuation of outcomes predicts that a patient prefers option A to option B, then one would expect this to be reflected by their behaviour when faced with genuine clinical choices. This is normally assessed through the use of multitrait–multimethod techniques,[2] which map the correlations between alternative approaches to measuring the same construct and between measures of different constructs.

As can be seen, the choice of an outcome measure is not always as straightforward as it may seem at first. In addition to considerations regarding the patient group, there are also important considerations regarding the psychometric properties of the instruments. Different outcome measures will have uses for differing patient groups. For example, a biomedical measure such as blood pressure alone might be considered suitable for comparing two similar drug regimens to assess 'best' control of blood pressure. However, a study that attempts to compare renal transplant with dialysis might also wish to consider a much broader picture and would be likely to require consideration of quality-of-life issues together with mortality as outcome measures.

It is extremely important to choose the right outcomes for the purpose in question, as different conclusions can be drawn from the application of different outcome measures in the same study. For example, a study of vascular patients compared exercise training with angioplasty for stable claudication with results expressed in terms of ankle–brachial pressure indices and walking distance.[3] In the short term, it was found that angioplasty improved the pressure but not the walking distance, while exercise improved the walking distance but not the pressure. This example shows that different outcome measures may not always change in the same direction and used in isolation could lead to opposite conclusions.

The following sections examine some of the issues involved in the evaluation and application of some common specific outcome measures.

Mortality

The mortality rate expresses the incidence of death in a population of interest over a given period of time. It is calculated by dividing the number of fatalities in the given population by the total population.

Mortality is often used as an outcome measure in studies as an indication of the effectiveness, or otherwise, of a treatment. It is often easily derived and as such represents a readily accessible outcome measure. While mortality can indeed provide much useful information, its use in reporting results should always be interpreted with caution. First, procedure- and diagnosis-related mortality rates often refer to inpatient deaths only or perhaps mortality over a given postoperative period, for example 30 days. Variations in short-term survival rates might simply reflect differing discharge practices between differing hospitals or settings. Longer-term survival rates are frequently reported for cancer and other chronic conditions. In interpreting these, it must be borne in mind that distortion may occur as a result of the starting point or choice of time frame. For example, survival may be longer in a screened population because there is an earlier starting point[4] and comparisons between surgical and medical treatments may be very sensitive to follow-up periods because of early excess operative mortality in surgical treatments, which may be offset by better long-term survival. For these reasons, it is often necessary to compare survival curves rather than total survival at a specific time point. This may raise further issues regarding the possible need for discounting, to take account of a preference for survival in the earlier years after treatment (see below).

Second, mortality can only be a partial measure of quality, and it is often not the most appropriate outcome measure for use in most situations. Many studies report mortality and tend to ignore other important outcomes such as morbidity and quality of life. These are more complex to quantify and are not routinely collected. Mortality is particularly limited in usefulness for studies investigating low-risk procedures. Accurate assessment of the quality of such procedures requires more sensitive measures.

It is also necessary to highlight the effect that differences in case mix can have on the mortality rate. For example, there is a tendency in studies relating workload to outcome for the results to be reported for the whole sample of patients. It is important to be aware that results reported in this way may be misleading as no account is taken of the diversity of patient characteristics that may be contained in such a sample. Both differences in severity of illness and in risk of adverse outcomes relating to comorbidity can significantly affect any interpretation of mortality rates. This problem is illustrated by Sowden and Sheldon, who discuss examples from coronary artery bypass grafting and intensive care to demonstrate the importance of adjusting for case mix.[5] For coronary artery bypass grafting, they report that the strength of the relationship between low volume and increased mortality is reduced in studies that adjust for differences in risk among patients receiving treatment. With adult intensive care, they cite a study by Jones and Rowan[6] in which the apparent higher mortality associated with smaller intensive care units ceased to be significant once the data were adjusted to reflect the fact that severity of illness was on average higher among patients admitted to small units. These examples clearly demonstrate that, in order to minimise bias in such studies, account must

be taken of any factors (beyond workload) that are likely to affect patient outcomes.

Condition-specific outcome measures

The term 'condition specific' describes instruments designed to measure health outcomes considered to be of specific interest to patients who incur health problems attributable to a particular disease or as the result of other processes. Such instruments are often referred to as 'disease specific', but this term is more general as it encompasses more diverse areas such as natural ageing, trauma and pregnancy, which are not diseases.[7]

The measurement of health status is not restricted to broad generic measures. There are many instances when researchers and clinicians are interested in assessing the health status of individuals with a certain condition or disease. As might be anticipated, many tools have been designed for this purpose and these are primarily aimed at measuring changes that are of importance to clinicians. For example, Spilker et al. identified over 300 such instruments in 1987 and many more are presently available.[8] Examples of such instruments include: measures for arthritis, such as the Arthritis Impact Measurement Scales;[9] measures for the heart, such as the Specific Activity Scale;[10] and measures that assess pain, such as the McGill Pain Questionnaire.[11] These instruments have a varying number of dimensions, differing numbers of items and are generally self-completion or interview, though some methods include professional assessment and clinical interview. Such questionnaires are usually scored in a simplistic fashion. Most have simple numerical scaling, such as from 1 to 5, and these scores are usually summed across the items for each dimension, or across all items.

Advantages of condition-specific measures include their relevance and their greater responsiveness to health change.[12] Disadvantages are that they often exclude items relevant to potential complications of treatment and symptoms that do not easily fit the medical model of disease. Generic measures have tended to be used in preference because they can be used to assess benefits for differing treatments or conditions, in a common and exchangeable currency. This enables decisions to be made on allocative efficiency between healthcare programmes within the total healthcare budget, rather than helping to establish the technical efficiency of producing health benefits for a specific condition.[7]

The measurement of pain

Pain is a common and important symptom of many medical conditions and deserves special consideration. While many generic and condition-specific instruments dedicate specific dimensions to the measurement of pain, there are also a number of instruments designed specifically to assess levels of pain. The measurement of pain cannot be directly assessed through clinical measures (e.g. blood samples) and, in the absence of such objective approaches, it is necessary to assess pain subjectively through the patient's own perceptions.

Subjective measures allow for reproducible results providing that the tools used to assess pain are measured appropriately. While subjective measures for the measurement of pain have many advantages over other instruments, there are problems in assessing subjects for whom communication is difficult. Examples include very young children and patients who are incapable of expressing how they feel. Those patients who are unconscious or who are terminally ill will continue to present particular difficulties for those attempting to assess levels of pain.

As with other outcome measures, options exist to use binary, categorical or visual analogue scales. Within this area, there are both pain-relief scales and pain-intensity scales to be considered. There are often occasions when it will be necessary to measure the state of the pain rather than the effect of a particular intervention or therapy, and in these circumstances pain-intensity scales will be appropriate. In situations where both pain-relief and pain-intensity scales are appropriate, a decision is required regarding which should be used. Pain-relief scales may well encompass more than an intensity scale, as any side-effects resulting from an intervention, such as dizziness, might be included in such judgements. Pain-relief scales also require the patient to make judgements about how the current pain now compares with remembered pain, before the intervention. This might make such scales more complicated for patients to grasp compared with intensity scales and this may raise doubts about validity.

Pain can manifest itself in a variety of qualities, and one of the most widely used tools is the McGill Pain Questionnaire.[11] This is a generic instrument, designed primarily for adults, which was developed to specify the qualities and intensities of pain; as such, it is intended to provide a quantifiable profile of pain. The questionnaire can be completed by the patient or administered in an interview. Completion takes roughly 15–20 minutes but becomes quicker on subsequent applications. The instrument contains 78 pain descriptor words, which are grouped into 20 subclasses, each of which contains two to five words that describe pain on an ordinal scale. These words are arranged to reflect three dimensions of pain: sensory, affective and evaluative. The questionnaire can yield three indices of pain: a pain-rating index based on the scale values of the words

chosen by the patient; a rank score using the rank values within each subgroup chosen; and the total number of descriptions chosen by the patient.

The McGill Pain Questionnaire has been thoroughly investigated in recent years and the instrument has proved to be the most reliable in applications to patients with moderate-to-severe chronic or acute pain. It has been shown to be particularly useful in disaggregating explained pain from unexplained pain. When the instrument was used in a cohort of cancer patients with lymphoedema, it proved to be more sensitive than categorical or analogue scales.[13]

Health-related quality of life

Recent years have witnessed quite an upsurge in interest in the measurement of health-related quality of life, much of which has no doubt been stimulated by the analytical demands of researchers and the need for outcome information as a basis for policy decisions.

Such health status measures are standardised questionnaires, or instruments, which are used to evaluate patient health across a broad range of areas. These areas include symptoms, physical functioning, mental well-being, work and social activities. Measures can be either generic or condition specific, and such measures can generate a profile of scores or a single index. These scores can be based upon people's preferences (e.g. EQ-5D) or, more usually, arbitrary scoring procedures (e.g. SF-36, assumes equal weighting for most items).[14] Three of the most frequently used instruments are discussed below in further detail.

EQ-5D

Of those instruments that generate a single index, EQ-5D has been rapidly adopted and widely used.[14] The measure was developed by a group of researchers from seven centres across five countries.[15] The present measure has five dimensions, whereas the original version had six. Patients are classified by the completion of a five-item questionnaire. The EuroQol is a brief, easy-to-use questionnaire of two pages. It can be made even simpler by using the one-page descriptive classification. Self-completion, or interview, usually only takes a matter of minutes, and response rates tend to be extremely high.[14] The five dimensions of the EQ-5D comprise mobility, self-care, usual activities, pain/discomfort and anxiety/depression. Each of the five questions has three levels; therefore combining the five questions defines 243 health states. In addition, the instrument contains a visual analogue scale: a thermometer scale calibrated from 0 (representing 'worst possible health state') to 100 (representing 'best imaginable health state').

The EQ-5D is now one of the most widely adopted methods for measuring health-related quality of life and is the method favoured by the National Institute for Health and Clinical Excellence (NICE) for deriving utility weightings for cost-effectiveness analysis (see below). It has been used in a wide variety of clinical areas, many pharmaceutical companies now include it as a standard outcome measure in clinical research, and the questionnaire has been translated into many different languages and validated in a number of different countries.[16]

SF-36

The SF-36 is a self-administered questionnaire composed of 36 items. It measures health across eight multi-item dimensions, covering functional status, well-being and overall evaluation of health. Responses within each of the dimensions are combined in order to generate a score from 0 to 100, where 0 represents 'worst health' and 100 indicates 'best health'. Dimension scores should not be aggregated into a single index score. The questionnaire takes about 5 minutes to complete, attains good response rates and is suitable for completion by the patients themselves or for administration by trained interviewers on a face-to-face or telephone basis.[17]

The questionnaire has been used in a variety of settings, administered on differing populations and exhibits good psychometric properties. Detailed information regarding the scoring process and computation are readily available, as are published data for comparative norms. The question complexity can be a problem in situations where the sample comprises individuals with low education levels, but otherwise the instrument is suitable for administration in a wide range of settings.[17]

Nottingham Health Profile

The Nottingham Health Profile (NHP) measures levels of self-reported distress. The instrument consists of two parts, each of which can be used independent of the other. Part 1, the most frequently used component, comprises 38 statements that are grouped into six sections: physical mobility, pain, sleep, social isolation, emotional reaction, and energy. The number of statements in each of these sections varies from three for the energy dimension to nine for emotional reaction. The second part of the instrument asks respondents to indicate whether or not their state of health influences activity in seven areas of everyday life: work, looking after the home, social life, home life, sex life, interests and hobbies, and holidays. Responses for both parts 1 and 2 are yes/no responses.[18]

Scoring is straightforward, with 0 assigned to a 'no' response and 1 to a 'yes' response. Scores for each of the sections range between 0 ('worst health') and 100 ('best health'). The NHP was designed for self-completion and can readily be used in postal surveys, although it can also be administered by an interviewer. Generally, the instrument takes around 5 minutes to complete.

Quality-adjusted life-years

QALYs were developed as an outcome measure to incorporate effects on both the quality and quantity of life. Each year of life is multiplied by a weighting factor reflecting quality of life.[19] An alternative to QALYs is healthy years equivalent (HYE), which is discussed below.

QALYs are estimated by assigning every life-year a weight between 0 and 1, where a weight of 0 reflects a health status that is valued as equal to being dead and a weight of 1 represents full health. For example, a patient receives a surgical intervention and can then be expected to live for an additional number of years. These additional years would be quality adjusted in some way by comparison with the 0–1 scale. Therefore, if the person who has undergone the surgery is calibrated (scored by raters) to be in a health state of 0.8, then each expected life-year will be assigned a QALY value of 0.8.

The QALY is frequently used by decision-makers or researchers to draw comparisons between differing types of health programme or intervention. The QALY can be used in economic evaluation: the number of additional QALYs that a new surgical intervention might yield can be compared with the costs of the new procedure, thus enabling cost per QALY ratios to be generated.[20] Such ratios have been used in so-called QALY league tables, whereby procedures or interventions are ranked on this basis. These tables might be seen as useful within the decision-making process, but caution should be exercised in making quick decisions regarding the allocation of resources based upon these comparative tables.[21–24]

More recently, HYEs have been developed as an alternative in order to address some of the suggested shortcomings of QALYs.[25] HYEs produce a hypothetical combination of the number of years in full health that equates to the individual's utility of living a number of years at a health state rated at less than full health. In effect, this can be considered as a lifetime profile of health and is often referred to as a stream of health states. In order to produce the values for the HYEs, a two-stage gamble procedure is used. There has, however, been criticism of the use of HYEs and at present the use of QALYs remains the most common method of performing cost-effectiveness analysis.[26,27] For the QALY to be a useful measure of outcome, it should reflect patient or individual preferences, which means that if an individual has a choice between two or more treatments or interventions then they should choose the treatment option that yields the most QALYs.

 QALYs remains the most common method of performing cost-effectiveness analysis.[26,27]

Utilities

Quality weights for use in QALYs can be obtained directly using one of three main methods – visual analogue scales (VAS), standard gamble and time trade-off – which are described in turn below. In addition to these direct methods of measurement, it is possible to obtain utilities through the mapping of health states derived from other quality-of-life measures onto valuations obtained from members of the general population.[28] The method for obtaining utility weightings is currently the subject of considerable research, and there is evidence that different values are obtained depending on the method of evaluation and framing of questions. In addition, there is considerable controversy as to whether the most appropriate utility values for economic evaluation are those of the general population or of patients with the particular conditions.[29]

Visual analogue scales

With the VAS approach, respondents are required to locate their present health state on a straight line chart, often a thermometer with fixed points, where the bottom of the thermometer is represented by 0, which is a health state equivalent to being dead, and the top of the thermometer is 1, which indicates full health. If thermometers ranging between 0 and 100 are used, these values are equated to 0–1, and the same assumptions regarding the health states hold. If, by way of an example, we wanted to measure the quality weight for being an amputee, and the respondent selects the health state at 55 on the thermometer scale of 0–100, then for that health state their quality weight is equivalent to 0.55. Advantages of VAS include their simplicity, but this can be counterbalanced by the fact that there is no choice to be made between health states and therefore it is not possible to observe any trade-offs that the individual might have between health states. Another problem with VAS is that it is uncertain whether the responses lie on a linear interval scale: it is questionable whether moving from 20 to 30 is equivalent to moving from 70 to 80. Given these reservations, it is difficult to use VAS methods to determine quality weights in a way that is consistent with the theoretical basis of utility measurement.[30]

Standard gamble

The second method routinely used to estimate quality weights is standard gamble. Under this approach, the quality weight of a health state can be constructed by comparing a specific number of years in the health state to a gamble with a probability (P) of achieving full health for the same number of years and a complementary probability ($1 - P$) of immediate death. The probability of full health is varied until the individual is indifferent between the alternatives, and the quality weight of the assessed health state is therefore equal to P. As an example, let us consider that we are comparing 10 years with heart disease with the gamble of full health for 10 years (probability P) or immediate death, with a complementary probability ($1 - P$). Here, let us assume that the individual is indifferent at a probability of 0.6 of full health. In practical terms, this means that the individual would consider a certainty of living 10 years with the heart disease to be equivalent to taking a gamble that gives a 60% chance of living 10 years in full health and a 40% chance of immediate death. The quality weight here would be 0.6 for the heart disease health state. The advantages of standard gamble include the fact that it is based on expected utility theory;[30] however, one of the major disadvantages is that respondents might find the concept difficult to understand because of the probabilities associated with the method. Another drawback is that the hypothetical choices used in such an approach are not representative of 'real' life, since choices between large improvements in health status and large mortality risks are seldom encountered, especially with the assumption that we will live for a certain number of years for sure.

Time trade-off

A third approach to estimating quality weights is time trade-off.[31] This method compares D years duration in the health state with X years in full health. The number of years in full health is varied until the individual is indifferent between their options; at this point, the quality weight of the health state is calculated by X/D. As an example, consider that we wish to calculate the quality weight for heart disease and that we assess the measurement for 10 years of heart disease. If the individual considers that 10 years of living with heart disease ($D = 10$) is equivalent to 6 years of full health ($X = 6$), then the quality weight is equal to 0.6 (6/10).

Obtaining utilities from health-related quality of life

The direct methods of obtaining utilities have a number of drawbacks. In particular, the VAS has a poor theoretical basis, and standard gamble and time trade-off methods may be complex to administer.[32] An alternative approach is to derive single index measures from generic or disease-specific health-related quality-of-life measures.[33,34]

One of the most widely adopted methods is derived from the EQ-5D, as described above.[34] The questionnaire generates a limited number of discrete health states depending upon the grading of the responses to each of the questions and previous research has used direct measurement methods to obtain a utility tariff associated with each of these states.[35] These tariffs have been widely used for cost-effectiveness analysis and alternative tariffs for different populations have also been developed.[16] Another generic measure that has been used to generate utilities is the SF-6D, a measure derived from the SF-36 questionnaire.[36] This has been extensively validated and compared with EQ-5D in a number of studies.[37]

In cases where information from generic scores is not available methods have been developed to derive utility weightings from disease-specific measures such as scoring systems for arthritis[38] or even from laboratory measures such as haemoglobin levels, used as a proxy for anaemia-related symptoms.[39] Disease-specific scores may be more sensitive to changes in symptoms for the condition in question but suffer from the disadvantage that they may fail to capture adverse events or other outcomes of treatment that are outside the main domains that are of interest in the specific disease so that comparability with other diseases may be questionable. There remains considerable controversy about the relative benefits of the use of generic and disease-specific measures to generate utilities.[40,41]

Costs, charges and resource use

From the above discussion, it can be seen that, from a health economist's perspective, there are several methods for assessing the benefits that might be accrued from a healthcare intervention within the context of an economic evaluation. Whichever approach is adopted within the economic evaluation, the method of identifying either the costs or the benefits is essentially the same for each of the approaches. In order to identify the relevant costs, it will be necessary to categorise all items of resource that will be utilised within the healthcare programme. Therefore, we need to identify which resources are required and which are not. Measurement requires an estimation of the amount of resources that are used within the programmes, and these should be measured using natural units of measurement. For example, to look specifically at staffing time, one would use units of time (such as hours) that are spent on activities relating to the programme and the specific grades of staff. For other categories of resource use, different units would be appropriate. One might look at drug use in units such as doses of specific drugs. Other examples of resource use and their relevant methods of measurement are outlined in Table 2.1.

Many of the items in Table 2.1 are readily identifiable and straightforward to value. Of these, staffing costs usually have the greatest impact upon healthcare costs, and these can be readily costed providing that we are aware of the staffing scale and can use wage rates or salary levels attached to the staff level. For example, to cost consultant time one would multiply the number of hours of consultant time in our study by their hourly pay, with added allowance to cover the costs of leave, sick pay and superannuation, etc. The majority of the other categories of resource use for health services identified in the table (consumables, overheads, capital, etc.) can be readily costed through the use of the market price.

Table 2.1 • Resource use and methods for measurement

Resource	Measurement	Valuation
Health services		
Staff time	Time (e.g. hours/days worked)	Salary levels
General consumables	Units/quantities used	Market price
Capital	Units/quantities used	Market price
Overheads	Units/quantities used	Market price/salary levels
Other services		
Community services	Units/quantities used	Market price
Ambulance services	Units/quantities used	Market price
Voluntary services	Units/quantities used	Estimated values for staff costs
Patients and their families		
Personal time	Hours of input	Salary levels
Expenses	Units/quantities used	Market price or cost of actual expenses
Time off work	Duration of time	Salary levels plus other imputed values

Elsewhere, community services, ambulance services and the expenses incurred by patients and their families would usually be costed in the same manner as health service resources.

Within the above, certain components are notoriously difficult to cost. For example, using patient or family leisure time incurs an opportunity cost, which is complex to measure as there are differing types of activity that are forgone in such situations. It is also complex to attach monetary values to activity involving voluntary care or time lost from housework. No accessible market value exists for either of these areas; therefore, it is customary to use a comparable market value from another market. As an example, Gerard used the wage rate for auxiliary nursing staff in order to cost the inputs by volunteers assisting with respite services for mentally handicapped adults.[42] However, there are occasions when comparable proxy market values are not readily accessible. This is often the case for the costing of 'time off usual activities', such as housework, which by its nature is not of routine duration and is often irregular in its occurrence, making comparison with other occupations virtually impossible. One approach that is advocated in such circumstances is to use average female labour costs as a relatively accurate reflection of the opportunity cost of housework.[43]

While costing might appear to be rather simplistic and straightforward, there are a number of considerations that need to be taken into account before embarking upon such an exercise.

Counting costs in base year

First, we should consider whether healthcare costs should be counted during the base year. By this, we mean that the costs should be adjusted in order to take account of inflation. If we assume that the annual inflation rate is running at 6% then £1060 would be required to purchase an item of medical equipment in a year's time that would currently cost £1000. The two values (both now and in 1 year's time) are considered to be equivalent in real terms, although of course they represent two different amounts of money. This problem becomes more acute if we are considering a comparison of two or more health programmes that have their costs spread at differing proportions over a different number of years. To illustrate this point, let us consider the following example taken from Auld et al.[43] where surgical and drug treatment options are considered for the same hypothetical condition (Table 2.2). We assume that each option has the same effect, but the cost streams are different between the two options, and the inflation rate is at 5% per annum. This rate means that a cost of £1050 in a year's time is equivalent to £1000 now (i.e. £1050/1.05), and likewise £1102.5 in 2 years time is also equivalent to £1000 now (i.e. £102.5/1.05^2). If we compare the costs between the different options in this example, we would conclude that surgery is the more efficient option when compared with the unadjusted drug option, since it is the least costly of the two but equally effective. However, it should be noted at this point that the drug therapy option is only greater in terms of cost owing to inflation. Therefore, if the costs are adjusted to take account of inflation, by adjusting costs to year 0 prices, then both therapies cost exactly the same, with the same effectiveness, and neither of the options could be considered superior to the other.

Discounting

Not all costs and benefits of healthcare programmes are observed to occur at the same point in time. For example, the costs associated with a vaccination programme are incurred very early in order to provide benefits to the individual, or society, in later life. In general, individuals prefer to reap the benefits sooner rather than later and prefer to incur the costs later rather than sooner. The most common method of allowing for such circumstances is to apply a discount rate to future costs and benefits.[44]

This leads us to consider whether the costs (and benefits) occurring at differing time points should be allocated equal weighting. There is not a consensus amongst health economists over what the appropriate discount rates are, or whether costs and benefits should be discounted at the same rate. Choosing the appropriate discount rate can have significant implications for the results of evaluations; the current recommended rates in England and Scotland are

Table 2.2 • Adjusting costs to base year (assuming 5% inflation)

| Options | Costs arising (£/person/year) | | | |
	Year 0	Year 1	Year 2	Total
Surgery	3000			
Drug (unadjusted for inflation)	1000	1050	1102.5	3125.5
Drug (adjusted to year 0 prices)	1000	1000	1000	3000

3.5%. Consequently, sensitivity analysis is essential to assess the implications of varying the discount rate. Recent convention dictates that costs should be discounted at the same rate as benefits,[45,46] though again this should be done in conjunction with sensitivity analysis to assess variations in such assumptions. Issues of discounting of costs and benefit may have a particularly dramatic effect on conclusions if different options have marked differences in the timing of expenditure or outcomes. This is particularly important when considering screening programmes and preventative treatments.

Marginal costing

The marginal cost is the cost incurred or saved from producing one unit more, or one unit less, of a healthcare programme. This is in contrast to the average cost, which is the total cost of a programme divided by the total units produced.

In calculating marginal costs the costs of treating an extra case, or moving from one programme to another, need to be assessed. For example, if there is currently a breast-screening programme for 50- to 65-year-old women and one wishes to consider whether breast screening is as cost-effective in women aged 40–50 years of age, this should be done by looking at the marginal costs and benefits of reducing the age at which screening is started rather than assessing average costs for the entire programme. The use of marginal rather than average costs has been found to be extremely important in screening programmes, where the marginal cost of screening an additional individual can be significantly lower than the average cost.[47]

Auld et al. illustrate this point with an example of hospital care.[43] Although it may well cost £25 000 per annum, on average, to care for an elderly person in hospital, it is extremely unlikely that this amount would be saved if one person less were admitted to the hospital. Similarly, this figure is unlikely to equate to an additional expense if one person more were admitted to the hospital. The reasoning behind this is that some costs, such as capital and overhead costs plus some staffing costs, will not differ with small incremental changes in the numbers of patients entering the hospital.

The use of full costs or marginal costs may depend upon the purpose of an economic evaluation and also the time scale of interest. For example, if one is considering making the most cost-effective use of limited resources then the issue may be one of opportunity costs in that a change in activity may be more or less cost-effective depending upon the activity that is displaced. Marginal costing depends upon an ability to distinguish between fixed and variable costs, and this can be difficult as it may depend upon time-scale and capacity issues. In the long term most resources can be altered in line with

activity, although there may be issues of economies of scale. In general the assessment of whether a new technology is considered a cost-effective use of resources will depend upon an assessment of the full costs that would be incurred; however, there may be special considerations where a particular resource has limited availability which could not be influenced by additional expenditure due to capacity constraints.[48]

Another issue which arises in addressing costs is the difference between the true cost of providing care or treatment and the charge that may be made for that treatment by the providing authority. In the UK in recent years the costs of treatment have been classified according to health resource groups that may cover a range of related procedures and/or diagnostic groupings. For these procedures, reference costs have been determined that represent the average costs of treatment within the NHS and a set of tariffs has been developed that determines the level of funding available to providers that deliver the services. In some cases these tariff rates or reference costs are used for economic analysis; however, they frequently cover a wide of range of procedures and case mix and may not represent true costs.[49]

Summary of cost analysis

This section highlights the importance of adhering to the appropriate methods when undertaking the costing component of an evaluation. Failure to do so might well lead to incorrect conclusions and to recommendations based upon flawed analysis. Clearly, not all studies that are published will have fully adopted the principles underlying the methods outlined in this section, and it is important when assessing the results from evaluations to consider whether appropriate analyses have been undertaken.

Economic evaluation

Within the healthcare sector, there will never be enough resources to allow the sufficient provision of healthcare to satisfy the demands of society. Quite simply, resources are scarce and choices need to be made about how best to distribute such resources. Such problems are further increased by the fact that healthcare is a mercurial environment with changing technology and population structures. This leads on to the concept of opportunity cost. Because of the scarcity of resources, choices need to be made regarding the best method for their deployment. It is therefore inevitable that choosing to use resources for one activity requires that their use in other activities must be forsaken. The benefits, often referred to as utility, that would have resulted from these forsaken activities are referred to as opportunity costs. In healthcare, the opportunity costs of the use of resources for a particular healthcare programme or intervention are equivalent to the benefits forsaken in the best alternative use of these resources.

It is necessary to identify from whose perspective the economic evaluation is undertaken. The perspective can be that of the individual patient, the NHS, the individual hospital or service provider, the government or society as a whole. If we considered the societal perspective, then we would seek to include all costs and benefits, no matter where they occur. In the UK, the methods recommended by NICE consider that the base case for cost-effectiveness analysis should include health and personal social service costs, but not all societal or costs incurred by patients, although other issues may be taken into account in evaluating technologies.

Within healthcare, economic evaluation is used as a general term to describe a range of methods that look at the costs and consequences of different programmes or interventions.[47] Each of the methods involves identifying, measuring and, where necessary, valuing all of the relevant costs and consequences of the programme or intervention under review.

There are four main approaches for undertaking economic evaluation: cost-minimisation analysis, cost-effectiveness analysis, cost–utility analysis and cost–benefit analysis. A summary of the features of these is given in Table 2.3 and each is discussed below, outlining their appropriate use in healthcare.

Cost-minimisation analysis

Cost-minimisation analysis is often considered to be a form of cost-effectiveness analysis but is treated here as a separate method of economic evaluation. This particular form of economic evaluation is appropriate in circumstances where, prior to investigation, there is no reason to expect that there will be any therapeutic difference in the outcomes of the procedures under consideration. For example, we might wish to consider two different forms of

treatment for varicose veins, such as day-case and inpatient treatment. Here, one might assume that there would be no expected differences in outcome between the two forms of treatment, and therefore the preferred option would involve choosing the treatment method that was the least costly of the two. Care should be taken in applying cost minimisation and it should be borne in mind that the lack of evidence regarding differences in outcomes is not the same as evidence that such differences do not exist. If there is potential for such differences then a safer approach is to carry out cost-effectiveness analysis with a sensitivity analysis to examine the effect of possible differences in outcome (see below). It is not unusual to find that plausible but unsubstantiated differences in outcome would outweigh the cost differences, which might have led to incorrect conclusions had analysis been confined to cost-minimisation techniques.

Cost-effectiveness analysis

Cost-effectiveness analysis should be used when the outcomes from the different programmes or interventions are anticipated to vary. The outcomes are expressed in natural units, though the appropriate measure to be used in such studies depends ultimately upon the programmes that are being compared. For interventions that would be expected to extend life, natural units such as life-years gained would be an appropriate measure. However, there might be a programme, such as the treatment for hypertension, where other measures might be considered appropriate, in this case for example unit reductions in blood pressure. Likewise, there might be a comparison of two different preventative treatments for coronary heart disease, where heart attacks avoided might be a suitable measure to use.

In order to assess the cost-effectiveness, or otherwise, of the interventions, cost is expressed per unit of outcome (cost-effectiveness ratios). The outcome of interest in the appraisal of two or more

Table 2.3 • Methods of economic evaluation

Type of economic evaluation	Units of measurement
Cost-minimisation analysis	Outcomes are the same between the different options; evaluation based upon cost
Cost-effectiveness analysis	Benefits are quantity or quality of life, which are measured in natural units (e.g. life-years gained, cases avoided, etc.)
Cost–utility analysis	Benefits are quantity and quality of life, which are measured using QALYs or HYEs
Cost–benefit analysis	Benefits are quantity and quality of life, which are measured in monetary terms such as human capital or willingness to pay

HYE, healthy years equivalent; QALY, quality-adjusted life-year.

interventions must be exactly the same for each of the alternatives that are considered. Therefore, the results from cost-effectiveness studies cannot often be generalised in order to assess the impact of interventions for differing conditions unless a unified measure that reflects both quantity and quality of survival is used (see cost–utility analysis). In conclusion, cost-effectiveness analysis is a useful tool for informing choices between alternatives where common outcomes have been used for the analysis.

As an example, one might assess the cost per stroke avoided in comparing the cost-effectiveness of a drug treatment for stroke prevention with that of carotid endarterectomy. However, such figures would be of little help in comparing the value of these treatments with that of a treatment for a different condition, such as joint replacement.

Cost–utility analysis

As has been discussed above, one of the potential limitations of cost-effectiveness analysis is that it does not allow for decisions to be made regarding different treatments for differing diseases or conditions if the units of outcome differ between disease areas.

Cost–utility analysis can be thought of as a special case of cost-effectiveness analysis where the outcomes are expressed in generic units that are able to represent the outcome for different conditions and treatments. Therefore, the units of outcome combine both mortality and morbidity information into a single unit of measurement (such as QALYs or HYEs). This two-dimensional outcome measure allows comparisons to be drawn between treatments for different therapeutic areas. These units of measurement are often expressed in terms of a universal unit, usually cost per QALY gained. Such units have resulted in league tables that compare the outcomes for treatments in different areas, and these will be discussed below.

 Cost–utility analysis expressed in terms of cost per QALY gained has become the predominant form of cost-effectiveness analysis in recent years.

Incremental cost-effectiveness ratios

In comparing the results of cost-effectiveness analysis for different treatments it is usual to report the incremental cost-effectiveness ratio (ICER). The ICER is the ratio between the additional cost that is incurred and the additional benefit (frequently measured in QALYs). Thus, for example, if a treatment produces 0.5 of a quality-adjusted life-year more than the next best treatment but costs an additional £5000, the incremental cost-effectiveness ratio would be £5000 divided by 0.5 or £10 000 per QALY. If the treatment that produces greater clinical benefit is less costly than the alternative then the ICER is negative and the treatment with better outcomes is said to 'dominate', thus being the preferred option in that it produces greater benefit at lower cost.

Where the ICER is positive it reflects the fact that the additional benefit comes at an additional cost and the ICER can be compared with other alternative uses for the available resources. Such calculations have been used to produce league tables to compare the cost of providing benefits by treatment in different clinical settings.

Cost-effectiveness league tables

Decision-makers face difficult decisions when asked how to allocate resources in healthcare. Such decisions are increasingly influenced by the relative cost-effectiveness of different treatments and by comparisons between healthcare interventions in terms of their cost per life-year or per QALY gained. The first compilation of such league tables was undertaken by Williams, who calculated the cost per QALY of a range of interventions and divided them into strong candidates for expansion and less strong candidates for expansion.[20] Advocates of such analyses argue that if properly constructed, these tables provide comprehensive and valid information to aid decision-makers.

There are, however, problems with the use of such tables and these can make interpretation and comparison between studies problematical.[50] First, the year of origin for the studies varies and, because of technological changes and shifts in relative prices, the ranking might not be truly reflective of the intervention under current practice. Second, differing discount rates have been used in the studies, some appropriately and others inappropriately, which impacts upon the results. Third, there have been a variety of preference values for health states, and currently it is difficult to determine which measure of quality of life has been used to derive the estimates concealed within the statistics presented in the league table. Clearly, if there is a high degree of homogeneity between the methods used to derive such estimates then these statistics might well aid decision-makers. Fourth, there is a wide range of costs used within the studies, and often costs are presented at an insufficient level of detail to allow recalculation to reflect local circumstances. In addition, many studies used in such league tables are often compared with differing programmes from which the incremental cost per QALY has been assessed. For example, some might compare with a 'do nothing' or 'do minimum' alternative, while other programmes would compare with the incremental cost per QALY of expanding services to other groups of patients. Finally, the setting of the study will prove important in drawing comparisons between the statistics in such tables, especially in situations where the studies are undertaken in different countries, requiring adjustments for exchange rates.

There has been a substantial amount of literature on the topic,[21–24] and while these tables might aid the decision-maker they also need to be interpreted with extreme caution as there is ample opportunity to mislead the casual observer.

Willingness-to-pay thresholds

A more common practice in recent years has been to compare incremental cost-effectiveness ratios against a 'willingness-to-pay' (WTP) threshold rather than directly against the ICER of other specific treatments. The WTP threshold is a figure that represents the amount that those who fund the healthcare consider is the maximum that should be paid to generate one unit of benefit, usually one QALY. This figure may be specific to local circumstances, depending upon the population and funding arrangements.

There has been much discussion in recent years about the appropriate level of WTP thresholds and the theoretical basis for the figure. On one hand it may be thought of as representing the amount that society is prepared to pay to generate additional healthcare benefit. An alternative interpretation is that if one assumes that the resources available to health are finite then additional expenditure on a new treatment will displace expenditure elsewhere. Assuming that healthcare provision was fully efficient, the WTP threshold would be the level of cost per additional QALY at which the activity displaced resulted in a net loss of health benefit that was equivalent to that produced by the new treatment. Thus any treatments that fell below the threshold would displace activities that produced less overall benefit, providing a net gain in health, whilst any treatment that was purchased above the threshold would be displacing greater health gain than was provided by the new treatment.

At present there is active empirical research to try to establish a realistic WTP threshold. In the UK setting NICE works with a threshold of £20 000–£30 000 per QALY,[51] although early empirical research suggests that this may be set rather high.[52,53]

Cost–benefit analysis

Cost–benefit analysis is a type of evaluation that places a single value, usually in monetary terms, upon the benefits and outcomes from differing programmes of healthcare, i.e. it determines the absolute benefit. In order to do this the health outcomes from treatment need to be measured in the same

units as cost. This can be carried out as an extension to cost–utility analysis where the costs and benefits are converted to the same units using the WTP threshold. For example, if one were to consider a treatment that produces one additional QALY then at a WTP threshold of £20 000 this may be considered equivalent to a £20 000 benefit. If the cost of providing that treatment were £10 000 the treatment would result in a net benefit of £10 000. However, at a cost of £30 000 the net benefit would be –£10 000, implying that there would be a net loss from providing the treatment (as, for example, if it were to displace a more cost-effective use of the available resources). An alternative way of presenting such analysis is in terms of net health benefit rather than economic benefit, so that the result is presented in terms of QALY rather than monetary terms (0.5 or –0.5 QALY in the above example).[54]

Choosing an evaluation method

The appropriate method of economic evaluation depends upon which choices need to be made and the context within which those choices need to be reached. If outcomes are expected to be the same then the choice is quite straightforward: cost-minimisation analysis may be used. The limitations of cost-effectiveness with disease-specific outcomes should be borne in mind. Cost–utility analysis has increased in popularity in an attempt to standardise and allow comparisons across different conditions and healthcare programmes. Cost–benefit analysis may offer decision-makers an alternative way of viewing such analysis but is dependent upon a predetermined WTP threshold.

Sensitivity analysis

Evaluations will always be subject to elements of uncertainty, be it in terms of resource use, costs or effectiveness. Sensitivity analysis is essential in such circumstances as it allows us to assess how sensitive the study results are to variations in key parameters or assumptions that have been used in the analysis. This allows us to assess whether changes in key parameters will result in savings or costs.

It is possible to undertake sensitivity analysis using as few or as many variables as desired. Commonly, variables such as production variables or discount rates will be used, or if statistical analysis of the variables has been undertaken one can carry out sensitivity analysis around known confidence intervals. Although sensitivity analysis is advocated for evaluations, a review by Briggs and Sculpher[45] found that only 39% of articles reviewed had taken at least an adequate account of uncertainty, while only 14% were judged to have provided a good account of uncertainty. In addition, 24% had failed to consider uncertainty at all. There are differing methods of sensitivity analysis, which are discussed below.

Simple sensitivity analysis

Simple sensitivity analysis, in which one or more parameters contained within the evaluation are varied across a plausible range, is widely practised. With one-way analysis, each uncertain component of the evaluation is varied individually in order to assess the separate impact that each component will have upon the results of the analysis. Multiway sensitivity analysis involves varying two or more of the components of the evaluation at the same time and assessing the impact upon the results. It should be noted that multiway sensitivity analysis becomes more difficult to interpret as progressively more variables are varied in the analysis.[45]

Threshold analysis

Threshold analysis involves the identification of the critical value of a parameter above or below which the conclusion of a study will change from one conclusion to another.[55] Threshold analysis is of greatest use when a particular parameter in the evaluation is indeterminate, for example a new drug with a price that has not yet been determined. A major limitation of threshold analysis is that it deals only with uncertainty in continuous variables, meaning that it is normally only useful for addressing uncertainty in analyses with data inputs.[45]

Analysis of extremes

In analysis of extremes, a base-case analysis is undertaken that incorporates the best estimates of the inputs and then further analyses consider extreme estimates of the relevant variables. For example, if two alternative treatment strategies are being compared, then both the high and low costs can be considered for both therapies and costs can be assessed for each of the options based upon combinations of these. Analysis of extremes can be particularly effective in situations where a base-case value is known together with a plausible range, but the actual distribution between the outer limits is unknown. However, a problem with this approach is that it does not consider how likely it is that the various scenarios will arise.[45]

Probabilistic sensitivity analysis

A final approach to dealing with uncertainty is through the use of probabilistic sensitivity analysis (PSA). This method allows ranges and distributions to be assigned to variables about which we are uncertain, thus allowing for combinations of items that are more likely to take place. For example, it is unlikely that all of the pessimistic factors regarding costs will occur in the evaluation. Techniques such as Monte Carlo simulations allow for the random simultaneous selection of items at designated values and undertake analysis based upon hypothetical patient cohorts. This approach allows the proportion of patients to be estimated for whom one of the options under evaluation is preferred; generally, proportions approaching 100% suggest that the intervention is nearly always preferable under a range of conditions. PSA is generally considered to be the most rigorous form of sensitivity analysis and is gaining widespread use.[56]

Value of information analysis

Value of information analysis is a recent development that is an extension of PSA. The method uses the results of PSA to consider the effect of reducing the uncertainty. Whilst PSA can provide a measure of the uncertainty around a prediction of cost-effectiveness, expected value of perfect information (EVPI) gives a measure that also incorporates the importance of such uncertainty.[57] Further developments of this may help to guide priorities for future research[58] or to help to design studies and estimate required sample size.[59]

Ethical issues

Any formal method for determining the costs and benefits of different treatments that may be used to allocate resources is likely to raise complex ethical issues. In particular, certain methods may create apparent discrimination against certain groups, such as the elderly or disabled, due to reduced capacity to gain from a particular treatment. Such methods may also fail to take into account other issues that are seen by society as being important in allocating resources, such as preferences relating to the process of care and issues such as equity.[60] It is important that such economic methods should not be used without considering these wider implications of the decisions which stem from such analyses.

Summary

Whether making individual or policy decisions regarding healthcare provision, it is becoming increasingly important for clinicians to take into account evidence about both the effectiveness and the cost-effectiveness of the treatment options. This requires that they examine the available evidence with particular attention to the appropriateness of the outcome measures used and of any techniques for economic analysis. In particular, there is a need for both clinicians and researchers to focus upon outcomes that are relevant to patients and truly represent their views about the relative values of the health states and events that they may encounter. Outcome research and economic evaluation are relatively new areas of healthcare research but they are progressing rapidly. An understanding of the methods used is a prerequisite for an adequate interpretation of the conclusions drawn from such work.

Key points

- The choice of outcome measure is important in assessing the results of surgical treatment and needs to be carefully considered.
- The measure used should be clinically relevant and preferably have been validated by previous research.
- Possible measures relevant to surgery include mortality, condition-specific measures, standard pain questionnaires and generic measures of health-related quality of life.
- Quality-adjusted life-years are a commonly used measure of outcome and there are several different ways to produce the weights (utilities) that are required to calculate these.
- The estimation of the cost of treatments should include a detailed analysis of the resources used and their valuation, and may require consideration of the timing of incurring various costs.
- There are several different methods of economic evaluation, including cost-minimisation, cost-effectiveness, cost–utility and cost–benefit analysis.
- The use of cost-effectiveness analysis may allow comparison of health benefits to be gained by expenditure on different treatments but is not without both technical and ethical problems in its application.

References

1. Collin C, Wade DT, Davies S et al. The Barthel ADL Index: a reliability study. Int Disabil Stud 1988; 10(2):61–3.

2. Campbell DT, Fiske DW. Convergent and discriminant validation by the multitrait–multimethod matrix. Psychol Bull 1959; 56(2):81–105.

3. Perkins JM, Collin J, Creasy TS et al. Exercise training versus angioplasty for stable claudication. Long and medium term results of a prospective, randomised trial. Eur J Vasc Endovasc Surg 1996; 11(4):409–13.

4. Stockton D, Davies T, Day N et al. Retrospective study of reasons for improved survival in patients with breast cancer in East Anglia: earlier diagnosis or better treatment. Br Med J 1997; 314(7079):472–5.

5. Sowden AJ, Sheldon TA. Does volume really affect outcome? Lessons from the evidence. J Health Serv Res Policy 1998; 3(3):187–90.

6. Jones J, Rowan K. Is there a relationship between the volume of work carried out in intensive care and its outcome? Int J Technol Assess Health Care 1995; 11(4):762–9.

7. Brazier J, Dixon S. The use of condition specific outcome measures in economic appraisal. Health Econ 1995; 4(4):255–64.

8. Spilker B, Molinek FR Jr, Johnston KA et al. Quality of life bibliography and indexes. Med Care 1990; 28(12, Suppl):DS1–77.

9. Meenan RF, Mason JH, Anderson JJ et al. AIMS2. The content and properties of a revised and expanded Arthritis Impact Measurement Scales Health Status Questionnaire. Arth Rheum 1992; 35(1):1–10.

10. Goldman L, Hashimoto B, Cook EF et al. Comparative reproducibility and validity of systems for assessing cardiovascular functional class: advantages of a new specific activity scale. Circulation 1981; 64(6):1227–34.

11. Melzack R. The McGill Pain Questionnaire: major properties and scoring methods. Pain 1975; 1(3):277–99.

12. Guyatt GH, Berman LB, Townsend M et al. A measure of quality of life for clinical trials in chronic lung disease. Thorax 1987; 42(10):773–8.

13. Carroll D, Rose K. Treatment leads to significant improvement. Effect of conservative treatment on pain in lymphoedema. Prof Nurse 1992; 8(1): 32–3, 35–6.

14. Brazier J, Deverill M, Green C et al. A review of the use of health status measures in economic evaluation. Health Technol Assess 1999; 3(9):i–iv, 1–164.

15. The EuroQol Group. EuroQol – a new facility for the measurement of health-related quality of life. The EuroQol Group. Health Policy 1990; 16(3):199–208.

16. Rabin R, de Charro F. EQ-5D: a measure of health status from the EuroQol Group. Ann Med 2001; 33(5):337–43.

17. Brazier JE, Harper R, Jones NM et al. Validating the SF-36 health survey questionnaire: new outcome measure for primary care. Br Med J 1992; 305(6846):160–4.

18. Hunt SM, McKenna SP, McEwen J. Measuring health status. London: Croom Helm, 1986.

19. Torrance GW. Measurement of health state utilities for economic appraisal. J Health Econ 1986; 5(1):1–30.

20. Williams A. Economics of coronary artery bypass grafting. Br Med J (Clin Res Ed) 1985; 291(6491):326–9.

21. Birch S, Gafni A. Cost-effectiveness ratios: in a league of their own. Health Policy 1994; 28(2):133–41.

22. Drummond M, Mason J, Torrance G. Cost-effectiveness league tables: think of the fans. Health Policy 1995; 31(3):231–8.

23. Drummond M, Torrance G, Mason J. Cost-effectiveness league tables: more harm than good? Soc Sci Med 1993; 37(1):33–40.

24. Mason J, Drummond M, Torrance G. Some guidelines on the use of cost effectiveness league tables. Br Med J 1993; 306(6877):570–2.

25. Mehrez A, Gafni A. Healthy-years equivalents versus quality-adjusted life years: in pursuit of progress. Med Decis Making 1993; 13(4):287–92.

26. Buckingham K. A note on HYE (healthy years equivalent). J Health Econ 1993; 12(3):301–9.

27. Johannesson M, Jonsson B, Karlsson G. Outcome measurement in economic evaluation. Health Econ 1996; 5(4):279–96.

28. Brazier J, Roberts J, Deverill M. The estimation of a preference-based measure of health from the SF-36. J Health Econ 2002; 21(2):271–92.

29. Johannesson M, O'Conor RM. Cost–utility analysis from a societal perspective. Health Policy 1997; 39(3):241–53.

30. von Neumann J, Morgenstern O. Theory of games and economic behaviour. New York: Wiley, 1967.

31. Torrance GW, Thomas WH, Sackett DL. A utility maximization model for evaluation of health care programs. Health Serv Res 1972; 7(2):118–33.

32. Hollingworth W, Deyo RA, Sullivan SD et al. The practicality and validity of directly elicited and SF-36 derived health state preferences in patients with low back pain. Health Econ 2002; 11(1):71–85.

33. Stein K, Fry A, Round A et al. What value health?: A review of health state values used in early technology assessments for NICE. Appl Health Econ Health Policy 2005; 4(4):219–28.

34. Rasanen P, Roine E, Sintonen H et al. Use of quality-adjusted life years for the estimation of effectiveness of health care: a systematic literature review. Int J Technol Assess Health Care 2006; 22(2):235–41.

35. Dolan P. Modeling valuations for EuroQol health states. Med Care 1997; 35(11):1095–108.

36. Brazier J, Usherwood T, Harper R et al. Deriving a preference-based single index from the UK SF-36 Health Survey. J Clin Epidemiol 1998; 51(11):1115–28.

37. Brazier J, Roberts J, Tsuchiya A et al. A comparison of the EQ-5D and SF-6D across seven patient groups. Health Econ 2004; 13(9):873–84.

38. Bansback N, Marra C, Tsuchiya A et al. Using the health assessment questionnaire to estimate preference-based single indices in patients with rheumatoid arthritis. Arth Rheum 2007; 57(6):963–71.

39. Wilson J, Yao GL, Raftery J et al. A systematic review and economic evaluation of epoetin alpha, epoetin beta and darbepoetin alpha in anaemia associated with cancer, especially that attributable to cancer treatment. Health Technol Assess 2007; 11(13):1–202, iii–iv.

40. Sculpher MJ, Price M. Measuring costs and consequences in economic evaluation in asthma. Respir Med 2003; 97(5):508–20.

41. Stolk EA, Busschbach JJ. Validity and feasibility of the use of condition-specific outcome measures in economic evaluation. Qual Life Res 2003; 12(4):363–71.

42. Gerard K. Determining the contribution of residential respite care to the quality of life of children with severe learning difficulties. Child Care Health Dev 1990; 16(3):177–88.

43. Auld C, Donaldson C, Mitton C et al. Economic evaluation. In: Detels R et al. (eds) Oxford textbook of public health, Vol. 2: The methods of public health. Oxford: Oxford University Press, 2002.

44. Drummond MF. Methods for the economic evaluation of health care programmes, 3rd edn. Oxford: Oxford University Press, 2005.

45. Briggs A, Sculpher M. Sensitivity analysis in economic evaluation: a review of published studies. Health Econ 1995; 4(5):355–71.

46. Cairns J. Discounting and health benefits: another perspective. Health Econ 1992; 1(1):76–9.

47. Drummond M, Maynard A. Purchasing and providing cost-effective health care. Edinburgh: Churchill Livingstone, 1993.

48. Hartwell D, Colquitt J, Loveman E et al. Clinical effectiveness and cost-effectiveness of immediate angioplasty for acute myocardial infarction: systematic review and economic evaluation. Health Technol Assess 2005; 9(17):1–99, iii–iv.

49. Baboolal K, McEwan P, Sondhi S et al. The cost of renal dialysis in a UK setting – a multicentre study. Nephrol Dial Transplant 2008; 23(6):1982–9.

50. Mason J, Drummond M. Reporting guidelines for economic studies. Health Econ 1995; 4(2):85–94.

51. Rawlins MD, Culyer AJ. National Institute for Clinical Excellence and its value judgments. Br Med J 2004; 329(7459):224–7.

52. Appleby J, Devlin N, Parkin D. NICE's cost effectiveness threshold. Br Med J 2007; 335(7616):358–9.

53. Martin S, Rice N, Smith P. The link between health care spending and health outcomes: evidence from English programme budgeting data. Centre for Health Economics Research Paper 24, University of York, 2007.

54. Stinnett AA, Mullahy J. Net health benefits: a new framework for the analysis of uncertainty in cost-effectiveness analysis. Med Decis Making 1998; 18(2, Suppl):S68–80.

55. Pauker SG, Kassirer JP. The threshold approach to clinical decision making. N Engl J Med 1980; 302(20):1109–17.

56. Claxton K, Sculpher M, McCabe C et al. Probabilistic sensitivity analysis for NICE technology assessment: not an optional extra. Health Econ 2005; 14(4):339–47.

57. Felli JC, Hazen GB. Sensitivity analysis and the expected value of perfect information. Med Decis Making 1998; 18(1):95–109.

58. Claxton KP, Sculpher MJ. Using value of information analysis to prioritise health research: some lessons from recent UK experience. Pharmacoeconomics 2006; 24(11):1055–68.

59. Ades AE, Lu G, Claxton K. Expected value of sample information calculations in medical decision modeling. Med Decis Making 2004; 24(2):207–27.

60. Ubel PA, DeKay ML, Baron J et al. Cost-effectiveness analysis in a setting of budget constraints – is it equitable? N Engl J Med 1996; 334(18):1174–7.

3

Day case surgery

Paul Baskerville

Introduction

One of the main aims of surgery is to return the postoperative patient to their home environment, in a safe and timely fashion. If, following a surgical procedure, the patient does not spend a few days in hospital, but returns home the same day, we describe that process as day case surgery. Why should this obvious and rather banal variation in length of hospital stay deserve a chapter of its own in a surgical textbook? The reason is that the development of successful day surgery practice, and the knowledge gained from studying its component parts, have been instrumental in improving the delivery of all surgical care in the last 30 years. It has helped all parties responsible for that delivery to understand how to introduce, create and then manage all surgical developments in a timely, safe, efficient and cost-effective manner.

Understanding how day surgery works, how traditional inpatient care can be successfully transferred to the day unit, and what is required to enable that to happen is a fundamental requirement for all those involved in the care of the surgical patient, be they surgeon or anaesthetist, nurse or manager, health purchaser or provider.

Day surgery has been described as the planned admission of a patient to hospital for a surgical procedure which, while requiring recovery from a bed or trolley, allows the patient to return home the same day. As a consequence, procedures not requiring full operating theatre facilities and/or general anaesthesia, procedures which can be performed in outpatient or endoscopic suites, are no longer called true 'day surgery'.

Successful and well-managed day surgery has the potential to improve the quality of care for patients by separating their elective treatment from the bustle of emergency surgical care, both of which are traditionally managed on the same wards. Most people would rather not stay in hospital longer than necessary, and short stays reduce the risks of hospital-acquired infections. Reducing length of stay also reduces costs and can improve efficiency, reasons that make day surgery attractive to all healthcare systems worldwide.

In the UK, the NHS plan proposed by the government in 2001 set the patient firmly at the centre of a framework for modernising the NHS.[1] The idea was to reduce waiting times, implement booking systems and introduce patient choice. However, the government was faced with capacity constraints and one solution to increase patient throughput was to reduce the length of patients' stay by focusing on a National Day Surgery Programme.

 The day surgery strategy was launched in 2002 with the broad aim of achieving 75% of all elective surgery in the UK to be performed on a day case basis by the year 2005.[2]

Day surgery now comprises over 70% of all elective surgery in the UK, over 80% in the USA and is likely to become the default method of treating most surgical patients in the next two decades. This growth has occurred over the last 30 years, most of it in the last 15. How has this come about? What are the main driving forces behind it? What are its strengths and weaknesses? This chapter covers those aspects of day surgery that are essential to good practice, and highlights some areas of current controversy.

The development of day surgery

The concept of day surgery is not new. In 1909, James Nicholl, a surgeon working at the Royal Hospital for Sick Children in Glasgow, reported on nearly 9000 children undergoing operations for conditions such as hernia and hair lip, all of whom went home on the day of surgery.[3] He described the benefits for parent and child of returning home the same day, but stressed the importance of suitable home conditions in the success of day surgery. A decade later, in 1919, Ralph Waters, an anaesthetist in Sioux City, Iowa, reported on the 'downtown anaesthesia clinic' where adults underwent minor surgical procedures, returning home within a few hours.[4]

The modern era of day surgery began in the years following World War II with the realisation that prolonged bed rest was associated with high rates of postoperative complications such as deep vein thrombosis.[5] The move towards early ambulation led to earlier discharge and, for the first time, the economic benefits of day surgery were noted.[6] In 1955, Eric Farquharson of Edinburgh described a series of 458 consecutive inguinal hernia repairs performed on a day case basis at a time when the average length of postoperative stay was approximately 2 weeks.[7] The medical benefits of early ambulation were recorded and the potential impact on surgical waiting times were considered.

Further development of day surgery occurred not in the UK but in North America, where cost savings associated with day surgery in privately run healthcare systems led to the early development of day units within hospitals, and by 1969 the first freestanding ambulatory surgical centre in Phoenix, Arizona. The huge commercial success of such units led to a significant shift in surgical care out of hospital inpatient beds, and forced surgeons, anaesthetists and hospital managers to study and improve the safety and efficiency of surgical care.

The UK, with its state-run NHS, was much slower to introduce day surgery. The few existing units were poorly utilised and there was little support for the expansion seen in the USA. In 1980 Paul Jarrett, in the day unit at Kingston Hospital, demonstrated once again the benefits of dedicated day surgery lists for hernias, including the rapid reduction of waiting times from 3 years to 3 months.[8] This time the government was quick to see the advantages, and supported day surgery expansion throughout the UK for a decade. In 1985 the Royal College of Surgeons of England published a report (revised in 1992) entitled *Guidelines for day case surgery*.[9] At that time, it was estimated that only 15% of elective surgery was performed on a day case basis and the report suggested 50% as an appropriate target. In 1989, the gathering momentum of day surgery demonstrated a need for a professional body to promote the specialty and set quality standards of care. The result was the British Association of Day Surgery (BADS) encompassing surgeons, anaesthetists, nurses and managers involved in day surgery. The same year the NHS Management Executive's value-for-money unit demonstrated that the cost of treating patients as day cases was significantly less than as inpatients.[10] By 1990, the Audit Commission had taken over the role of external auditors within the NHS and it introduced the concept of a 'basket' of 20 surgical procedures suitable for day case surgery to allow benchmarking between health authorities.[11] The audit figures also demonstrated wide variations between hospitals.

By 1991, the Audit Commission Report *Measuring quality: the patient's view of day surgery* found that 80% of day case patients preferred this mode of treatment to traditional inpatient treatment, adding further impetus to the development of day surgery.[12] In 1993 the national Day Surgery Task Force suggested that 60% of elective surgery should be performed on a day case basis nationally.[13]

By the end of the decade, the introduction of newer surgical and anaesthetic techniques to the day unit and the loss of others to the outpatient department forced a reassessment of the surgical basket to reflect modern day case activity. Changing practice and fiscal rationing made several of the procedures on the original list poor comparators of day surgery. At the same time, more advanced day units were already performing more complex procedures on a day surgery basis and in 1999, continuing the supermarket analogy, the BADS recommended an additional 20 operations to form a 'trolley' of procedures suitable for day surgery in the more experienced day unit (Box 3.1). The trolley included major operations such as laparoscopic cholecystectomy, thoracoscopic sympathectomy, partial thyroidectomy and laser prostatectomy. The concept of the trolley is that a target of 50% of these procedures on a day case basis would be realistic.

By 2001 the Audit Commission had updated its basket of procedures (Box 3.2), reflecting the lead taken by BADS, and included procedures such as laparoscopic cholecystectomy and haemorrhoidectomy;

Box 3.1 • British Association of Day Surgery 'trolley' of procedures 1999, of which 50% should be suitable for day case surgery

Laparoscopic hernia repair
Thoracoscopic sympathectomy
Submandibular gland excision
Partial thyroidectomy
Superficial parotidectomy
Wide excision of breast lump with axillary clearance
Haemorrhoidectomy
Urethrotomy
Bladder neck incision
Laser prostatectomy
Transcervical resection of endometrium
Eyelid surgey
Arthroscopic meniscectomy
Arthroscopic shoulder decompression
Subcutaneous mastectomy
Rhinoplasty
Dentoalveolar surgery
Tympanoplasty
Laparoscopic cholecystectomy
Bunion operations

Box 3.2 • Audit Commission basket of 25 procedures 2001

Orchidopexy
Circumcision
Inguinal hernia repair
Excision of breast lump
Anal fissure dilatation or excision
Haemorrhoidectomy
Laparoscopic cholecystectomy
Varicose vein stripping or ligation
Transurethral resection of bladder tumour
Excision of Dupuytren's contracture
Carpal tunnel decompression
Excision of ganglion
Arthroscopy
Bunion operations
Removal of metalware
Extraction of cataract with or without implant
Correction of squint
Myringotomy
Tonsillectomy
Submucous resection
Reduction of nasal fracture
Operation for bat ears
Dilatation and curettage/hysteroscopy
Laparoscopy
Termination of pregnancy

this was incorporated into the Department of Health's *Day surgery: operational guide* published to support the National Day Surgery Programme to achieve a 75% day case rate for elective surgery by 2005.[2] The continual drive to improve the delivery of healthcare means that day surgery practice will continue to evolve.

How does it work for the patient?

Facilities for day surgery

The organisation of day surgery services differs from traditional inpatient surgery. Patients arrive at the hospital on the day of surgery, fully assessed with the results of investigations already checked. Following operation, patients recover in the day unit and are discharged home, accompanied by their carer. The entire admission episode is preplanned and the routine nature of the hospital visit ensures quality care. Any error in the system results in an unnecessary overnight admission and it is therefore not surprising that the facilities for day surgery differ from inpatient surgery.

Initially, day surgery was attempted from the inpatient ward, but this environment is a mixture of emergency admissions, unwell elective surgery patients and the 'well' elective day surgery patient. Quality of care for the day case patient suffered as busy ward staff naturally concentrated on the acutely ill. There was also no incentive to ensure the day patient was able to go home the same evening. In the UK, the patient's procedure was often cancelled on the day of admission as their projected bed had been occupied overnight by an emergency admission.

Self-contained day units or dedicated day wards were therefore developed and unplanned overnight admission rates dropped dramatically from 14% on an inpatient ward to 2.4% in a dedicated day unit.[2] These units may be free-standing or integrated within the main hospital where they benefit from the full range of available support services. The self-contained unit should have its own day surgery theatre within the day surgery suite, performing dedicated day case lists.

Dedicated lists require appropriate staffing levels to be allocated as there is a greater intensity of work for theatre staff if several day cases are to be treated rather than a single major case. Experience has shown that the most effective units unite all managerial as well as nursing and operative functions under the same roof. Further efficiencies are made if the day unit can be accessed directly from the street or car park, and if day patients have their own dedicated car parking facilities.

The day surgery cycle

In traditional inpatient surgery, the patient is admitted either from the waiting list or directly from the surgical outpatient clinic if the patient is classified as urgent. In day surgery, the processes are different (**Fig. 3.1**). In many hospitals the patient is seen in the outpatient clinic and then sent directly for preassessment. While this has the advantage of a single hospital visit, some patients become overwhelmed with the amount of information they are given in a short space of time. Therefore some patients find it convenient to come back for preassessment at a later date.

A few hospitals accept fast tracking by general practitioners, who refer patients directly for preassessment to the day unit. In this case, the surgeon will not see the patient until the morning of operation and, for obvious reasons, the process is only suitable for the young, fit patient with a straightforward surgical problem.

Patient selection

Patient selection addresses the suitability of the patient for day surgery. Factors that influence this selection include the risk of major complications, social conditions and medical fitness including obesity. There are no upper limits on age or body mass index (BMI), although each patient is judged on an individual basis. Social factors rarely restrict admission and American Society of Anesthesiologists (ASA) class III patients are accepted. In any hospital, over 75% of traditional inpatient procedures can be performed on a day case basis.[2]

Social factors

The effects of general anaesthesia on cerebral function, affecting judgement and coordination, are well recognised. After day surgery, all patients must be accompanied home by a responsible and physically able adult, who should be present for the first 24 hours following operation. Patients themselves must not drive home and preferably should avoid public transport. Greater travelling times are associated with increased discomfort and nausea,[14] and patients should reside within an hour's journey from the hospital in case of emergency. The patient's home conditions should be sufficient to allow them to recover in comfort. In general, they should have access to a telephone in case of emergency, there should be adequate toilet facilities and household stairs should be minimal, but each set of circumstances requires individual judgement.

Age

Biological age is more important than chronological age, although many day units arbitrarily and illogically apply upper limits of 65 or 70 years of age. Whilst the older patient is more likely to suffer from respiratory and cardiovascular disease and the carer may also be in an elderly age group, with careful preoperative evaluation, the elderly patient can benefit from day surgery through a rapid return to familiar home circumstances and less postoperative confusion.

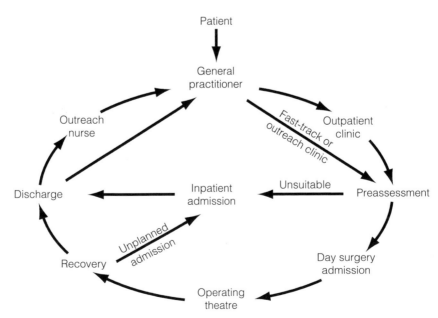

Figure 3.1 • The day surgery cycle.

Body mass index

Obesity is measured by BMI (in kg/m^2) and height–weight charts are used as 'ready reckoners' to calculate it (**Fig. 3.2**). Obesity is defined as a BMI equal to or greater than 30.[15] The prevalence of obesity has doubled in the 1990s, with 24% of adults in England now fulfilling the definition.[16] The very obese were excluded from day surgery because of delayed recovery related to the absorption of volatile anaesthetic agents into body fat, but this is less of a problem with modern total intravenous anaesthetic agents such as propofol.[17] The problems that do occur with the obese patient are related to comorbidity, the surgical procedure and the anaesthetic. Obesity is associated with cardiac disease, diabetes mellitus, hiatus hernia, hypertension and sleep apnoea, and it may be the comorbidity factor that excludes an obese patient from day surgery rather than the obesity itself. Operating on the obese patient is often more technically demanding, and the complication rate is often higher, with increased rates of postoperative haematoma formation and pain as a result of the need for greater surgical access. Anaesthetic problems include problems of venous access, intubation and airway control. Operating on patients early in the day is advisable to ensure that any minor postoperative complications can be corrected and do not prevent the patient from returning home.

 The upper safe BMI limit for day surgery remains controversial. While some day units still remain at a restrictive BMI of 30, others have safely increased this upper limit to 35, 37 and even 40.[18]

Smoking

Smokers undergoing surgery have increased intraoperative complications such as impaired gas exchange and increased secretions, with postoperative problems consisting of an increased incidence of bronchospasm, chest infection and wound complications.[19] Advice at preassessment regarding cessation of smoking depends on whether the patient would like to stop permanently or else temporarily suspend their habit in the perioperative period. For those attempting permanent cessation, this should commence 6–8 weeks before surgery since this is the minimum time required for lung function to improve significantly.[20] The least effective time of smoking cessation is in the week before surgery when the effects of withdrawal are maximal.[21] For those who intend continuing their habit, temporary cessation 12 hours before surgery confers a reduction in circulating carboxyhaemoglobin, thereby improving perioperative lung function.

Medical factors

 In 1991 the ASA classified surgical patients into five classes of physical fitness (Table 3.1), which has provided a framework for patient selection in day surgery.[22]

While ASA class I or class II patients are generally accepted for day surgery, the suitability of patients in the ASA class III group is less clear. While hypertension, chronic lung disease and symptomatic heart disease increase the risk of complications, this is not evident with asthma or insulin-dependent diabetes mellitus.

 Stable ASA class III patients have the same risk of unplanned overnight admissions as lower ASA status patients,[23] and any increase in complications with ASA class III patients is related to the surgical procedure rather than comorbidity.

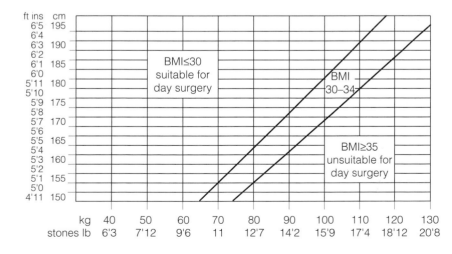

Figure 3.2 • Assessment chart for body mass index (BMI).

Table 3.1 • Adaptation of the American Society of Anesthesiologists' classification of physical status

Class I	A healthy patient
Class II	Mild-to-moderate systemic disease caused by the surgical condition to be treated or by another disease process, with no functional limitation, controlled hypertension, mild diabetes, mild asthma
Class III	Severe systemic disease with some functional limitation plus diabetes with complications, severe asthma, myocardial infarction >6 months
Class IV	Severe systemic disease that is a constant threat to life plus unstable angina, severe cardiac, pulmonary, renal, hepatic or endocrine insufficiency
Class V	Moribund patient not expected to survive 24 hours even with surgical intervention

Diabetes mellitus

Patients with diabetes mellitus can undergo successful day surgery. Type I diabetic patients are more difficult to manage in the perioperative period than type II patients and are more liable to unplanned admission. Stability of the disease in the months before surgery is central to success of the admission, especially in the type I patient. A glycosylated haemoglobin (HbA_{1c}) result of less than 8% suggests that the patient is suitable for day surgery. Most intermediate surgical procedures, such as those in the Audit Commission basket of 25 (Box 3.2), can be safely undertaken in adult diabetic patients with the occasional exception of laparoscopic cholecystectomy due to the increased risk of postoperative nausea and vomiting.

Where possible, the patient should be managed with local or regional anaesthesia as this may remove the need for the patient to starve preoperatively. However, if general anaesthesia is required, diabetic medication is omitted on the morning of surgery, the procedure is scheduled as early as possible on the list and the normal regimen is resumed as soon as possible.[24] Well-controlled non-insulin-dependent diabetics present few problems but insulin-dependent diabetics require intensive monitoring throughout the day surgery process.

Cardiac disease

The risk of myocardial ischaemia during anaesthesia is increased in the hypertensive patient, and elevated blood pressure is one of the most common reasons for 'on the day' cancellation: the blood pressure has either not been accurately measured at preoperative assessment or it has not been adequately treated (see 'Preoperative assessment'). Preoperative sedation can lower a marginally elevated blood pressure but the underlying cause requires further investigation. Many patients with significant cardiovascular disease can still undergo day surgery procedures provided exercise tolerance is good.

> The specific blood pressure that is unsafe for the patient undergoing day surgery remains unclear but a systematic review and meta-analysis of 30 observational studies found little evidence for an association between admission arterial pressure and perioperative complications if systolic and diastolic pressures are less than 180 and 110 mmHg respectively.[25]

Asthma

The younger asthmatic using an inhaler and with good exercise tolerance is suitable for day surgery. Only those with steroid-controlled asthma are excluded or require investigation before proceeding. Non-steroidal anti-inflammatory drugs (NSAIDs) can be administered safely for pain relief to 95% of asthmatics.[26] A history of previous administration without bronchial spasm, usually from over-the-counter preparations, is often available.

Preoperative assessment

The admission, operation and discharge of a patient within a day requires accurate forward planning, with the procedure occurring on a scheduled day at a scheduled time. Day surgery pioneered the role of preoperative assessment, performed up to 6 weeks prior to surgery. As a result nursing, anaesthetic and surgical assessment on the day of admission is both rapid and minimal. Preassessment of patients also ensures that 'on the day' cancellation for clinical reasons is rare. Cancellations not only waste hospital resources but cause distress to patients and their families and often disrupt work commitments.

While strict assessment criteria ensure patient safety, identifying these criteria at preassessment allows for timely correction of some of these factors, therefore enabling the patient to undergo day surgery safely. The most common treatable exclusion factors are hypertension and identifying an overnight carer for patients living on their own. Assessment also allows the patient a second chance to discuss anxieties that may not have been considered at initial outpatient consultation. Involvement of the patient at this early stage permits flexibility and choice regarding their operating date and improves non-attendance rates.

Day surgery preassessment is best performed by trained nurses in nurse-based preassessment clinics. The availability of a consultant anaesthetist to deal immediately with some queries and concerns further improves efficiency.

To maximise day surgery throughput, a cultural change is required from an 'opt-in' policy such as 'Is this patient suitable for day surgery?' to an 'opt-out' policy such as 'Is there any reason this patient cannot be treated as a day case?' The design of day surgery preassessment may be accomplished by:

- automatic assignment for day surgery of all patients undergoing a procedure included in the BADS's trolley of procedures (Box 3.1) or the Audit Commission's updated basket of procedures (Box 3.2);
- hospital-wide preassessment for all elective surgical procedures (with procedure-specific exclusions for major surgical procedures such as major bowel resection and aortic aneurysm repair).

Preassessment clinics use a patient questionnaire to screen for social and medical problems. Nurse-based assessment allows the patient adequate consultation time and nursing colleagues are also more adept at the assessment of the patient's social situation. Most questionnaires follow a standard format to screen and triage the suitability of patients for day surgery. Questionnaires should address the generic status of the health of the patient, but additional questions may be added for specific surgical specialties (e.g. ophthalmology; ear, nose and throat; orthopaedics).

Patient information leaflets should be available covering both general day surgery information and information specific to the proposed operation. These may have been issued at the outpatient consultation where first-stage consent is usually obtained. The later preassessment visit allows the patient to ask questions which may have arisen since their consultation, and subsequent discussion leads to better understanding by the patient and family, and may reduce anxiety levels.

Investigations

Routine investigations are unnecessary in the asymptomatic day surgery patient[27] and preoperative testing should be limited to circumstances in which the results will affect patient treatment and outcomes. Investigations should not be prescriptive but should be tailored to the individual's needs because most investigations required can be predicted from the history alone. Even when minor abnormalities are found they rarely entail cancellation. A full blood count is only required if there is a risk of anaemia, chronic renal disease, rectal bleeding or haemorrhage. Similarly, analysis for urea and electrolytes is only indicated if the patient has renal disease or is taking diuretics. Urinalysis is often routinely performed as part of the preoperative routine but, again, unsuspected disease is more likely to be picked up on history alone. In Oxford, routine urine testing of more than 30 000 day case admissions resulted in only one cancellation, caused by unsuspected diabetes mellitus.[17]

The incidence of electrocardiographic (ECG) abnormalities increases with age but minor preoperative ECG abnormalities do not predict adverse cardiovascular perioperative events in day surgery.[28] The only indications for preoperative ECG include chest pain, palpitations and dyspnoea, but these patients have often already been excluded from day surgery by other comorbidity. A chest X-ray examination is also unnecessary. If required, then the patient is probably unsuitable for day surgery in the first place.

Testing for sickle cell disease is more controversial. Patients with sickle cell disease usually present in childhood with chronic haemolytic anaemia. Preoperative screening in adults is unlikely to identify a patient with previously unknown sickle cell disease but will, of course, identify those with sickle cell trait. However, the 'at-risk' population (those of African, Asian and Mediterranean origin) is often difficult to define in Britain today as a result of ethnic mixing. Furthermore, those factors which precipitate sickling (hypotension, hypoxaemia and acidosis) are unlikely to occur during day case surgery.

Day of surgery admission

On arrival at the day unit on the prearranged day of operation, most documentation is already complete and bureaucracy is minimised. Any change of circumstance, either social or medical, should be noted since the time of preassessment, and the preoperative surgical visit by the person performing the operation need only consist of verification of the consent and marking the appropriate operation site. The final anaesthetic assessment is performed at this time and not in the anaesthetic room where levels of anxiety are already high. Many day surgery units have successfully introduced staggered admission times for patients, which is more convenient for both patient and the day unit. In most centres, the 12-hour fasting ritual has now been replaced by regimens of no solids within 4–6 hours and up to 300 mL of clear fluid within 2 hours of surgery.

Patient discharge

Discharge after inpatient surgery for procedures suitable for day surgery usually occurs at least 18–24 hours after its completion. By then, there is little concern regarding postoperative complications or the adverse effects of the anaesthetic. In contrast, discharge on the day of surgery must address strict discharge criteria if complications are to be avoided. Before returning home, patients may be seen by the surgeon and anaesthetist involved in their care, but the final decision to discharge is usually nurse

Box 3.3 • Discharge criteria

Vital signs stable for at least 1 hour
Correct orientation as to time, place and person
Adequate pain control and supply of oral analgesia
Understanding the use of oral analgesia supplied, supported by written information
Ability to dress, walk (if appropriate)
Minimal nausea, vomiting or dizziness
Oral fluids taken
Minimal bleeding (or wound drainage)
Has passed urine (if appropriate)
Has a responsible escort for the homeward journey
Has a carer at home for next 24 hours
Written and verbal instructions given about postoperative care
Knows when to return for follow-up (if appropriate)
Emergency contact number supplied

initiated, based on discharge guidelines. Some units adhere to strict scoring systems which address vital signs, patient activity, postoperative nausea and vomiting (PONV), pain and bleeding,[29] but whether such regimented protocols offer any advantage over the checklist of criteria outlined in Box 3.3 is debatable. Generic criteria have their limitations. For example, the criterion of being able to 'walk unaided' from the day unit may be inappropriate following orthopaedic surgery to the foot. Common sense in such situations is clearly required and the individual surgical procedure or type of surgery undertaken may prompt additional specific criteria.[30]

How do we do it?

Developing and maintaining good practice in day surgery requires attention to detail in all aspects of anaethetic and surgical care. Special considerations apply to management of children in the day unit.

Anaesthesia

Day surgery may be performed under four basic anaesthetic techniques: sedation, local, regional or general anaesthesia, with or without premedication. Where local or regional anaesthetic techniques can be applied safely advantages arise both for the patient and for the efficient running of the service.

Premedication

In day surgery, premedication relates to any drugs administered in the day unit before the patient leaves for surgery and they are usually administered orally or rectally. There is a widely held belief that premedication sedatives for anxiety are unnecessary in day surgery and, if given, recovery time may be prolonged. In most cases this is true, but up to 19% of patients suffer significant anxiety and these may benefit from sedative premedication.[31]

Other premedication drugs commonly used in day surgery include oral ranitidine 150 mg for known acid reflux and NSAIDs for postoperative pain if the procedure is of short duration. In addition, the patient's normal drug therapy, including antihypertensive agents, should be given as normal.

Sedation

Sedation, commonly used in dental and endoscopy practice, may be defined as 'a technique in which the use of a drug or drugs produces a state of depression of the central nervous system enabling treatment to be carried out, but during which verbal contact with the patient is maintained'.[32] Standards of monitoring for sedation in gastrointestinal endoscopy were published in 1991 and address safety issues such as the availability of resuscitation equipment and the safe use and administration of benzodiazepines.[33] Patient responses to sedative agents vary considerably and they should be titrated to the desired clinical effect to minimise overdose. Ideally, the sedationist should be an experienced anaesthetist. Monitoring during the procedure is mandatory and consists of pulse oximetry to measure oxygen saturation, an assessment of the patient's level of consciousness and ECG and blood pressure monitoring, especially for patients with a history of ischaemic heart disease or cardiac arrhythmias. Oxygen supplementation is provided by oxygen mask or nasal cannulae.

In surgical practice, intravenous sedation should be kept simple and consists in adults of midazolam at a titrated dose of 0.07 mg/kg. Dosage is reduced in the elderly patient because hypotension and respiratory depression can occur. It is a better amnesic drug than diazepam and its solubility has reduced the incidence of pain on injection or phlebitis. As it has a short half-life of 2–4 hours, 'hangover' effects are reduced. If overdose occurs, the competitive benzodiazepine antagonist flumazenil is given, but as its half-life is only approximately 1 hour, it is important to recognise that re-sedation may occur and premature discharge of the patient must be avoided.

Sedo-analgesia is a combination of a benzodiazepine and an analgesic agent such as pethidine (meperidine) or morphine. It is often used in the more painful endoscopic procedures such as colonoscopy. The longer-acting traditional opioids are often now replaced by the more rapid onset short-acting agents such as fentanyl (50–200 µg i.v.), alfentanil and remifentanil, which act within several minutes.

Local and regional anaesthesia

As with sedation, perioperative monitoring is required and should include pulse oximetry, with ECG and blood pressure monitoring in the elderly

Table 3.2 • Dosage and application of local anaesthetic agents

Agent	Dose (mg/kg) Alone	Dose (mg/kg) With adrenaline	Application
Cocaine	–	–	Topical
Amethocaine (tetracaine)	–	Topical	
Prilocaine	5	7	Intravenous regional anaesthesia
Lignocaine (lidocaine)	3	5	Infiltration nerve blocks
Bupivacaine	1–2	1–2	Infiltration nerve blocks, spinal/epidural
Ropivacaine	1–2	1–2	Infiltration nerve blocks, spinal/epidural

or cardiovascularly unfit. Several local anaesthetic agents are available (Table 3.2) but toxic reactions can occur in overdosage. Toxic blood levels lead to circumoral tingling, tinnitus and dizziness. Serious overdosage is reflected in loss of consciousness, convulsions or cardiac dysrhythmia. Dosage levels therefore need to be controlled. Higher dosage can be administered if it is given with adrenaline (epinephrine; 1:200 000), which causes vasoconstriction. This assists haemostasis, slow absorption and prolongs anaesthesia. The administration of adrenaline is contraindicated in end-artery procedures such as in the penis or in the digits of the hand or feet.

Local or regional anaesthesia may be used alone, with sedation or with general anaesthesia to prolong pain relief after completion of the procedure. Cocaine, which also has vasoconstrictor properties, may be topically applied to the nasal mucosa prior to nasal surgery. Amethocaine (tetracaine), which is systemically toxic, is mainly used for topical anaesthesia in ophthalmology. Prilocaine is short acting, has less toxic levels in the blood and is useful in intravenous regional anaesthesia such as Bier's block. Field infiltration with local anaesthetic and adrenaline may be used for the removal of minor 'lumps and bumps'. Bupivacaine (and the newer ropivacaine) has a long duration of action, lasting several hours, but can take up to 30 minutes to achieve simple nerve block. It is therefore a useful adjunct for wound infiltration or nerve block in association with general anaesthesia.

Spinal anaesthesia is not widespread in UK day surgery practice, in contrast to many other parts of the world. The main advantage of spinal anaesthesia is for operations below the waist such as arthroscopic surgery on the knee, foot surgery, haemorrhoidectomy or other minor rectal surgery, neurological surgery and inguinal hernia repair. The principal reasons for selecting spinal anaesthe-

sia are in the obese or those with cardiorespiratory disease who would otherwise be excluded from day surgery.[34]

General anaesthesia

The techniques and drugs used in general anaesthesia today permit up to 90 minutes of anaesthetic time for day surgery. The use of the laryngeal mask rather than the endotracheal tube has changed anaesthetic practice in day surgery since its introduction in 1988. Muscle relaxants are not required with its insertion, which is quicker and easier, and it is tolerated in light anaesthesia, allowing rapid patient turnaround. The introduction of total intravenous anaesthesia using propofol for induction and maintenance of anaesthesia has major advantages over inhalation agents; these include reduced PONV, early recovery and rapid control of the depth of anaesthesia, making it ideal for day case surgery. PONV after surgery is best prevented rather than treated, but is more likely if surgery lasts more than 1 hour or involves laparoscopy, dental procedures, squint surgery or correction of bat ears.

 Adequate hydration reduces PONV and intravenous fluid should be administered during longer procedures. Intravenous fluids at a dose of 20 mL/kg significantly reduce the incidence of postoperative drowsiness and dizziness.[35]

Pain management during anaesthesia is based on a concept of multimodal analgesia, which is a combination of two or more analgesic agents or analgesic techniques to minimise side-effects. A common strategy is to use an NSAID or short-acting opioid in combination with regional or local anaesthesia. The administration of stronger opiates such as morphine and pethidine at this stage is to be avoided as its longer-lasting effects may lead to unplanned overnight admission. Administration of analgesia in recovery and on the day ward before discharge should be given before 'breakthrough' pain occurs and is based on the accurate measurement of pain by the patients themselves.

Surgery

The safe, effective and efficient surgery required for a day case procedure demands the competence of a trained surgeon, a consultant or an experienced specialist registrar. In the past, the day surgery list of intermediate procedures was delegated to the most junior surgical trainee to perform without supervision. Not surprisingly, this led to prolonged operating times, patient cancellations, increased complications (such as bleeding or haematoma formation) and an inevitable rise in the unplanned overnight admission rate. As surgical trainees may no longer work unsupervised, such poor-quality practices should be features of the past. Nevertheless, some consultant surgeons' attitudes towards day surgery remain lukewarm, mainly because many have never considered the importance of their role in the overall delivery of patient care and the need for them to be more actively involved in the process of care through the hospital system. A frequent excuse was that the surgery itself was mundane and lacked the technical challenge of complex major procedures. With the introduction of more major minimal access procedures into the field of day surgery, this excuse no longer holds true. Indeed, many day surgery experts would contend that any intermediate or major surgery performed on a day case basis is a true surgical challenge if morbidity is to be maintained at near zero levels.

Day surgery rates for specific procedures vary between hospitals and between individual surgeons. The reasons for such variations are complex and remain largely unexplained. Patient preference must always be considered but it is accepted that only 5–10% of patients are actively opposed to day surgery. Patients in rural areas living more than 1 hour's travel from the hospital are also more likely to require overnight admission. Large teaching hospitals tend to attract complex tertiary referrals and therefore day surgery accounts for a smaller percentage of their overall activity, but some maintain very high rates of over 80%. Population demographics might also explain why day case activity can be low in hospitals that serve a large geriatric population. Medical personnel may also have strong views for or against day surgery which will influence local day surgery rates.

Whilst these variations were understandable in the development phase of day surgery, they become increasingly difficult to justify as we move to a genuine National Healthcare system, with equal access to treatment for all. A new generation of surgeons

and anaesthetists who are more familiar with the skills and techniques necessary to provide high-quality day surgery should ensure that most of these extreme variations disappear over the next few years.

Surgical practice: controversies

Haemorrhoidectomy

Only 24% of all haemorrhoidectomies in the UK are currently performed as day cases, although the percentage recommended as safe in the BADS Directory is 65%.[36] It is possible to perform the traditional Milligan–Morgan technique on a day case basis but the raw rectal surface created by the procedure often results in unacceptable postoperative pain. The newer haemorrhoid techniques such as Ligasure haemorrhoidectomy[37] and stapled anopexy[38] are less invasive and are associated with a reduction in operative pain when compared with conventional techniques and may therefore be more suitable for day surgery. Spinal or caudal anaesthesia[34] may also confer an advantage for the day surgery patient. After-care consists of non-constipatory analgesia, pre-emptive laxatives to avoid unnecessary hospital stay until the bowels open, glyceryl trinitrate ointment for local pain relief and metronidazole antibiotics to reduce incidents of pain and secondary haemorrhage in the days following the procedure.[39]

Laparoscopic cholecystectomy

The day case rate for laparoscopic cholecystectomy in the UK is 6.4% and has changed little over the last few years, but varies from none in half of all hospitals to 60% in a few.[40] The reasons for this relate to fears about reactionary haemorrhage, delayed haemorrhage and bile leak. Reactionary haemorrhage occurs within 4–6 hours after surgery and can be addressed within the ordinary working day if the surgery is performed before noon. Delayed haemorrhage usually occurs 3–4 days after cholecystectomy and even if the patient had undergone their operation as an inpatient, they would still have gone home before the secondary haemorrhage was apparent. Bile leaks rarely become apparent before 48 hours after surgery: accessory duct injury is often insidious, diathermy injury to the biliary tree may take days to leak and cystic duct stump leakage likewise. Again, if the patient had undergone inpatient surgery the likelihood is that they would already have been discharged home. It is therefore more important to warn these patients of possible delayed complications and that they should seek medical review in the first few days after discharge if alarm symptoms such as abdominal pain, nausea and vomiting occur. The NHS Institute published a clinical pathway in 2007 which noted that 70% of laparoscopic cholecystectomies could be safely performed as day cases[40] and this target has been recommended to NHS commissioners as part of the 18-week programme.[41]

Successful day case laparoscopic cholecystectomy relies on rigorous patient selection, accepting only well-motivated and non-obese patients, and attention to detailed surgical technique. Patients require approximately 6 hours of recovery time and the procedure is best performed early in the

 Age greater than 50 and ASA class II and III are poor prognostic indicators.[42,43]

operating day.

Good operative technique is also relevant when creating the pneumoperitoneum, as carbon dioxide inadvertently placed in the extraperitoneal space can cause considerable discomfort. Shoulder tip pain from diaphragmatic irritation has been related to the size of the gas bubble under the diaphragm[44] and attempts should therefore be made to expel as much gas as possible at the end of the procedure. Blood in the peritoneal cavity is irritant and liver bed haemostasis and peritoneal lavage before exiting the abdomen are worthwhile. While much of the postoperative pain in laparoscopic cholecystectomy is deep in nature, laparoscopy port sites should always be infiltrated with a long-acting local anaesthetic (such as bupivacaine). There appears to be little difference between infiltration at the beginning or the end of the procedure.[45]

Prostatectomy

Patients requiring prostatectomy tend to be older and less fit and many have previously been excluded from day surgery by comorbidity. Conventional transurethral resection of the prostate (TURP) can be performed as a day case but postoperative haemorrhage remains a problem. Over the last 5 years, laser prostatectomy day case programmes have been developed,[46,47] with the patients discharged with a catheter in situ, returning to the day unit approximately 1 week later for trial without catheter. Some units now perform over 90% of prostatectomies as day cases.[48]

Tonsillectomy

 In the UK, 6% of tonsillectomies are performed on a day case basis due to worries about reactionary haemorrhage. This risk is small and in a recent series of 668 adults and children undergoing day case tonsillectomy in Salisbury, the reactionary haemorrhage rate was 0.3% occurring within the first 6–8 hours after the operation while the patient was still on the day unit.[49]

Secondary haemorrhage occurs in approximately 1% of post-tonsillectomy patients and occurs several days after discharge, but may cause rapid airway obstruction at home with fatal consequences. The Salisbury Unit has a high readmission rate of 6% and reflects their policy of readmitting even minor bleeds for 24 hours in case they herald a more major bleed.

Bariatric surgery

Bariatric or weight loss surgery is increasingly performed in the UK, as a result of the growing number of morbidly obese in the population who fail to respond to dietary methods or exercise. Obesity is a risk factor for any surgery,[15] but shorter, minimal access procedures such as laparoscopic gastric banding has been performed successfully as a day case procedure,[50] the limiting criteria being the 150-kg weight limit of most operating trolleys. Of greater significance is perhaps the implied message that BMI should no longer be seen as a limiting factor in the delivery of day surgery generally.

Recovery

Upon completion of anaesthesia at the end of a surgical procedure, the patient is transferred to the operating theatre recovery area known as 'first-stage recovery'. Formerly, patients remained here for a predetermined period, commonly 30 or 60 minutes. However, the development of short-acting anaesthetic agents, the introduction of minimally invasive surgical techniques and individual patient variability meant that patients were often ready for transfer to 'second-stage recovery' before their predetermined time. Therefore 'time-based recovery' is no longer necessary and has in many units been superseded by 'criteria-based recovery', where discharge is determined by the observations of stable vital signs, return of protective reflexes and the ability to obey commands. 'Second-stage recovery' occurs back in the ward or trolley area of the day unit itself, where patients recover sufficiently to allow safe discharge home. Certain patients may be suitable for direct transfer to second-stage recovery from the operating theatre itself (**Fig. 3.3**) and include patients who have received local or regional anaesthesia with or without minimal sedation.

Postoperative complications

Precise patient selection should ensure that postoperative morbidity is minimised, but complications do occur and can be classified into major and minor problems (Box 3.4).[51] Major complications occur less often than anticipated in the day surgery patient population,[52] with an incidence of 1 in 1455, and are independent of ASA status.

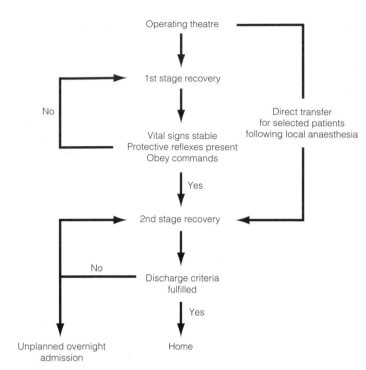

Figure 3.3 • Staged patient recovery.

Operating theatre

1st stage recovery

No

Vital signs stable
Protective reflexes present
Obey commands

Direct transfer
for selected patients
following local anaesthesia

Yes

2nd stage recovery

No

Discharge criteria
fulfilled

Yes

Unplanned overnight
admission

Home

Box 3.4 • Postoperative morbidity after day surgery

Major complications

Unrecognised visceral damage
Severe postoperative haemorrhage
Myocardial infarction
Pulmonary embolus
Cerebrovascular accident
Respiratory failure
(Death)

Minor complications

Pain
Postoperative nausea and vomiting
Drowsiness/dizziness
Sore throat/hoarseness
Headache
Minor bleeding
Infection

Mortality is low and varies between 1 in 66 500 and 1 in 11 273.

Minor complications are more common and may precipitate unplanned overnight admission; these range from 0.1% to 5% depending on case mix.[53] Postoperative morbidity is usually related to the procedure undertaken and the anaesthetic used rather than the ASA status, which predicts complications in major inpatient surgery but not in day surgery patients. Surgical causes account for 60–70% of unplanned admissions and are usually the result of the surgeon embarking on a more extensive procedure than planned rather than surgical misadventure. Day surgery lists require careful planning, with the more major surgical procedures performed earlier in the day to allow adequate recovery time. Failure to adhere to this policy often leads to unplanned admissions.[54] The more lengthy and invasive surgical procedures tend to increase postoperative pain, PONV and drowsiness, and preclude safe discharge. Even once the patient has returned home, PONV may return and last up to 5 days in 35% of patients[55] and is often severe. Readmission rates are similar to unplanned admission rates (0.7–3.1%) and again are most often from surgically related causes.

Before leaving the day unit, patients require specific information regarding their medication, wound care and when they are able to bath or shower, arrangements for suture removal or dressing renewal, when they can resume normal activities and arrangements for follow-up (if appropriate). It is also important to offer a contact telephone number for emergency purposes on the night of discharge. In addition, patients must be clearly instructed not to drive a motor vehicle for at least 24 hours. After groin or limb surgery, patients are advised only to drive when they can safely perform an emergency stop, usually 1 week later.

The most common reason for a patient visiting their general practitioner after day surgery is to obtain certification for time off work. The second commonest reason, usually in an unplanned manner, relates to worries about their wound. After discharge, many day surgery units offer outreach or telephone follow-up for their patients 24 hours later. This can be an effective evaluation tool, where any identified actual or potential problems can be highlighted to the day surgery team for action. This may only be necessary after specialised surgery (e.g. cataract surgery, where a change of dressing can be combined with outreach follow-up) or after the introduction of an unfamiliar procedure to the unit.

Paediatric day surgery

Children find surgery and hospital visits a daunting and stressful prospect and are therefore treated both separately and differently from adults. In 1991, the National Association for the Welfare of Children in Hospital published quality standards for care of paediatric day cases and suggested that children should be managed by staff trained in their care, in a child-safe and child-friendly environment with open access to the conscious child for the parents.[56] Ideally, paediatric day surgery should be performed in a dedicated paediatric day unit, but this is only achievable in specialised children's hospitals. In non-specialised hospitals where the availability of anaesthetists and surgeons with appropriate paediatric training and registered children's nurses is limited, it is savings efficient to plan 'children's days' in the day unit, for example one day per week. At the very least, on these lists children should have their operation on the first part of the list and in the ward be separated from adults and nursed in a paediatric area with play facilities available.

Most children are fit and healthy ASA class I patients. ASA class II and III patients are not excluded but an anaesthetist with paediatric expertise is recommended. ASA class III children include those with stable asthma, epilepsy or minor corrected congenital heart problems. Procedures for children with respiratory infections should be postponed for 2–4 weeks depending on severity, but after measles or whooping cough this should be extended to 6 weeks because of irritability of the respiratory tract.[57] In many units, children under the age of 6 months are considered unsuitable for day surgery, but if specialist facilities are available, full-term neonates are acceptable provided inpatient neonatal care is available. Premature babies are excluded up to 60 weeks after conception because of the risk of postoperative apnoea.[58] Many units also exclude children who are less than 5 kg because of the risk of hypothermia or hypoglycaemia associated with their physical status.

Psychosocial factors also determine a child's fitness for day surgery, and preparation begins with the preadmission visit to the day unit, the anaesthetic room and theatre recovery area, to allay the fears of both child and parents. At these so-called 'Saturday Clubs', routine information is given to the parents about day surgery, the procedure and preoperative fasting. Formal preassessment or preoperative investigation is not usually required. Very timid children, especially with overly anxious parents, may find the day surgery episode with all the associated unfamiliarity totally unacceptable and should be excluded. Single parents with many children and little help similarly cannot cope with a child's recovery.

Therefore, while the range of surgical procedures undertaken is similar to adult day surgery, in children it is often confined to a more restricted list (Box 3.5).

On the day of admission, sedative premedication is required for selected cases only, where the child is very anxious, has a needle phobia or has had a previous traumatic experience with anaesthetic induction. In the anaesthetic room, venous access is obtained after the application of topical local anaesthetic 1 hour before; parental presence in the anaesthetic room is useful, especially in the preschool group. Postoperative pain relief is obtained first through adjunctive local or regional anaesthesia. NSAIDs cannot be given to children under 1 year of age or 10 kg in weight because of their immature kidneys, but paracetamol is effective if given in a premedication dose of 20 mg/kg. Before discharge, the parents require clear instructions regarding pain control, wound care, mobilisation and resumption of normal activities.

Box 3.5 • Paediatric day surgery procedures

General surgery

Herniotomy, hydrocele excision, examination under anaesthesia, anal stretch, excision of minor lumps and bumps, ingrowing toenail treatment, endoscopy, biopsy (rectal, skin, lymph node)

Urology

Circumcision and associated procedures, orchidopexy

ENT

Myringotomy/grommets, adenoidectomy, tonsillectomy

Dental

Extractions

Ophthalmology

Correction of squint

Orthopaedic

Change of plaster cast

What will happen next?

The shift of elective surgery from the inpatient setting to short stay and eventually day care is now inexorable and will continue to be driven by three factors. The first and most important is the natural dislike in most people of in-hospital stays, particularly amongst those born since the 1960s; most people prefer to be at home, and as soon as a day surgery procedure can be shown to be performed as safely and effectively as in the traditional inpatient setting, most of us will opt for the former. In recent years, this move has been accelerated by the growing fear of acquired infections amongst inpatients, a problem not seen in stand-alone day units.

The second drive for change is the continued growth of minimal access techniques, including the use of robotics and the development of natural orifice transluminal endoscopic surgery (NOTES).[59] These techniques are associated with less surgical trauma and reduced postoperative pain both in the short and medium term, and have led to the concept of 'fast-track' surgery for inpatient procedures.[60] The concomitant development of better anaesthetic and pain-relieving techniques will further reduce the need for inpatient postoperative care. The third factor driving change is that of healthcare costs. By dispensing with inpatient hotel costs including staffing, procedures performed as day cases offer significant cost savings to healthcare providers and purchasers, even though high-quality day surgery may require greater expenditure on the day than is customary for inpatient care.

Nevertheless, the 2005 target of 75% of day case rates for all elective activity has not yet been achieved by all hospitals and there are several strategies that can be adopted for the further expansion of day surgery in those departments seeking further improvements:

- **Preassessment.** Preassessment should be nurse led, and the preassessment team, rather than the surgeon, should make the final decision regarding the suitability of the patient for true day surgery, 23-hour surgery or inpatient stay. The system should implement an 'opt out' rather than an 'opt in' policy (i.e. 'Is there any reason this patient *cannot* be a day case?').
- **Expand patient selection criteria.** Accept biological rather than chronological age and abandon formal upper age limits. Consider patients with a BMI up to 40 but with caution in laparoscopic surgery. Evaluate patients with stable ASA class III for day surgery suitability. Liaise with outreach nurses and social workers for patients with difficult social situations.

- **Consider alternative anaesthetic methods.** Local and regional anaesthetic methods reduce PONV and uncontrolled pain, which are factors contributing to unplanned overnight admissions. In many patients with major comorbidity, the use of methods other than general anaesthesia can convert the patient to day surgery. By using local and regional anaesthesia in inguinal hernia repair, 80–90% of patients can undergo day surgery.
- **Adopt new surgical procedures.** Several of the original Audit Commission 'basket' of procedures are now outpatient or office-based procedures. The introduction of new technology is often a catalyst for converting a traditional inpatient procedure to day case procedures. Examples include laparoscopic rather than open cholecystectomy, newer and less invasive techniques for haemorrhoidectomy, and the introduction of laser technology for prostatectomy.
- **Organisational redesign.** Maximising elective surgery on a day case basis requires resolute planning of operating lists for both patients and staffing. The more major day surgery procedures should be scheduled at the beginning of the day's list and the intermediate procedures later. If it is an all-day list, then intermediate procedures performed under local anaesthesia or regional block can be scheduled late in the afternoon and the patients can still return home that evening. For mixed inpatient and day surgery lists, it seems obvious to schedule day surgery procedures first on the list before the more major inpatient cases. All too often traditional surgical practice commences with the most major surgery of the day, finishing the list with the day surgery cases and risking an unplanned overnight admission. Reduction in junior doctors' hours and the resultant patterns of shift work indicate that many surgeons will be operating without a surgical trainee. Many hospitals have introduced non-medical practitioners to help with the task of assistance and they now form permanent and valuable members of the surgical team.
- **Lengthen the day surgery day.** Increase the traditional 12-hour day to 14 or even 16 hours. This increases the time available for recovery and maximises use of theatre time even allowing

day case procedures to be performed late in the afternoon. Alternatively, consider 'hotel' facilities, where the patient remains overnight but without medical or nursing supervision. This is certainly useful for patients who travel long distances or where the facilities at home are inadequate. Finally, if clinical overnight observation is required, then the day may be extended to 23 hours with the creation of an extended day surgery unit, allowing more surgical procedures to be performed on an ambulatory basis.[61]

Key points

- The government targeted 75% of all elective surgery to be performed on a day case basis by the end of 2005.
- All elective surgical patients should be preassessed by a nurse preassessment team who make the decision to allocate to 12-hour, 23-hour or inpatient surgery.
- Day surgery should be independent and separate from the inpatient infrastructure as successful day surgery depends on day of surgery admission, preassessment and nurse-led discharge.
- Regional and local anaesthetic block techniques are ideal for day surgery but are currently underutilised.
- Major surgical procedures, such as laparoscopic cholecystectomy, TURP, bilateral varicose vein surgery and arthroscopic procedures, can now be performed safely and routinely as day cases.

References

1. Department of Health. The NHS plan: a plan for investment, a plan for reform. London: Department of Health, 2000.

2. Department of Health. Day surgery: operational guide. London: Department of Health, 2002.

   The Department of Health operational guide for day surgery helps day surgery units achieve 75% elective surgery on a day case basis and covers aspects of patient selection, day surgery activity, day surgery accommodation, management and staffing.

3. Nicholl JH. The surgery of infancy. Br Med J 1909; ii:753–6.

4. Waters RM. The down-town anesthesia clinic. Am J Surg 1919; 33(Suppl):71–3.

5. Asher RAJ. The dangers of going to bed. Br Med J 1947; ii:967–8.

6. Palumbo LT, Laul RE, Emery FB. Results of primary inguinal hernioplasty. Arch Surg 1952; 64:384–94.

7. Farquharson EL. Early ambulation with special references to herniorrhaphy as an outpatient procedure. Lancet 1955; ii:517–19.

8. Baskerville PA, Jarrett PEM. Day case inguinal hernia repair under local anaesthetic. Ann R Coll Surg Engl 1983; 65:224–5.

9. Royal College of Surgeons of England. Report of the working party for day case surgery. London: RCS, 1992.

10. NHS Management Executive. A study of the management and utilisation of operating departments. London: HMSO, 1989.

11. Audit Commission. A short cut to better services: day surgery in England and Wales. London: HMSO, 1990.

12. Audit Commission. Measuring quality: the patient's view of day surgery. London: HMSO, 1991.

13. NHS Management Executive. Day surgery: report by the Day Surgery Task Force. London: NHS Health Publications Unit, 1993.

14. Fogg KJ, Saunders PRI. Folly! The long distance day surgery patient. Ambul Surg 1995; 3:209–10.

15. National Institutes of Health. Clinical guidelines on the identification, evaluation, and treatment of overweight and obesity in adults – evidence report. Obesity Res 1998; 6(Suppl 2):515–2095.

16. Department of Health. Annual health statistics. London: Department of Health, 2008.

17. Miller JM. Selection and investigation of adult day cases. In: Miller JM, Rudkin GE, Hitchcock M (eds) Practical anaesthesia and analgesia for day surgery. Oxford: BIOS Scientific, 1997; pp. 5–16.

18. Davies KE, Houghton K, Montgomery J. Obesity and day case surgery. Anaesthesia 2001; 56:1090–115.

19. Myles PS, Iacono GA, Hunt JO et al. Risks of respiratory complications and wound infection in patients

undergoing ambulatory surgery: smokers versus non-smokers. Anesthesiology 2002; 97:842–7.

20. Buist AS, Sexton GJ, Magy JM et al The effect of smoking cessation and modification on lung function. Am Rev Respir Dis 1976; 114:115–22.

21. Stechman MJ, Healy J, McMillan R et al. Is current advice on smoking prior to day surgery in the UK appropriate? J One Day Surg 2004; 14:5–8.

22. American Society of Anesthesiology. ASA classification of surgical patients. Chicago: American Society of Anesthesiology, 1991.

A definitive classification of comorbidity by the American Society of Anesthesiology that has become universally accepted to assess fitness for anaesthesia.

23. Ansel GL, Montgomery J. Outcome of ASA III patients undergoing day case surgery. Br J Anaesth 2004; 92:71–4.

24. Watson B, Smith I, Jennings A et al. Day surgery and the diabetic patient. London: British Association of Day Surgery, 2002.

25. Howell SJ, Sear JW, Foex P. Hypertension, hypertensive heart disease and perioperative cardiac risk. Br J Anaesth 2004; 92:570–83.

A systematic review and meta-analysis of 30 observational studies demonstrated no association between admission arterial pressure when less than 180 mmHg systolic and 110 mmHg diastolic and perioperative complications. This evidence indicates that patients whose blood pressure is elevated within these limits can undergo routine safe surgery without cancellation.

26. Committee on Safety of Medicines. Avoid all NSAIDs in aspirin sensitive patients. Curr Prob Pharmacovig 1993; 19:8.

27. Carlisle J. Guidelines for pre-operative testing. J One Day Surg 2004; 14:13–16.

28. Gold BS, Young ML, Kinman JL et al. The utility of preoperative electrocardiograms in the ambulatory surgical patient. Arch Intern Med 1992; 152:301–5.

29. Aldrete BA. The Post-anaesthesia Recovery Score revisited. J Clin Anesth 1995; 7:89–91.

30. Cahill H, Jackson I, McWhinnie D. Ready to go home? London: British Association of Day Surgery, 2000; pp. 1–8.

31. Mackenzie JW. Day case anaesthesia and anxiety. Anaesthesia 1989; 44:437–40.

32. Wylie report. Report of the Working Party on Training in Dental Anaesthesia. Br Dent J 1981; 151:385–8.

33. Bell GD, McCloy RF, Charlton JE et al. Recommendations for standards of sedation and patient monitoring during gastrointestinal endoscopy. Gut 1991; 32:823–7.

34. Watson B, Allen J, Smith I. Spinal anaesthesia: a practical guide. London: British Association of Day Surgery, 2004.

35. Yogendran S, Asokumar B, Cheng DC et al. A prospective randomised double blinded study of the effect of intravenous fluid therapy on adverse outcomes on outpatient surgery. Anaesth Analg 1995; 80:682–6.

Two hundred ASA grade I–III ambulatory surgical patients were prospectively randomised into two groups to receive high (20 mL/kg) or low (2 mL/kg) prospective isotonic infusion over 30 minutes preoperatively. The incidence of thirst, drowsiness and dizziness was significantly lower in the high-infusion group 60 minutes after surgery, confirming an advantage to routine perioperative intravenous fluid administration.

36. General surgery recommended lengths of stay. In: BADS directory of procedures, 2nd edn, 2007; pp. 8–9.

37. Jayne DG, Botterill I, Ambrose NS et al. Randomised clinical trial of Ligasure versus conventional diathermy for day case haemorrhoidectomy. Br J Surg 2002; 89:428–32.

38. Rowsell M, Bello M, Hemingway DM. Circumferential mucosectomy (stapled haemorrhoidectomy) versus conventional haemorrhoidectomy: randomised controlled trial. Lancet 2000; 355:779–81.

39. Carapeti EA, Kamm M, McDonald PJ et al. Double blind randomised controlled trial of effect of metronidazole on pain after day case haemorrhoidectomy. Lancet 1998; 351:169–72.

40. Focus on: Cholecystectomy. NHS Institute for Innovation and Improvement, 2007.

41. Tackling hospital waiting: the 18 week patient pathway. London: Department of Health 2006.

42. Robinson TN, Biffl WL, Moore EE. Predicting failure of outpatient laparoscopic cholecystectomy. Am J Surg 2002; 184:515–18.

43. Lau H, Brookes DC. Predictive factors for unanticipated admission after ambulatory laparoscopic cholecystectomy. Arch Surg 2001; 136:1150–3.

44. Jackson SA, Lawrence AS, Hill JC. Does post laparoscopy pain relate to residual carbon dioxide? Anaesthesia 1996; 51:485–7.

45. Mjaland O, Raeder J, Aasboe V et al. Outpatient laparoscopic cholecystectomy. Br J Surg 1997; 84:958–61.

46. Keoghane SR, Millar JM, Cranston DW. Is day case prostatectomy feasible? Br J Urol 1995; 76:600–3.

47. Gomez Sancha F, Bachmann A, Choi BB et al. Photoselective vaporization of the prostate (Greenlight PV): lessons learnt after 3500 procedures. Prostate Cancer Prostatic Dis 2007; 10(4):316–22.

48. Urological recommended lengths of stay. BADS directory of procedures, 2nd edn, 2007; pp. 16–17.

49. Dennis S, Georgallow M, Elcock L et al. Day case tonsillectomy: the Salisbury experience. J One Day Surg 2004; 14:17–22.

50. Dunsire MF, Patel AG, Awad N et al. Laparoscopic gastric banding for morbid obesity in the day surgery setting. J One Day Surg 2007; 17:1.

51. Natof HE. Complications. In: Wetcher BV (ed.) Anaesthesia for ambulatory surgery. Philadelphia: Lippincott, 1985; p. 321.

52. Hitchcock M. Postoperative morbidity following day surgery. In: Millar JM, Rudkin GE, Hitchcock M (eds) Practical anaesthesia and analgesia for day surgery. Oxford: BIOS Scientific, 1997; pp. 205–11.

53. Levy ML. Complications: prevention and quality assurance. Anesth Clin North Am 1987; 5:137–66.

54. Twersky RS, Abiona M, Thorne AC et al. Admissions following ambulatory surgery: outcome in seven urban hospitals. Ambul Surg 1995; 3:141–6.

55. Carrol NV, Miederhoff P, Cox FM et al. Postoperative nausea and vomiting after discharge from outpatient surgery centres. Anesth Analg 1995; 80:903–9.

56. Thornes R. Just for the day. London: National Association for the Welfare of Children in Hospital, March 1991.

57. McEwan AI, Birch M, Bingham R. The preoperative management of the child with a heart murmur. Paediatr Anaesth 1995; 5:151–5.

58. Steward DJ. Preterm infants are more prone to complications following minor surgery than are term infants. Anesthesiology 1982; 56:304–6.

59. Buyske J. Natural orifice transluminal endoscopic surgery. J Am Med Assoc 2007; 298:1560–1.

60. Kehlet H, Wilmore DW. Fast track surgery. Br J Surg 2005; 92:3–4.

61. Phillips D, Healy J, McWhinnie D et al. Extended day surgery. J One Day Surg 1999; 8:5–6.

4

Abdominal hernias

Andrew C. de Beaux

Introduction

A hernia is defined as an abnormal protrusion of a cavity's contents, through a weakness in the wall of the cavity, taking with it all the linings of the cavity, although these may be markedly attenuated. The anterior abdominal wall can be divided into two structural/functional zones: the upper 'parachute area' aiding respiratory movement and a lower 'belly support' area.[1] Functional failure in the abdomen may lead to epigastric and umbilical hernia in the upper zone and to inguinal and femoral hernia in the lower zone. The external abdominal hernia is the commonest form of hernia, the most frequent varieties being the inguinal (75%), femoral (8.5%) and umbilical (15%).

Hernias can be described as reducible, incarcerated or strangulated. A reducible hernia is one in which the contents of the hernial sac can be manually introduced back into the abdomen while, conversely, an irreducible or incarcerated hernia cannot be manipulated back into the abdomen. A strangulated hernia occurs when the vascular supply to the contents contained within the hernia is compromised, resulting in ischaemic and gangrenous tissue.

Aetiology

Multiple factors contribute to the development of hernias. Hernias are associated with a number of medical conditions, including connective tissue disorders such as Ehlers–Danlos syndrome, as well as a number of abnormal collagen-related disorders such as varicose veins and arterial aneurysm. In essence, hernias can be considered design faults, either anatomical or through inherited collagen disorders, although these two aetiological factors probably work together in the majority of patients. Anatomical design faults could be considered at any site where structures within the cavity exit through an opening in the wall of the cavity such as blood vessels, bowel or the spermatic cord. This is typical, for example, around the oesophagus and in the groin. However, not everyone develops a groin hernia so other factors must be important. The fascia and surrounding tissues which cover muscle, acting to hold the muscle bundles together, may appear relatively avascular, but it remains a complex and living structure. The genetic code for fascia is coded on DNA, and within fibroblasts the sequence is messenger RNA, transfer RNA, peptide formation, with fusion of peptides into approximately 1000-amino-acid polypeptides called alpha chains. The endoplasmic reticulum converts these to procollagen. Procollagen is the large building block of collagen, comprised of triple-helix strands, stabilised by hydroxylation of proline and lysine, which is vitamin C dependent. These triple-helix strands form microfibrils, then fibrils, then fibres and finally bundles. These collagen bundles surrounded by extracellular matrix comprise fascia. The control of this process is mediated through matrix metalloproteinases, which in turn are controlled by tissue inhibitory metaloproteinases. If this is not complex enough, there is also control by collagen-interacting proteins and receptors such as fibronectin, tenasin and collagen receptor discoidin domain receptor 2. Fascia and tendon are made up of type I and type III collagen (type II is found in cartilage and type IV in the basement membrane of cells). In cross-section, there is a bimodal distribution of bundle size. The larger bundles are type I collagen, imparting the strength to the fascia or tendon. The type III collagen bundles are smaller and are thought to provide elastic recoil following stretch when the tissues have been loaded. The type I to III collagen ratio varies between individuals but is constant in all the fascia of a particular individual.

A clinical observation was made by surgeons in the late 1960s that the anterior rectus sheath some distance from the hernial defect was thinner than normal, especially in those patients with direct hernias.[2] Since then, research has demonstrated a variety of defects in collagen sythesis in such patients.[3,4] The current notion is that the majority of hernias are a disease of collagen metabolism. One of the key factors in this is the type I to III collagen ratio. The lower this ratio, from an average of around 5, the more likely the individual is to develop a hernia. Currently, collagen typing is not used in clinical practice to help decide perhaps which patients merit a mesh as opposed to a suture repair, but this may well be a development in the near future.

 Hernias are a collagen disease, with reduced collagen type I to III ratio.[3,4]

Mesh

Much will be mentioned about mesh repairs of hernias in the remainder of this chapter, but this section gives a brief overview of mesh and its science.

Many companies produce a variety of mesh for hernia repair. These are either synthetic (man made) or biological (preparations from animal or human tissue). The majority of synthetic meshes are woven from either polypropylene or polyester. Biological meshes are typically animal collagen, either from skin or bowel, but there are also human preparations. Biological meshes tend to be much more expensive and are thus reserved for specialist use and will not be discussed further.

It goes without saying that any mesh should have the usual properties of any implant, including being non-allergenic, non-carcinogenic, have good incorporation into tissue and mimic the tissue it is replacing or reinforcing. The abdominal wall is not a rigid structure, but regularly copes with increases in abdominal pressure on coughing and sneezing, etc. of up to 200 mmHg. The abdominal wall elasticity is greater in women than in men and is greater in the craniocaudal direction than transversely or obliquely. The traditional standard weight polypropylene mesh, of around 100 g/m^2, is significantly over-engineered with a burst strength at least an order of magnitude greater than the anterior abdominal wall and an elasticity of much less.[5] There are now many polypropylene meshes on the market of lighter weight. There are no strict definitions of light weight and heavy weight but a reasonable guideline is that mesh of 40–80 g/m^2 is medium weight and <40 g/m^2 is light weight. However, it is not just the weight of the mesh that imparts elasticity and flexibility. Pore size or the size of the large holes in the mesh is also important. Fibrosis will occur around each strand of the mesh. If the strands are close together, the fibrosis around each strand will coalesce together, forming a solid scar plate. As the scar plate matures it will shrink, reducing the overall size of the mesh. The minimum pore size should be about 1 mm^2 but many meshes have pore sizes around 3–5 mm. Increasing the macroporosity of the mesh produces a scar net, rather than a scar plate, with normal tissue in between the fibre/scar complex, reducing mesh/scar shrinkage and improving flexibility (**Fig. 4.1**). In addition to the macropore size, mesh also has micropores within the mesh material itself. These should be at least 10 μm in size. If the micropore size is smaller, bacteria can harbour in the pores out of reach of the larger inflammatory cells.

The majority of synthetic meshes in the UK are polypropylene. Gortex and other polytetrafluoroethylene (PTFE)-based meshes have some popularity. PTFE has no macropores so will be encapsulated by fibrous tissue with minimal tissue ingrowth. Polyester-based meshes are gaining popularity and have some advantages over polyproplyene but are multifilament rather than monofilament. The multifilament arrangement increases the developed surface of the mesh (around 2000 mm^2 per cm^2 mesh as compared to 200 mm^2 per cm^2 for polypropylene) and thus improves tissue incorporation. As a result, the peel strength (the effort required to separate the mesh from the tissues once it is incorporated) is greater, in the region of 190 N as compared to 160 N for a polypropylene mesh (**Fig. 4.2**).

There is increasing evidence that lightweight, large pore mesh is of benefit to the patient.[6] There are some reports that the recurrence rate may be higher[7] when such mesh is used, but it is likely that this is for technical regions. Fixation sutures on such mesh should be placed at least 1 cm in from the edge of the mesh and slightly larger meshes may need to be used.

 Preferred mesh should be lightweight (<80 g/m^2), large pore (>1 mm) and macroporous (>10 μm).[6]

Figure 4.1 • **(a)** Micrograph of a macropore mesh of <0.5 mm pore size showing scar plate formation and contraction/distortion of the mesh. **(b)** Micrograph of a macropore mesh of 0.8 mm pore size showing minimal scar bridging and no distortion of the mesh. **(c)** Micrograph of a macropore mesh of 3 mm pore size showing scar net formation and no contraction/distortion of the mesh. Micrographs used by permission of Covidien UK.

Figure 4.2 • Micrograph of a polyester mesh fibre. There is evidence of fibrosis around the fibre bundle as well as fibrous ingrowth around each strand. Micrograph used by permission of Covidien UK.

Traditional meshes placed within the abdominal cavity have a high rate of adhesions of the omentum and bowel to the mesh. This can result in bowel fistulation or make subsequent laparotomy more difficult, with increased risk of bowel perforation and thus the need for bowel resection during the process of re-entering the abdominal cavity.[8] A number of tissue-separating meshes are available, where the intra-abdominal side of the mesh is coated with a product to minimise adhesion formation. It would be fair to say that such coatings do reduce adhesion formation, but in the majority of patients significant adhesion to such coatings still occur. The main points of adhesion appear to be the edge of the mesh and to the points of fixation, either sutures, tacks or staples. Nevertheless, it is likely that these products will improve in the future, as meshes become more physiological, perhaps with impregnated growth hormones and other biologically active molecules to improve the mesh/tissue integration.

Epigastric hernia

An epigastric hernia is defined as a fascial defect in the linea alba between the xiphoid process and the umbilicus. The true incidence is unknown but autopsy studies have suggested a prevalence of 0.5–10% in the general population. There is a male preponderance, with a male to female ratio of approximately 4:1, with the diagnosis usually being made in the third to fifth decades.

Aetiology

The aetiology is related to the functional anatomy of the 'parachute area'. The anterior abdominal wall aponeurosis consists of tendinous fibres that lie obliquely in aponeurotic sheets, allowing for changes in the shape of the abdominal wall, for example during respiration. However, the midline can change only in length and breadth, an increase in one necessitating a decrease in the other. During abdominal distension, the linea alba must increase in both dimensions, the resulting tearing of fibres possibly leading to the development of an epigastric hernia.

Clinical presentation

The majority of epigastric hernias (probably 75%) are asymptomatic. Typical symptoms, if present, include vague upper abdominal pain and nausea associated with epigastric tenderness. The symptoms tend to be more severe when the patient is lying down, attributed to traction on the hernial contents. Pain on exertion localised to the epigastrium is also a common symptom. Incarceration is common, while strangulation of preperitoneal fat or omentum results in localised pain and tenderness. Incarceration or strangulation of intra-abdominal viscera is extremely rare, the symptoms depending on the incarcerated organ.

The presence of a midline mass on physical examination usually confirms the diagnosis. In obese patients, palpation of the mass may be difficult and confirmation of the diagnosis by ultrasound or computed tomography may be helpful.

Management

Epigastric hernias are rare in infants and children, and asymptomatic hernias in children under the age of 10 years may resolve spontaneously. The decision for surgical intervention depends on the presence and severity of symptoms.

Operative details

Small solitary defects may be approached with either a vertical or transverse incision in the midline, centred over the hernia. For larger hernias, if the defects are multiple or in the emergency setting when a strangulated viscus is suspected, a vertical incision is preferred. The hernia and its contents are dissected free of the surrounding tissues and, if present, the hernial contents examined and dealt with appropriately. If the defect is small (<2 cm), repair by primary suture closure with non-absorbable sutures is usually sufficient. The orientation of the suture closure remains controversial, some surgeons preferring a vertical closure and others a horizontal orientation. There are very few data to support one technique over the other and probably the direction resulting in the least tension is the most appropriate. If the defect is large (>6 cm²), or occurs within a divarification of the recti, the hernia should be repaired with prosthetic mesh. This technique is described later in the chapter when considering incisional hernias. The technique applied to intermediate-sized hernias is controversial and either suture or mesh techniques are currently deemed acceptable. Laparoscopic repair of epigastric hernias[9] was first described in 1992 and the technique has grown in popularity. The author prefers an open technique under local anaesthetic whenever possible for smaller hernias (defect <2 cm), suture or mesh depending on the quality of the tissues, and the laparoscopic approach for larger, multiple, recurrent or hernias in the obese. At laparoscopic repair, it is important to take down the falciform ligament and remove any preperitoneal fat above the linea alba, otherwise the 'hernia' may still be palpable following alleged repair.

Complications

Complication rates are low and most are the usual complications associated with abdominal wall incisions (haematoma, infection). There are very few data on recurrence rates, historical series reporting rates around 7%.[10] In perhaps 50% of patients, however, the recurrence probably represents the persistence of a second hernia or area of weakness overlooked at the initial procedure. The laparoscopic technique avoids this problem because all fascial defects are visible laparoscopically if adequate dissection is carried out.

Umbilical and paraumbilical hernias

There are several distinct types of hernia that occur around the umbilicus: congenital (omphalocele), infantile, paraumbilical and adult umbilical hernias.

Congenital umbilical hernias

A congenital umbilical hernia occurs when the abdominal viscera herniate into the tissue of the umbilical cord. Normally, the gut returns to the abdominal cavity at 10 weeks of gestation. If this fails to occur, normal rotation and fixation of the intestine are prevented, the umbilicus is absent and a funnel-shaped defect in the abdominal wall is present through which viscera protrude into the umbilical cord. The abdominal wall defect may vary in size from no larger than an umbilical stump to a defect that appears to involve the entire abdominal wall. Congenital umbilical hernia occurs in 1 in 5000 births and is associated with other serious congenital anomalies.

Clinical presentation

Congenital umbilical hernia may be diagnosed in utero or at birth. On ultrasound examination, fetal abdominal wall defects are not subtle and may be visualised as early as 15 weeks of gestation.

The management is surgical correction and one of the most important contributors to the morbidity and mortality of isolated abdominal wall defects is the delay between delivery and appropriate surgical repair. Antenatal knowledge of the existence of a congenital hernia can allow for the birth of the child at a tertiary care institution with the appropriate neonatal and paediatric surgical expertise (see also Chapter 12).

Management

Surgical correction should only be undertaken in specialised centres. If the diagnosis is made prenatally, the mother should be transferred to such a centre for delivery. If the diagnosis only becomes apparent at birth, the baby should be kept warm and hydrated, and the sac handled with care to avoid rupture or twisting of the sac. The sac should be wrapped in moist sterile gauze and covered with impervious plastic sheeting or aluminium foil. Mother and baby should then be transferred as soon as feasible to a tertiary centre for further management.

Infantile umbilical hernias

Infantile umbilical hernias occur when the umbilical vessels fail to fuse with the urachal remnant and umbilical ring. It presents with a protrusion of the umbilicus, usually at the superior margin of the ring. The infantile hernia, as opposed to the congenital type, is always covered by skin. It is the third most common surgical disorder in children, occurring in approximately one in five live births.

Clinical presentation

Clinically, the commonest presenting 'symptom' is the cosmetic appearance, the hernia resulting in a cone-like protrusion of the umbilicus that bulges every time the child cries or strains. Infantile umbilical hernias rarely enlarge over time and 90% disappear by the time the child is 2 years of age, although they are unlikely to close spontaneously if they persist to the age of 5 years.[11] Spontaneous resolution of umbilical hernias appears to be directly influenced by the size of the umbilical ring. If, at the age of 3 months, the hernia has a fascial ring of <0.5 cm, 96% heal spontaneously within 2 years. Defects that have a fascial diameter >1.5 cm are unlikely to heal spontaneously. Complications of umbilical hernias are rare, occurring in approximately 5%, and include strangulation of the omentum, strangulation of the intestine and evisceration.

Management

Management of the infant with an umbilical hernia is expectant. The majority will resolve spontaneously without surgical correction. The indications for surgery in children less than 2 years of age are the development of complications or tenderness over the site of the hernia. There is no consensus on the appropriate timing of herniorrhaphy in older children but generally repair is performed before school/nursery to avoid the child becoming self-conscious of the umbilical protrusion.

Operative details

Elective repair of infantile umbilical hernia is performed on an outpatient basis under general anaesthesia. A curvilinear incision is made within a skin fold on the inferior aspect of the hernia. The sac is then encircled by blunt dissection. If there is any concern regarding the contents of the sac, the sac should be opened on its caudal aspect, as abdominal contents usually adhere to the fundus of the sac. Once dealt with appropriately, the contents should be reduced and the incision continued to the cephalic aspect of the sac. If the sac is empty, the fundus may simply be disconnected from the umbilicus and reduced intact. Repair is by simple fascial apposition using horizontal mattress sutures of absorbable material. While the Mayo ('vest-over-pants') technique of umbilical hernioplasty is frequently taught, there is no evidence that the results are any better than simple apposition of the fascial edges. The umbilicus is refashioned by leaving a small button of the fundus of the sac attached to the inner surface of the cicatrix and tacking it down to the area of fascial repair.

Complications

Complications of umbilical hernioplasty are rare, but include seroma or haematoma formation and infection. Recurrence is possible if large defects are closed under tension or if an associated paraumbilical hernia is overlooked.

Paraumbilical hernias

Paraumbilical hernias are acquired hernias and occur in all age groups. They occur secondary to disruption of the linea alba and generally occur above the umbilical cicatrix. Aetiological factors include stretching of the abdominal wall by obesity, multiple pregnancy and ascites. Paraumbilical hernias are more common in patients over the age of 35 years and are five times more common in females.

Clinical presentation

Clinically, paraumbilical hernias are frequently symptomatic. Patients complain of intermittent abdominal pain (possibly caused by dragging on the fat and peritoneum of the falciform ligament) and, when the hernial sac contains bowel, colic resulting from intermittent intestinal obstruction.

The hernia tends to progress over time and intertrigo and necrosis of the skin may occur in patients with large dependent hernias.

Management

It is important to distinguish paraumbilical hernias from true umbilical defects as the latter may resolve spontaneously in the young, whereas the former require surgical correction. Umbilical hernias classically produce a symmetric bulge with the protrusion directly under the umbilicus. This is in contrast to paraumbilical hernias where about half the fundus of the sac is covered by the umbilicus and the remainder is covered by the skin of the abdomen directly above or below the umbilicus. Paraumbilical hernias do not resolve spontaneously and have a high incidence of incarceration and strangulation; therefore, surgical repair is nearly always indicated.

Operative details

For solitary hernias separated from the umbilicus, a transverse incision over the hernia produces the best exposure. In patients with a paraumbilical and umbilical hernia, a midline incision may provide better access. Similarly, if multiple fascial defects are present or there is concern about the integrity of visceral contents of the sac, a vertical incision may be better employed. If the defect simply contains preperitoneal fat, this may be reduced. In patients with strangulated or infected preperitoneal fat, it is best excised. If there is a sac present, it should be dissected free from the fascial edges, opened and the contents examined. Once the contents have been dealt with appropriately, they may be reduced and redundant sac excised. There is no requirement to close the peritoneum but some authors recommend transfixing the neck of the sac once the contents have been reduced. Repair is performed by fascial apposition either transversely or longitudinally, depending on the defect and the direction of least tension. As this is an acquired defect, non-absorbable sutures are recommended. Indeed, the author usually creates a preperitoneal pocket, inserting a 5 cm × 5 cm square (minimum size – bigger if necessary) mesh and closing the fascia over this. For larger paraumbilical hernias, with a neck size >3 cm (or smaller hernias in an obese patient), it is the author's preference to repair these laparoscopically and very large hernias with a neck size >8 cm by an open sublay technique (described later).

Adult umbilical hernias

Umbilical hernias in adults represent a spectrum of conditions from the partially unfolded cicatrix to huge dependent sacs. The umbilicus may become partially unfolded in patients with acute abdominal distension. Persistent elevation of intra-abdominal pressure eventually results in the umbilical cicatrix giving way and the development of an umbilical hernia. Although uncommon, causes include ascites from cirrhosis, congestive cardiac failure or nephrosis. Patients undergoing peritoneal dialysis also have a high incidence of these hernias. Management should be non-operative where possible, as the majority of these patients have serious underlying pathology. Operative repair is not indicated unless the hernia incarcerates or becomes extremely large and the overlying skin is thinned down to such an extent that spontaneous rupture is possible.

Umbilical hernias in adults do not represent persistence of infantile hernias but are indirect herniations through an umbilical canal, which is bordered by umbilical fascia posteriorly, the linea alba anteriorly and the medial edges of the two rectus sheaths on each side. They have a tendency to incarcerate and strangulate and do not resolve spontaneously. Umbilical hernias in adults have a high morbidity and mortality. Over 90% occur in females and almost all patients are obese and multiparous.

Clinical presentation

Clinically, the diagnosis is usually obvious. The hernias are usually large and complete reduction is not possible because of the adherence of omentum to the fundus of the sac. Adult umbilical hernias can be painful because, as they enlarge, they have a tendency to sag downwards, causing traction on the stomach and transverse colon. Attacks of intermittent colicky pain may be caused by episodes of incomplete intestinal obstruction. Surgery is usually indicated in these circumstances as the hernias are often incarcerated with a relatively small hernia neck size.

Management

Operative details

Umbilical hernias in high-risk adult patients are generally operated on using regional or local anaesthesia. In smaller umbilical hernias, a subumbilical incision may be used, but with large hernias, and particularly incarcerated hernias, a large midline incision may be necessary. The sac is isolated and the entire mass of fat and sac elevated while the neck of the sac is incised. The incarcerated contents must be evaluated and treated as required. The sac is frequently loculated and Richter-type hernias may occur within one or more of the loculi. After the contents are dealt with, the peritoneal sac is repaired and an edge-to-edge fascial closure performed in the direction of least tension, which may be either transverse or vertical. For small hernias (<2 cm in diameter), primary edge-to-edge apposition with non-absorbable sutures of appropriate size is sufficient. The classic Mayo approach[12] was to overlap the edges, but there has never been any demonstration that the bursting strength of the wound is improved by imbrication and may actually be impaired to a degree proportional to the amount of overlapping and tension. In larger hernias (>4 cm diameter), it is important to obtain closure without tension. If the fascial edges can be brought together with ease, the repair is reinforced with prosthetic mesh placed either extraperitoneally or retromuscularly, behind the rectus muscle (anterior to the posterior rectus sheath). If the fascial edges cannot be apposed easily, mobilisation of the lateral abdominal muscles will be required before placement of mesh in the retromuscular space (sublay). Only rarely, when the defect cannot be closed, should a mesh be placed to bridge the defect in the extra peritoneal space, with an overlap of the fascial edges of at least 5 cm. The mesh should be secured with interrupted non-absorbable sutures.

The overlying umbilical skin need not be excised unless it is macerated or infected, although the cosmetic appearance is often enhanced by judicious removal of excess skin and subcutaneous fat. All patients should be warned that it might be necessary to excise the umbilicus. If a new umbilicus is to be created, care should be taken as recurrences may occur at the point on the linea alba where the new umbilicus is fixed to the fascia.

Laparoscopic repair of such hernias is becoming popular. A small hernia in a thin patient can easily be done under local anaesthetic as a day case. But as the hernias and/or the patient increases in size, or the hernia is recurrent, laparscopic hernia repair becomes more attractive.[13]

Complications

Complications include the development of seromas, haematomas and infection. Sealed suction drains may be employed in the retromuscular and subcutaneous planes to avoid the development of large seromas. In addition to local problems, these patients often have respiratory and cardiovascular complications and may require prolonged hospitalisation.

Inguinal hernias

Anatomy

The anatomy of the inguinal region is complex. The inguinal canal is approximately 4 cm in length and is located just above the inguinal ligament between the internal and external rings. The inguinal canal allows passage of the spermatic cord into the scrotum, along with the testicular, deferential and cremasteric vessels. The superficial ring is a triangular aperture in the aponeurosis of the external oblique and lies about 1 cm above the pubic tubercle. The ring is bounded by a superomedial and an inferolateral crus joined by the criss-cross intercrural fibres. Normally, the ring will not admit the tip of the

little finger. The deep ring is a U-shaped condensation of the transversalis fascia and it lies about 1 cm above the inguinal ligament, midway between the pubic tubercle and the anterior superior iliac spine. The transversalis fascia is the fascial envelope of the abdomen and the competency of the deep inguinal ring depends on the integrity of this fascia.

The anterior boundary of the inguinal canal comprises mainly the external oblique aponeurosis with the conjoined muscle laterally. The posterior boundary is formed by the fascia transversalis and the conjoined tendon (internal oblique and transversus abdominus medially). The inferior epigastric vessels lie posteriorly and medially to the deep inguinal ring. The superior boundary is formed by the conjoined muscles (internal oblique and transversus) and the inferior boundary by the inguinal ligament.

Definition

An indirect hernia travels down the canal on the outer (lateral and anterior) side of the spermatic cord. A direct inguinal hernia comes out directly forwards through the posterior wall of the inguinal canal. While the neck of an indirect hernia is lateral to the epigastric vessels, the direct hernia usually emerges medial to these vessels, except in the saddlebag or pantaloon type, which has both a lateral and a medial component.

Inguinal hernia in infants and children (see also Chapter 12)

Repair of congenital inguinal hernia is the most frequently performed operation in the paediatric age group. Although inguinal hernias can present at any age, the peak incidence is during infancy and childhood. About 3–5% of full-term infants may be born with a clinical inguinal hernia.[14] Between 80% and 90% of paediatric hernias occur in boys, about one-third of the hernias presenting in the first 6 months of life. Congenital inguinal hernias have a 15% bilateral presentation.

Clinical presentation

Examination of the inguinal area for a hernia may show an obvious bulge at the site of the external ring or within the scrotum which can often be gently reduced. However, the bulge may only be seen during severe straining, such as with crying or defecation. If the infant is old enough to stand, he or she should be examined in both the supine and standing positions. If not, the parent can hold the infant upright so that the surgeon can closely observe the inguinoscrotal area. It is essential to make sure that the testis is within the scrotal sac to avoid mistaking a retractile testis for a hernial bulge. The presence of an empty scrotum should alert the examining surgeon to a possible undescended or ectopic testis, which is associated with an inguinal hernia more than 90% of the time. Although routine orchidopexy is usually delayed until the child is 1 year of age, a coexisting symptomatic hernia should be promptly repaired and orchidopexy accomplished at the same time.

Inguinal hernias are prone to incarcerate, the overall rate being 12%.[15] Incarceration is most common in the first 6 months of life, when more than half of instances are observed. An incarcerated hernia usually presents as an acute tender mass in the inguinal canal. The mass may protrude beyond the external inguinal ring or into the scrotum. The skin over the mass may be discoloured, oedematous, erythematous or blue. Strangulation, characterised by abdominal distension, vomiting, failure to pass faecal material, tachycardia and radiological evidence of small-bowel obstruction, demands emergency operative intervention for relief of obstruction, intestinal salvage and hernia repair. In contrast to the adult with an incarcerated hernia, in children, testicular ischaemia is far more common than intestinal ischaemia, and it is therefore appropriate to be aggressive about reducing the hernia (see Chapter 12).

Management

In general, hernias in children and particularly infants should be managed by experienced paediatric surgeons (see also Chapter 12). However, this is not always possible depending on geography and availability. In these circumstances the general surgeon on-call may be required to manage these patients. As most (80%) incarcerated hernias in children may be managed initially by non-operative measures, which include sedation, and then gentle reduction when the baby is quiet, exploration may be safely delayed for about 24–48 hours, allowing, if possible, a more experienced paediatric surgeon to become involved. However, if the hernia remains irreducible at this stage, emergency repair is indicated. The complication rate is approximately 20 times greater after emergency repair for incarcerated hernia than after elective procedures.[15] It is therefore worthwhile to reduce the hernia whenever possible and perform an elective procedure within 24–48 hours of the reduction. The high risk of incarceration in the paediatric age group makes the presence of an inguinal hernia an indication for surgical repair.

Operative details

Surgical access is achieved through a short (2–3 cm) transverse incision in the lowest inguinal skin crease. The superficial fascia (Scarpa's fascia) is incised and the external oblique fascia identified. The aponeurosis is traced laterally to identify the inguinal ligament and the exact location of the external inguinal ring identified. Although some surgeons advocate

repair through the external ring (Mitchell Banks technique[16]), an alternative approach is to incise the external oblique fascia in the long axis of its fibres, perpendicular to the external inguinal ring. This exposes the cremasteric muscle and fascia, which envelop the cord structures.

The hernial sac is always located in an anteromedial position in relation to the cord and gentle blunt dissection of the cremasteric fibres usually brings the sac into view. The sac is elevated with a haemostat and the cremasteric fibres carefully freed from the anterior and lateral aspects. Retraction of the sac medially allows identification of the spermatic vessels and vas deferens, and these structures may be carefully teased away from the sac in a posterolateral direction. Injection of 1–2 mL of saline into the cord may help to define the planes of separation. The vas itself should not be grasped and the floor of the canal not disturbed. Once the end of the sac has been freed, the dissection of the sac is carried superiorly to the level of the deep inguinal ring. If the sac extends down into the scrotum, it may be divided once the cord structures are identified and protected. The base of the sac may then be gently twisted to reduce any fluid or viscera into the peritoneal cavity. The base of the sac should be suture ligated with an absorbable suture and, once the suture is cut, the peritoneal stump should retract proximally through the deep inguinal ring. Free ties should not be used because of the risk of them becoming dislodged if abdominal distension occurs. Absolute haemostasis is essential to prevent postoperative haematoma formation. The position of the testis within the scrotum should be confirmed to avoid iatrogenic entrapment within the inguinal canal. There is an increasing role for laparoscopic hernia repair in infants and young children.[17]

An emergency operation is required for patients with an incarcerated hernia, with toxicity and obvious intestinal obstruction or after failed attempts at reduction. After appropriate resuscitation, prophylactic antibiotics and insertion of a nasogastric tube, the operation begins with preparation of the whole abdomen in case laparotomy is required. An inguinal incision is utilised and the incarcerated intestine carefully inspected for viability once the obstruction at the internal ring is relieved. A rapid return of pink colour, sheen, peristalsis and palpable or visible pulsations at the mesenteric border should be observed. If there is any question regarding intestinal viability, resection and anastomosis should be carried out and hernial repair accomplished.

In certain circumstances, the incarcerated intestine may reduce during surgical manipulation, before the intestine has been visualised. However, such spontaneous reduction of infracted bowel is very rare. Laparoscopy through the hernial sac can be undertaken if there are serious concerns regarding bowel viability. Surgery for incarcerated hernia may be difficult because of oedema, tissue friability and the presence of the mass, which may obscure the anatomy. The gonad should be carefully inspected because it may become infarcted by vascular compression caused by the incarcerated intestine. The undescended testis is more vulnerable to this complication in the presence of incarcerated intestine.

Complications

Complications may be divided into intraoperative and postoperative categories. Intraoperative complications include: division of the ilioinguinal nerve, which can be avoided if the external oblique fascia is elevated before incision; division of the vas deferens, which should be repaired with interrupted 7–0 monofilament sutures; and bleeding, which is usually secondary to needle-hole injury and can usually be controlled with withdrawal of the suture and the application of pressure.

Postoperative complications include wound infection, scrotal haematoma, postoperative hydroceles and recurrence. The wound infection rate is low (1–2%) and recurrence rates of less than 1% are reported; 80% of recurrences are noted within the first postoperative year. The major causes of recurrence in infants and children include: (i) a missed hernial sac or an unrecognised tear in the peritoneum; (ii) a broken suture ligature at the neck of the sac; (iii) injury to the floor of the inguinal canal, resulting in the development of a direct inguinal hernia; (iv) severe infection in the inguinal canal; and (v) increased intra-abdominal pressure, as is noted in patients with ascites after ventriculoperitoneal shunts, in children with cystic fibrosis, after previous operation for incarceration and in patients with connective tissue disorders. Although failure to repair a large internal inguinal ring is a possible (and very occasional) cause of recurrence, attempts to tighten the internal ring at the time of the first repair by approximating the transversalis fascia medial to the inferior epigastric vessels risks compromising the blood supply to the testicle and should be avoided where possible. Simple excision of the sac is all that is required in most patients. Re-operations for recurrent inguinal hernia may be a technical challenge and a preperitoneal approach is an extremely useful alternative for recurrent hernias.

Adult inguinal hernias

Inguinal hernias are more frequent in males, with a male to female ratio of 12:1. The peak incidence is in the sixth decade and 65% are indirect in type. Right-sided inguinal hernias are slightly more common than left-sided, 55% occurring on the right. Bilateral hernias are four times more common in direct than indirect forms.

Aetiology

The pathogenesis of groin hernias is multifactorial. It was initially believed that persistence of a patent processus vaginalis into adult life was the predisposing factor for inguinal hernia formation. However, postmortem studies have shown that 15–30% of adult males without a clinically apparent inguinal hernia have a patent processus vaginalis.[18] Similarly, review of the contralateral side in infantile inguinal hernias reveals a patent processus vaginalis in 60% of neonates and a contralateral hernia in 10–20%. During 20 years of follow-up after infantile hernia repair, only 22% of men will develop a contralateral hernia.

It is therefore apparent that the problem of indirect inguinal hernia is not simply one of a congenital defect. The high frequency of indirect inguinal hernia in middle-aged and older people suggests a pathological change in connective tissue of the abdominal wall to be a contributory factor,[2] as discussed earlier.

Management

The essential goal of hernia repair is to restore the functional integrity of the laminar musculo-aponeurotic structure of the groin region and the musculo-aponeurotic fenestration, which allows the vessels to the genitalia to penetrate this structure. It is beyond the scope of this chapter to review the history of the various repair techniques that have been previously employed and are now mainly historical. However, **Fig. 4.3** illustrates how the popularity of suture and mesh techniques has changed in the Lothian region of Scotland in the last 20 years. Only the latest techniques (i.e. prosthetic repairs) will be considered here.

Tension-free prosthetic mesh repair

Lichtenstein first described the technique of tension free repair of groin hernia, which now bears his name.[19] Tension-free repair of primary groin hernias may be performed as an outpatient procedure under local anaesthesia, although in the UK open mesh repair is still more commonly performed under general anaesthetic.

Once the local anaesthesia has been administered (typically a mixture of 0.5% bupivocaine and 1% lignocaine) along the line of the proposed incision, a cut is made in the groin-crease and a window established through the subcutaneous tissues including Scarpa's fascia at the lateral end of the wound, exposing the external oblique aponeurosis. The window is increased in size to expose the medial end of the external oblique aponeurosis, the inguinal ligament and the superficial ring. Additional anaesthetic is then injected under the external oblique aponeurosis, following which a small incision is made in the external oblique along the line of the fibres, approximately 2 cm above the inguinal ligament. The edges are carefully lifted with haemostats to avoid damage to the ilioinguinal nerve. The external oblique

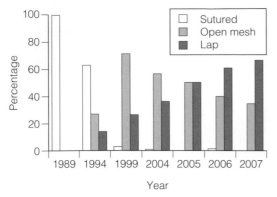

Figure 4.3 • Changing patterns in suture, mesh and laparoscopic inguinal hernia repair in the Lothian Region, Scotland.

aponeurosis is then opened along a line from the incision to the superficial ring and the contents of the inguinal canal gently separated from it. After a self-retaining retractor has been inserted under the edges of the external oblique aponeurosis, the spermatic cord is mobilised utilising the avascular space between the pubic tubercle and the cord itself to avoid damage to the floor of the canal, injury to the testicular blood flow and crushing of the genital nerve, which always lies in juxtaposition to the external spermatic vessels.

In order to thin out the spermatic cord and remove any lipoma present (**Fig. 4.4**), the cremaster fibres are incised longitudinally at the level of the deep ring. Complete excision of the cremaster fibres from the spermatic cord is unnecessary and may result in damage to the vas deferens, increasing the likelihood of postoperative neuralgia and ischaemic orchitis. Indirect hernial sacs are opened and digital exploration performed to detect any other defects or the presence of a femoral hernia. Lichtenstein states that the sac may be simply inverted into the abdomen without excision, suture or ligation, which he feels is unnecessary and may contribute to postoperative discomfort.[19] However, it is the author's practice to suture ligate any but the smallest hernial sacs at the level of the deep ring and excise any redundant peritoneum. To prevent postoperative hydrocele formation, complete scrotal sacs are transected at the midpoint of the canal, with the distal section left in place and open. Handling of the sac can cause pain and often further local anaesthetic to the sac area in the region of the deep ring is required.

In the event of a large direct hernia, the sac (transversalis fascia) is invaginated with an imbricating suture to achieve a flat surface over which to lay the prosthetic mesh. The external oblique aponeurosis is separated from the underlying internal oblique muscle at a point high enough to accommodate a mesh measuring around 10 cm × 6 cm. This size

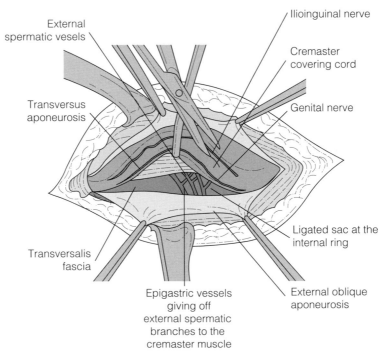

Figure 4.4 • Elevation of cord. Reproduced from Lichtenstein IL, Shulman AG, Amid PK. The tension-free repair of groin hernias. In: Nyhus LM, Condon RE (eds) Hernia. Philadelphia: JB Lippincott, 1995; pp. 237–49. With permission from Lippincott, Williams & Wilkins.

will vary depending on the size of the patient and the size of the hernial defect.

The mesh is trimmed as appropriate so that the patch overlaps the internal oblique muscle and aponeurosis by at least 2 cm above the border of the Hesselbach triangle. The medial portion of the mesh is rounded to the shape of the medial corner of the inguinal canal. The mesh is sutured to the aponeurotic tissue over the pubic bone, overlapping the bone to prevent any tension or weakness at this critical point, but ensuring the periosteum is not caught in the suture as this is believed to be a good source of chronic pain. The medial part of the mesh should extend at least 2 cm medial to the pubic tubercle to reduce the risk of medial recurrence. The same suture is continued along the lower edge, attaching the mesh to the shelving portion of the inguinal ligament to a point just lateral to the deep ring with a continuous suture (**Fig. 4.5a**).

A slit is made at the lateral end of the mesh, creating a wider tail above the cord and a narrower one below the cord. This manoeuvre positions the cord between the two tails of the mesh and avoids the keyhole opening, which is less effective at preventing recurrence. The upper edge of the patch is sutured to the internal oblique aponeurosis using a few interrupted sutures or widely spaced continuous suture. Sharp retraction of the upper leaf of the external oblique aponeurosis from the internal oblique muscle is important because it provides the appropriate amount of laxity for the patch. When the retraction is released, a true tension-free repair is taken up when the patient strains on command during the operation or resumes an upright position afterwards. Using a single non-absorbable monofilament suture, the lower edges of the two tails are fixed to the shelving margin of the inguinal ligament just lateral to the completion knot of the lower continuous suture. This creates a new deep ring of mesh (Fig. 4.5b). Some surgeons simply suture the lower edge of the upper tail to the upper edge of the lower tail and this is becoming the standard now.

The excess patch is trimmed on the lateral side, leaving 3–4 cm beyond the deep ring. This is tucked underneath the external oblique aponeurosis and the external oblique aponeurosis closed with a continuous suture. Unrestricted activity is encouraged and patients are expected to return to their normal activity 2–7 days after surgery.

In the past few years, there has been an explosion in different mesh types for the open repair of inguinal hernias. The plug and patch utilises a cone-shaped mass of mesh which can be inserted, tip side inwards, into either the deep or superficial rings, depending on the type of hernia. A flat mesh is then placed over the plug akin to the Lichtenstein technique. The prolene hernia system is two flat meshes secured together by a small cyclinder of mesh. The aim is to insert one mesh into the preperitoneal space and the other is secured akin to the Lichtenstein technique. There is also the open preperitonel approach with the Kugel patch, for example. All these alternatives report good results in the hands of experts, but the open flat mesh technique in its various forms, akin to the Lichtenstein technique, remains the commonest technique in Western countries to date. It is also the author's prejudice that if a mesh is to be inserted into the preperitoneal space, it makes sense to do this under direct vision using a laparoscope rather than use a digital, less well-visualised technique.

Laparoscopic repair

The alternative to an open operation is a laparoscopic approach. Ger is credited with the first laparoscopic approach to hernia, repairing indirect hernias with a stapling instrument developed for this purpose.[20,21] In parallel, Gazayerli described a suture repair technique through a transabdominal approach, approximating the transversus abdominis aponeurotic arch and the iliopubic tract.[22] After the repair is completed, the peritoneum is reapproximated. Since the early 1990s, laparoscopic hernia repair has evolved from simple closure of a small indirect hernia, through the placement of mesh plugs and a small mesh patch over the internal ring, to the current use of large pieces of prosthetic mesh to reinforce the lower abdominal wall.

The rationale for the use of large mesh sheets placed into the preperitoneal space was based on the surgical experience of the open preperitoneal hernia repair, especially in the treatment of recurrent hernias.[23,24] Although a variety of laparoscopic repairs have been described, they can be categorised in general according to the approach used to expose the defect. Three exposures are used: the intraperitoneal approach, in which the prosthesis is placed as an onlay graft over the peritoneum; the transabdominal preperitoneal prosthetic (TAPP) repair; and the totally extraperitoneal prosthetic (TEP) repair.

Intraperitoneal repair

In the intraperitoneal repair with an onlay graft, the prosthesis is placed within the peritoneal cavity. The technique is well described by Toy and Smoot.[25] Compared to the TAPP and TEP approaches, it has the advantages of being less time-consuming to perform and requires less dissection of the preperitoneal space. It has the disadvantage of leaving the prosthetic material exposed within the peritoneal cavity and has a higher recurrence rate. It is the author's view that this operation is very much an operation of last resort, when other open or laparoscopic techniques have failed. It is possible that when better non-stick meshes become available, combined with glue fixation, this technique may gain in popularity.

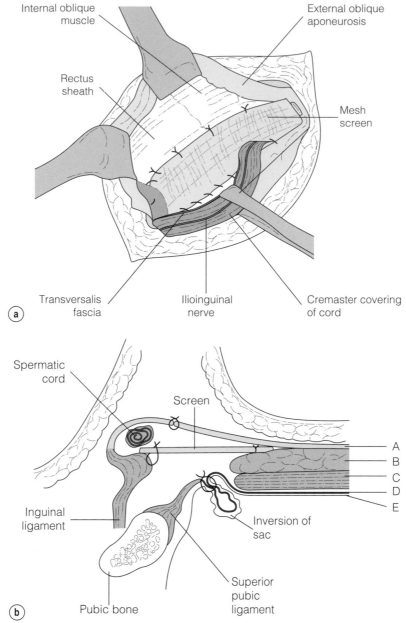

Figure 4.5 • Use of a prosthetic mesh. **(a)** The mesh sutured in place. **(b)** The implanted mesh in parasagittal section: A, external oblique aponeurosis; B, internal oblique muscle; C, transverse muscle and aponeurosis; D, transversalis fascia; E, peritoneum. Reproduced from Lichtenstein IL, Shulman AG, Amid PK. The tension-free repair of groin hernias. In: Nyhus LM, Condon RE (eds) Hernia. Philadelphia: JB Lippincott, 1995; pp. 237–49. With permission from Lippincott, Williams & Wilkins.

Transabdominal preperitoneal prosthetic repair

TAPP repair is one of the most popular approaches used for laparoscopic herniorrhaphy, particularly in Europe. The abdomen is insufflated with carbon dioxide and the laparoscope introduced through an umbilical incision. Two accessory trocars, placed well above and slightly medial to the anterior superior iliac spines, are used to provide access for the

dissecting instruments and the stapler. After both groins have been inspected, a second incision is made in the pelvic peritoneum several centimetres above the hernia defect, typically in line with the level of the anterior iliac spine, and the peritoneum then peeled away to expose the hernia defect. The peritoneum is dissected bluntly away from the abdominal wall, allowing the hernia sac to be inverted and dissected free of adherent tissue. Preperitoneal fat is removed to allow identification of the transversus abdominis arch, the pubic tubercle, the iliopubic tract and Cooper's ligament. A prosthetic mesh of approximately 10 cm × 15 cm is inserted and fixed in place with staples or sutures so that it covers the entire myopectineal orifice. The peritoneum is closed over the mesh with staples or sutures. This approach has the advantage of permitting inspection of the abdomen in general, and of the opposite side in particular, enabling bilateral repairs to be performed if necessary. In addition, exposure is usually excellent. The disadvantage is that a wider dissection is required to accommodate the mesh than is used in the intraperitoneal onlay procedure. In addition, the intra-abdominal incision presents the possibility of injury to intraperitoneal structures and a second peritoneal incision in the groin increases the potential for adhesion formation and late bowel obstruction.

Totally extraperitoneal prosthetic repair

TEP repair is a laparoscopic adaptation of the open posterior preperitoneal approach first described by Annandale.[26] The laparoscope is introduced into the preperitoneal space through a paraumbilical incision. The preperitoneal space is dissected towards the symphysis pubis, Cooper's ligament and the iliac vessels with a blunt instrument or balloon. Carbon dioxide is insufflated into the preperitoneal space to maintain exposure. Care must be taken to avoid entering the peritoneum; if this occurs, loss of pressure in the preperitoneal space can result, making exposure more difficult. A venting Verres needle in the right iliac fossa will usually resolve this problem, or alternatively a structural balloon attached to the umbilical port helps to keep the preperitoneal space open. Direct hernial sacs usually reduce with ease, but an indirect hernial sac may need more work. The key landmark here is the vas. The indirect hernial sac lies above and lateral to the vas, taking the dissection away from the iliac vessels, preventing their inadvertent injury. A mesh of minimum size 10 cm × 15 cm is used to cover all the inguinal and femoral myopectineal orifices, ensuring good cover laterally and superiomedially. There is now good evidence that suturing, tacking or stapling of mesh does not reduce the risk of hernia recurrence but is a cause of postoperative chronic pain.[27] The author does occasionally tack the mesh, confined mainly to the patient with a very large direct hernial defect or when there has been more bleeding than usual, especially patients on aspirin. In all circumstances tacks are placed medial to the inferior epigastric vessels and superior to the pubic bone only. The TEP approach avoids the risks of entering the peritoneal cavity and subsequent intraperitoneal adhesion formation.

There is little evidence to support TEP versus TAPP and the technique used is largely down to the individual surgeon. The author's preference is the TEP approach, with the TAPP approach reserved for recurrence after a previous TEP or open perperitoneal operation.

Laparoscopic repair of inguinal hernias causes less acute and chronic pain, thus earlier return to work, less infection, fewer wound complications and less numbness than the open operations. It is currently the preferred technique recommended by the National Institute for Clinical Excellence (NICE) for recurrent inguinal hernias and bilateral primary inguinal hernias and an alternative operation for primary unilateral hernias.[28]

Complications

Complications of herniorrhaphy include recurrence, urinary retention, ischaemic orchitis and testicular atrophy, wound infection and nerve injuries (neuromas of the ilioinguinal or genitofemoral nerves). A wide variation in recurrence rates is reported in the literature, depending on both the surgical technique employed and the method and length of follow-up (questionnaire, physical examination, etc.). In general, papers comparing mesh to a suture repair note lower recurrence rates in the mesh group.[29] Nevertheless, the percentage of recurrent to primary hernia repair has remained largely constant in Lothian, Scotland over the past 30 years at around 10%. Perhaps the only role for suture repairs remains in the adolescent age group, where perhaps a herniotomy alone is insufficient and the risks of mesh insertion not merited. There has been a suggestion that mesh repairs in the groin can affect fertility in males.[30] This is a very controversial area, as the occurrence of a hernia per se in the young is associated with reduced fertility. There is no convincing evidence to support the view that a mesh repair affects fertility except when there is obviously direct trauma to the vas or vessels to the testicle.

The complication that is becoming the benchmark for comparing hernia repairs is the incidence of chronic pain, rather than recurrence rate. Risk factors for chronic pain include nerve damage, preoperative pain in the hernia, young age, pain at other sites of the body, postoperative complications and psychosocial features.[31,32]

Suture, mesh or laparoscopic repair?

The Shouldice technique using suture repair rather than mesh is still carried out in many centres worldwide and numerous publications have reported recurrence rates of 1–2%.[33]

To date, the Lichtenstein tension-free repair has the largest number of published repairs with the lowest recurrence rates. Lichtenstein and colleagues published a multicentre series of 22 300 hernioplasties performed by this technique with a recurrence rate of 0.77%.[34]

The 2004 NICE report commented on 37 randomised controlled trials that compared laparoscopic with open mesh repair of inguinal hernias in a total of 5560 participants.[28] The report summarised these results stating that the laparoscopic repair as compared to an open repair was associated with less acute pain and thus a quicker return to daily activites and work, fewer wound complications such as haematoma, seroma and infection, and less risk of chronic pain. There was a similar recurrence rate and a similar risk of major vessel, bowel or bladder injury (except for a slightly higher risk for the TAPP repair). However, the laparoscopic repair took longer to perform and was a more expensive option. The cost of open surgery has to be set against the price of open surgery for the patient and society, namely more acute and chronic pain, more time off work and more wound complications. This is borne out by a cost–benefit analysis using the same data for the 2004 NICE report.[35] Unilateral hernia open flat mesh repair was the least costly option, but it provided less quality-adjusted life-years compared to both TAPP and TEP. Also, laparoscopic repair for bilateral hernias reduces both operating times and convalescence period, equating to a greater cost-effectiveness. In addition, repair of an occult hernia on the other side may also be performed, enhancing the benefit of the laparoscopic procedure.

Mesh repair using the Lichtenstein technique has the lowest worldwide recurrence rate for primary inguinal hernias. The laparoscopic repair is associated with less early and late pain, earlier return to normal activities and work but is more expensive. It is, however, the preferred technique for the repair of recurrent and bilateral hernias.[28,35]

Recent publications now demonstrate that laparoscopic repairs, whether unilateral or bilateral, can be performed more quickly laparoscopically as compared to open surgery.[36,37] The only downside to laparoscopic hernia surgery is the need for general anaesthesia. While small numbers have been done under local or regional techniques, these have been confined to young fit patients, for whom avoidance of a general anaesthetic is not necessary. Nevertheless, in many Western countries open inguinal hernias are still predominantly repaired under general anaesthetic.

Contralateral repair

Inguinal hernia arises as a design fault, both anatomically and at the level of collagen metabolism, so there is every reason why it should be a bilateral disease. Furthermore, clinical assessment of bilateral or unilateral hernia has a false positive and negative rate of around 10%. The rate of development of a contralateral inguinal hernia following open repair is around 25% at 10 years.[29] The Edinburgh experience is that time from first repair to contralateral repair in the laparoscopic era is about half the time compared to open hernia repair. It could be argued that the larger mesh inserted laparoscopically places more strain on the contralateral side. An alternative hypothesis is that patients following laparoscopic repair are more likely to volunteer for repair of the contralateral side as the operation is less painful. It is thus the author's practice to offer the majority of patients a bilateral laparoscopic repair, unless the laparoscopic approach is contraindicated and the patient unfit or elderly.

Recurrent inguinal hernias

The repair of recurrent inguinal hernia remains a common operation and there is now some evidence to suggest that the increasing use of mesh may be having a small reduction in the number of recurrent hernia repairs.[29,38] As a result there is little role now for suture repair of recurrent inguinal hernias, and a re-recurrence rate of 30% for the Bassini technique has been reported.[39] The McVay procedure and transversalis repair are not commonly employed and the results are probably of historic interest only. In centres where alloplastic material is unavailable or too expensive for routine use, the Shouldice technique is probably the technique of choice.[40]

Prosthetic mesh repair of recurrent inguinal hernias

The Lichtenstein repair remains the commonest operation for recurrent inguinal hernias. Rate of re-recurrence depends to an extent on the length of follow-up, but is typically under 10%. Since its introduction, excellent results have been reported with the mesh plug method.[41] The transinguinal preperitoneal prosthetic repair/Rives procedure tends to be reserved for selected cases and is not indicated for the majority of recurrent inguinal hernias.[42] When an open preperitoneal approach is used with preperitoneal mesh implantation, the re-recurrence rate ranges between 0.5% and 25% after an observation period of up to 10 years, suggesting that this technique may require a degree of surgical experience for success.[43,44] Divergent results are also reported for the Stoppa technique, with re-recurrence rates varying between 1% and 12%.[45,46] The most likely explanation for this wide variation is that the size and type of recurrence probably varied between the reporting centres.

Laparoscopic repair of recurrent inguinal hernias

The 2004 NICE[28] report acknowledges that after a previous open repair, laparoscopic repair is the preferred technique. The advantages of the laparoscopic approach include: elimination of one of the commonest causes of recurrence, the missed hernia; allowing the surgeon to identify those patients with complex hernias; and covering the entire myopectineal orifice, buttressing the intrinsic collagen deficit, thereby overcoming one of the causes of late recurrence. The complication rate is low, and the majority of such repairs are as easy as primary laparoscopic repair. The type of surgery following recurrence after a previous laparoscopic repair is less well defined, and is more governed by surgeon preference and expertise. It is the author's opinion that an open mesh repair is the best option following a failed TAPP repair, and a TAPP repair for a failed TEP repair. The TAPP approach allows assessment as to why the TEP repair failed, and maintains the speedier recovery of the laparoscopic approach over open repair. However, the significant adhesions following a TAPP make a redo TAPP much more difficult, but still possible in experienced hands.

The asymptomatic hernia

Traditional teaching was that once an inguinal hernia was detected, it merited repair to prevent hernia-related complications unless the patient was not fit for such surgery. However, increasing awareness of complications following hernia repair, particularly chronic pain, has questioned this approach. Two randomised trials have reported similar results but come to different conclusions.[47,48] In essence, chronic pain on follow-up is similar between the operation groups and the watchful waiting group. Significant numbers in the watchful waiting group cross over to the surgery arm because of increasing symptoms, but it is likely that such patients would tolerate complications of surgery better than if they were asymptomatic at the time of the surgery. However, the risk of incarceration or strangulation is much lower than previously thought. Thus, following informed consent, surgery or watchful waiting for an asymptomatic hernia is appropriate. The younger the patient, or less fit the patient on presentation, then perhaps the earlier surgery should be offered, with suitable informed consent of the risks, benefits and alternatives to the proposed surgery.

 Repair of an asymptomatic hernia does not increase the incidence of chronic pain as compared to a wait and see policy. Either treatment option is acceptable with appropriate informed consent.[47,48]

Femoral hernia

Femoral hernia represents the third commonest type of primary hernia. It accounts for approximately 20% of hernias in women and 5% in men, strangulation being the initial presentation in 40%.

Anatomy

The femoral canal occupies the most medial compartment of the femoral sheath, extending from the femoral ring above to the saphenous opening below. It contains fat, lymphatic vessels and the lymph node of Cloquet. It is closed above by the septum crurale, a condensation of extraperitoneal tissue pierced by lymphatic vessels, and below by the cribriform fascia. The femoral ring is bounded anteriorly by the inguinal ligament and posteriorly by the iliopectineal (Cooper) ligament, the pubic bone and the fascia over the pectineus muscle. Medially, the boundary is the edge of the lacunar ligament, while laterally it is separated from the femoral vein by a thin septum.

Aetiology

Femoral hernias are considered to be acquired, possibly as a result of increased abdominal pressure. A postulated mechanism is the insinuation of fat into the femoral ring secondary to raised intra-abdominal pressure. This bolus of fat drags along pelvic peritoneum to develop a peritoneal sac. Once the peritoneal sac has moved the short distance down the canal and out of the femoral orifice, the sac becomes apparent. The hernia not only becomes visible and palpable, but the contents of the sac become at risk of incarceration and strangulation. The incidence of femoral herniation increases with age, and a potential mechanism for this involves the muscle bulk adjacent to the distal femoral canal. Normally, the iliopsoas and pectineus muscle bundles encroach on the canal and thus act as a barrier to the development of a femoral hernia. With the natural atrophy of muscle tissue that occurs with senescence, the actual volume of muscle within the canal decreases, allowing positive intra-abdominal pressure to push the peritoneum into the canal. This would explain the high rate of femoral hernia among elderly women as well as men. In women of all ages, the muscle mass is not as great as in men. Consequently, women are predisposed to femoral hernias with any condition that increases intra-abdominal pressure, such as pregnancy or obesity.

Management

The treatment of femoral hernia is surgical repair due to the invariable presence of incarceration and the associated risk of strangulation. Several operative approaches have been described: the low approach

(Lockwood), the high approach (McEvedy) and the inguinal approach (Lothiessen). To these can now be added the laparoscopic approach.

Operative details

The low approach (Lockwood)

The low approach is based on a groin crease incision and dissection of the femoral hernia sac below the inguinal ligament. The anatomical layers covering the sac should be peeled away and the sac opened to inspect its contents. Once empty, the neck of the sac is pulled down, ligated as high as possible and redundant sac excised. The neck then retracts through the femoral canal and the canal is closed with a plug or cylinder of polypropylene mesh, anchored to the inguinal ligament and iliopectineal ligament with non-absorbable sutures. Suturing of the iliopectineal ligament to the inguinal ligament may result in tension due to the rigidity of these structures and may predispose to recurrence.

Transinguinal approach (Lothiessen)

Techniques of femoral repair that open the posterior inguinal wall for exposure and repair (the inguinal approaches of Lothiessen, Bassini, Shouldice, McVay–Cooper, Halsted and Andrews) should rarely be used. This technique usually involves ligation and division of the inferior epigastric vessels at the medial border of the internal inguinal ring followed by incision of the transversalis fascia to expose the extraperitoneal space and the femoral hernia sac. This is reduced and the defect closed by either suture (as in the original description) or, increasingly, mesh. However, the need to incise the natural fascial barrier in Hasselbach's triangle for exposure results in this technique being inferior to either the low or high approach, both of which leave the inguinal floor intact.

High approach (McEvedy)

The high approach was classically based on a vertical incision made over the femoral canal and continued upwards above the inguinal ligament. This has now been replaced with a transverse 'unilateral' Pfannenstiel incision, which can be extended to form a complete Pfannenstiel incision if a formal laparotomy is required. The dissection is continued through the subcutaneous tissue to the anterior rectus sheath. This can either be divided transversely or longitudinally, following which transversalis fascia is incised, the rectus muscle retracted medially and the preperitoneal space entered. The femoral hernia sac is identified medial to the iliac vessels and reduced by traction. If the hernia is incarcerated, the sac may be released by incising the insertion of the iliopubic tract into Cooper's ligament at the medial margin of the femoral ring. The sac is then opened, the contents dealt with appropriately and the sac ligated at its neck. The hernioplasty may then be completed

by either suturing the iliopubic tract to the posterior margin of Cooper's ligament or by insertion of a prosthetic mesh, either as a sheet covering the whole of the myopectineal opening or as a mesh plug. The wound is closed in layers. This technique is particularly useful in the presence of strangulated femoral hernias as it is easy to convert to laparotomy for bowel resection.

Laparoscopic approach

The laparoscopic approach is the same as for inguinal hernias and may employ the TAPP or TEP technique. The femoral ring is easily seen during either of these approaches and, indeed, visualisation of the whole of the myopectineal opening is frequently quoted as one of the advantages of laparoscopic herniorrhaphy. Small series of laparoscopic femoral hernia surgery have been reported with excellent results on short-term follow-up.[49,50]

Incisional hernia

Aetiology

Incisional hernias are unique in that they are the only hernia to be considered iatrogenic. The cause of wound complications after laparotomy is multifactorial, conditioned by local and systemic factors and by preoperative, perioperative and postoperative factors. Several factors including advanced age, pulmonary disease, morbid obesity, malignancy and intra-abdominal infection are associated with impaired wound healing and predispose patients to serious wound complications such as wound dehiscence, wound infection and incisional herniation. Prospective trials in the 1990s showed burst abdomen rates of 1–3%, wound infection rates of 10–15% and incisional hernia rates of 4–21%.[51] Technical factors influencing wound complications include surgical technique and suture material.

 A higher incidence of incisional hernia rate was reported when absorbable sutures were employed in three trials.[52–54] Several trials of continuous versus interrupted suture closure have failed to show any difference in the rate of wound dehiscence or incisional hernia.[52,55]

The continuous method has the advantages of being quicker, cheaper and adjusts to some degree the tension in the tissues along the line of closure, so that tissues are less ischaemic than when they are approximated comparably with multiple interrupted sutures.

There is also a difference in wound complication rates when the skill of the surgeon is taken into account. Gislason[51] compared the results of experienced surgeons performing the same type of procedures and found wound failure rates ranging from 3.9% to 20%. When surgeons expressing an interest in the field of abdominal wall closure performed similar procedures, much lower complication rates were reported (wound dehiscence <0.5%, incisional hernia 3%, wound infection 3–4%).

The final technical consideration is the ratio of suture length to wound length (SL:WL) when using a continuous technique. This ratio depends on the stitch interval, the amount of tissue included in the stitches and the tension on the suture. A strong correlation between the SL:WL ratio and the development of incisional hernia has been found. With an SL:WL ratio of at least 4, the wound tension seems to be distributed in such a way that the suture-holding capacity of the tissues is not exceeded. The incisional hernia rate is lower if the SL:WL ratio is 4 or more, and suturing with a lower ratio is associated with a threefold increase in the rate of incisional hernia.[56] However, the SL:WL ratio should not be higher than 5 since this has been associated with a higher rate of both wound infection and incisional hernia, probably because a large amount of tissue other than fascia is then included in the suture. An SW:LW ratio of 4 equates to 1-cm bites of tissue on each side of the incision taken at 1-cm intervals along the length of the incision.

Management

The large number of surgical procedures described in the literature to repair incisional hernias illustrates that no single technique has stood out as being effective. While 50% of incisional hernias occur within 1 year after primary operation, 10–18% are diagnosed more than 5 years after laparotomy. Any study reporting re-recurrence rates following incisional hernia repair should therefore ideally have at least 5 years of follow-up data for analysis. Unfortunately, prospective randomised trials comparing different types of incisional hernia repair are lacking and the majority of studies are retrospective. However, recurrence rates ranging from 6% to 46% for primary closure are documented.[57] The results for the Mayo ('vest-over-pants') procedure are no better (overall recurrence rate 33%).[57]

As a consequence of the disappointing data on mesh-free repair of incisional hernias, meshes were introduced to strengthen the abdominal wall repair. Several different techniques were developed: inlay, onlay and sublay (**Fig. 4.6**). Mesh implantation as an inlay does not achieve any strengthening of the abdominal wall and is essentially a suture repair at the muscle/mesh interface. It has the highest recurrence rate of the three techniques. The results of randomised trials comparing mesh to suture repair demonstrate a clear advantage for mesh repair, even for small hernias.[58,59] However, incisional hernia should be considered an incurable disease, mesh just increasing the time from repair to recurrence.[60] Although suture repair is now rarely indicated, it might still have a role in young women who wish repair of an incisional hernia but are also contemplating further pregnancy.

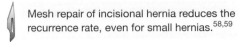

Mesh repair of incisional hernia reduces the recurrence rate, even for small hernias.[58,59]

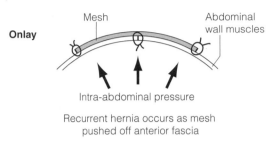

Onlay

Recurrent hernia occurs as mesh pushed off anterior fascia

Inlay

Recurrent hernia occurs as mesh / abdominal wall 'suture' repair fails

Sublay

Recurrent hernia minimised as intra-abdominal pressure pins the mesh against the abdominal wall

Figure 4.6 • Cross-sectional appearance of techniques of incisional hernia repair. Reproduced from Schumpelick V, Klinge V. Immediate follow-up results of sublay polypropylene repair in primary or recurrent incisional hernias. In: Schumpelick V, Kingsnorth AN (eds) Incisional hernia. Berlin: Springer-Verlag, 1999; pp. 312–26. With permission from Springer.

Mesh repair

The onlay technique remains the commonest technique in the West, largely because it is relatively easy to perform. The technique is dependent on adequate fixation of the mesh to the fascia and a minimum overlap of 5–8 cm is recommended. If the connection between the mesh and the fascia is lost, a buttonhole hernia develops at the edge of the mesh. Good results can be reported with attention to detail, namely wide overlap of the mesh, and obliteration of large skin flaps with fibrin glue.[61] However, for many surgeons the relatively high rate of hernia recurrence, seroma formation and mesh infection make this operation a poor option for the patient.

The sublay technique is the procedure favoured by the author. A mesh in the sublay position is not only sutured into position but is also held in place by the intra-abdominal pressure. Mesh in this position is therefore able to strengthen the abdominal wall both by mechanical sealing and by the induction of strong scar tissue. Several authors have compared the recurrence rate in a single institution where all three techniques have been used.[62,63] Both these studies clearly demonstrate the superior results achieved by the sublay technique.

Open sublay repair

The sublay operation begins by excising the old scar and performing a laparotomy. Adhesions tend to be maximal at the neck of the sac, so entering the abdominal cavity through the hernia sac is usually straightforward. It is helpful to mobilise adhesions off the underside of the anterior abdominal wall. It is not the author's routine practice to mobilise all the bowel adhesions unless there is a good history of recurrent episodes of obstruction. The sublay space is then developed, which is the space anterior to the posterior rectus sheath, although this becomes preperitoneal below the semi-arcuate line. Care should be taken to mobilise the inferior epigastric vessels up with the belly of the rectus muscle to minimise bleeding. It is also important to preserve as many of the intercostal nerves as possible to minimise muscle denervation (**Fig. 4.7**). The preperitoneal space can be developed behind the pelvis, akin to a TEP repair, especially if the hernia arises in a Pfannensteil incision. Superiorly, the sublay space can be developed behind the xiphisternum if necessary. The posterior rectus sheath is divided on either side close to the linea alba to expose the area known as the fatty triangle (**Fig. 4.8**). The posterior rectus sheath is approximated with an absorbable suture. The mesh is cut to size, aiming to have at least a 6-cm overlap in all directions. This mesh is sutured to the posterior rectus sheath with interrupted absorbable sutures, avoiding any obvious nerves. These sutures are purely to hold the mesh flat until it is encased in fibrous tissue. A suction drain is often left anterior to the mesh. Any futher redundant skin and hernial sac is excised and the anterior rectus sheath closed with an absorbable suture, as is the skin, minimising any subcutaneous dead space. The cross-sectional appearance is illustrated in **Fig. 4.9**. If an abdominoplasty is performed at the same time, then further drains are placed to the subcutaneous space.

 The open sublay technique for incisional hernia repair has a lower recurrence rate and wound complication rate compared to onlay or inlay repair techniques.[62,63]

Figure 4.7 • Fresh cadaveric dissection of the retromuscular space for sublay incisional hernia. Used with permission of Dr J Conze, Aachen, Germany.

Figure 4.8 • Fresh cadaveric dissection demonstrating the fatty triangle by division of the posterior rectus sheath as it attaches to the linea alba. This allows development of the sublay space behind the xiphisternum. Used with permission of Dr J Conze, Aachen, Germany.

Laparoscopic repair

The laparoscopic (intraperitoneal) approach has also been applied to incisional hernias. The laparoscopic approach has the advantages of shorter hospital stay, lower analgesic requirements, fewer wound complications and an earlier return to normal activities over open surgery. However, the cosmetic result for larger hernias is often less good. The laparoscopic approach makes no attempt to approximate divaricated muscle and there is no abdominoplasty. The author reserves the laparoscopic approach for smaller incisional hernias, with a hernial neck size less than 10 cm. The method of fixation remains controversial. Transfascial sutures are believed by some to be essential. However, these are a source of chronic pain postsurgery. The author prefers a double crown tack technique. The recent introduction of absorbable tacks may reduce the risk of chronic pain and bowel adhesion

Skin
Subcutaneous fat
Anterior rectus sheath
Rectus muscle
Posterior rectus sheath
Preperitoneal fat
Peritoneum
Mesh

Skin
Subcutaneous fat
Anterior rectus sheath
Rectus muscle
Posterior rectus sheath
Preperitoneal fat
Peritoneum
Mesh

Figure 4.9 • (a) Cross-sectional appearance of peritoneum closure showing the sublay position of the mesh, which is fixed to the posterior sheath of the rectus muscle with an interrupted absorbable suture. **(b)** The anterior and posterior rectus sheath is closed continuously with an absorbable suture.

to the tacks. Centring the mesh over the hernial defect is important to minimise hernia recurrence. The mesh can be centred with a central stitch,[64] although two or four corner sutures are probably more accurate. Only one randomised trial comparing open to laparoscopic surgery has been published[65] at the time of writing, although a number of multicentre trials are currently ongoing. This study reported that the laparoscopic group had a shorter operative time, a shorter period of hospital admission, fewer wound infections and a faster return to work. A number of comparative series have been published, suggesting that the outcome for laparoscopic incisional hernia repair is at least equivalent to open surgery.[66,67]

One of the main risks of the laparoscopic repair of incisional hernias is the placement of the mesh in direct contact with the intra-abdominal structures. As mentioned earlier, the use of meshes which have one side coated with a relatively non-adhesive material will help reduce adhesion formation to the mesh. The other main risk is infection of the mesh, which is nearly always due to contamination from a bowel injury. Care should be taken with any adhesiolysis to minimise bowel injury with thermal sources such as diathermy and ultracision dissection kept to a minimum. The current consensus is that if the colon is injured, then it should be repaired, laparoscopically or open, according to the skills of the surgeon and no mesh inserted at this time. The patient can return in a number of months for a

further attempt at repair. If the small bowel is injured with minimal contamination, then laparoscopic repair, washout and mesh insertion is acceptable. If there is significant small-bowel injury and risk of failure of the bowel repair, then no mesh should be inserted. The patient should be observed in hospital and if they remain well 4–5 days later, then it is appropriate to re-laparoscope the patient and if no continuing contamination/infection is observed, the laparoscopic mesh repair is completed. The use of antibiotic-impregnated mesh may allow a change to this policy with placement of such a mesh at the same time as bowel injury and repair.[68]

Emergency hernia surgery

Much of what has been mentioned above is applicable to hernia repair in the emergency situation. However, there are a few dilemmas which occur more frequently in the emergency setting. Patients who present as an emergency but have no bowel compromise can be treated as per elective hernia surgery. When bowel is compromised, especially when there has been significant contamination, current opinion is that synthetic mesh should not be used. However, there is little in the way of evidence apart from anecdote to support such a view and this view has been challenged.[69] For those who support the laparoscopic approach, it is not unreasonable to offer this in the emergency setting and laparoscope the patient with an irreducible hernia. If the bowel can be reduced and is viable, then convert the operation to a TEP and place mesh as usual. If the bowel is compromised, then resect the bowel through a small incision and return 6 weeks later for a TEP. In the emergency incisional hernia setting, if the hernia is large, then proceed directly to open sublay mesh repair. If the hernia is smaller, then laparoscopy and intra-abdominal mesh are appropriate if there is no bowel compromise. If there is bowel ischaemia, then convert to the open sublay repair. The use of mesh in the sublay space in the emergency setting should not be associated with an increase in mesh infection as it lies external to the peritoneal cavity, but clearly each case will need to be assessed individually.

Emergency hernia surgery remains a high-risk surgical procedure, with the main risk factor for postoperative mortality being infarcted bowel.[70,71] Such operations should not be left to junior members of the surgical and anaesthetic teams. Appropriate resuscitation, followed by timely and appropriate surgery, may save lives. Occasionally, the techniques of damage limitation surgery (see Chapter 13) may be appropriate.

Bowel infarction is the main risk factor for mortality in emergency hernia surgery.[70,71]

Port-site hernia

This is a hernia with an increasing incidence associated with the increase in laparoscopic surgery. Insertion of larger ports through the midline as opposed to more laterally appear to be a significant risk factor. This is especially true in the presence of a divarification of the recti or an unrecognised umbilical hernia. There is little evidence to support closure of the fascia except when a cut-down is performed for the first port. The use of dilating rather than cutting trocar tips may reduce the incidence of port-site hernia formation.

Antibiotic prophylaxis in hernia surgery

In general, elective hernia surgery to the groin and ventral regions does not require antibiotic prophylaxis.[72,73] However, as the risk of bowel injury is always present in incisional hernia surgery, it would be reasonable to give routine antibiotic prophylaxis for such surgery. Patients at increased risk of infection, including the immunocompromised, skin conditions with higher bacterial carriage such as psoriasis and in the emergency setting, all merit antibiotic prophylaxis.

All theatres have bacteria (called colony-forming units) in the circulating theatre air. It therefore makes sense to open the mesh just before it is required during the operation. Changing to fresh gloves before the handling of the mesh, minimising mesh contact with the skin and inserting the mesh deep to the subcutaneous tissues may all help reduce the risk of mesh contamination. The author uses a gentamycin solution (240 mg gentamycin in 250 mL normal saline) to irrigate larger meshes following insertion, although there is no evidence-based medicine to support this manoeuvre. Methicillin-resistant *Staphylococcus aureus* (MRSA) bacteria have been found on mesh several years after insertion, so prophylaxis to MRSA is appropriate if a previous repair has been complicated by MRSA infection.

Prophylatic hernia surgery

The topic of prophylactic mesh insertion to minimise subsequent hernia formation in high-risk groups of patients remains controversial. One study reduced the incidence of incisional hernia following open gastric bypass surgery from 21% to 0% by the prophylactic insertion of a polypropylene mesh in the sublay position.[74] Another study reduced the incidence of parastomal hernia following permanent end colostomy from 50% to 5% by the prophylactic insertion of a polypropylene mesh in the sublay position.[75] Both studies have small patient numbers, but no increase in morbidity was noted in the prophylactic mesh group. It is likely that prophylactic mesh to minimise subsequent hernia formation will become more mainstream practice. This may be supported by preoperative collagen type I/III ratio typing.

Management of an infected mesh

In general, an infected mesh has to be removed or exposed to the surface. If the mesh is lying in a pool of pus with no adherence to the patient, then the only option is removal of the mesh. If the mesh is partly embedded in tissue, then if there is adequate drainage through an open wound, many infected meshes will slowly granulate over and remain sound. However, sometimes chronic sinuses will develop and the only option is excision of these along with as much of the visible mesh as possible. Not all patients who require mesh removal will develop a hernia recurrence, although the majority probably will at some stage in the future.[76] It is the author's opinion that it is best to remove as much of the mesh foreign body as possible, control the sepsis and return at a later date for further repair. The use of biological mesh in a contaminated field is rarely indicated. The use of vacuum-assisted dressing to control the fluid exudates from the wound may aid wound care in such patients.

Key points

- Herniorrhaphy is one of the commonest operations performed.
- Techniques advanced considerably during the 1990s.
- The use of prosthetic mesh should now be considered for the repair of all hernias.
- The laparoscopic approach may be more appropriate than a traditional open approach.
- Recurrent hernias may be best managed in specialist centres or by surgeons with a specialist interest in hernia surgery who are technically competent to perform both open and laparoscopic procedures.
- A multidisciplinary approach, including plastic surgeons, may be appropriate for complex, multiply recurrent hernias.

References

1. Devlin B. Functional anatomy. In: Schumpelick V, Kingsnorth AN (eds) Incisional hernia. Berlin: Springer-Verlag, 1999; pp. 32–44.

2. Wagh PV, Leverich AP, Sun CN et al. Direct inguinal herniation in men: a disease of collagen. J Surg Res 1974; 17:425–33.

3. Si Z, Rhanjit B, Rosch R et al. Impaired balance of type I and type III procollagen mRNA in cultured fibroblasts of patients with incisional hernia. Surgery 2002; 131:324–31.

4. Junge K, Klinge U, Rosche R et al. Decreased collagen typeI/III in patients with recurring hernia after implantation of alloplastic prostheses. Langenbeck's Arch Surg 2004, 389:17–22.

5. Junge K, Klinge U, Prescher A et al. Elasticity of the anterior abdominal wall and impact for reparation of incisional hernias using mesh implants. Hernia 2001; 5:113–18.

6. Cobb WS, Kercher KW, Heniford BT. The argument for lightweight polypropylene mesh in hernia repair. Surg Innov 2005; 12:63–9.

7. Akolekar D, Kumar S, Khan LR et al. Comparison of recurrence with lightweight composite polypropylene mesh and heavyweight mesh in laparoscopic totally extraperitoneal inguinal hernia repair: an audit of 1232 repairs. Hernia 2008; 12:39–43.

8. Holm JA, de Wall LC, Steyerberg EW et al. Intraperitoneal polypropylene mesh hernia repair complicates subsequent abdominal surgery. World J Surg 2007; 31:423–9.

9. LeBlanc KA, Booth WV. Laparoscopic repair of incisional abdominal hernias using expanded polytetrafluoroethylene: preliminary findings. Surg Laparosc Endosc 1993; 3:39–41.

10. Askar OM. Aponeurotic hernias: recent observations upon paraumbilical and epigastric hernias. Surg Clin North Am 1984; 64:315–29.

11. Sibley WL III, Lynn HB, Harris LE. A 25-year study of infantile umbilical hernias. Surgery 1964; 55:462–70.

12. Mayo WJ. An operation for the radical cure of umbilical hernia. Ann Surg 1901; 34:276–8.

13. Goodney PP, Birkmeyer CM, Brikmeyer JD. Short-term outcomes of laparoscopic and open ventral hernia repair: a meta analysis. Arch Surg 2002; 137:1161–5.

14. Holder TM, Ashcroft KW. Groin hernias and hydroceles. In: Holder TM, Ashcroft KW (eds) Pediatric surgery. Philadelphia: WB Saunders, 1980; pp. 594–608.

15. Rowe MI, Clatworthy HW Jr. Incarcerated and strangulated hernias in children. Arch Surg 1970; 101:136–43.

16. Kurlan MZ, Web PB, Piedad OH. Inguinal herniorrhaphy by the Mitchell Banks technique. J Pediatr Surg 1972; 7:427–31.

17. Schier F. Laparoscopic inguinal hernia repair – a prospective personal series of 542 children. J Pediatr Surg 2006; 41:1081–4.

18. Hughson W. The persistence or performed sac in relation to oblique inguinal hernia. Surg Gynecol Obstet 1925; 41:610–14.

19. Lichtenstein IL, Shulman AG, Amid PK et al. The tension-free hernioplasty. Am J Surg 1989; 157:188–93.

20. Ger R. The management of certain abdominal hernias by intra-abdominal closure of the neck. Ann R Coll Surg Engl 1982; 64:342–5.

21. Ger R, Monroe K, Duvivier R et al. Management of indirect inguinal hernias by laparoscopic closure of the neck of the sac. Am J Surg 1990; 159:370–6.

22. Gazayerli MM. Anatomical laparoscopic hernia repair of direct or indirect inguinal hernias using the transversalis fascia and iliopubic tract. Surg Laparosc Endosc 1992; 2:49–52.

23. Nyhus LM, Pollak R, Bombeck CT et al. The preperitoneal approach and prosthetic buttress repair for recurrent hernia. Ann Surg 1988; 203:733–8.

24. Rignault DP. Properitoneal prosthetic inguinal hernioplasty through a Pfannenstiel approach. Surg Gynecol Obstet 1986; 163:465.

25. Toy FK, Smoot RT Jr. Laparoscopic herniorrhaphy update. Laparoendosc Surg 1992; 2:197–9.

26. Annandale T. Case in which a reducible oblique and direct inguinal and femoral hernia existed on the same side and were successfully treated by operation. Edinb Med J 1876; 27:1087–9.

27. Taylor C, Layani L, Liew V et al. Laparoscopic inguinal hernia repair without mesh fixation, early results of a large randomized clinical trial. Surg Endosc 2008; 22:757–63.

28. National Institute for Clinical Excellence. Laparoscopic surgery for inguinal hernia repair. Technology Appraisal Guidance 83. London: NICE, 2004. Available at www.nice.org.uk/TA083guidance.

   An excellent meta-analysis of open versus laparoscopic inguinal hernia repair.

29. van Veen RN, Wijsmuller AR, Vrijland WW et al. Long term follow up of a randomized clinical trial of non-mesh versus mesh repair of primary inguinal hernia. Br J Surg 2007; 94:506–10.

30. Fitzgibbons RJ. Can we be sure polypropylene mesh causes infertility. Ann Surg 2005; 241:559–61.

31. Franneby U, Sandblom G, Nordin P et al. Risk factors for long-term pain after hernia surgery. Ann Surg 2006; 244:212–9.

32. Kehlet H. Chronic pain after groin hernia repair. Br J Surg 2008; 95:135–6.

33. Bendavid R. The Shouldice repair. In: Nyhus LM, Condon RE (eds) Hernia. Philadelphia: Lippincott, 1995; pp. 217–36.

34. Shulman AG, Amid PK, Lichtenstein IL. The safety of mesh repair for primary inguinal hernias. Am Surg 1992; 58:255–9.

35. McCormack K, Wake B, Perez J et al. Laparoscopic surgery for inguinal hernia repair: systematic review of effectiveness and economic evaluation. Health Technol Assess 2005; 9:1–203.

   Cost analysis of laparoscopic compared to open surgery using the same data that were used for the 2004 NICE report (Ref. 28 above).

36. Duff M, Mofidi R, Nixon SJ. Routine laparoscopic repair of primary unilateral inguinal hernias – a viable alternative in the day surgery unit? Surgeon 2007; 5:209–12.

37. Eklund A, Rudberg C, Smedberg S et al. Short-term results of a randomized clinical trial comparing Lichtenstein open repair with totally extraperitoneal laparoscopic inguinal hernia repair. Br J Surg 2006; 93: 1060–8.

38. Atkinson HDE, Nicol SG, Purkayastha S et al. Surgical management of inguinal hernia: retrospective cohort study in southeastern Scotland 1985–2001. BMJ 2004; 329:1315–16.

39. Herzog U. Das Leistenhernienrezidiv. Schweiz Rundsch Med Prax 1990; 79:1166–9.

40. Wantz GE. The Canadian repair: personal observations. World J Surg 1989; 13:516–21.

41. Shulman AG, Amid PK, Lichtenstein IL. The plug repair of 1402 recurrent inguinal hernias: 20-year experience. Arch Surg 1990; 125:265–7.

42. Bendavid R. The rational use of mesh in hernias: a perspective. Int Surg 1992; 77:229–31.

43. Fong Y, Wantz GE. Prevention of ischaemic orchitis during inguinal hernioplasty. Surg Gynecol Obstet 1992; 174:399–402.

44. Schaap HM, van de Pavoordt H, Bast TJ. The preperitoneal approach in the repair of recurrent inguinal hernias. Surg Gynecol Obstet 1992; 174:460–4.

45. Beets GL, Dirkoen CD, Go PM et al. Open or laparoscopic mesh repair for recurrent inguinal hernia. A randomised controlled trial. Surg Endosc 1999; 13:323–7.

46. Langer I, Herjog U, Schuppisser JP et al. Preperitoneal prosthesis implantation in surgical management of recurrent inguinal hernia. Retrospective evaluation of our results 1989–1994. Chirurg 1996; 67:394–402.

47. O'Dwyer PJ, Norrie J, Alani A et al. Observation or operation for patients with an asymptomatic inguinal hernia. A randomized clinical trial. Ann Surg 2006; 244: 167–73.

   The first randomised trial on surgery versus no surgery in the asymptomatic hernia.

48. Fitzgibbons RJ, Giobbie-Hurder A, Gibbs JO et al. Watchful waiting vs repair of inguinal hernia in minimally symptomatic men. A randomized clinical trial. JAMA 2007; 295:285–92.

49. Yalamarthi S, Kumar S, Stapleton E et al. Laparoscopic totally extraperitoneal mesh repair for femoral hernia. J Laparoendosc Adv Surg Tech A 2004; 14:358–61.

50. Hermandez-Richter T, Schardey HM, Rau HG et al. The femoral hernia. An ideal approach for the transabdominal preperitoneal technique (TAPP). Surg Endosc 2000; 14:736–40.

51. Gislason H. Closure of the abdomen in acute wound failure. In: Schumpelick V, Kingsnorth AN (eds) Incisional hernia. Berlin: Springer-Verlag, 1999; pp. 253–7.

52. Wissing J, van Vroonhoven TJMV, Schattenkerk ME et al. Fascia closure after midline laparotomy: results of a randomised trial. Br J Surg 1987; 74:738–45.

53. Bucknall TE, Ellis H. Abdominal wound closure: a comparison of monofilament nylon and polyglycolic acid. Surgery 1981; 89:672–5.

54. Brolin RE. Prospective, randomised evaluation of midline fascial closure in gastric bariatric operations. Am J Surg 1996; 172:328–31.

55. Sahlin S, Ahlberg J, Granstrom L et al. Monofilament versus multifilament absorbable sutures for abdominal closure. Br J Surg 1993; 80:322–4.

    A good summary of the evidence for type of suture used in abdominal wall closure.

56. Cameron AEP, Gray RCF, Talbot RW et al. Abdominal wound closure: a trial of Prolene and Dexon. Br J Surg 1980; 67:487–91.

57. Decurtins M. Significance of fascia doubling in the management of incisional hernia. In: Schumpelick V, Kingsnorth AN (eds) Incisional hernia. Berlin: Springer-Verlag, 1999; pp. 287–93.

58. Luijendijk RW, Hop WC, van den Tol MP et al. A comparison of suture repair with mesh repair for incisional hernia. N Engl J Med 2000; 343: 392–8.

    The first randomised trial to demonstrate the benefit of mesh in reducing recurrence in incisional hernia repair.

59. Burger JW, Luijendijk RW, HopWC et al. Long term follow up of a randomized controlled trial of suture versus mesh repair of incisional hernia. Ann Surg 2004; 240:578–83.

60. Flum DR, Horvath K, Koepsell T. Have outcomes of incisional hernia repair improved with time. Ann Surg 2003; 237:129–35.

61. Kingsnorth AN, Shahid MK, Valliattu AJ et al. Open onlay mesh repair for major abdominal wall hernias with selective use of component separation and fibrin sealant. World J Surg 2008; 32: 26–30.

62. Langer C, Liersch T, Kley C et al. Twenty five years of experience in incisional hernia surgery. A comparitive retrospective study of 432 incisional hernia repairs. Chirurg 2003; 74:638–45.

63. de Vries Reilingh TS, van Geldere D, Langenhorst BLAM et al. Repair of large midline incisional hernias with polypropylene mesh: comparison of three operative techniques. Hernia 2004; 8:56–9.

64. Motson RW, Engledow AH, Medhurst C et al. Laparoscopic incisional hernia repair with a self-centring suture. Br J Surg 2006; 93:1549–53.

65. Olmi S, Scaini A, Cesana GC et al. Laparoscopic versus open incisional hernia repair: an open randomized controlled study. Surg Endosc 2007; 21:555–9.

66. Sains PS, Tilney HS, Purkayastha S et al. Outcomes following laparoscopic versus open repair of incisional hernia. World J Surg 2006; 30:2056–64.

67. Lomanto D, Lyer SG, Shabbir A et al. Laparoscopic versus open ventral hernia mesh repair: a prospective study. Surg Endosc 2006; 20:1030–5.

68. LeBlanc KA, Elieson MJ, Corder JM. Enterotomy and mortality rates of laparoscopic incisional and ventral hernia repair: a review of the literature. JSLS 2007; 11:408–14.

69. Kelly ME, Behrman SW. The safety and efficacy of prosthetic hernia repair in clean-contaminated and contaminated wounds. Am Surg 2002; 68:524–9.

70. Nilsson H, Stylianidis G, Haapamaki M et al. Mortality after groin hernia surgery. Ann Surg 2007; 245:656–60.

71. Derici H, Unalp HR, Bozdaq AD. Factors affecting morbidity and mortality in incarcerated abdominal wall hernia. Hernia 2007; 11:341–6.

72. Sanchez-Manuel FJ, Lozano-Garcia J, Seco-Gil JL. Antibiotic prophylaxis for hernia repair. Cochrane Database Syst Rev 2007; CD003769.

    The latest meta-analysis on this topic.

73. Antibiotic prophylaxis in surgery. Guideline 45, 2000; www.sign.ac.uk.

    This guideline is under review with expected publication date in 2009. The SIGN website allows all guidelines produced to date to be downloaded for free. An excellent reference source on current best practice in a variety of medical and surgical conditions.

74. Strzelczyk JM, Szymanski D, Nawicki ME et al. Randomised trial of post operation hernia prophylaxis in open bariatric surgery. Br J Surg 2006; 93:1347–50.

75. Janes A, Cenqiz Y, Israelsson LA. Preventing parastomal hernia with a prophylactic mesh. Arch Surg 2004; 139:1356–8.

76. Fawole AS, Choperala RP, Ambrose NS. Fate of the inguinal hernia following removal of infected prosthetic mesh. Hernia 2006; 10:58–61.

5

Organisation of emergency general surgical services and the early assessment and investigation of the acute abdomen

Simon Paterson-Brown

Introduction

The management of emergency surgery has traditionally been an area which has been poorly resourced, tacked on to the end of the working day and very much the Cinderella specialty of 'general surgery'. Despite recognition from the Senate of Surgery in 1994 that the care of emergency surgical admissions was one of the most important aspects of general surgical practice,[1] elective work, until recently, has usually continued in tandem with the team's on-call commitments. As such, getting timely surgical intervention on all but the sickest emergency patient was difficult, resulting in delayed operations, usually going on late into the night and often carried out by junior surgical trainees. Thankfully over the last few years, due to a number of factors, this has all now changed and undoubtedly for the better. The increased number of surgical admissions to many hospitals,[2] partly due to current and proposed regional reorganisation of surgical services[3,4] and the associated workload this brings;[5] the reduced experience of surgical trainees, due to the reduction in junior doctors hours and training period;[6] and the recognition that early assessment by experienced senior surgeons with timely surgical intervention,[7] preferably by someone with an interest in that condition; has led in a large number of hospitals to the separation of elective and emergency general surgical care, not just in the UK but increasingly more wider afield.

Organisation of emergency general surgical services

On-call surgical team

Where in the past the continuity of care for surgical patients was maintained by the 'middle grade' surgical team, the new rotas currently being put into place are increasingly of a shift pattern where the maximum time worked per week is 48 hours and consultants found they were rarely working with the same trainees.[8] One solution to this problem is the establishment of the 'emergency team' where the whole surgical team (consultant and supporting junior staff) have no elective commitments and are on call for a more extended period of time. Although there will have to be some change of juniors because of the European Working Time Directive (EWTD), these can be kept to a minimum by allocating juniors to emergency activities for a defined period of time, perhaps a week, perhaps longer. Their subsequent attachment to elective activity then no longer suffers from the disruption associated with on-call shifts, a state of affairs which enhances both emergency and elective training opportunities. This 'emergency team' system, with many adaptations according to local requirements, has now been adopted in many units throughout the UK since it was first introduced in Edinburgh in 1997.[9]

The emergency team undoubtedly improves the ability of the consultant general surgeon, as well as the middle grade team, to provide safe and effective emergency care, but requires other conditions to be met if this is to be both efficient and cost-effective, not only in terms of lost elective activity for the consultant but also training opportunities for the surgical trainees. These include easy access to radiological imaging, a dedicated emergency operating theatre with full (and senior) anaesthetic support available 24 hours each day,[10] enough surgical admissions to make the system worthwhile, and a distinct and dedicated admission area for emergency patients to be assessed.

Many patients have equivocal signs and symptoms of acute appendicitis and the value of 'active observation' with reassessment after 2–3 hours by the same surgeon, repeated thereafter as necessary, is well established[11] and should be routine in all units. This is only really possible if all acute admissions remain in a single identifiable area.

Separation of elective and emergency surgery

The concept of the emergency surgeon of the day[12] is not new, but when combined with an emergency theatre and dedicated 'emergency team' it has been shown to be associated with significant improvements in overall patient care.[9]

The benefits of separating elective and emergency general surgery have now been widely recognised, and the Royal College of Surgeons of England has recently produced a consensus document supporting the separation of elective and emergency surgical care.[13] A summary of their recommendations for practice is shown in Box 5.1.

Clearly, how the 'emergency team' is structured and delivers its care will vary from hospital to hospital and region to region, depending very much on local pressures and resources. What remains clear, however, is that where there is a dedicated emergency general surgical team, there must also be protected theatre time[10] with appropriate anaesthetic support and early access to radiological imaging (and intervention), in addition to adequate critical care support.

Subspecialisation in emergency general surgery

Along with the recognition that emergency surgery deserves more attention and support has also come the recognition that specialist conditions are often better treated by surgeons with a particular interest

Box 5.1 • Summary of recommendations for separation of emergency and elective surgical care

1. A physical separation of services, facilities and rotas works best, although a separate unit on the same site is preferable to a completely separate location.
2. The presence of senior surgeons for both elective and emergency work will enhance patient safety and the quality of care, and ensure that training opportunities are maximised.
3. The separation of emergency and elective surgical care can facilitate protected and concentrated training for junior surgeons providing consultants are available to supervise their work.
4. Creating an 'emergency team', linked with a 'surgeon of the week', is a good method of providing dedicated and supervised training in all aspects of emergency and elective care.
5. Separating emergency and elective services can prevent the admission of emergency patients (both medical and surgical) from disrupting planned activity and vica versa, thus minimising patient inconvenience and maximising productivity for the Trust (hospital). The success of this will largely depend on having sufficient beds and resources for each service.
6. Hospital-aquired infections can be reduced by the provision of protected elective wards and avoiding admissions from the emergency department and transfers from within/outside the hospital.
7. The improved use of IT (information technology) solutions can assist with separating workloads (for example, scheduling systems for appointments and theatres, telemedicine, picture archiving and communication systems, etc.), although it is recognised that developments in IT for the NHS are generally behind schedule.
8. High-volume specialties are particularly suited to separating two strands of work. Other specialties can also benefit by having emergencies seen by senior surgeons – this can help to reduce unnecessary admissions, deal with ward emergencies and facilitate rapid discharge.

and experience in that subspecialty. This has of course been recognised for some time in the elective performance of a number of surgical procedures, including oesophagectomy, gastrectomy, abdominal aortic aneurysm repair, lung lobectomy, cardiac surgery and colectomy,[14,15] and although mainly thought to be related to hospital and surgeon volumes,[16] specialisation of the surgical team is also an important factor.[17] However, there are now data available to support similar improvements in patient outcomes for emergency conditions, such as acute gallstone disease,[18,19] peptic ulcer disease[20] and acute colorectal disorders.[21] This is not surprising considering the worldwide subspecialisation that has occurred in general surgery over the last decade,[22] with consultant surgeons now being expected to deal with surgical conditions in the emergency situation which they no longer see in their elective practice. Early reports of the separation of upper and lower elective and emergency gastrointestinal (GI) services in one region of Scotland have been encouraging.[23] The challenge now for all those surgeons involved in the development and provision of emergency surgical care is to produce on-call rotas which allow, where possible, patients with specific subspecialty conditions to be treated and operated upon by surgeons with a specific interest in that area. This will undoubtedly involve reorganisation of regional emergency surgical services, bringing together a wider group of surgeons for the on-call rota, with the ability to provide both upper and lower GI cover. The political hurdles of closing some emergency services in some hospitals in order to provide these larger emergency surgical units in other hospitals must be overcome if the undoubted improvements in patient care associated with dedicated emergency surgical services delivered by surgical teams with appropriate subspecialty expertise are to be realised, while at the same time providing robust junior doctor rotas which comply with the appropriate working time directives.

Early assessment

Attempts to improve preoperative diagnosis and early management of patients with acute abdominal pain are continuingly being sought; this chapter discusses all the current available techniques and the evidence for their incorporation into emergency surgical practice. For the purposes of most studies looking at acute abdominal pain, the broad definition is taken as 'abdominal pain of less than 1 week's duration requiring admission to hospital, which has not been previously treated or investigated'. However, this must be accepted as a fairly loose definition.

For an emergency team system to work efficiently the surgical team must have rapid access to diagnostic blood tests and appropriate imaging, which should include plain and contrast radiology, both diagnostic and interventional (percutaneous drainage and biopsy), ultrasound (US) and computed tomography (CT). Furthermore, plain radiography evaluated by senior radiologists substantially enhances senior surgical assessment of patients with acute abdominal pain, resulting in reduced surgical admissions.[24] All these modalities are discussed below.

Conditions associated with abdominal pain

Many studies have looked at the spectrum of patients admitted to hospital with acute abdominal pain and the approximate percentage represented by each condition is now well understood. Figures from one study[25] appear to be fairly representative (Box 5.2). In this study the 30-day mortality in 1190 emergency admissions was 4%, with a perioperative mortality of 8%. Not surprisingly, the mortality rate was age related, with perioperative mortality in patients below 60 years being 2%, rising to 12% in those 60–69 years and reaching 20% in patients over the age of 80 years. Laparotomy for irresectable disease was the most common cause of perioperative mortality (28%), with ruptured abdominal aortic aneurysm (23%), perforated peptic ulcer (16%) and colonic resections (14%) all being associated with significant perioperative mortality.

What stands out from all the studies on acute abdominal pain published over the last few decades is the high incidence of non-specific abdominal pain (NSAP), with published figures of 40% or more.[26] NSAP usually reflects a failure of diagnosis, as many of these patients do have a cause for the pain and it has been shown that further investigations, such as laparoscopy, can reduce the overall incidence of NSAP to around 27%.[27]

Box 5.2 • Conditions that may present with acute abdominal pain

Non-specific abdominal pain (NSAP) (35%)
Acute appendicitis (17%)
Intestinal obstruction (15%)
Urological causes (6%)
Gallstone disease (5%)
Colonic diverticular disease (4%)
Abdominal trauma (3%)
Abdominal malignancy (3%)
Perforated peptic ulcer (3%)
Pancreatitis (2%)

Conditions contributing 1% or less

Exacerbation of peptic ulcer
Ruptured abdominal aortic aneurysm
Gynaecological causes (these may go unnoticed as NSAP)
Inflammatory bowel disease
Medical conditions
Mesenteric ischaemia
Gastroenteritis
Miscellaneous

Reproduced from Irvin TT. Abdominal pain: a surgical audit of 1190 emergency admissions. Br J Surg 1989; 76:1121–5. © British Journal of Surgery Society Ltd. Reproduced with permission. Permission is granted by John Wiley & Sons Ltd on behalf of the BJSS Ltd.

Some authors have examined this diagnosis of NSAP further and describe a certain number of alternative conditions that could be related (Box 5.3),[26] including abdominal wall pain[28] and rectus nerve entrapment.[29] In some cases of NSAP, detection of abdominal wall tenderness (increased abdominal pain on tensing the abdominal wall muscles) may be a useful diagnostic test.[30] Possible causes of abdominal wall pain are also given in Box 5.3. The major problem with making a diagnosis of NSAP is in missing serious underlying disease, and the late Tim de Dombal demonstrated that 10% of patients over the age of 50 years who were admitted to hospital with acute abdominal pain were subsequently found to have intra-abdominal malignancy.[31] Half of these patients had colonic carcinoma and the major concern was that 50% of the patients who were subsequently proved to have intra-abdominal cancer were discharged from hospital with a diagnosis of NSAP.

Acute gynaecological conditions such as pelvic inflammatory disease and ovarian cyst accidents are another group of diagnoses that may often be included under the umbrella of NSAP, simply because of failure to take a good history or examination or even perform a thorough pelvic examination, whether digitally, ultrasonographically or at operation. In one study from a general surgical unit, gynaecological causes represented 13% of all diagnoses in a consecutive series of all emergency admissions (both male and female) initially presumed to be 'surgical' in origin.[32] As many of these patients present with 'query appendicitis', accurate assessment is essential if unnecessary operations are to be avoided, and even then the diagnosis may remain hidden unless the surgeon examines the pelvic organs once a normal appendix has been found. However, with the increased use of diagnostic laparoscopy, discussed later in this chapter, these conditions are now being recognised by the emergency surgeon with much greater frequency. Early recognition and appropriate treatment of pelvic inflammatory disease may help to avoid potentially serious long-term sequelae and must be encouraged.[33] Indeed, the condition of Curtis–Fitz-Hugh syndrome, when transperitoneal spread of pelvic inflammatory disease produces right upper quadrant pain due to perihepatic adhesions, is now well recognised and care must be taken to differentiate this from acute biliary conditions.[34]

Although much is made of possible 'medical' causes of acute abdominal pain in surgical textbooks, the incidence of conditions such as myocardial infarction, lobar pneumonia and some metabolic disorders is extremely small, though many still masquerade as NSAP. However, the possibility of such conditions must still be borne in mind during the clinical assessment of all patients with acute abdominal pain: one study has shown that 19 of 1168 children (1.6%) admitted to hospital with acute abdominal pain had pneumonia as the sole cause of symptoms.[35] It is therefore still extremely important to recognise these medical conditions when they do present, before exploratory surgery, as the mortality can be significantly increased.[36]

History and examination (including computer-aided diagnosis)

In the early 1970s, de Dombal et al.[37] in Leeds and Gunn[38] in Edinburgh developed a computer program based on Bayesian reasoning that produced a list of probable diagnoses for individual patients with acute abdominal pain. They demonstrated that the accuracy of clinical diagnosis could be improved by around 20%, and since then a multicentre study has confirmed this finding.[39] Furthermore, these studies have shown that there is a reduction in the unnecessary laparotomy rate and in bad management errors (patients whose surgery is incorrectly delayed). When the reasons for the improvement in diagnostic accuracy associated with the use of computer-aided diagnosis (CAD) are examined, there appear to be three main factors involved: (i) peer review and audit, which is invariably associated with improved results in most aspects of medical management;[40] (ii) an educational factor related to feedback;[41] and (iii) probably of greatest significance, the use of structured data sheets onto which the history and examination findings are documented before being entered into the computer program. One study demonstrated that the diagnostic accuracy of junior doctors improved by nearly 20% when they used structured data sheets alone, without going on to use the CAD program.[42] The same study also demonstrated that medical students assessing patients with the structured data sheets and then using the CAD program reached similar levels of diagnostic accuracy. Other studies have since confirmed similar improvements in clinical decision-making following the introduction of these data sheets.[43]

Box 5.3 • Causes of non-specific abdominal pain[26]

Viral infections
Bacterial gastroenteritis
Worm infestation
Irritable bowel syndrome
Gynaecological causes
Psychosomatic pain
Abdominal wall pain[28]

- Iatrogenic peripheral nerve injuries
- Hernias
- Myofascial pain syndromes
- Rib tip syndrome
- Nerve root pain
- Rectus sheath haematoma

The message from all these studies is clear: a good history and examination remain essential for both diagnostic accuracy and good clinical decision-making, and the use of a structured data sheet helps the clinician to achieve this objective.[39,42,43]

The aim of both the history and examination is to determine a diagnosis and clinical decision. There are undoubtedly specific features associated with all acute abdominal conditions that are well established; however, it remains the ability to identify the presence or absence of peritoneal inflammation that probably has the greatest influence on the final surgical decision. In other words, the presence or absence of guarding and rebound tenderness, and a history of pain on coughing, correlates well with the presence of peritonitis.[44] The differential diagnosis of acute appendicitis from NSAP is always difficult, particularly in children, and both guarding and rebound tenderness are significantly more likely to be present in acute appendicitis.[45] There has always been great store taken from tenderness elicited on rectal examination during the assessment of patients with suspected acute appendicitis. However, when rebound tenderness is detected in the lower abdomen, as evident by pain on gentle percussion, further examination by rectal examination has been shown to provide no new information.[46] Rectal examination can therefore be avoided in such cases and reserved for those patients without rebound tenderness or where specific pelvic disease needs to be excluded. Measurement of temperature has also been shown to be relatively non-discriminatory in the early assessment of the acute abdomen.[47] Urgent urinary microscopy should be carried out on anyone with any symptoms that could relate to the urinary tract and it is a good principle to dip test the urine on admission of every patient with acute abdominal pain. A recent study has reported a reliable urine dip test for acute pancreatitis that detects trypsinogen-2.[48]

Initial blood investigations and early decision-making

After the initial assessment (history and examination) of patients with acute abdominal pain, steps should be taken towards resuscitation, pain relief and further diagnostic tests as required.

There is now good evidence to support the early administration of opiate analgesia in patients with acute abdominal pain.[49] This has been clearly shown to have no detrimental effect on subsequent clinical assessment;[50] on the contrary, because the patient becomes more comfortable, further assessment may actually be facilitated. The cruel practice of withholding analgesia until the emergency surgeon has examined the patient with acute abdominal pain must be condemned.

Once the initial assessment has been completed, the surgeon will reach a differential diagnosis and, perhaps more importantly, a clinical decision: early operation definitely required, early operation definitely not required or need for early operation uncertain. Clearly, further investigations in the first category are unlikely to influence management, with the exception of a serum amylase level, which may reveal acute pancreatitis.[51] Further investigations in the group in which the surgeon considers early operation is not required can be organised on a more leisurely basis, and it is not surprising that it is in the group in which the surgeon is uncertain as to whether early operation is required that most difficulty exists.[52] Most of the uncertainty relates to 'query appendicitis', particularly in the young female, but also involves patients with intestinal obstruction and the elderly patient, in whom the diagnosis of mesenteric ischaemia must always be considered.[53]

Early diagnosis in patients with mesenteric ischaemia is particularly important as survival after surgery is much better in those with venous thrombosis than those with arterial thrombosis.[54]

In the assessment of the role of subsequent investigations in the acute abdomen, it is important to identify their potential influence on clinical decision-making rather than evaluating them purely on diagnostic potential.

Although blood tests are often useful as a baseline, their influence on the diagnosis of acute abdominal pain remains unclear, with the exception of serum amylase for acute pancreatitis.[55] As already mentioned, a quick and reliable dip test has recently been developed to confirm acute pancreatitis[48] and may complement testing of serum amylase levels, particularly if they are equivocal. Studies examining the influence of white cell concentration,[56] C-reactive protein[57] and skin temperature in the right iliac fossa[58] in patients with 'query appendicitis' have concluded that serial white cell counts are useful (compared with a single measurement), while measurement of skin temperature over the right iliac fossa is of little value. Although isolated C-reactive protein levels may also be fairly non-discriminatory, when they are interpreted with white cell count and both are normal, acute appendicitis is unlikely.[59,60]

Overall, inflammatory markers are poor discriminators of conditions such as appendicitis when looked at individually, but when combined and used with history and clinical findings of peritoneal irritation they achieve a high discriminatory power.[59] Thus routine measurement of the white cell count in patients with acute abdominal pain can be justified, not just for a baseline with which to compare subsequent levels depending on clinical progress, but also to be interpreted along with all other clinical and biochemical findings.

Liver function tests are of course an essential investigation in the early assessment of the acute abdomen where acute biliary disease is suspected.[61]

The other area that has attracted great interest in the role of blood tests for aiding diagnosis in the acute abdomen is intestinal ischaemia, whether from strangulated obstruction or mesenteric ischaemia and infarction. Estimation of acid–base status to assess the degree of metabolic acidosis is often a late change and measurement of serum phosphate, lactate, kinase, creatine, lactate dehydrogenase, alkaline phosphatase, diamine oxidase and porcine ileal peptide have all been shown to be unreliable.[54]

Radiological investigations

With advances in technology and improved radiological techniques, the radiologist is playing an ever-important role in the diagnosis of patients with acute abdominal pain. Furthermore, abdominal ultrasonography and plain radiography evaluated by senior radiologists substantially enhances senior surgical assessment of patients with acute abdominal pain, resulting in reduced surgical admissions.[62]

Plain radiology

The role of plain radiology in the investigation of the acute abdomen has been extensively examined. Until recently there was general consensus that the erect chest radiograph was the most appropriate investigation for the detection of free intraperitoneal gas, with use of the lateral decubitus film if either the erect chest film could not be taken (due to the patient's condition) or was equivocal. This no longer seems to be true following a report from Taiwan, where ultrasonography was shown to be superior to the erect chest radiograph, with a sensitivity of 92% in the detection of pneumoperitoneum compared with only 78% for plain radiology.[63] Undoubtedly there will be operator dependence and for now the erect chest radiograph should still be the initial test for suspected perforation. Failure to detect free gas under the diaphragm in a patient with suspected intestinal obstruction can then be further investigated by US, CT or contrast radiology, as discussed below.

This has also been questioned and is still carried out unnecessarily in a large number of patients,[64] although could be significantly reduced if attempts are made to limit its use to those patients where it might provide some diagnostic help, such as patients with suspected intestinal obstruction, suspected perforation and exacerbation of colitis.[65]

The use of the supine abdominal radiograph should be limited to patients with suspected intestinal obstruction, suspected perforation and exacerbation of colitis, as indicated in the guidelines produced by the Royal College of Radiologists.[66]

Similar controversy exists in the use of erect abdominal radiographs for the assessment of patients with suspected intestinal obstruction. Most surgeons still prefer both views (erect and supine) on the basis that in those patients in whom the supine radiograph is normal or equivocal the erect film may be helpful.[67]

Contrast radiology

It has been recognised for many years that gastrointestinal contrast studies can be used to evaluate acute gastrointestinal conditions.[68] Its main function remains the assessment of both large- and small-bowel obstruction and possible gastrointestinal perforation. However, with the increasing availability of multislice CT (see below) this role is rapidly dwindling.

Perforated peptic ulcer

Although the erect chest radiograph is recognised as the most appropriate first-line investigation for a suspected perforated peptic ulcer, in approximately 50% of patients no free gas can be identified on the radiograph.[69] This leaves the emergency surgeon with three options: (i) to review the diagnosis, such as reconsidering acute pancreatitis; (ii) to proceed to laparotomy based on the clinical findings alone; or (iii) particularly if there are reasonable grounds for uncertainty, to arrange a water-soluble contrast study. This test will confirm or refute the presence of perforation (**Fig. 5.1**) but will not differentiate between the patient without a perforation and one in whom the perforation has sealed. The addition of ultrasonography,[63] as already discussed, and increasingly multislice CT in this scenario may help by revealing free abdominal air and fluid in the patient whose perforation has sealed spontaneously. As has been well understood for quite some time now, many patients with perforated peptic ulcers can be managed non-operatively;[70] with this knowledge, the assessing surgeon has plenty of time to resuscitate the patient and make efforts to confirm or refute the diagnosis before rushing to emergency surgery. Patients who might be considered for non-operative treatment of their perforation should have a contrast meal to confirm spontaneous sealing of the perforation. This topic is discussed in more detail in Chapter 6.

Figure 5.1 • Supine abdominal radiograph taken 20 minutes after the oral administration of 50 mL of water-soluble contrast material in a patient with a suspected perforated peptic ulcer in whom the erect chest radiograph was normal. Note the small trickle of contrast through the perforation. These findings were confirmed at laparotomy. Reproduced from Hamilton Bailey's emergency surgery, 13th edn. With permission from Hodder Murray.

Small-bowel obstruction

Surgery for small-bowel obstruction is performed for one of two reasons: first, there has been failure of non-operative management or, second, there is clinical suspicion of impending strangulation. Although plain abdominal radiographs are useful in establishing the diagnosis of small-bowel obstruction, they cannot differentiate between strangulated and non-strangulated gut. The criteria on which strangulated intestine must be suspected are well established: peritonism, fever, tachycardia and leucocytosis.[71] However, even when the diagnosis is suspected, the changes at operation are often irreversible and resection required. Some workers have looked at serum markers such as phosphate and lactate concentrations[53] to help identify patients with possible strangulation in order to allow earlier surgery, but unfortunately they are unreliable. As in other areas of acute abdominal imaging, ultrasonography also appears to be able to contribute to the diagnosis of intestinal obstruction,[72] but the problem of detecting early ischaemic changes in small-bowel obstruction remains largely unsolved. There is little doubt that water-soluble contrast studies in patients with small-bowel obstruction are useful in detecting those patients who are not likely to settle with non-operative management.[73] A recent randomised trial comparing water-soluble contrast follow-through versus conventional management in patients with suspected adhesive small-bowel obstruction demonstrated a significantly shorter time to surgery and therefore overall hospital stay in the group receiving the contrast study.[74] Water-soluble contrast material also allows quicker resolution of symptoms.[75] In general, failure of water-soluble contrast to reach the caecum by 4 hours strongly suggests that surgical intervention is likely to be required, and better sooner than later (**Fig. 5.2**). Water-soluble contrast follow-through is also useful in the assessment of early postoperative obstruction in order to identify those patients with an ileus from those with mechanical obstruction who need re-operation.[76]

 In patients with small-bowel obstruction early administration of a water-soluble contrast material should be considered as it allows those patients who require surgery to be identified sooner and those that will settle non-operatively to do so quicker than patients managed conventionally.[74,75]

More detailed information on the surgical management of small-bowel obstruction is provided in Chapter 9.

Large-bowel obstruction

The management algorithm for large-bowel obstruction has now become well established following the more widespread recognition that colonic pseudo-obstruction could not be distinguished from mechanical obstruction on plain radiographs alone (**Fig. 5.3**a,b).[77] The decision that all patients with suspected large-bowel obstruction should now undergo a contrast enema (**Fig. 5.3**c,d) before laparotomy has probably been the most important factor in reducing not only the unnecessary operation rate for pseudo-obstruction, but also the associated mortality. Patients with acute colonic pseudo-obstruction present with similar history and clinical signs to the patient with a mechanical obstruction. Although factors recognised as precipitating pseudo-obstruction, such as dehydration, electrolyte abnormalities, pelvic and spinal surgery, acid–base imbalance and so on, may alert the clinician as to the possible cause, it cannot be confirmed without further investigation. As the treatment for one is non-operative and for the other is usually operative, accurate assessment is essential.

 All patients with a suspected large-bowel obstruction should undergo some form of contrast examination to exclude pseudo-obstruction.[76]

The surgical management of both large-bowel obstruction and the next topic, acute diverticulitis, is covered in Chapter 10.

Acute diverticulitis

The majority of patients who present with symptoms and signs of acute diverticulitis can be managed non-operatively, with the exception of those patients who have overt peritonitis from perforation. Although ultrasonography in experienced hands might identify a thickened segment of colon, perhaps with an associated paracolic collection of fluid, invariably there is too much gas for adequate assessment and quite significant collections can go unnoticed. For this reason clinicians have attempted to evaluate other modalities, such as water-soluble contrast radiology and CT.[78] The former has the ability to identify a 'leak', the latter a collection. Both of these pieces of information may be of use to the surgeon in reaching a decision to operate, even though the ultimate decision must be based on clinical rather than radiological criteria. Overall, CT is no more specific than a contrast enema but does allow guided percutaneous drainage to be carried out if a collection is identified.[79]

Ultrasonography (US)

The use of US is now one of the mainstays of investigation of the acute abdomen. Accurate detection of small amounts of intraperitoneal fluid associated with conditions such as perforated peptic ulcer, acute cholecystitis, acute appendicitis, strangulated bowel and ruptured ovarian cysts can be very helpful in alerting the clinician to the possible severity of the patient's symptoms. Furthermore, reports on the accuracy of US in the detection of specific conditions such as acute cholecystitis and appendicitis are impressive (see Chapter 8). The presence of free fluid, gallstones, a thickened gallbladder wall and a positive ultrasonographic Murphy's sign are all good indicators of acute cholecystitis.[80] US is the first-line investigation for acute biliary disease, with a sensitivity greater than 95% for the detection of acute cholecystitis.[81] As the most appropriate management of these patients is now laparoscopic cholecystectomy during the same admission, and if possible within 48 hours,[82] early US examination on any patient with suspected acute biliary disease should be undertaken soon after admission.

In experienced hands US has been shown to be able to detect an acutely inflamed non-perforated appendix with a sensitivity of 81% and specificity of 100%.[83] Because the technique relies on visualising a non-compressible swollen appendix, the sensitivity for perforated appendicitis was much lower (29%). When a scoring system is used for both clinical diagnosis and ultrasonographic findings, the addition of the latter increases the diagnostic accuracy for acute appendicitis.[84,85] Clearly, it would be inappropriate to scan everyone with suspected appendicitis, but where the diagnosis is uncertain, particularly in women, the case for ultrasound scanning is strong, as many alternative diagnoses can be detected.[86]

Figure 5.2 • Supine abdominal radiograph taken 90 minutes **(a)** and 4 hours **(b)** after oral administration of 50 mL of water-soluble contrast material. Note failure of contrast to reach the caecum and the obvious small-bowel obstruction. These findings were not obvious on plain radiographs. Laparotomy confirmed small-bowel obstruction due to adhesions.

Figure 5.3 • Supine abdominal radiographs in two patients with large-bowel obstruction. **(a)** Patient A has pseudoobstruction. **(b)** Patient B has mechanical obstruction. **(c,d)** Water-soluble contrast enema confirmed pseudo-obstruction in patient A **(c)** and an obstructing carcinoma of the sigmoid colon in patient B **(d)**.

Other areas where US is specifically used to assess the acute abdomen are abdominal aortic aneurysms, renal tract disease and acute gynaecological emergencies. US may also have a role to play in the diagnosis of strangulated small-bowel obstruction, by detecting dilated non-peristaltic loops of bowel in association with free intraperitoneal fluid.[87] US can also be useful in detecting acute abdominal wall problems, such as rectus sheath haematoma, and differentiating them from intra-abdominal pathology.[88] US also has a role in the early assessment of patients with blunt abdominal trauma,[89] and this is covered in detail in Chapter 13.

Computed tomography (CT)

The place of CT in the early assessment of the acute abdomen has received wide attention over the last few years following the introduction of multislice CT and recognition of the excellent images that can be produced, especially if intravenous contrast is used. Its role in the investigation of severity of acute diverticulitis has already been discussed[78,79] and it can also be used to identify miscellaneous intra-abdominal collections resulting from other conditions. Attempts to improve the diagnostic accuracy of acute appendicitis using CT have been impressive, with a 98% accuracy in 100 consecutive patients with suspected appendicitis, of whom 53 had acute appendicitis.[90] However, irrespective of the cost and availability issue, care must be taken to ensure that such techniques of investigation are used to complement rather than to replace the clinical assessment of patients with suspected appendicitis.[91] A randomised study from Cambridge that examined the effect of early CT (within 24 hours of admission) on patients with acute abdominal pain demonstrated a significant reduction in missed serious diagnoses.[92] In addition to its overall role in the investigation of the acute abdomen,[93] CT is also extremely useful specifically in both the detection of gastrointestinal obstruction (**Fig. 5.4**), perforations (**Fig. 5.5a,b**), along with indications of the site of perforation[94] and intestinal ischaemia.[95] Multislice CT with intravenous and rectal contrast can also be useful in the detection and differentiation of different types of colitis, including ulcerative, Crohn's, pseudomembranous and *Clostridium difficile* colitis.[96] Despite the relatively high diagnostic accuracy of CT in the assessment of the acute abdomen, and particularly acute appendicitis, the main drawbacks remain cost and radiation exposure.[97] As a result the role of CT in the early assessment of patients with acute abdominal pain should probably be limited to those in whom there remains uncertainty as to either diagnosis or decision to operate after initial assessment.

Magnetic resonance imaging (MRI)

With the increased use of CT in the investigation of the acute abdomen it was only a matter of time before attention turned to the role of MRI, which is not asso-

Figure 5.4 • Multislice CT with intravenous contrast demonstrating small-bowel obstruction due to an incarcerated inguinal hernia. With thanks to Dr Dilip Patel, Consultant Radiologist, Royal Infirmary, Edinburgh.

ciated with the radiation exposure of CT. MRI can undoubtedly differentiate an acutely inflamed appendix from a normal one[98] and therefore is useful in pregnant patients where the diagnosis of acute appendicitis can be difficult.[99] However, in a recent review of academic centres in North America, radiologists

Figure 5.5 • **(a)** Sagittal view of a multislice CT with intravenous contrast demonstrating free intraperitoneal gas from a perforated peptic ulcer. Note the free air anterior to the liver. **(b)** Axial view of the same patient showing free air above the liver. With thanks to Dr Dilip Patel, Consultant Radiologist, Royal Infirmary, Edinburgh.

still preferred CT to MRI in the second and third trimester to investigate acute abdominal pain.[100]

Fine catheter peritoneal cytology

Fine catheter peritoneal cytology[101] involves the
insertion of a venous cannula into the peritoneal
cavity under local anaesthesia through which a fine
umbilical catheter is inserted. Peritoneal fluid is aspirated back, placed on a slide, stained and examined
under a light microscope for percentage of polymor-
phonuclear cells. A value greater than 50% suggests
a significant underlying inflammatory process but
obviously cannot identify the exact cause. This procedure can be carried out at the bedside or even in the
accident and emergency department in all patients
with acute abdominal pain or just acute appendicitis, where the sensitivity and specificity have been
reported as 91% and 94% respectively.[102] Although
rarely used now, it still has an occasional use in those
patients with unexplained sepsis in the intensive care
unit considered too unstable for transfer to CT, in
whom bedside abdominal US has been unable to
exclude a possible intra-abdominal source.

Laparoscopy

Laparoscopy is now established as an essential
modality for both diagnosis and treatment of acute
abdominal conditions. Many studies have demonstrated that laparoscopy significantly improves
surgical decision-making in patients with acute
abdominal pain when it is used as a diagnostic
tool,[103] particularly when the need for operation is
uncertain.[43] With the increasing use of laparoscopic
appendicectomy (see Chapter 9), most patients with
suspected appendicitis can now undergo diagnostic
laparoscopy followed by laparoscopic appendicectomy if the diagnosis of acute appendicitis is confirmed (**Fig. 5.6**). Even if a policy of laparoscopic
appendicectomy is not followed, all females with
suspected acute appendicitis should still undergo
diagnostic laparoscopy because the diagnostic error
is more than twice that of males,[104] usually due to
underlying gynaecological conditions (**Figs 5.7** and
5.8). When used as a diagnostic tool in patients
admitted to hospital with suspected acute non-
specific abdominal pain, some of whom of course
subsequently turn out to have a surgical cause, early
laparoscopy versus observation has been shown to
be of benefit. Two randomised studies[105,106] have
demonstrated that the associated improved diagnostic accuracy in the patients undergoing laparoscopy
converts to a reduced hospital stay, and in one of
the studies[105] an improved quality of life (assessed 6
weeks after discharge from hospital).

The decision on what to do if a normal appendix is
seen at laparoscopy is discussed in detail in Chapter 9,

and there are differing arguments for and against its
removal. What is essential is that the patient must
be clearly told the diagnosis made at laparoscopy
and the precedure performed. It has been shown

Figure 5.6 • Laparoscopy showing an acutely inflamed
appendix with pelvic peritonitis.

Figure 5.7 • Laparoscopic view of a torsion of the right
fallopian tube with ischaemia of the distal tube and ovary.

Figure 5.8 • Laparoscopic view of a haemorrhagic
ovarian cyst.

that around 27% of patients undergoing laparoscopy for acute abdominal pain could either not remember what had happened or their recall was incorrect.[107] This included knowedge as to whether the appendix had been removed or not.

It is clear that there is now overwhelming evidence in support of the use of diagnostic laparoscopy in the management of patients with acute abdominal pain in whom the need for surgery is uncertain and in women with suspected appendicitis.[102,104,105]

Key points

- The art of good management of patients with acute abdominal pain lies in an accurate history, careful examination and logical decision-making, taking into account results from all appropriate and available investigations.
- Regular reassessment of patients is an essential part of this process and emergency surgeons who do not make use of the investigative options discussed in this chapter are in danger of falling short of providing the standards of care which patients with acute abdominal pain now have a right to expect.
- The ability to provide adequate emergency surgical care, with careful observation and reassessment, is best provided by dedicated emergency surgical teams without elective commitments.
- Swift access to investigations and an emergency theatre must be made available.
- Although emergency subspecialisation has great attractions for the overall care of the emergency patient with complex problems, this area of development will depend very much on local resources, requirements and workload.

References

1. Senate of the Royal Surgical Colleges of Great Britain and Ireland. Consultant practice and surgical training in the UK. London: Royal Surgical Colleges, 1994.

2. Hobbs R. Rising emergency admissions. Br Med J 1995; 310:207–8.

3. Senate of Surgery of Great Britain and Ireland. Reconfiguration of surgical, accident and emergency and trauma services in the UK, 2004; www.rcsg.ac.uk/recreport.htm

4. Black A. Reconfiguration of surgical, accident and emergency and trauma services in the UK. Br Med J 2004; 328:178–9.

5. Watkin DFL, Layer GT. A 24-hour snapshot of emergency general surgery in the UK. Ann R Coll Surg Engl 2002; 84(Suppl):194–9.

6. Campling EA, Devlin HB, Hoile RW et al. Report of the National Confidential Enquiry into Perioperative Deaths 1990. London: HMSO, 1992.

7. Beecham L. New Scottish CMO criticises training reforms. Br Med J 1996; 313:947.

8. Hilton JR, Shiralkar SP, Samsudin A et al. Disruption of the on-call surgical team. Ann R Coll Surg Engl 2002; 84(Suppl):50–3.

9. Addison PDR, Getgood A, Paterson-Brown S. Separating elective and emergency surgical care (the emergency team). Scot Med J 2001; 46:48–50.

10. Calder FR, Jadhav V, Hale JE. The effect of a dedicated emergency theatre facility on emergency operating patterns. J R Coll Surg Edinb 1998; 43:17–19.

11. Thomson HJ, Jones PF. Active observation in acute abdominal pain. Am J Surg 1986; 152:522–5.

12. Kelly MJ. Off-duty for consultants in the week? It can be done! Ann R Coll Surg Engl 1995; 77(Suppl):257–9.

13. The Royal College of Surgeons of England. Separating emergency and elective surgical care: recommendations for practice, 2007; www.rcseng.ac.uk/publications/doc

14. Halm EA, Lee C, Chassin MR. Is volume related to outcome in health care? A systematic review and methodologic critique of the literature. Ann Intern Med 2002; 137:511–20.

15. Hannan EL, Radzyner M, Rubin D et al. The influence of hospital and surgeon volume on in-hospital mortality for colectomy, gastrectomy and lung lobectomy in patients with cancer. Surgery 2002; 131:6–15.

16. Paterson-Brown S. Surgical volume and clinical outcome. Br J Surg 2007; 94:523–4.

17. Smith JAE, King PM, Lane RHS et al. Evidence of the effect of 'specialisation' on the management of surgical outcome and survival from colorectal cancer in Wessex. Br J Surg 2003; 90:583–92.

18. Mercer SJ, Knight JS, Toh SKC et al. Implementation of a specialist-led service for the management of gallstone disease. Br J Surg 2004; 91:504–8.

19. Simpson DJ, Wood AM, Paterson HM et al. Improved management of acute gallstone disease after regional surgical subspecialisation. World J Surg 2008; 32:2690–94.

20. Robson AJ, Richards JMJ, Nixon SJ et al. The effect of surgical subspecialisation on outcomes in peptic ulcer disease complicated by perforation and bleeding. World J Surg 2008; 32:1456–61.

21. Darby CR, Berry AR, Mortensen N. Management variability in surgery for colorectal emergencies. Br J Surg 1992; 79:206–10.

22. Dawson EJ, Paterson-Brown S. Emergency general surgery and the implications for specialisation. Surgeon 2004; 2:165–70.

23. Elson DW, Sa'adedin F, Partridge R et al. The separation of upper and lower gastrointestinal surgery: implications for emergency surgery. Br J Surg 2004; 91(Suppl):62.

24. Cochrane RA, Edwards AT, Crosby DL et al. Senior surgeons and radiologists should assess emergency patients on presentation: a prospective randomised controlled trial. J R Coll Surg Edinb 1998; 43:324–7.

25. Irvin TT. Abdominal pain: a surgical audit of 1190 emergency admissions. Br J Surg 1989; 76:1121–5.

26. Gray DWR, Collin J. Non-specific abdominal pain as a cause of acute admission to hospital. Br J Surg 1987; 74:239–42.

27. Paterson-Brown S. The acute abdomen: the role of laparoscopy. In: Williamson RCN, Thompson JN (eds) Baillière's clinical gastroenterology: gastro-intestinal emergencies, Part 1. London: Baillière Tindall, 1991; pp. 691–703.

28. Gallegos NC, Hobsley M. Abdominal wall pain: an alternative diagnosis. Br J Surg 1990; 77:1167–70.

29. Hall PN, Lee APB. Rectus nerve entrapment causing abdominal pain. Br J Surg 1988; 75:917.

30. Gray DWR, Seabrook G, Dixon JM et al. Is abdominal wall tenderness a useful sign in the diagnosis of non-specific abdominal pain? Ann R Coll Surg Engl 1988; 70:233–4.

31. de Dombal FT, Matharu SS, Staniland JR et al. Presentation of cancer to hospital as 'acute abdominal pain'. Br J Surg 1980; 67:413–16.

32. Paterson-Brown S, Eckersley JRT, Dudley HAF. The gynaecological profile of acute general surgery. J R Coll Surg Edinb 1988; 33:13–15.

33. Pearce JM. Pelvic inflammatory disease. Br Med J 1990; 300:1090–1.

34. Shanahan D, Lord PH, Grogono J et al. Clinical acute cholecystitis and the Curtis–Fitz-Hugh syndrome. Ann R Coll Surg Engl 1988; 70:45–7.

35. Ravichandran D, Burge DM. Pneumonia presenting with acute abdominal pain in children. Br J Surg 1996; 83:1706–8.

36. Blidaru P, Blidaru A, Popa G. False acute abdomen in emergency surgery. Br J Surg 1996; 83(Suppl 2):61–2.

37. de Dombal FT, Leaper DJ, Staniland JR et al. Computer-aided diagnosis of acute abdominal pain. Br Med J 1972; 2:9–13.

38. Gunn AA. The diagnosis of acute abdominal pain with computer analysis. J R Coll Surg Edinb 1976; 21:170–2.

39. Adams ID, Chan M, Clifford PC et al. Computer aided diagnosis of acute abdominal pain: a multi-centre study. Br Med J 1986; 293:800–4.

A large study involving eight centres, 250 doctors and 16 737 patients demonstrated an improvement in diagnostic accuracy, reduction in the incidence of perforated appendicitis and bad management errors associated with the use of the computer.

40. Batstone GF. Educational aspects of medical audit. Br Med J 1990; 301:326–8.

41. Marteau TM, Wynne G, Kaye W et al. Resuscitation: experience without feedback increases confidence but not skill. Br Med J 1990; 300:849–50.

42. Lawrence PC, Clifford PC, Taylor IF. Acute abdominal pain: computer aided diagnosis by non-medically qualified staff. Ann R Coll Surg Engl 1987; 69:233–4.

This paper demonstrates that medical students assessing patients with acute abdominal pain using a structured proforma and then CAD have the same diagnostic accuracy as medical staff who use the proforma but not CAD.

43. Paterson-Brown S, Vipond MN, Simms K et al. Clinical decision-making and laparoscopy versus computer prediction in the management of the acute abdomen. Br J Surg 1989; 76:1011–13.

The addition of structured patient proformas without CAD significantly improved clinical decision-making and laparoscopy.

44. Bennett DH, Tambeur LJMT, Campbell WB. Use of coughing test to diagnose peritonitis. Br Med J 1994; 308:1336–7.

45. Williams NMA, Johnstone JM, Everson NW. The diagnostic value of symptoms and signs in childhood abdominal pain. J R Coll Surg Edinb 1998; 43:390–2.

46. Dixon JM, Elton RA, Rainey JB et al. Rectal examination in patients with pain in the right lower quadrant of the abdomen. Br Med J 1991; 302:386–8.

47. Howie CR, Gunn AA. Temperature: a poor diagnostic indicator in abdominal pain. J R Coll Surg Edinb 1984; 29:249–51.

48. Kylanpaa-Back M-L, Kemppainen E, Puolakkainen P et al. Reliable screening for acute pancreatitis with rapid urine trypsinogen-2 test strip. Br J Surg 2000; 87:49–52.

49. Attard AR, Corlett MJ, Kidner NJ et al. Safety of early pain relief for acute abdominal pain. Br Med J 1992; 305:554–6.

Assessment of patients with acute abdominal pain is not affected adversely by early analgesia.

50. Thomas SH, Cheema F, Reisner A et al. Effects of morphine analgesia on diagnostic accuracy in emergency department patients with abdominal pain: a prospective randomized trial. J Am Coll Surg 2003; 196:18–31.

This was a randomised study of 74 patients who received either morphine or placebo. The diagnostic accuracy was not affected by morphine.

51. Clavien PA, Burgan S, Moossa AR. Serum enzymes and other laboratory tests in acute pancreatitis. Br J Surg 1989; 76:1234–43.

52. Paterson-Brown S, Eckersley JRT, Sim AJW et al. Laparoscopy as an adjunct to decision-making in the acute abdomen. Br J Surg 1986; 73:1022–4.

53. Bradbury AW, Brittenden J, McBride K et al. Mesenteric ischaemia: a multi-disciplinary approach. Br J Surg 1995; 82:1446–59.

54. Schoots IG, Koffeman DA, Levi M et al. Systematic review of survival after acute mesenteric ischaemia according to disease aetiology. Br J Surg 2004; 91:17–27.

Data from 45 observational studies including 3692 patients were reviewed. Prognosis after acute mesenteric venous thrombosis is better than for arterial ischaemia, and that for arterial embolism is better than that for arterial thrombosis.

55. Thompson MM, Underwood MJ, Dookeran KA et al. Role of sequential leucocyte counts and C-reactive protein measurements in acute appendicitis. Br J Surg 1992; 79:822–4.

56. Davies AH, Bernau F, Salisbury A et al. C-reactive protein in right iliac fossa pain. J R Coll Surg Edinb 1991; 36:242–4.

57. Middleton SB, Whitbread T, Morgans BT et al. Combination of skin temperature and a single white cell count does not improve diagnostic accuracy in acute appendicitis. Br J Surg 1996; 83:499.

58. Gronroos JM, Gronroos P. Leucocyte and C-reactive protein in the diagnosis of acute appendicitis. Br J Surg 1999; 86:501–4.

59. Andersson REB. Meta-analysis of the clinical and laboratory diagnosis of appendicitis. Br J Surg 2004; 91:28–37.

Systematic Medline search of 28 diagnostic variables in 24 studies.

60. Sengupta A, Bax G, Paterson-Brown S. White cell count and C-reactive protein measurement in patients with possible appendicitis. Annals RCS Engl (in press).

61. Peng WK, Sheikh Z, Paterson-Brown S et al. Role of liver function tests in predicting common bile duct stones in acute calculous cholecystitis. Br J Surg 2005; 92:1241–7.

62. Cochrane RA, Edwards AT, Crosby DL et al. Senior surgeons and radiologists should assess emergency patients on presentation: a prospective

randomised controlled trial. J R Coll Surg Edinb 1998; 43:324–7.

63. Chen S-C, Yen Z-S, Wang H-P et al. Ultrasonography is superior to plain radiology in the diagnosis of pneumoperitoneum. Br J Surg 2002; 89:351–4.

64. Anyanwu AC, Moalypour SM. Are abdominal radiographs still overutilised in the assessment of acute abdominal pain? A district general hospital audit. J R Coll Surg Edinb Irel 1998; 43:267–70.

65. Bell DJ, Woo EK. Are abdominal radiographs still overutilised in the assessment of acute abdominal pain? (letter). Surgeon 2006; 4:60–1.

66. Royal College of Radiologists working party. Making the best use of a department of clinical radiology: guidelines for doctors, 5th edn. London, 2003.

67. Traill ZC, Nolan DJ. Imaging of intestinal obstruction. Br J Hosp Med 1996; 55:267–71.

68. Ott DJ, Gelfand DW. Gastrointestinal contrast agents: indications, uses and risks. JAMA 1983; 249:2380–4.

69. Wellwood JM, Wilson AN, Hopkinson BR. Gastrografin as an aid to the diagnosis of perforated peptic ulcer. Br J Surg 1971; 58:245–9.

70. Crofts TJ, Park KGM, Steele RJC et al. A randomized trial of non-operative treatment for perforated peptic ulcer. N Engl J Med 1989; 320:970–3.

71. Stewardson RH, Bombeck CT, Nyhus LM. Critical operative management of small bowel obstruction. Ann Surg 1978; 187:189–93.

72. Ogata M, Mateer JR, Condon RE. Prospective evaluation of abdominal sonography for the diagnosis of bowel obstruction. Ann Surg 1996; 223:237–41.

73. Brochwocz MJ, Paterson-Brown S, Murchison JT. Small bowel obstruction: the water-soluble follow-through revisited. Clin Radiol 2003; 58:393–7.

74. Lee JF-Y, Meng WC-S, Leung K-L et al. Water soluble contrast follow-through in the management of adhesive small bowel obstruction: a prospective randomized trial. Ann Coll Surg HK 2004; 8:120–6.

A randomised prospective trial of 150 patients with suspected adhesive small-bowel obstruction demonstrated that the group given water-soluble contrast studies received surgery significantly sooner (42 vs. 65h) and had a significantly shorter hospital stay (5 vs. 7 days) than the group treated conventionally. The incidence of surgical intervention in both groups was the same.

75. Burge J, Roadley G, Donald J et al. Randomised controlled trial of gastrografin in adhesive small bowel obstruction. Aust NZ J Surg 2005; 75:672–4.

A randomised trial of 40 patients with suspected adhesive small-bowel obstruction treated conventionally or given gastrografin. Four patients in each group required surgery. Time to resolution of symptoms was significantly quicker in the group given gastrografin.

76. Sajja SBS, Schein M. Early postoperative small bowel obstruction. Br J Surg 2004; 91:683–91.

77. Dudley HAF, Paterson-Brown S. Pseudo-obstruction. Br Med J 1986; 292:1157–8.

Leading article which provides the history of pseudo-obstruction and the relevant papers in relation to diagnosis and treatment.

78. Shrier D, Skucas J, Weiss S. Diverticulitis: an evaluation by computer tomography and contrast enema. Am Coll Gastroenterol 1991; 86:1466–71.

79. McKee RF, Deignan RW, Krukowski ZH. Radiological investigation in acute diverticulitis. Br J Surg 1993; 80:560–5.

80. Laing FC, Federie MP, Jeffrey RB et al. Ultrasonic evaluation of patients with acute right upper quadrant pain. Radiology 1981; 140:449–55.

81. Samuels BL, Freitas JE, Bree RL et al. A comparison of radionuclide hepatobiliary imaging and real-time ultrasound for the detection of acute cholecystitis. Radiology 1983; 47:207–10.

82. Peng WK, Sheikh Z, Nixon SJ et al. Role of laparoscopic cholecystectomy in the early management of acute gall bladder disease. Br J Surg 2005; 92:586–91.

83. Puylaert IBCM, Rutgers PF, Lalisang RI et al. A prospective study of ultrasonography in the diagnosis of appendicitis. N Engl J Med 1987; 317:666–9.

84. Gallego MG, Fadrique B, Nieto MA et al. Evaluation of ultrasonography and clinical diagnostic scoring in suspected appendicitis. Br J Surg 1998; 85:37–40.

85. Douglas CD, Macpherson NE, Davidson PM et al. Randomised controlled trial of ultrasonography in diagnosis of acute appendicitis, incorporating the Alvarado score. Br Med J 2000; 321:919–22.

86. McGrath FP, Keeling F. The role of early sonography in the management of the acute abdomen. Clin Radiol 1991; 44:172–4.

87. Ogata M, Mateer JR, Condon RE. Prospective evaluation of abdominal sonography for the diagnosis of bowel obstruction. Ann Surg 1996; 223:237–41.

88. Klingler PJ, Wetscher G, Glaser K et al. The use of ultrasound to differentiate rectus sheath hematoma from other acute abdominal disorders. Surg Endosc 1999; 13:1129–34.

89. Stengel D, Bauwens K, Sehouli J et al. Systematic review and meta-analysis of emergency ultrasonography for blunt abdominal trauma. Br J Surg 2001; 88:901–12.

90. Rao PM, Rhea JT, Novelline RA et al. Effect of computed tomography of the appendix on treatment of patients and use of hospital resources. N Engl J Med 1998; 338:141–6.

91. McColl I. More precision in diagnosing appendicitis. N Engl J Med 1998; 338:190–1.

92. Ng CS, Watson CJE, Palmer CR et al. Evaluation of early abdominopelvic computer tomography in patients with acute abdominal pain of unknown cause: prospective randomised study. Br Med J 2002; 325:1387–9.

93. Leschka S, Alkadhi H, Wildermuth S et al. Multidetector computed tomography of acute abdomen. Eur Radiol 2005; 15(12):2435–47.

94. Imatu M, Awai K, Nakayama Y et al. Multidetector CT findings suggesting a perforation site in the gastrointestinal tract: analysis in surgically confirmed 155 patients. Radiat Med 2007; 25(3):113–18.

95. Chou CK, Mak CW, Tzeng WS et al. CT of small bowel ischemia. Abdom Imaging 2004; 29(1):18–22.

96. Thoeni RF, Cello JP. CT imaging of colitis. Radiology 2006; 240(3):623–38.

97. Old JL, Dusing RW, Yap W et al. Imaging for suspected appendicitis. Am Fam Physician 2005; 71(1):71–8.

98. Nitta N, Takahashi M, Furukawa A et al. MR imaging of the normal appendix and acute appendicitis. J Magn Reson Imaging 2005; 21(2):156–65.

99. Pedrosa I, Levine D, Eyvazzadeh AD et al. MR imaging evaluation of acute appendicitis in pregnancy. Radiology 2006; 238(3):891–9.

100. Jaffe TA, Miller CM, Merkle EM. Practice patterns in imaging of the pregnant patient with abdominal pain: a survey of academic centers. Am J Roentgenol 2007; 189(5):1128–34.

101. Baigrie RJ, Saidan Z, Scott-Coombes D et al. Role of fine catheter peritoneal cytology and laparoscopy in the management of acute abdominal pain. Br J Surg 1991; 78:167–70.

102. Caldwell MTP, Watson RGK. Peritoneal aspiration cytology as a diagnostic aid in acute appendicitis. Br J Surg 1994; 81:276–8.

103. Paterson-Brown S. Emergency laparoscopic surgery. Br J Surg 1993; 80:279–83.

Review article showing the overwhelming evidence in support of diagnostic laparoscopy in the assessment of patients with acute abdominal pain, particularly when the diagnosis and decision to operate is in doubt.

104. Paterson-Brown S, Thompson JN, Eckersley JRT et al. Which patient with suspected appendicitis should undergo laparoscopy? Br Med J 1988; 296:1363–4.

105. Decadt B, Sussman L, Lewis MPN et al. Randomised clinical trial of early laparoscopy in the management of acute non-specific abdominal pain. Br J Surg 1999; 86:1383–6.

A randomised trial which demonstrated the improvements in diagnostic accuracy and subsequent quality of life in the group undergoing laparoscopy.

106. Morino M, Pellegrino L, Castagna E et al. Acute non-specific abdominal pain: a randomized, controlled trial comparing early laparoscopy versus clinical observation. Ann Surg 2006; 244:881–8.

107. Murphy SM, Donnelly M, Fitzgerald T et al. Patients' recall of clinical information following laparoscopy for acute abdominal pain. Br J Surg 2004; 91:485–8.

Perforations of the upper gastrointestinal tract

Enders Ng

Introduction

Foregut perforations are challenging surgical emergencies. This chapter reviews current evidence concerning the investigation and therapeutic options for perforations in different parts of the upper gastrointestinal tract. Owing to the potential implication in prognosis and planning of management, perforations are conventionally classified according to the anatomical position and causative mechanism.

Gastroduodenal perforation

Diagnosis

The most common cause of gastroduodenal perforation relates to peptic ulcer disease; the estimated lifetime risk of perforation in peptic ulcer disease ranges from 2% to 10%.[1-3] Typical presentation includes a sudden onset of epigastric pain which rapidly generalises to other parts of the abdomen. Some patients may report a history of dyspepsia or peptic ulcer, but such a finding is absent in about one-third of patients.[4] 'Board-like rigidity' is the most commonly coined physical sign, which refers to the diffuse peritonitis revealed on abdominal examination. However, in the elderly and the critically ill who develop ulcer perforation during hospitalisation, the presentation can be atypical and subtle. Diagnosis under such circumstances requires a high index of suspicion. Though subdiaphragmatic free gas on a plain erect chest X-ray (**Fig. 6.1**) is diagnostic (see also Chapter 5), it is seen in no

more than 70% of patients.[5] A lateral decubitus abdominal X-ray, ultrasound scan and computed tomography (CT) are thus invaluable investigations when the diagnosis is dubious. However, it has been suggested that the role of CT may be limited if the onset of symptoms is less than 6 hours before the imaging investigation.[6] Pneumogastrogram was once advocated by some surgeons as being able to increase the diagnostic yield from 66% on plain erect chest X-ray to 91%.[7] However, such a practice is now being condemned because forceful insufflations of air into the stomach are likely to reopen

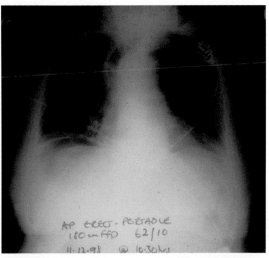

Figure 6.1 • Erect chest radiograph showing right subphrenic gas associated with a perforated peptic ulcer.

some of the perforations that have already sealed off spontaneously. For patients with profound peritoneal signs, a laparoscopy or laparotomy is indeed the most efficient investigation because immediate therapeutic intervention can be offered once the diagnosis of ulcer perforation is confirmed.

Prognosis

Perforation accounts for the majority of deaths related to peptic ulcer disease.[8,9] Spillage of gastroduodenal content through the perforation initiates a severe chemical peritonitis, which will be superimposed by bacterial infection if left untreated. Systemic inflammatory response syndrome and multiorgan dysfunction are the most feared consequences of the bacterial translocation across the peritoneal surface. Despite surgical intervention, mortality rates remain around 5–15%.[10,11] The prognostic factors for ulcer perforation have been widely studied, yet most published series consisted of relatively small numbers of patients with marked heterogeneity in demographics and treatment methods.

Before the era of laparoscopic surgery, Boey et al. reported significantly higher rates of mortality among patients having ulcer perforation admitted with major medical illness, preoperative shock and long-standing perforation (more than 24 hours). Those with no, one, two and all three risk factors at presentation were noted to have mortality rates of 0%, 10%, 45.5% and 100% respectively.[12] Similar findings have been reported by other multivariate analyses. Some have also identified that age >65 years and perforation during hospital stay are additional predictive factors of death.[13,14] In 2001, Lee et al. compared the Acute Physiology and Chronic Health Evaluation (APACHE) II score with Boey's parameters in order to determine the postoperative outcome in a cohort of over 400 patients.[15] An APACHE II score >5 was found to have predictive value for increasing postoperative complications and mortality, whereas the Boey score only predicted mortality but not morbidity. Interestingly, in the same study, a higher Boey score was found to be associated with an increased chance of conversion when laparoscopic repair was attempted. Albeit a precise and useful tool for research purpose, the APACHE II system is cumbersome to employ in daily practice, not to mention that the calculated score may vary with different time points of assessment.

Patient comorbidity, age >65 years, the presence of preoperative shock and long-standing perforation are associated with an increase in mortality and morbidity following perforated peptic ulcer.

Treatment

Some 50% of perforated peptic ulcers are spontaneously sealed off upon admission.[16] Such an observation has led to the sporadic advocacy of non-operative management, initially for older patients with poor premorbid status.[17,18] However, the non-operative approach in general has not been widely accepted with the exception of a few centres. Donovan et al. were among the first to advocate the use of diatrizoate meglumine (Hypaque) water-soluble contrast meal for confirmation of spontaneous sealing of the perforation.[19] In the absence of duodenal scarring and extravasation of contrast, patients with subphrenic free gas were managed non-operatively with nasogastric suction and intravenous antibiotics. By implementing this preset policy, these authors were able to report an overall mortality rate of only 4.6% in a series of 249 patients.[20]

The non-operative approach to the treatment of perforated peptic ulcers has been studied in a randomised trial consisting of 83 patients, of whom 40 were assigned to non-operative management while the rest underwent immediate laparotomy.[21] After 12 hours, 28% of the patients in the non-operative group failed to improve and required surgery. Though mortality rates were comparable between the two approaches, the incidence of intra-abdominal collections and sepsis was much higher in the non-operative group. Most strikingly, patients over 70 years of age were found to be less responsive to the non-operative approach when compared to the younger patients. In concluding the study, the authors did not recommend routine use of non-operative management for patients with duodenal ulcer perforation. However, they recognised that the results suggested that patients (a) did not need to be rushed to the operating theatre and time could be more usefully spent in better preoperative resuscitation, and (b) in selected patients the non-operative approach has a role to play.

Though the majority of surgeons now advocate immediate surgical intervention for perforated peptic ulcers, there remains debate as to what constitutes the most appropriate operation. The omental patch repair first described by Graham in 1938 is a quick and effective way to manage the perforation,[22] but for a time was associated with a high ulcer relapse rate in most of the follow-up studies.[23–25] This resulted in the popularity of adding a definitive acid-reducing procedure which was shown to be effective in lowering ulcer relapse.[26–29] In a prospective follow-up study, 107 selected patients with perforated pyloroduodenal ulcers undergoing omental patch closure and parietal cell vagotomy were evaluated up to 21 years later. The operative mortality was only 0.9% and the recurrent ulcer rate by life table analysis was 7.4%, with a re-operative rate of only 1.9%.[30] As a result, emergency vagotomy was once a standard of care recommended for peptic ulcer perforation. However, that has all changed over the last 15 years.

While the addition of a truncal or highly selective vagotomy may have caused little early morbidity or mortality apart from prolonging the time of anaesthesia, resectional surgery in the form of distal gastrectomy has been shown to increase the risk of mortality in patients undergoing surgery for perforated peptic ulcers.[31]

Following better understanding as to the pathogenesis of peptic ulcer diease, this has all changed. Most surgeons now prefer a much less aggressive 'damage control' approach when treating ulcer perforations.[32,33] The availability of *Helicobacter pylori* eradication regimens and potent proton-pump inhibitors provide excellent means to alleviate ulcer diathesis without the need of a definitive acid-reducing procedure. A simple omental patch repair and thorough peritoneal toileting are the key manoeuvres for treating the majority of patients. The only exception is probably those suffering from a giant duodenal perforation, which is not amenable to a simple repair.[34]

The majority of patients with a perforated peptic (pyloroduodenal) ulcer should be managed by simple omental patch closure, thorough peritoneal lavage, and subsequent treatment with proton inhibitors and eradication of *Helicobacter pylori* as necessary.

Role of *Helicobacter pylori* and non-steroidal anti-inflammatory drugs (NSAIDs)

While the relationship between *Helicobacter pylori* infection and uncomplicated peptic ulcers is indisputable, the role of the bacteria in ulcer perforation was once enigmatic. Reported infection rates in earlier series varied markedly from 0% to 100%.[35–38] The difference in the number, timing and types of diagnostic tests used to diagnose *H. pylori* infection in these studies may have accounted for the widely different findings. Furthermore the frequency of NSAID intake can be an important confounding factor. In a consecutive series of 73 patients with perforated duodenal ulcers, intraoperative antral biopsies for rapid urease test and histopathology were taken. These revealed an *H. pylori* infection rate of 70%,[39] the figure rising to 80% if NSAID users were excluded. Some studies have also reported a high proportion of NSAID use among patients with perforated gastric ulcers, especially in those without

H. pylori infection, suggesting that these drugs may represent a factor of relevance to *H. pylori*-negative ulcer perforation.[40,41]

The more affirmative evidence confirming a causal relationship between *H. pylori* infection and non-NSAID peptic ulcer perforation comes from long-term follow-up studies. A large study of 163 consecutive patients with perforated peptic ulcer managed by simple closure confirmed the strong association between persistent *H. pylori* infection and ulcer.[42] Of the 163 patients, 47.2% were found to have *H. pylori* infection during endoscopy at a mean follow-up of 6 years. Male gender and *H. pylori* infection were the only two independent predictive factors of ulcer relapse in the study.

In a randomised study, 99 patients with perforated duodenal ulcers and confirmed *H. pylori* infection received either 1 week of anti-*Helicobacter* therapy or 4 weeks of omeprazole.[43] Endoscopic surveillance after 1 year showed that ulcer recurrence rate decreased significantly from 38% in the control group to 4.8% in the eradication group. This confirms that medical eradication of *H. pylori* results in resolution of ulcer diathesis without the need for long-term antacid therapy or definitive surgery in patients who have undergone simple omental patch closure for perforated duodenal ulcer.[43]

Laparoscopic versus open repair

As the ulcer diathesis is readily corrected by *H. pylori* eradication and cessation of NSAID usage, most patients with ulcer perforation can now be treated with a simple repair together with a thorough peritoneal washing. These operations used to mandate a midline laparotomy in the past, but recent developments in minimally invasive surgery have revolutionised the surgical approach. The first laparoscopic closure of peptic ulcer perforation was reported in 1992.[44] Since then several series have been published.[45–48] Interpretation of these data, however, is difficult due to the marked heterogeneity in the study designs, patients' demographics and laparoscopic techniques used. With the exception of the two truly randomised trials from Hong Kong,[49,50] all the others are either single-centre series or non-randomised comparative studies. Most have shown significantly better, albeit marginal, outcomes in the laparoscopic group, which is likely, in part, to be related to publication bias.

In a systematic review of 13 publications comprising 658 patients, a significantly lower analgesic requirement and decreased wound infection rate were observed in the laparoscopic group when compared to the open repair group, but the overall success rate (following laparoscopic repair) was only 87%.[51] Another systematic review of 15 studies again demonstrated that laparoscopic closure was associated with significantly less analgesic use, shorter hospital stay, less wound infection and lower mortality rate.[52] However, shorter operating time and less suture-site leakage were clear advantages of the open method. In light of the evidence available, the laparoscopic approach is recommended mainly for patients with a low anaesthetic risk and short duration of perforation before surgery.

The role of cyclo-oxygenase-2 (COX-2)-specific inhibitors

Selective COX-2 inhibitors have been approved for symptomatic treatment of arthritis for nearly a decade. In contrast to conventional NSAIDs, COX-2 inhibitors provide anti-inflammatory effects without suppressing synthesis of prostaglandins essential for maintenance of mucosal integrity.[53] In the Celecoxib Long-term Arthritis Safety Study (CLASS), a double-blind randomised controlled trial, selective COX-2 inhibitor was confirmed to be associated with a significantly lower annualised incidence of peptic ulcer complications when compared to non-selective NSAIDs (0.44% vs. 1.27%, $P = 0.04$).[54] However, such a protective effect was negated if the patient used aspirin concomitantly.[54,55] In another population-based study, a 44% increase in the annual number of prescriptions for NSAIDs (both selective and non-selective) had been recorded since the introduction of COX-2 inhibitors, but the annual hospitalisation rates for perforated peptic ulcer decreased from 17 per 100 000 person-years to 12 per 100 000 person-years during the study period.[56]

The impact of COX-2 inhibitors and traditional NSAIDs on perforation-related death was recently determined in a population cohort study. While the observed 30-day mortality of the entire cohort of 2061 patients with ulcer perforation was 25%, that among NSAID and COX-2 inhibitor users was much higher, amounting to 35%.[57] The increase in mortality associated with use of COX-2 inhibitors was similar to that of traditional NSAIDs, with an adjusted mortality rate ratio (compared to non-users of NSAIDs) of 2.0 and 1.7 respectively. COX-2 inhibitors, albeit being able to reduce the overall incidence of perforated ulcers, do not confer any advantage in clinical outcomes if perforating complication occurs.

Perforated gastric ulcers

Reports pertaining to gastric ulcer perforation only are scarce.[58] On a statistical basis, gastric perforation tends to cluster among the elderly and is more likely to be associated with use of NSAIDs, but other causes include carcinoma, lymphoma and gastrointestinal stromal tumours. Perforation in the older age group carries a less favourable prognosis, partly related to their impaired physiological response to the septic insult, and more so to the delay in presentation, which is not uncommon. While a simple omental patch remains the best option, many surgeons prefer an ulcer excision if this can be carried out easily and without compromise to the stomach. Formal gastric resection is not indicated unless either of these options are not possible. Because a small minority are malignant,[59] and the possibility of gastric lymphoma needs to be remembered here, it is essential to biopsy the ulcer edge, if is not being excised. Definitive surgery, if then required, can be carried out at a later date once the pathology has been reviewed, full staging investigations carried out, and after a full and frank discussion undertaken with the patient regarding prognosis and alternative treatment options. Gastric resection for a perforated gastric cancer will invariably be palliative and gastric lymphoma can now be managed almost entirely by chemotherapy, radiotherapy or a combination of the two. (The reader is referred to the *Oesophagogastric Surgery* volume in this Companion to Specialist Surgical Practice series for more detailed information.)

 Simple omental patch closure with biopsies of the ulcer edge or ulcer excision is the best option for perforated gastric ulcers. The former works surprisingly well, even for large tumours, and is to be preferred where possible over resection. Gastric resection, often at night, in difficult circumstances on a sick patient and increasingly by surgeons who may not be experienced upper gastrointestinal surgeons should only be undertaken as a last resort, when all other methods of closure have failed.

Oesophageal perforation

Classification

Perforation of the oesophagus can be broadly classified into iatrogenic and spontaneous. Most iatrogenic perforations are related to endoscopic instrumentation, while some are related to para-oesophageal operations, such as fundoplication, cardiomyotomy, bariatric operations, etc. The reported incidence of perforation for rigid oesophagoscopy is 0.11% and for fibre-optic endoscopy varies from 0.018% to 0.03%.[60–62] Therapeutic endoscopy is associated with a much higher frequency of perforation (1–10%).[63,64] Other less common causes include foreign body penetration, traumatic endotracheal intubation, nasogastric catheterisation and swallowing of corrosives. Spontaneous rupture of the oesophagus (Boerhaave's perforation) is rare but tends to occur after forceful retching or vomiting, and is usually related to an episode of binge eating and/or drinking. It is typically located just proximal to the oesophagogastric junction and more commonly opens into the left pleural space.

Diagnosis

Diagnosis of oesophageal perforation can be difficult. The presentation is often non-specific and may easily be confused with other disorders such as spontaneous pneumothorax/pneumomediastinum, myocardial infarction, acute pancreatitis and pneumonia. The essential attribute is the maintenance of a high index of suspicion. Pain is the most common symptom, which may occur anywhere from the neck to the abdominal region, depending on the location, the cause and the time lapse between onset and presentation. Less often, dysphagia, odynophagia, dyspnoea, cyanosis and fever are other possible complaints. A preceding history of forceful vomiting, oesophageal instrumentation, paraoesophageal surgery and chest trauma should always be taken into consideration. Physical examination may reveal surgical emphysema over the neck and upper chest wall. Hydrothorax or pneumothorax may also be found on erect chest X-ray. Hamman's sign (a crunching sound heard on chest auscultation) is found less commonly than suggested in textbooks.

The role of ancillary investigations for oesophageal perforation depends largely on the condition of the patient. If a patient is relatively stable and requires no endotracheal intubation, a water-soluble contrast swallow is a relatively easy way to confirm the diagnosis, determine the location and assess the severity of the perforation. However, for patients with profound sepsis mandating intubation and ventilatory support, a contrast-enhanced CT scan of the suspected region will be required to establish the diagnosis. A careful flexible oesophagoscopy is a very useful technique when the diagnosis remains in doubt after these other investigations (**Fig. 6.2**).

Management

The management of oesophageal perforation starts with aggressive resuscitation and appropriate monitoring of the physiological parameters. Further contamination of the mediastinum is minimised by putting the patient on nil by mouth. Although insertion of a nasogastric tube reduces potential for ongoing leakage from refluxed gastric contents, in the presence of a perforation which might be managed non-operatively (see below), this will need to be inserted either under direct vision (endoscopically)

Figure 6.2 • Endoscopic view of a Boerhaave perforation. The grey substance is necrotic mucosa and the pink lung.

or using X-ray guidance. Vigorous intravenous fluid replacement and broad-spectrum antibiotics are prescribed for control of systemic infection. Chest drainage should be established if there is hydrothorax or hydropneumothorax. Most patients require intensive care support. Subsequent management should be based on the clinical features, the underlying cause, the location of perforation, and sometimes the time lapse between perforation and diagnosis.

Non-operative management

Candidates for non-operative treatment, as defined by Cameron et al. in 1979, include those with a small perforation without pleural involvement, accompanied by minimal symptoms and no evidence of systemic sepsis.[65,66] Preferably the perforation is accompanied by a re-entry of extravasated contrast medium back into the oesophageal lumen. Any sympathetic pleural effusion has to be drained, with the effluent regularly inspected to exclude enteric contents suggesting fistulation. Nutritional support, either by parenteral route or through a surgically inserted feeding jejunostomy, is commenced early to avoid excessive catabolic activity.

It has been shown that patients who truly respond to non-operative management are those with small cervical tears following oesophagoscopy or traumatic intubation, well-circumscribed intramural dissection following pneumatic dilatation for achalasia, and small anastomotic leaks following oesophageal operation.[67,68] An important adjunct now available in dealing with these 'minor' perforations is endoluminal stenting.[69,70] The recent development of a retrievable type of silicone-coated stent has shown some promising results. In a prospective series of 18 patients with iatrogenic perforation of the oesophagus, 17 were treated with the Polyflex (Boston Scientific, Natick, Mass, USA) stent in addition to chest drainage.[71] Except for one patient with a persistent leak who required operative repair, the remaining 16 had successful resolution of their leak as confirmed by oesophagram. Most of the patients were able to resume oral intake in 72 hours, and the mean time before the stent was removed was 52 days. Alternatively elderly and frail patients who suffer perforation following attempted dilatation of a malignant stricture can be managed by insertion of a covered permanent stent (**Fig. 6.3**).

Surgical repair

Non-operative treatment of spontaneous rupture (Boerhaave's syndrome) and iatrogenic perforation of the thoracic oesophagus with pleural breach and leak into the pleural cavity are almost all bound to fail. Furthermore it has been suggested that surgical intervention is required in as many as 43% of patients initially selected for non-operative management.[72] Except for those who are at extreme risk of surgery, early surgical intervention is recommended in the majority of patients with thoracic oesophageal perforation.[73] In addition to thorough drainage of the mediastinum and the pleural cavity, three surgical manoeuvres for control of leakage may be applied:

1. Isolation and diversion (cervical oesophagostomy) followed by delayed staged reconstruction.

2. Primary repair of the perforation, with or without reinforcement, and drainage.

3. Immediate oesophagectomy.

Oesophageal exclusion and diversion

The technique of oesophageal exclusion and diversion was described several decades ago. It involves division and closure of the oesophagus proximal and distal to the site of injury, with creation of an end-cervical oesophagectomy. Subsequently it has evolved to a side-cervical oesophagostomy for proximal diversion of saliva and a staple transection of the oesophagogastric junction to prevent reflux of gastroduodenal content back to the oesophageal lumen. Nevertheless, such an incomplete diversion often ends up with continuous soiling in the mediastinum, leading to persistent thoracic sepsis. With time, it proves to be a suboptimal treatment and is now reserved mainly for patients who are too unstable to undergo definitive repair or resection.

Primary repair

Primary repair is an appropriate option for perforations occurring less than 24 hours after diagnosis, because the surrounding tissues are neither excessively inflamed nor ischaemic. As the laceration on the mucosal side can be much longer/wider than is appreciated from the adventitial surface, a cautious longitudinal extension of the muscular defect is often

Figure 6.3 • Contrast radiography of the oesophagus. **(a)** Barium swallow demonstrating a tight malignant stricture. **(b)** Water-soluble contrast swallow after dilatation demonstrating a perforation. **(c)** Water-soluble contrast study in the same patient following insertion of an expandable metal stent, demonstrating no further leak.

required for better assessment of the extent of the mucosal injury. Following careful debridement of the necrotic tissues along the perimeter of the perforation, the edges are then closed with interrupted absorbable sutures. It may be possible, in very early perforations with very healthy tissue, to close the defect wound in two layers: first the mucosa/submucosal layer, followed by the muscular layer. However, in the majority of circumstances a single all-layer suture is adequate. Enrolment of a reinforcing autogenous vascular pedicle flap (intercostals muscle) remains controversial.[74,75] Most advocates of reinforcement flaps suggest an onlay patch rather than a wrap, to minimise the possibility of stricture at the repair site. A major concern with the wrap technique is the induction of an obstructive component distal to the repair site, rendering it more prone to leakage.

Though technically feasible, primary repair is associated with a high failure rate and many surgeons now advocate insertion of a T-tube into the perforation, which is closed around it (after debridement), producing a controlled fistula. This can be removed at a later date, often many weeks/months later, once the patient has recovered and surrounding leakage (managed by appropriately placed chest drains) has subsided.

Immediate resection

Several series have pointed out that primary repair results in greater morbidity and even mortality than immediate oesophageal resection.[76–78] However, this may well relate to the underlying cause of perforation and whether the cause remains. In a series of 41 patients, of whom 25 underwent surgical repair of oesophageal perforation,[79] about one-third had continued swallowing difficulty which mandated regular oesophageal dilation after an average of 3.7 years.

Oesophagectomy is therefore a reasonable option (if the surgeon is experienced in this procedure) in patients with underlying disease (including carcinoma, if the lesion was considered operable before the perforation occurred) if the diagnosis has been made early and the patient is in a good condition. Occasionally it may also be required in patients presenting late in whom simple closure over a T-tube is not possible. This scenario is, however, very uncommon. (The reader is referred to the *Oesophagogastric Surgery* volume in this Companion to Specialist Surgical Practice series for more detailed information.)

 Primary repair with or without T-tube drainage is the best option for management of oesophageal perforations depending on time from occurrence to diagnosis. Patients with an underlying condition related to the perforation, in whom the diagnosis has been made early (<24 hours) and who are in a good condition, can be considered for resection if the appropriate surgical experience is available.

Corrosive perforation

Corrosive injury to the upper gastrointestinal tract is a notoriously difficult situation associated with dreadful rates of morbidity and mortality. While more than 80% of accidental corrosive ingestion occurs in children, injuries in adults are usually intentional, and thus more severe in extent.[80] The mortality rate ranges from 10% to 78% in cases of attempted suicide.[81,82] The severity of damage depends on the type, concentration, volume, and duration of contact of the agent with the mucosal surface. Making a distinction between acid and alkali as to the extent and severity of oesophagogastric damage has been elusive. It is well known that acid induces a coagulating burn injury, which tends to self-limiting with the coagulum formation. In contrast, alkali causes a liquefactive necrosis to the tissue, leading to dissolution of protein and collagen, saponification of fats, and thrombosis of blood vessels. All these incur a deeper damage and even transmural perforation.

The acute management of corrosive ingestion entails a quick and efficient assessment of the patient's vital signs. Laryngeal oedema can be life threatening and establishment of a patent airway is of paramount importance. Either an early endotracheal intubation or tracheostomy may be required in difficult cases before further resuscitation and management. It is generally agreed that early gentle endoscopic examination is of value for both prognostic consideration and decision making.[83,84] Surgical intervention, such as thoracotomy, drainage, mediastinal debridement, proximal diversion of saliva and exclusion from gastric reflux are better performed early if signs of full thickness perforation are detected on radiological or endoscopic investigations. Reconstruction should be deferred until sepsis has subsided. More often than not, reconstruction is carried out by fashioning a jejunal or colonic interposition loop through an extra-anatomical plane (e.g. the substernal or presternal routes).

Perforation after endotherapy for mucosal/submucosal tumours

Since its introduction in the 1980s, endoscopic mucosal resection (EMR) has been increasingly practised for upper gastrointestinal lesions identified at early stages.[85–87] With the snaring technique, en bloc resection used to be a challenging task as the average size of lesion removed is limited (<15 mm in diameter).[88] The recent development of new endoscopic accessories, such as the insulated-tip knife and hook knife, has opened up a new horizon for such purposes.[89–91] The novel endoluminal procedure, namely endoscopic submucosal dissection (ESD), has virtually no limitation on the size of resection, provided that the lesion is superficial with a low chance of nodal spread.[92] However, ESD is a technically demanding procedure with a significantly higher risk of perforation compared with conventional EMR.[93–95] As most ESD-induced perforations can be recognised intraoperatively, attempts to close the defect by various techniques have been reported.[96] Fujishiro et al. described a 100% success rate for closing ESD perforations using endoscopic clips.[97] The average duration of hospital stay was only 12 days and none of the 27 patients in the series required surgical salvage. More importantly, as reported in an intermediate-term follow-up study by Ikehara et al., perforation during ESD for early oesophageal and gastric cancers has not been associated with increased risk of dissemination of the malignancy.[98]

Perforation during endoscopic retrograde cholangiopancreatography (ERCP)

Visceral perforations due to ERCP are not uncommon, with reported incidence ranging between 0.5% and 2.1%.[99,100] Risk factors for ERCP-related perforation are older age of patients, suspected sphincter of Oddi dysfunction, a dilated duct, performance of a sphincterotomy and longer duration of the procedure.[101] ERCP-related perforation can be further subclassified according to the causative mechanism and location, which is useful as the management strategy may vary accordingly. Perforations of the oesophagus, stomach or duodenum during ERCP are often related to insertion and positioning of the side-viewing duodenoscope. Vulnerability further increases if there is anatomical

deformity. Another prominent risk factor for 'scope' perforation is a history of previous Billroth II gastrectomy, because retrograde insertion of the endoscope along the afferent loop may overstretch and rupture the jejunum around the relatively fixed duodenojejunal flexure. The reported incidence under such circumstances amounts to 10% even in expert centres.[102,103] This kind of perforation tends to be intraperitoneal with sizeable defects and early operative repair is necessary.

In contrast, perforations resulting from endoscopic sphincterotomy or guidewire insertion are mostly retroperitoneal with small size of leakage, and therefore more amenable to non-operative therapy. Although some perforations can be identified at the time of the ERCP, many are not suspected until after the procedure. Clearly early suspicion is raised by the presence of abdominal pain postprocedure, but the observation of paraduodenal or perinephric gas shadows on plain abdominal radiographs are suggestive of a retroperitoneal perforation. In such cases, and even if the plain X-rays are unremarkable, a CT scan of the abdomen with oral and intravenous contrast should be organised to confirm the diagnosis and extent of the perforation. Small perforations with minimal extravasation of contrast can be successfully managed by non-operative means, including nasogastric drainage, antibiotics and parenteral nutrition. However, extensive extravasation will require surgical repair and drainage. This can be a formidable undertaking and is associated with significant morbidity and mortality. Thankfully they are relatively rare, but when they occur each patient will need to be managed according to first priciples: debridement of ischaemic and damaged tissue, primary repair of the defect if possible, diversion of biliary contents (by means of a T-tube) and consideration given to duodenal exclusion (closure of pylorus and gastroenterostomy). In such circumstances a feeding jejunostomy should also be inserted for long-term nutritional support.

 It has been shown in various series that one of the key prerequisites for successful non-operative management of ERCP perforations is the early recognition and diagnosis of the situation.[104,105]

Key points

- Perforations of the upper gastrointestinal tract are either spontaneous or iatrogenic.
- Early surgery is generally required for the majority of perforations as delay in diagnosis and treatment is associated with increased morbidity and mortality.
- For perforated duodenal ulcers omental patch repair followed by postoperative therapy with proton-pump inhibitors and eradication of *Helicobacter pylori*, if present, is the treatment of choice.
- For perforated gastric ulcers, either ulcer excision (if feasible) or omental patch repair and biopsy of the ulcer is all that is required. Gastric resection should not be carried out without histology unless closure cannot be achieved using these other techniques.
- Management of oesophageal perforations depends largely on whether the pleura has been breached. It can be a challenging condition and surgical strategies will depend on the expertise available. These include non-operative management, stent insertion (both permanent and removable), repair (with or without T-tube drainage) and occasionally oesophageal resection.
- Early endoscopy is a very useful technique to assess many oesophageal emergencies including corrosive injury.
- ERCP perforations vary from simple to extensive and management depends on early diagnosis and accurate assessment as to the degree of extravasation.

References

1. Coggon D, Lambert P, Langman MJ. 20 years of hospital admissions for peptic ulcer in England and Wales. Lancet 1981; 1:1302–4.

2. Walt R, Katschinski B, Logan R et al. Rising frequency of ulcer perforation in elderly people in the United Kingdom. Lancet 1986; 1(8479):489–92.

3. Svanes C, Lie RT, Kvåle G et al. Incidence of perforated ulcer in western Norway, 1935–1990: cohort- or period-dependent time trends? Am J Epidemiol 1995; 141:836–44.

4. Bornman PC, Theodorou NA, Jeffery PC et al. Simple closure of perforated duodenal ulcer: a prospective evaluation of a conservative management policy. Br J Surg 1990; 77:73–5.

5. Chen CH, Yang CC, Yeh YH. Role of upright chest radiography and ultrasonography in demonstrating free air of perforated peptic ulcers. Hepatogastroenterology 2001; 48:1082–4.

6. Grassi R, Romano S, Pinto A et al. Gastro-duodenal perforations: conventional plain film, US and CT findings in 166 consecutive patients. Eur J Radiol 2004; 50:30–6.

7. Lee CW, Yip AW, Lam KH. Pneumogastrogram in the diagnosis of perforated peptic ulcer. Aust NZ J Surg 1993; 63:459–61.

8. Svanes C. Trends in perforated peptic ulcer: incidence, etiology, treatment and prognosis. World J Surg 2000; 24:277–83.

9. Robson AJ, Richards JM, Ohly N et al. The effect of surgical subspecialization on outcomes in peptic ulcer disease complicated by perforation and bleeding. World J Surg 2008; 32(7):1456–61.

10. Kujath P, Schwandner O, Bruch HP. Morbidity and mortality of perforated peptic gastroduodenal ulcer following emergency surgery. Langenbeck's Arch Surg 2002; 387:298–302.

11. Egberts JH, Summa B, Schulz U et al. Impact of preoperative physiological risk profile on postoperative morbidity and mortality after emergency operation of complicated peptic ulcer disease. World J Surg 2007; 31:1449–57.

12. Boey J, Choi SK, Poon A et al. Risk stratification in perforated duodenal ulcers. A prospective validation of predictive factors. Ann Surg 1987; 205:22–6.

13. Kocer B, Surmeli S, Solak C et al. Factors affecting mortality and morbidity in patients with peptic ulcer perforation. J Gastroenterol Hepatol 2007; 22:565–70.

14. Sillakivi T, Lang A, Tein A et al. Evaluation of risk factors for mortality in surgically treated perforated peptic ulcer. Hepatogastroenterology 2000; 47:1765–8.

15. Lee FY, Leung KL, Lai BS et al. Predicting mortality and morbidity of patients operated on for perforated peptic ulcers. Arch Surg 2001; 136:90–4.

16. Donovan AJ, Berne TV, Donovan JA. Perforated duodenal ulcer: an alternative therapeutic plan. Arch Surg 1998; 133:1166–71.

17. Dascalescu C, Andriescu L, Bulat C et al. Taylor's method: a therapeutic alternative for perforated

gastroduodenal ulcer. Hepatogastroenterology 2006; 53:543–6.

18. Bucher P, Oulhaci W, Morel P et al. Results of conservative treatment for perforated gastroduodenal ulcers in patients not eligible for surgical repair. Swiss Med Wkly 2007; 137:337–40.

19. Donovan AJ, Vinson TL, Maulsby GO et al. Selective treatment of duodenal ulcer with perforation. Ann Surg 1979; 189:627–36.

20. Berne TV, Donovan AJ. Nonoperative treatment of perforated duodenal ulcer. Arch Surg 1989; 124:830–2.

21. Crofts TJ, Park KG, Steele RJ . A randomized trial of nonoperative treatment for perforated peptic ulcer. N Engl J Med 1989; 320:970–3.

This randomised trial disproved the recommendation of non-operative treatment for older patients. The higher incidence of intra-abdominal sepsis and prolonged hospital stay are additional discouraging factors for conservative management in patients with peptic ulcer perforation.

22. Graham RR. Technical surgical procedures for gastric and duodenal ulcer. Surg Gynecol Obstet 1938; 66:269–87.

23. Drury JK, McKay AJ, Hutchison JS et al. Natural history of perforated duodenal ulcers treated by suture closure. Lancet 1978; 2:749–50.

24. Griffin GE, Organ CH. The natural history of the perforated duodenal ulcer treated by suture placation. Ann Surg 1976; 183:382–5.

25. Bornman PC, Theodorou NA, Jeffery PC et al. Simple closure of perforated duodenal ulcer: a prospective evaluation of a conservative management policy. Br J Surg 1990; 77:73–5.

26. Tanphiphat C, Tanprayoon T, Na Thalang A. Surgical treatment of perforated duodenal ulcer: a prospective trial between simple closure and definitive surgery. Br J Surg 1985; 72:370–2.

27. Christiansen J, Andersen OB, Bonnesen T et al. Perforated duodenal ulcer managed by simple closure versus closure and proximal gastric vagotomy. Br J Surg 1987; 74:286–7.

28. Boey J, Lee NW, Koo J et al. Immediate definitive surgery for perforated duodenal ulcers: a prospective controlled trial. Ann Surg 1982; 196:338–44.

29. Ceneviva R, de Castro e Silva Júnior O, Castelfranchi PL et al. Simple suture with or without proximal gastric vagotomy for perforated duodenal ulcer. Br J Surg 1986; 73:427–30.

30. Jordan PH Jr, Thornby J. Perforated pyloroduodenal ulcers. Long-term results with omental patch closure and parietal cell vagotomy. Ann Surg 1995; 221:479–86.

31. Noguiera C, Silva AS, Santos JN et al. Perforated peptic ulcer: main factors of morbidity and mortality. World J Surg 2003; 27:782–7.

32. Gilliam AD, Speake WJ, Lobo DN et al. Current practice of emergency vagotomy and Helicobacter pylori eradication for complicated peptic ulcer in the United Kingdom. Br J Surg 2003; 90:88–90.

33. Liu CC, Lee CL, Chan CC et al. Maintenance treatment is not necessary after Helicobacter pylori eradication and healing of bleeding peptic ulcer: a 5-year prospective, randomized, controlled study. Arch Intern Med 2003; 163:2020–4.

34. Gupta S, Kaushik R, Sharma R et al. The management of large perforations of duodenal ulcers. BMC Surg 2005; 5:15.

35. Reinbach DH, Cruickshank G, McColl KE. Acute perforated duodenal ulcer is not associated with Helicobacter pylori infection. Gut 1993; 34:1344–7.

36. Matsukura N, Onda M, Tokunaga A et al. Role of Helicobacter pylori infection in perforation of peptic ulcer: an age- and gender-matched case–control study. J Clin Gastroenterol 1997; 25(Suppl 1):S235–9.

37. Sebastian M, Chandran VP, Elashaal YI et al. Helicobacter pylori infection in perforated peptic ulcer disease. Br J Surg 1995; 82:360–2.

38. Mihmanli M, Isgor A, Kabukcuoglu F et al. The effect of H. pylori in perforation of duodenal ulcer. Hepatogastroenterology 1998; 45:1610–12.

39. Ng EK, Chung SC, Sung JJ et al. High prevalence of Helicobacter pylori infection in duodenal ulcer perforations not caused by non-steroidal anti-inflammatory drugs. Br J Surg 1996; 83:1779–81.

40. Gisbert JP, Legido J, García-Sanz I et al. Helicobacter pylori and perforated peptic ulcer prevalence of the infection and role of non-steroidal anti-inflammatory drugs. Dig Liver Dis 2004; 36:116–20.

41. Bobrzynski A, Konturek PC, Konturek SJ et al. Helicobacter pylori and nonsteroidal anti-inflammatory drugs in perforations and bleeding of peptic ulcers. Med Sci Monit 2005; 11:CR132–5.

42. Chu KM, Kwok KF, Law SY et al. Helicobacter pylori status and endoscopy follow-up of patients having a history of perforated duodenal ulcer. Gastrointest Endosc 1999; 50:58–62.

43. Ng EK, Lam YH, Sung JJ. Eradication of Helicobacter pylori prevents recurrence of ulcer after simple closure of duodenal ulcer perforation: randomized controlled trial. Ann Surg 2000; 231:153–8.

This is the first randomised trial showing significant reduction in ulcer recurrence after eradication of Helicobacter pylori in patients undergoing simple omental repair of perforated duodenal ulcer.

44. Nathanson LK, Easter DW, Cuschieri A. Laparoscopic repair/peritoneal toilet of perforated duodenal ulcer. Surg Endosc 1990; 4:232–3.

45. Druart ML, Van Hee R, Etienne J et al. Laparoscopic repair of perforated duodenal ulcer. A prospective multicenter clinical trial. Surg Endosc 1997; 11:1017–20.

46. Katkhouda N, Mavor E, Mason RJ et al. Laparoscopic repair of perforated duodenal ulcers:

outcome and efficacy in 30 consecutive patients. Arch Surg 1999; 134:845–8.

47. Lau WY, Leung KL, Zhu XL et al. Laparoscopic repair of perforated peptic ulcer. Br J Surg 1995; 82:814–16.

48. Lam PW, Lam MC, Hui EK et al. Laparoscopic repair of perforated duodenal ulcers: the"three-stitch" Graham patch technique. Surg Endosc 2005; 19:1627–30.

49. Lau WY, Leung KL, Kwong KH et al. A randomized study comparing laparoscopic versus open repair of perforated peptic ulcer using suture or sutureless technique. Ann Surg 1996; 224:131–8.

50. Siu WT, Leong HT, Law BK et al. Laparoscopic repair for perforated peptic ulcer: a randomized controlled trial. Ann Surg 2002; 235:313–19.

51. Lau H. Laparoscopic repair of perforated peptic ulcer: a meta-analysis. Surg Endosc 2004; 16:1013–21.

    This is the first meta-analysis evaluating the role of laparoscopic repair in patients with peptic ulcer perforation. The laparoscopic approach confers superior short-term benefits in terms of postoperative pain and wound morbidity, and more importantly it is as safe and effective as open repair.

52. Lunevicius R, Morkevicius M. Systematic review comparing laparoscopic and open repair for perforated peptic ulcer. Br J Surg 2005; 92:1195–207.

53. Goldstein JL, Silverstein FE, Agrawal NM et al. Reduced risk of upper gastrointestinal ulcer complications with celecoxib, a novel COX-2 inhibitor. Am J Gastroenterol 2000; 95:1681–90.

54. Silverstein FE, Faich G, Goldstein JL et al. Gastrointestinal toxicity with celecoxib vs nonsteroidal anti-inflammatory drugs for osteoarthritis and rheumatoid arthritis: the CLASS study: a randomized controlled trial. Celecoxib Long-term Arthritis Safety Study. JAMA 2000; 284:1247–55.

55. García Rodríguez LA, Barreales Tolosa L. Risk of upper gastrointestinal complications among users of traditional NSAIDs and COXIBs in the general population. Gastroenterology 2007; 132(2): 498–506.

56. Christensen S, Riis A, Nørgaard M et al. Introduction of newer selective cyclo-oxygenase-2 inhibitors and rates of hospitalization with bleeding and perforated peptic ulcer. Aliment Pharmacol Ther 2007; 25(8):907–12.

57. Thomsen RW, Riis A, Munk EM et al. 30-day mortality after peptic ulcer perforation among users of newer selective COX-2 inhibitors and traditional NSAIDs: a population-based study. Am J Gastroenterol 2006; 101(12):2704–10.

58. Wysocki A, Biesiada Z, Beben P et al. Perforated gastric ulcer. Dig Surg 2000; 17:132–7.

59. Madiba TE, Nair R, Mulaudzi TV et al. Perforated gastric ulcer – reappraisal of surgical options. S Afr J Surg 2005; 43:58–60.

60. Wesdorp IC, Bartelsman JF, Huibregtse K et al. Treatment of instrumental oesophageal perforation. Gut 1984; 25:398–404.

61. Michel L, Grillo HC, Malt RA. Operative and non-operative management of esophageal perforation. Ann Surg 1981; 194:57–63.

62. Jones WG, Ginsberg RJ. Esophageal perforation: a continuing challenge. Ann Thorac Surg 1992; 53:534–43.

63. Adamek HE, Jakobs R, Dorlars D et al. Management of esophageal perforations after therapeutic upper gastrointestinal endoscopy. Scand J Gastroenterol 1997; 32:411–14.

64. Fry LC, Mönkemüller K, Neumann H et al. Incidence, clinical management and outcomes of esophageal perforations after endoscopic dilatation. Z Gastroenterol 2007; 45:1180–4.

65. Cameron JL, Kieffer RF, Hendrix TR et al. Selective nonoperative management of contained intrathoracic esophageal disruptions. Ann Thorac Surg 1979; 27:404–8.

66. Shaffer HA Jr, Valenzuela G, Mittal RK. Esophageal perforation. A reassessment of the criteria for choosing medical or surgical therapy. Arch Intern Med 1992; 152:757–61.

67. Molina EG, Stollman N, Grauer L et al. Conservative management of esophageal nontransmural tears after pneumatic dilation for achalasia. Am J Gastroenterol 1996; 91:15–18.

68. Michel L, Grillo HC, Malt RA. Operative and non-operative management of esophageal perforations. Ann Surg 1981; 194:57–63.

69. Hünerbein M, Stroszczynski C, Moesta KT et al. Treatment of thoracic anastomotic leaks after esophagectomy with self-expanding plastic stents. Ann Surg 2004; 240:801–7.

70. Siersema PD, Homs MY, Haringsma J et al. Use of large-diameter metallic stents to seal traumatic nonmalignant perforations of the esophagus. Gastrointest Endosc 2003; 58:356–61.

71. Freeman RK, Van Woerkom JM, Ascioti AJ. Esophageal stent placement for the treatment of iatrogenic intrathoracic esophageal perforation. Ann Thorac Surg 2007; 83:2003–7.

72. Amir AI, van Dullemen H, Plukker JT. Selective approach in the treatment of esophageal perforations. Scand J Gastroenterol 2004; 39:418–22.

73. Richardson JD. Management of esophageal perforations: the value of aggressive surgical treatment. Am J Surg 2005; 190:161–5.

74. Wright CD, Mathisen DJ, Wain JC et al. Reinforced primary repair of thoracic esophageal perforation. Ann Thoracic Surg 1995; 60:245–8.

75. Gouge T, Depan H, Spencer F. Experience with the Grillo pleural wrap procedure in 18 patients with perforation of the thoracic esophagus. Ann Surg 1989; 209:612–17.

76. Orringer MB. Esophagectomy for esophageal disruption. Ann Thorac Surg 1990; 49:35–42.

77. Altorjay A, Kiss J, Voros A. The role of esophagectomy in the management of esophageal perforations. Ann Thorac Surg 1998; 65:1433–6.

78. Salo JA, Isolauri JO, Heikkila LJ et al. Management of delayed esophageal perforation with mediastinal sepsis; esophagectomy or primary repair? J Thorac Cardiovasc Surg 1993; 106:1088–91.

79. Iannettoni MD, Vlessis AA, Whyte RI et al. Functional outcome after surgical treatment of esophageal perforation. Ann Thorac Surg 1997; 64:1606–9.

80. Gumaste VV, Dave PB. Ingestion of corrosive substances by adults. Am J Gastroenterol 1992; 87:1–5.

81. Ertekin C, Alimoglu O, Akyildiz H et al. The results of caustic ingestions. Hepatogastroenterology 2004; 51:1397–400.

82. Sugawa C, Lucas CE. Caustic injury of the upper gastrointestinal tract in adults: a clinical and endoscopic study. Surgery 1989; 106:802–6.

83. Poley JW, Steyerberg EW, Kuipers EJ et al. Ingestion of acid and alkaline agents: outcome and prognostic value of early upper endoscopy. Gastrointest Endosc 2004; 60:372–7.

84. Rigo GP, Camellini L, Azzolini F et al. What is the utility of selected clinical and endoscopic parameters in predicting the risk of death after caustic ingestion? Endoscopy 2002; 34:304–10.

85. Hirao M, Masuda K, Asanuma T et al. Endoscopic resection of early gastric cancer and other tumors with local injection of hypertonic saline–epinephrine. Gastrointest Endosc 1988; 34:264–9.

86. Inoue H, Takeshita K, Hori H et al. Endoscopic mucosal resection with a cap-fitted panendoscope for esophagus, stomach, and colon mucosal lesions. Gastrointest Endosc 1993; 39:58–62.

87. Akiyama M, Ota M, Nakajima H et al. Endoscopic mucosal resection of gastric neoplasms using a ligating device. Gastrointest Endosc 1997; 45:182–6.

88. Korenaga D, Haraguchi M, Tsujitani S et al. Clinicopathological features of mucosal carcinoma of the stomach with lymph node metastasis in eleven patients. Br J Surg 1986; 73:431–3.

89. Ohkuwa M, Hosokawa K, Boku N et al. New endoscopic treatment for intramucosal gastric tumors using an insulated-tip diathermic knife. Endoscopy 2001; 33:221–6.

90. Kodashima S, Fujishiro M, Yahagi N et al. Endoscopic submucosal dissection for gastric neoplasia: experience with the flex-knife. Acta Gastroenterol Belg 2006; 69:224–9.

91. Chiu PW, Chan KF, Lee YT et al. Endoscopic submucosal dissection used for treating early neoplasia of the foregut using a combination of knives. Surg Endosc 2008; 22:777–83.

92. Takeuchi Y, Uedo N, Iishi H et al. Endoscopic submucosal dissection with insulated-tip knife for large mucosal early gastric cancer: a feasibility study (with videos). Gastrointest Endosc 2007; 66:186–93.

93. Gotoda T. Endoscopic resection of early gastric cancer. Gastric Cancer 2007; 10:1–11.

94. Oda I, Saito D, Tada M et al. A multicenter retrospective study of endoscopic resection for early gastric cancer. Gastric Cancer 2006; 9:262–70.

95. Oka S, Tanaka S, Kaneko I et al. Advantage of endoscopic submucosal dissection compared with EMR for early gastric cancer. Gastrointest Endosc 2006; 64:877–83.

96. Minami S, Gotoda T, Ono H et al. Complete endoscopic closure of gastric perforation induced by endoscopic resection of early gastric cancer using endoclips can prevent surgery. Gastrointest Endosc 2006; 63:596–601.

97. Fujishiro M, Yahagi N, Kakushima N et al. Successful nonsurgical management of perforation complicating endoscopic submucosal dissection of gastrointestinal epithelial neoplasms. Endoscopy 2006; 38:1001–6.

98. Ikehara H, Gotoda T, Ono H et al. Gastric perforation during endoscopic resection for gastric carcinoma and the risk of peritoneal dissemination. Br J Surg 2007; 94:992–5.

99. Freeman ML, Nelson DB, Sherman S et al. Complications of endoscopic sphincterotomy. N Engl J Med 1996; 335(13):909–18.

100. Cotton PB, Lehman G, Vennes J et al. Endoscopic sphincterotomy complications and their management: an attempt at consensus. Gastrointest Endosc 1991; 37(3):383–93.

101. Enns R, Eloubeidi MA, Mergener K et al. ERCP-related perforations: risk factors and management. Endoscopy 2002; 34:293–8.

102. Faylona JM, Qadir A, Chan AC et al. Small-bowel perforations related to endoscopic retrograde cholangiopancreatography (ERCP) in patients with Billroth II gastrectomy. Endoscopy 1999; 31:546–9.

103. Bagci S, Tuzun A, Ates Y et al. Efficacy and safety of endoscopic retrograde cholangiopancreatography in patients with Billroth II anastomosis. Hepatogastroenterology 2005; 52:356–9.

104. Assalia A, Suissa A, Ilivitzki A et al. Validity of clinical criteria in the management of endoscopic retrograde cholangiopancreatography related duodenal perforations. Arch Surg 2007; 142:1059–64.

105. Martin DF, Tweedle DE. Retroperitoneal perforation during ERCP and endoscopic sphincterotomy: causes, clinical features and management. Endoscopy 1990; 22:174–5.

7

Acute non-variceal upper gastrointestinal bleeding

Colin J. McKay

James Lau

Introduction

A major audit of upper gastrointestinal (UGI) bleeding in England reported an incidence of 103 cases per 100 000 adults per year.[1] An audit from the West of Scotland reported a higher incidence of 172 cases per 100 000,[2] citing regional differences in deprivation or *Helicobacter pylori* prevalence as possible explanations. Whatever the actual incidence at regional level, UGI bleeding remains a significant health problem and in Scotland alone accounts for approximately 7000 hospital admissions each year. Overall mortality from an episode of UGI bleeding was 14% in the English study[1] and 8% in the study from the West of Scotland,[2] and both demonstrated a marked increase in mortality if bleeding occurred following hospitalisation with another complaint (33% and 44% in the respective studies). These studies suggest little improvement in overall mortality over earlier reports, despite widespread introduction of endoscopic haemostasis protocols. During this period, reports from single institutions commonly claimed mortality figures of 2–6%,[3–6] suggesting that improvements in management may not have been universally applied. In the major English audit study[1] there was a marked variation in outcome between hospitals, but much of this variation disappeared when figures were corrected for appropriate risk factors, highlighting the difficulty in comparing crude mortality statistics for such patients and the inherent problems in comparing units where each one treats relatively few patients. A further problem in interpretation

of these data is that death from haemorrhage was not clearly distinguished from death due to comorbidity. The typical patient with severe peptic ulcer bleeding is now elderly, often suffering medical comorbidity and taking antiplatelet therapy. Such patients are at greater risk of death despite skilled intervention and are less able to withstand surgery should this be necessary. The failure to improve overall mortality must therefore be interpreted with care. Despite the uncertainty surrounding any actual improvements in outcome, there is now an abundance of high-quality evidence to guide best practice in the management of UGI bleeding and most hospitals will now have local protocols in place.

Aetiology

In the Rockall study,[1] only 4% of patients had UGI bleeding due to varices, with the majority (35%) being attributed to peptic ulcer disease. Of some concern was the 25% of patients in this study where no cause for bleeding was identified, particularly as this group had a mortality of 20%. Very similar figures were reported in the Scottish study.[2] Of those patients with a diagnosis, approximately 25% were due to duodenal ulcer and 25% to peptic ulcers in the stomach, oesophagus or a combination of sites. The remainder were due to a number of other conditions, including oesophagitis, gastritis and duodenitis, with 10% of cases explained by malignancy or Mallory–Weiss syndrome (Table 7.1).

Table 7.1 • Aetiology of UGI haemorrhage

Aetiology	% of cases
No diagnosis	25
Peptic ulcer	35
Malignancy	4
Varices	4
Mallory–Weiss	5
Gastritis/duodenitis	11
Oesophagitis	10
Other	6

Reproduced from Rockall TA, Logan RFA, Devlin HB et al. Incidence of and mortality from acute upper gastrointestinal hemorrhage in the United Kingdom. Br Med J 1995; 311(6999): 222–6.[1] With permission from the BMJ Publishing Group.

Initial assessment and triage

Patients with acute UGI bleeding present with haematemesis, melaena or a combination of the two. Haematemesis may be defined as the vomiting of blood from the upper gastrointestinal tract and is indicative of significant bleeding from a site in the oesophagus, stomach or duodenum. Melaena is the passage of black, tarry stools and usually indicates a bleeding site in the upper gastrointestinal tract, although bleeding from the small bowel or even the right colon may present in a similar way. Coffee-ground vomiting (the vomiting of black, particulate material that tests positive for blood) is not indicative of active bleeding. Presentation with haematemesis is associated with an increased risk of mortality compared with melaena or coffee-ground vomiting.[2] Patients with upper gastrointestinal blood loss may occasionally present with frank rectal bleeding (haematochezia), but this is indicative of major blood loss and is associated with an increased need for transfusion, surgery and, not surprisingly, of mortality.[7] An example of this might be an aorto-duodenal fistula.

Scoring systems

Many patients with UGI haemorrhage have trivial bleeding, require no intervention and can safely be discharged early. Others, however, have catastrophic bleeding and many lie between these two extremes. On initial assessment, differentiation between patients can sometimes be difficult. Two separate studies have assessed the initial, pretreatment risk factors in an attempt to enable triage of patients to appropriate early endoscopy, observation or even non-admission. Rockall and colleagues identified risk factors for mortality[8] in the cohort of patients included in the English audit discussed above. Patients with an initial score of zero (i.e. age <60, no tachycardia, no hypotension and no comorbidity) had very low mortality, but in a subsequent study 18% of patients with an initial Rockall score of zero required further intervention. Assessment of re-bleeding risk requires the full Rockall score, necessitating endoscopic assessment.

In contrast, a scoring system was developed in the West of Scotland, the aim being to allow early assessment of the need for intervention rather than risk of death.[2] The Blatchford score performed significantly better than the Rockall score at predicting the need for intervention. In addition, a simplified screening tool was developed identifying a low need for intervention if at admission blood urea was less than 6.5 mmol/L, haemoglobin more than 130 g/L for men or 120 g/L for women, systolic blood pressure 110 mmHg or higher, and pulse less than 100 beats per minute. There is therefore the potential for this score to be used to allow outpatient treatment of a proportion of patients with UGI bleeding, but the authors themselves point to the need for external validation of these results before this becomes standard practice.[2]

Full assessment of mortality risk demands endoscopic determination of the cause of bleeding and assessment of the appearance of any ulcer present. These findings are incorporated into the full Rockall score. The Rockall system has been validated in prospective studies[9–11] but is more accurate in predicting mortality than risk of re-bleeding[9,11] (Table 7.2).

The full Rockall score combines the pre-endoscopy score with points for diagnosis and endoscopic stigmata, giving a total score of 0–11. A Rockall score of less than 3 identifes a group of patients with a low risk of re-bleeding (4%) and negligible risk of death, who may be considered suitable for early discharge.[8]

 A full Rockall score should be calculated for all patients with UGI bleeding following initial endoscopic assessment.[8–11]

Initial management

While it may be appropriate to consider discharge for young patients with no haemodynamic compromise and a Blatchford/Rockall score of zero, particularly where there has been no witnessed frank haematemesis, most patients will be admitted for observation and endoscopy. This will entail insertion of a large-bore cannula, administration of prewarmed crystalloid or colloid as required and immediate blood samples taken for crossmatch,

Table 7.2 • Rockall score for predicting risk of re-bleeding or death in non-variceal UGI haemorrhage

Component	0	1	2	3
Age (years)	<60	60–79	≥80	
Shock	Pulse <100 SBP ≥100 mmHg	Pulse ≥100 SBP ≥100 mmHg	SBP <100 mmHg	
Comorbidity			IHD, cardiac failure, other major comorbidity	Renal failure, liver failure, disseminated malignancy
Diagnosis	Mallory–Weiss, no lesion, no SRH	All other diagnoses		
Stigmata of recent haemorrhage	No stigmata or dark spot		Blood in UGI tract, adherent clot, visible or spurting vessel	

IHD, ischaemic heart disease; SBP, systolic blood pressure; SRH, stigmata of recent haemorrhage.
Reproduced from Rockall TA, Logan RFA, Devlin HB et al. Variation in outcome after acute upper gastrointestinal hemorrhage. Lancet 1995; 346(8971):346–50.[8] With permission from Elsevier.

biochemistry, full blood count, coagulation screen and arterial blood gases. There is some evidence that admission to a dedicated UGI bleeding unit is associated with a reduction in mortality.[12] Such a unit requires a 24-hour on-call service for immediate endoscopy if required and early (within 24h), consultant-led endoscopy for all patients. Indications for urgent (out-of-hours) endoscopy vary but the main factor determining the degree of urgency is the necessity for endostasis. Therefore patients with evidence of continuing haemorrhage, declared either by continuing haematemesis or haemodynamic instability despite initial fluid resuscitation, require emergency endoscopy with a view to endostasis. Repeated 'coffee-ground' vomiting or melaena in a haemodynamically stable patient are of less urgent concern. Most stable patients will undergo UGI endoscopy within 24h (usually on the morning after admission). In such patients the purpose of endoscopy is twofold: firstly, patients with minor bleeds undergo full diagnostic assessment and if considered at low risk of re-bleeding can be discharged; secondly, to identify the group of patients who have significant lesions and who require endoscopic therapy to reduce the risk of re-bleeding. This will be discussed in the next section.

Massive haemorrhage

In those patients who have evidence of haemodynamic compromise, initial resuscitation should follow the appropriate guidelines.[13] Initial volume expansion should be with prewarmed crystalloid or colloid and not blood or blood products.

A Cochrane review of 55 trials found no evidence of benefit of crystalloid over colloid resuscitation in critically ill patients.[14] As colloid solutions are more expensive, initial resuscitation with appropriate crystalloids is recommended.

Use of blood and blood products

Red cell replacement is likely to be required when 30% or more blood volume is lost. This can be difficult to assess, particularly in young patients, and clinical assessment of blood loss, coupled with the response to initial volume replacement, must guide the decision on the necessity of transfusion. Haemoglobin levels are a poor indicator of the degree of acute blood loss. It should very rarely be necessary to administer unmatched blood to such patients, but group-specific blood may be required in life-threatening haemorrhage. In the majority of patients there is usually sufficient time to allow full compatibility testing before transfusion. In patients with evidence of continuing haemorrhage, however, arrangements for emergency endoscopic intervention must be made in parallel with resuscitation.

Administration of platelets should aim to maintain a platelet count of more than 50×10^9/L, but in practice a platelet transfusion should be triggered by a count of less than 75×10^9/L in a patient with ongoing haemorrhage, and may be anticipated in a patient who has required more than two blood volumes of fluid/blood replacement. Platelet therapy may be required in the presence of a normal platelet count where a patient has been receiving antiplatelet therapy.

Coagulation factors are likely to be required when more than one blood volume has been lost. These are most commonly given in the form of fresh frozen plasma (FFP). The use of platelets, FFP and other agents such as recombinant factor VIIa should be guided by local protocols and early involvement of a haematologist.

Early pharmacological treatment

Upper gastrointestinal endoscopy is the mainstay of investigation and management of UGI bleeding, but there may also be a role for early treatment with acid suppression therapy. In vitro studies have shown that at pH < 6, platelet aggregation and plasma coagulation are markedly reduced,[15] a situation exacerbated by the presence of pepsin. It is therefore reasonable to expect acid suppression therapy to promote clot formation and stabilisation. Five randomised trials comparing pre-endoscopy proton-pump inhibitor (PPI) therapy with histamine-2 receptor antagonist or placebo were analysed in a Cochrane review.[16] No significant impact of PPI therapy was demonstrated on mortality, surgery or re-bleeding rates. There was, however, a reduction in the proportion of patients with stigmata of recent haemorrhage at the time of endoscopy. In a large, single-centre, randomised study, pre-endoscopy intravenous omeprazole infusion was associated with a reduction in the incidence of active bleeding and significant reduction in the necessity for endoscopic intervention. No difference was observed for re-bleeding, surgery or mortality rates, but these were seen in 3%, 2% and 2% of patients respectively. It therefore seems reasonable to propose pre-endoscopic PPI therapy in patients admitted with UGI bleeding, but this should not delay or act as a substitute for early endoscopic intervention. There is no evidence to support the use of other agents such as somatostatin or octreotide in the pre-endoscopy setting.

Pre-endoscopy treatment with PPIs is recommended as it reduces the risk of active bleeding at the time of endoscopy and may reduce the need for endoscopic intervention.[16]

Endoscopy

Upper gastrointestinal endoscopy is required for any patient with significant UGI bleeding. Patients with haemodynamic instability or evidence of continuing haemorrhage require emergency endoscopy, whereas the majority of patients will undergo endoscopy within 24 h of admission. In a study from Hong Kong, 70 patients aged less than 60 years with a clean ulcer base and stable vital signs were safely discharged on the same day as endoscopy. A systemic review of the literature supports a policy of early endoscopy, as this allows the safe discharge of patients with low-risk haemorrhage and improves outcome for patients with high-risk lesions.[17,18]

Early endoscopy is recommended for all patients with UGI haemorrhage.[18]

Endoscopic technique

Endoscopy for UGI bleeding requires the support of a dedicated endoscopic unit with trained nursing staff, availability of additional endoscopes and equipment, ready access to anaesthetic staff and operating theatre and, increasingly, access to interventional radiology services. These procedures are not ideal for the unsupervised trainee and should be performed or supervised by experienced consultant staff.

For the majority of stable patients, procedures can be safely carried out using standard diagnostic endoscopes. In the unstable patient or where continuing haemorrhage is suspected, the twin-channel or large (3.7-mm) single-channel endoscope is preferable and allows better aspiration of gastric contents as well as more flexibility with regard to the use of heater probes and other instruments. In some cases, the use of a pharyngeal overtube and gastric lavage tube is necessary to remove blood and clot from the stomach before adequate visualisation of the bleeding site can be achieved. Water is poured down the lavage tube via a funnel, which is then placed in a bucket at floor level, allowing siphoning of gastric contents. This, however, can be a time-consuming, unpleasant and messy experience, and in the presence of continuing bleeding should not be allowed to delay endostasis. The use of a tilting trolley allows repositioning of the patient, which can facilitate visualisation of the proximal stomach when obscured by blood and clot. Initially, placing the patient in an upright position may suffice, and if necessary rolling the patient into a right lateral and upright position may be needed for complete visualisation of the gastric fundus. In general, lavage is more successful in achieving visualisation than aspiration, as endoscope working channels rapidly block with clot. Lavage can be achieved using repeated flushes of saline down the endoscope working channel or with the use of the powered endoscopic lavage catheters such as that provided with the heater probe. With experience, it should rarely be necessary to proceed to surgery or angiography because of inability to visualise the bleeding site due to blood and clot in the stomach or duodenum.

Careful attention must be given to the most likely sites of ulcer bleeding. Bleeding gastric ulcers are most likely within the antrum or at the incisura (77%), or less commonly higher on the lesser curve (15%), with ulcers at other sites within the stomach being rare. Ulcers at the incisura can be readily overlooked unless the endoscope is retroflexed within the gastric antrum. The most common site for a bleeding duodenal ulcer is the posterior wall, sometimes with involvement of the inferior and superior walls of the first part of duodenum. Superficial anterior duodenal wall ulcers can ooze, but usually these ulcers perforate. Ulcers elsewhere in the duodenum are seen in less than 10% of patients.[19] The presence of active bleeding at the time of endoscopy and the size of the ulcer, rather than its anatomical site, are the main endoscopic determinants of the risk of therapeutic failure.[19]

Management of bleeding due to causes other than peptic ulceration

Gastritis/duodenitis

Bleeding due to gastritis or duodenitis may be associated with non-steroidal anti-inflammatory drug (NSAID) therapy or ingestion of alcohol. It may also be due to *Helicobacter pylori* and can be severe enough to cause superficial erosions. Such bleeding, however, is almost always self-limiting in the absence of bleeding disorders and therapeutic intervention is not required at the time of endoscopy. Treatment with appropriate acid suppression therapy and early discharge is usually appropriate in the absence of other comorbid illness.

Mallory–Weiss syndrome

Mallory–Weiss syndrome was first described in 1929 and refers to haematemesis following repeated or violent vomiting or retching. It is caused by a linear tear of the mucosa close to the oesophagogastric junction. It accounts for approximately 5% of patients with UGI haemorrhage and most will settle without the need for therapeutic intervention. However, if bleeding is seen at the time of endoscopy, several approaches have been described. The simplest and most readily available technique is the injection of 1:10 000 adrenaline, as for bleeding peptic ulcers, which is sufficient in the great majority of patients.[20] Mechanical methods of endostasis such as endoscopic band ligation or clip application have not been shown to be superior to adrenaline injection alone[20,21] but are appropriate alternatives, particularly where major bleeding or shock has occurred or where adrenaline injection fails to achieve endostasis.

Oesophagitis

Gastro-oesophageal reflux disease is responsible for approximately 10% of cases of UGI haemorrhage and is rarely severe. Treatment is with oral PPI therapy.

Neoplastic disease

Major bleeding is occasionally associated with oesophageal, gastric or duodenal tumours. Gastrointestinal stromal tumours may present with bleeding which can be severe in very occasional cases. Malignancies of the UGI tract commonly cause occult, chronic bleeding but major bleeding

can occur and may be difficult to control endoscopically. Management will be dependent on the specific circumstances and may include endoscopic techniques such as argon plasma coagulation, angiographic embolisation or surgical resection.

Dieulafoy's lesion

This rare cause of UGI bleeding is due to spontaneous rupture of a submucosal artery, usually in the stomach and often within 3 cm of the oesophagogastric junction. The characteristic endoscopic appearance is of a protruding vessel with no evidence of surrounding ulceration. They are commonly missed due to their small size and relatively inaccessible position. Endoscopic clip application or band ligation offers durable and definitive treatment when the lesion is identified. In a small randomised trial,[22] haemoclip application was associated with a lower rate of re-bleeding than adrenaline injection, although both achieved similar rates of initial haemostasis.

Endoscopic management of bleeding peptic ulcers

Endoscopy has a central role in the management of non-variceal UGI bleeding. It enables an early diagnosis and allows for risk stratification. Endoscopic signs or stigmata of bleeding are of prognostic value and in patients with actively bleeding ulcers or stigmata associated with high risk of recurrent bleeding, endoscopic therapy stops ongoing bleeding and reduces re-bleeding.[23] When compared to placebo in pooled analyses, endoscopic therapy has been shown not only to reduce recurrent bleeding, but also the need for surgery and mortality.[24,25]

Endoscopic stigmata of bleeding

Forrest et al.[26] categorised endoscopic findings of bleeding peptic ulcers into those with active bleeding, stigmata of bleeding and clean base. A modified nomenclature has been in common use in the endoscopy literature. Laine and Peterson[27] summarised published endoscopic series of ulcer appearances in which endoscopic therapy was not used and provided crude figures in both the prevalence and rate of recurrent bleeding associated with these stigmata of bleeding. In ulcers that are actively bleeding (**Fig. 7.1**) or exhibit a non-bleeding visible vessel (NBVV; **Fig. 7.2**), endoscopic treatment should be offered. There has been observer variation in the interpretation of endoscopic signs.[28] The National Institutes of Health Consensus Conference[29] defined an NBVV as 'protuberant discoloration' (Fig. 7.2). The endoscopist should search the ulcer base diligently in patients judged to have bled significantly

Figure 7.1 • Bleeding vessel in base of ulcer.

Figure 7.2 • Visible vessel.

Figure 7.3 • Adherent clot.

angiographic embolisation without clot elevation and possible provocation of bleeding may be a better option. Ulcers with flat pigmentation and clean base (**Fig. 7.4**) are associated with minimal risk of recurrent bleeding. Stable patients with such ulcers can be discharged home early (Table 7.3).

 Endoscopic therapy should be applied where there is active bleeding or a non-bleeding visible vessel in the ulcer base.[23] Adherent clot should be removed and endoscopic therapy applied to the underlying vessel.[30–32]

Endoscopic treatment

Modalities of endoscopic treatment can be broadly categorised into: injection, thermocoagulation and the use of mechanical devices.

or when there is circumstantial evidence of ongoing or recent bleeding, e.g. presence of fresh blood or coffee-ground materials in the gastroduodenal tract. There has been until recently a controversy whether to wash adherent clot overlying an ulcer (**Fig. 7.3**). Endoscopists vary in their vigour in clot irrigation before declaring a clot adherent. There have been several randomised studies and a pooled analysis indicating that recurrent bleeding would be less following clot elevation and treatment to the underlying vessel when compared to medical therapy alone.[30–32] Techniques for clot elevation include target irrigation using a heat probe and cheese-wiring using a snare with or without pre-injection with diluted adrenaline. One should, however, be cautious in elevation of clots overlying large deep bulbar and lesser curve ulcers. Some of these may have eroded into larger arteries. A recourse to

Figure 7.4 • Ulcer with clean base.

Table 7.3 • Prevalence and outcomes of ulcers based on endoscopic appearance[27]

Endoscopic signs	Prevalence (%)	Further bleeding (%)	Surgery (%)	Death (%)
Clean base	42	5	0.5	2
Flat spot	20	10	6	3
Adherent clot	17	22	10	7
Non-bleeding visible vessel	17	43	34	11
Active bleeding	18	55	35	11

Data from Laine L, Peterson WL. Bleeding peptic ulcer. N Engl J Med 1994; 331(11):717–27.[27]

Injection

Injection therapy has been widely used because of its simplicity. Injection therapy works principally by volume tamponade. Aliquots (0.5–1 mL) are injected near the bleeding point at four quadrants using a 21- or 23-gauge injection needle. Adrenaline has an added local vasoconstrictive effect. A sclerosant should probably not be used as there have been fatal case reports of gastric necrosis following its injection. The added injection of a sclerosant such as polidocanol or sodium tetradecyl sulphate after pre-injection of diluted adrenaline does not confer any advantage over injection of diluted adrenaline alone. For the same reason, injection of absolute alcohol (which rapidly dehydrates tissue) is to be discouraged. Injection of fibrin or thrombin has been shown to be effective in some studies.[33] In a large study that randomised patients into three groups (polidocanol, single injection of fibrin sealant and daily endoscopy with fibrin sealant injection to remaining stigmata), fibrin sealant injection was statistically better than polidocanol only when injected on a daily basis. Treatment failure occurred in 34 (13%) of 261 in the polidocanol group, 34 (12.4%) of 274 in the single fibrin injection group and 21 (7.7%) of 274 patients in the repeated fibrin injections group. Because of its cost, fibrin sealant is not routinely used.[34]

Thermal methods

In a canine mesenteric artery model, contact thermocoagulation is superior to injection therapy and non-contact coagulation such as laser photocoagulation in securing haemostasis. Contact thermocoagulation using a 3.2-mm probe consistently seals arteries up to 2 mm in diameter in ex vivo models. Johnston and colleagues emphasised the need for firm mechanical tamponade before sealing of the artery with thermal energy,[35] introducing the term 'coaptive thermocoagulation'. Mechanical compression alone stops bleeding, reduces heat sink effect and dissipation of thermal energy. The footprint after treatment provides a clear end-point to therapy. Non-contact thermocoagulation in the form of laser photocoagulation is no longer used as a laser unit is bulky and difficult to be transported. At least in animal experiments, non-contact coagulation in the form of laser photocoagulation is not as effective as contact thermocoagulation. There has also been interest in the use of argon plasma thermocoagulation, with two randomised trials comparing argon plasma thermocoagulation to injection sclerotherapy or heat probe treatment respectively.[36] Neither demonstrated any significant difference in treatment outcome.

Mechanical methods

Haemoclips are commonly used. Their application may be difficult in awkwardly placed ulcers such as those on the lesser curvature of the stomach and the posterior bulbar duodenum. In a meta-analysis of 15 studies with 390 patients[37] that compared haemoclipping versus injection and thermocoagulation, successful application of haemoclips (81.5%) was superior to injection alone (75.4%) but comparable to thermocoagulation (81.2%) in producing definitive haemostasis. In this pooled analysis, haemoclipping also led to reduced need for surgery when compared to injection alone.

Single versus combined methods

Soehendra introduced the concept of combination treatment that involved pre-injection with adrenaline allowing a clear view of the vessel, which then allowed targeted therapy using a second modality to induce thrombosis. In a meta-analysis of 16 studies and 1673 patients,[38] adding a second modality after adrenaline injection further reduces bleeding from 18.4% to 10.6% (odds ratio (OR) 0.53, 95% CI 0.4–0.69), emergency surgery from 11.3% to 7.6% (OR 0.64, 95% CI 0.46–0.90) and mortality from 5.1% to 2.6% (OR 0.51, 95% CI 0.31–0.84). In an independent meta-analysis of 22 studies (2472 patients),[39] dual therapy was shown to be superior to injection alone. However, treatment outcomes following combination treatments were not better than either mechanical or thermal therapy alone. Based on the above pooled analyses, adrenaline alone should no longer be considered an adequate treatment for bleeding peptic ulcers. The current evidence suggests that after initial adrenaline injection, the vessel should either be clipped or thermocoagulated. In ulcers with a clear view to the vessel, direct clipping or thermocoagulation should yield similar results.

> Endoscopic therapy for bleeding peptic ulcers should use dual therapy or mechanical therapy rather than adrenaline injection alone in order to reduce the risk of re-bleeding.[37–39]

Limit of endoscopic therapy

As mentioned previously, size of the bleeding artery is a critical determinant in the success of endoscopic treatment. In an ex vivo model, a vessel size of 2 mm could be consistently sealed by a 3.2-mm contact thermal device. In clinical studies which examined factors that might predict failure of endoscopic treatment, ulcer size greater than 2 cm, ulcers on the lesser curvature and ulcers on the superior or posterior wall of bulbar duodenum were consistently identified as major risk factors to recurrent bleeding.[23] These ulcers erode into large artery complexes such as the left gastric and the gastroduodenal artery, which are usually sizeable. Consideration should be given to prophylactic measures against recurrent bleeding in these ulcers judged to be at significant risk of re-bleeding.

Second-look endoscopy

Many endoscopists re-scope their patients the next morning and re-treat ulcers with remaining stigmata of bleeding. In a pooled analysis on the role of second-look endoscopy,[40] the authors found a modest 6.2% reduction in the absolute risk of re-bleeding (number needed to treat (NNT) to reduce one episode of recurrent bleeding). The NNT for reduction of surgery and surgery was 58 and 97 respectively. In many of these trials, adrenaline injection alone was used. With improved index treatment, the risk reduction associated with second-look endoscopy is even lower. With aggressive first endoscopic treatment, the risk of complications, especially perforation, with second treatment is substantial. With improved pharmacotherapy and endoscopic treatment, routine second-look endoscopy can no longer be recommended. However, in selected patients with subtle signs of recurrent bleeding or in whom results from first treatment are uncertain, second-look endoscopy seems more rational.

> Second-look endoscopy is not indicated as a routine if primary optimum endoscopic haemostasis has been performed.[40]

Pharmacological management of bleeding peptic ulcers

Acid suppression

It has been shown in an in vitro study that platelet aggregation is dependent on plasma pH. It is thought that a pH of 6 is critical for clot stability and an intragastric pH above 4 inactivates stomach pepsin, preventing the digestion of clots.[15] To raise intragastric pH consistently above 6, a high-dose PPI given intravenously is required. The antisecretory effect of histamine receptor antagonists, due to tolerance, is less reliable than PPIs. In a study from the Hong Kong group,[41] a 3-day course of high-dose omeprazole infusion given after endoscopic therapy to bleeding ulcers reduced the rate of recurrent bleeding from 22.5% to 6.7% at day 30. The majority of recurrent bleeding occurred within the first 3 days of endoscopic treatment. This trial demonstrated the importance of early endoscopic triage selecting only the high-risk ulcers for aggressive endoscopic treatment followed by profound acid suppression. In a Cochrane systematic review of 24 controlled trials and 4373 patients,[42] PPI treatment was shown to reduce re-bleeding (pooled rate of 10.6% vs. 17.3%, OR 0.49, 95% CI 0.37–0.65) as well as surgery (pooled rate of 6.1% vs. 9.3%, OR 0.61, 95% CI 0.48–0.78) when compared with placebo or histamine-2 receptor antagonist. There was no evidence of an effect on all-cause mortality, although when the analysis was confined to patients with high-risk stigmata (active bleeding or visible vessels) there was an associated reduction in mortality with PPI therapy. There remain controversies over the dose, route of PPI treatment and the timing of PPI administration.

> High-dose intravenous PPI therapy (80 mg omeprazole followed by 8 mg/h for 72 h) is recommended for patients with active bleeding or visible vessels at the time of endoscopy.[42]

Surgical management of bleeding peptic ulcers

The National United Kingdom audit revealed a mortality of 24% in those patients (251 of 2071, 12%) who required surgery for bleeding peptic ulcers.[1] However, in 78% of these patients, no previous attempt at endoscopic haemostasis had been made. Modern emergency ulcer surgery is associated with high mortality, principally because the population presenting with UGI bleeding is old. In some patients with severe comorbid illnesses and bleeding peptic ulcer, disease is an agonal event. Bleeding ulcers that fail endostasis are typically 'difficult' ulcers – larger chronic ulcers that erode into major arterial complexes. The decline in elective ulcer surgery also means the atrophy of surgical techniques in dealing with these ulcers. Ideally a specialist team with an experienced upper gastrointestinal surgeon should be involved in managing these patients.

Although emergency ulcer surgery has diminished significantly, it has an important gatekeeping role in the management algorithm. The clear indication for surgery is loosely defined as 'failure of endoscopic treatment'. In a patient with massive bleeding that cannot be controlled by endoscopy, immediate surgery should obviously follow. Similarly, in a patient with bleeding controlled at endoscopy, most clinicians would adopt a medical approach. However, the difficulty lies in deciding the exact role of surgery in ulcers judged to have a high risk of recurrent bleeding (e.g. >2 cm and at difficult locations), in whom endoscopic haemostasis has been initially successful.

Choice of surgical procedure for bleeding peptic ulcers

The choice of surgical procedure for bleeding peptic ulcers, when required, has not been adequately examined in the era following routine eradication of *Helicobacter pylori* and high-dose PPI therapy. Many surgeons maintain that under-running of ulcers alone combined with acid suppression using high-dose PPI therapy is safer than definitive surgery by either gastric resection or vagotomy. Two randomised studies looking at the different surgical procedures used to control bleeding peptic ulcers have been reported,[43,44] but both predate the PPI and routine *H. pylori* eradication era and therefore their results must be interpreted with considerable caution. One of these was a multicentre study comparing minimal surgery (under-running the vessel or ulcer excision alone plus intravenous histamine receptor antagonist) versus definitive ulcer surgery (vagotomy and pyloroplasty or partial gastrectomy) in patients with gastric and duodenal ulcers.[43] In 62 patients assigned to minimal treatment (59 under-running and three ulcer excisions), seven re-bled and six of these died. Of the 67 patients who underwent conventional ulcer surgery (25 partial gastrectomy and 42 vagotomy and drainage), four re-bled and none died. All re-bleeds had had vagotomy and under-running of their ulcers. The overall mortality was similar in both groups (26% after minimal surgery and 19% after conventional surgery). The trial was terminated, however, because of the high rate of fatal re-bleeding in the conservative group when compared to the conventional surgery group (6 vs. 0, $P = 0.02$).[43]

The other trial was carried out by the French Association of Surgical Research and included only bleeding duodenal ulcers.[44] The patients in this trial were randomly assigned to either under-running plus vagotomy and drainage (58 patients) or partial gast-

rectomy (60 patients). Recurrent bleeding occurred in 10 of 58 patients (17%) after under-running and vagotomy, six of whom required conversion to Billroth II gastrectomy. Five of these six patients went on to develop duodenal stump dehiscence. In the group assigned to partial gastrectomy, only two patients (3%) re-bled and both recovered without the need for further surgery. In the 60 patients assigned to gastrectomy, Billroth I reconstruction was performed in 18, Billroth I and vagotomy in six, Billroth II in 20 and Billroth II and vagotomy in 16 patients. No duodenal leak occurred in any of the 26 patients after Billroth I reconstruction. Among the 36 patients who received Billroth II reconstruction, duodenal stump leaks occurred in eight (22%). The overall rate of duodenal stump leak in the gastrectomy group was 8 in 60 (13%). When the results were analysed on an intention-to-treat basis, and those with duodenal leaks after re-operations for re-bleeding in the under-running and vagotomy group were included, duodenal leak rate was similar in both groups (7/58 vs. 8/60). The mortality in both groups was similar (22% after vagotomy and 23% after gastrectomy). The authors concluded that to avoid duodenal dehiscence, a Billroth I type reconstruction is preferred. In the group of patients who underwent vagotomy and drainage, proper ligation of the gastroduodenal artery complex including the right gastroepiploic artery is needed to avoid recurrent bleeding (Table 7.4).

Table 7.4 • Outcomes following under-running and vagotomy or gastric resection in ulcers at the duodenal bulb (the French Association of Surgical Research randomised trial)

	Oversewing and vagotomy $n = 58$	Gastric resection $n = 60$
Bleeding recurrences*	10	2
Duodenal leaks		
Per protocol	2	8[†]
Intention to treat	7	8
Re-operations	8	1
For re-bleeding	6	0
For duodenal leaks	2	1
Deaths after re-operations	4	1
Deaths	13	14

* $P < 0.05$, †$P < 0.01$.
Modified from Millat B, Hay JM, Valleur P et al. Emergency surgical treatment for bleeding duodenal ulcer: oversewing plus vagotomy versus gastric resection, a controlled randomized trial. French Association for Surgical Research. World J Surg 1993; 17(5):568–73.[44] With kind permission from Springer Science and Business Media.

Surgical technique

In a survey of UK surgeons, more than 80% of respondents rarely or never perform vagotomy for bleeding peptic ulcer.[45] Despite the absence of recent randomised evidence, it seems that surgeons have adopted a more conservative approach. With improvements in endoscopic therapy and the increasing age and comorbidity of patients, the risks of definitive ulcer surgery may outweigh any potential benefit from reduction in re-bleeding. For duodenal ulcer haemorrhage, longitudinal duodenotomy is carried out and control of bleeding achieved by digital pressure or by grasping the posterior duodenal wall in tissue forceps. If possible, preservation of the pylorus is preferred, but extension of the duodenotomy to include the pylorus may be required if access is difficult. Control of bleeding may be aided by mobilisation of the duodenum (Kocher's manoeuvre), allowing pressure to be applied posteriorly. In the majority of patients, simple under-running of the bleeding vessel can be achieved using 0 or 1/0 absorbable sutures above and below the bleeding point, ensuring deep enough tissue penetration to completely occlude the vessel. Due to the variation in anatomy of the gastroduodenal artery, four or five sutures should be placed to ensure enduring haemostasis (**Fig. 7.5**). The duodenotomy can then be closed longitudinally or converted into a formal pyloroplasty if the pylorus has been divided.

In cases of massive duodenal ulcer, it may be necessary to exclude the ulcer, perform a distal gastrectomy and close the distal duodenum. This can be a challenging procedure in an elderly, unstable patient, particularly where duodenal thickening and scarring prevent safe stump closure. In this situation it may be better to anticipate a controlled duodenal fistula by closing the duodenal stump around a Foley catheter rather than attempting more complex closures, such as with the Bilroth I reconstruction.

In the case of surgery for a bleeding gastric ulcer, the common scenario is for the ulcer to be located high on the lesser curve of stomach. Anterior gastrotomy, identification of the bleeding site and simple under-running of the ulcer (with biopsy of the ulcer edge) is the procedure of choice, and is also suitable for rare cases of Mallory–Weiss tear or a Dieulafoy lesion that does not respond to endoscopic management. In the rare case of a distal gastric ulcer that does not respond to endoscopic therapy, there may occasionally be a case for ulcer excision or even distal gastrectomy, but it is difficult to justify in the hands of a non-specialist surgeon, and simple under-running should be the aim in the majority of patients.

 The choice of operation in patients with bleeding peptic ulcers who have failed endoscopic treatment should involve, where possible, simple under-running of the bleeding ulcer, without either vagotomy or gastric resection.

Managing of recurrent bleeding

The decision on management of patients who re-bleed after initial endoscopic control can be difficult. In a randomised study that compared endoscopic re-treatment to surgery in such patients,[46] endoscopic re-treatment secured bleeding again in 75% of patients. With intention-to-treat analysis, complications following endoscopic re-treatment were significantly less when compared to those who received surgery. The gastrectomy rate in the surgery group was 50%. In a subgroup analysis, those re-bleeding in hypotensive shock from ulcers greater than 2 cm were less likely to respond to a repeat endoscopic treatment. It is therefore suggested that a selective approach can be used in re-bleeding patients. Patients with smaller ulcers and subtle signs of re-bleeding should be re-endoscoped and therapy repeated, often with successful outcome. If not successful, surgery should obviously follow. It remains probable that patients with large chronic ulcers and in shock are better treated by expeditious

Figure 7.5 • The anatomy of the gastroduodenal (GD) artery complex with confluence of several branches into the artery itself. RGE, right gastroepiploic artery; SPD, superior pancreatico-duodenal artery; TP, transverse pancreatic. Reproduced from Berne CJ, Rosoff L. Peptic ulcer perforation of the gastroduodenal artery complex: clinical features and operative control. Ann Surg 1969; 169:141–4. With permission from Lippincott, Williams & Wilkins.

surgery without recourse to endoscopic re-treatment. Some of these patients may benefit from early 'elective/pre-emptive' surgery.

 Management of re-bleeding following successful endostasis will depend on the specific circumstances. Further endoscopic haemostasis may be appropriate for many patients but high-risk ulcers, particularly those where good endostasis was difficult to achieve at the first procedure, may be better considered for surgery or even transarterial angiographic embolisation (see below).

The role of selective mesenteric embolisation

Transarterial angiographic embolisation (TAE) is an alternative rescue procedure. The technique has been in use for over two decades. In the 1980s, there were reports of visceral infarcts[47,48] following TAE, and its use was restricted to a small group of patients with refractory bleeding considered unfit for surgical intervention. With advances in embolisation techniques and specifically the use of superselective coiling, the success rate in the control of bleeding has been reported to be between 64% and 91% and mortality between 5% and 25%.[49–55] These small cohort studies therefore provide evidence that TAE may be considered as a reasonable option where endoscopic intervention has failed. In the only prospective non-randomised study comparing TAE to surgery, no difference was found between the TAE and surgery groups in incidence of recurrent bleeding (29% vs. 23%), need for additional surgery (16% vs. 30.8%) and death (25.8% vs. 20.5%).[53] In this study, patients who underwent TAE were significantly older (mean of 75.2 vs. 63.3, $P < 0.001$). The lack of difference and the more advanced age in the TAE group suggested that TAE may be at least as good an option as surgery in the management of refractory ulcer bleeding. Re-bleeding following surgery should now probably be treated by TAE in the first instance.

A randomised controlled study comparing surgery and TAE in this group of patients would be of great interest. Similarly, the role of semi-elective TAE following successful endostasis in patients considered at high risk of re-bleeding or death has not been studied but is another area where further research may be interesting (Table 7.5).

 Transarterial embolisation should be considered in patients who re-bleed following surgery for bleeding peptic ulcers and as an alternative to surgery when endoscopic haemostasis has failed, provided appropriate facilities and expertise are available. This may be particularly useful in elderly patients with medical comorbidity.

Helicobacter eradication

A Cochrane review of seven studies including 578 patients[56] concluded that *H. pylori* eradication was associated with a significant reduction in the risk of re-bleeding compared with no *H. pylori* eradication from 20% to 2.9%. If antisecretory therapy was continued the risk was 5.6%, still significantly higher than achieved with *H. pylori* eradication. The overall risk of re-bleeding following *H. pylori* eradication was less than 1% per year. It is therefore of concern that in a UK review of consultant behaviour, fewer than 60% routinely tested patients for *H. pylori* following treatment for complicated peptic ulcer.[45]

 Following treatment for bleeding duodenal ulcer, patients should be tested for *H. pylori* and receive eradication therapy where appropriate. Patients should have further testing to ensure successful eradication.[56]

Table 7.5 • Angiographic embolisation in bleeding peptic ulcers

First author, year	No. of patients	Haemostasis (*n*, %)	Death (*n*, %)
Holme, 2006[50]	40	26, 65%	10, 25%
Ripoll, 2004[53]	31	22, 71%	8, 26%
Ljungdahl, 2002[52]	18	15, 83%	1, 5%
De Wispelaere, 2002[49]	28	18, 64%	Not reported
Toyoda, 1996[55]	30	24, 80%	Not reported
Toyoda, 1995[54]	11	10, 91%	1, 9.9%
Lang, 1992[51]	57	52, 91%	Not reported

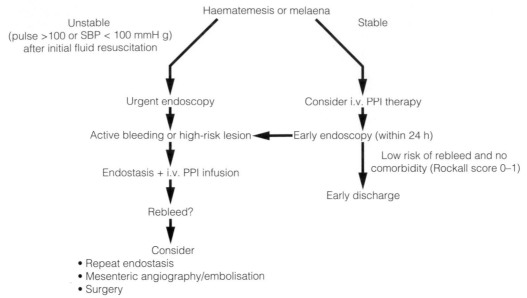

Figure 7.6 • Management algorithm. SBP, systolic blood pressure.

Use of NSAIDs

There is a clear association between NSAID use and increased risk of ulcer disease. The risk of ulcer bleeding is highest in patients with a history of complicated ulcer disease, the risk lasting for 2 months after cessation of treatment. In a study from Hong Kong, patients with UGI bleeding and *H. pylori* infection who required NSAID therapy were randomised to receive a 1-week course of *H. pylori* eradication therapy or 20 mg of omeprazole daily. The study demonstrated that *H. pylori* eradication alone is sufficient for the prevention of re-bleeding in patients taking low-dose aspirin but that PPI therapy was superior for patients taking other NSAIDs.

Summary

The challenge posed by peptic ulcer bleeding has altered with the increasing age of the population at risk and the increasing availability of skilled therapeutic endoscopy. Failure of endoscopic haemostasis is increasingly uncommon but the surgical challenge presented by the elderly patient with refractory bleeding from a large ulcer is considerable. Successful management of UGI bleeding will involve the close cooperation of a multidisciplinary team, aided by local protocols based on evidence-based best practice (**Fig. 7.6**).

Key points

- A full Rockall score should be calculated for all patients with UGI bleeding following initial endoscopic assessment.
- Pre-endoscopy treatment with PPIs is recommended as it reduces the risk of active bleeding at the time of endoscopy and may reduce the need for endoscopic intervention.
- Early endoscopy should be performed on all patients with UGI bleeding/haemorrhage.
- Endoscopic therapy should be applied where there is active bleeding or a non-bleeding visible vessel in the ulcer base. Adherent clot should be removed and endoscopic therapy applied to the underlying vessel.

- Endoscopic therapy for bleeding peptic ulcers should involve use of dual therapy or mechanical therapy rather than adrenaline injection alone in order to reduce the risk of re-bleeding.
- High-dose intravenous PPI therapy (80 mg omeprazole followed by 8 mg/h for 72 h) is recommended for patients with active bleeding or visible vessels at the time of endoscopy.
- The choice of operation in patients with bleeding peptic ulcers who have failed endoscopic treatment should involve, where possible, simple under-running of the bleeding ulcer, without either vagotomy or gastric resection.
- Management of re-bleeding following successful endoscopic haemostasis will depend on the specific circumstances. Further endoscopic haemostasis may be appropriate for many patients but for high-risk ulcers, particularly those where good endostasis was difficult to achieve at the first procedure, may be better considered for surgery or even transarterial angiographic embolisation.
- Following treatment for bleeding duodenal ulcer, patients should be tested for *H. pylori* and receive eradication therapy where appropriate. Patients should have further testing to ensure successful eradication.

References

1. Rockall TA, Logan RFA, Devlin HB et al. Incidence of and mortality from acute upper gastrointestinal hemorrhage in the United Kingdom. Br Med J 1995; 311(6999):222–6.

2. Blatchford O, Davidson LA, Murray WR et al. Acute upper gastrointestinal haemorrhage in west of Scotland: case ascertainment study. Br Med J 1997; 315(7107):510–14.

3. Carter R, Anderson JR. Randomized trial of adrenaline injection and laser photocoagulation in the control of haemorrhage from peptic ulcer. Br J Surg 1994; 81(6):869–71.

4. Choudari CP, Palmer KR. Endoscopic injection therapy for bleeding peptic ulcer; a comparison of adrenaline alone with adrenaline plus ethanolamine oleate. Gut 1994; 35(5):608–10.

5. Chung SC, Leung JW, Leong HT et al. Adding a sclerosant to endoscopic epinephrine injection in actively bleeding ulcers: a randomized trial. Gastrointest Endosc 1993; 39(5):611–15.

6. Jaramillo JL, Carmona C, Galvez C de la MM et al. Efficacy of the heater probe in peptic ulcer with a non-bleeding visible vessel. A controlled, randomised study. Gut 1993; 34(11):1502–6.

7. Wilcox CM, Alexander LN, Cotsonis G. A prospective characterization of upper gastrointestinal hemorrhage presenting with hematochezia. Am J Gastroenterol 1997; 92(2):231–5.

8. Rockall TA, Logan RFA, Devlin HB et al. Variation in outcome after acute upper gastrointestinal hemorrhage. Lancet 1995; 346(8971):346–50.

9. Church NI, Dallal HJ, Masson J et al. Validity of the Rockall scoring system after endoscopic therapy for bleeding peptic ulcer: a prospective cohort study [see comment]. Gastrointest Endosc 2006; 63(4):606–12.

10. Sanders DS, Carter MJ, Goodchap RJ et al. Prospective validation of the Rockall risk scoring system for upper GI hemorrhage in subgroups of patients with varices and peptic ulcers. Am J Gastroenterol 2002; 97(3):630–5.

11. Vreeburg EM, Terwee CB, Snel P et al. Validation of the Rockall risk scoring system in upper gastrointestinal bleeding. Gut 1999; 44(3):331–5.

12. Sanders DS, Perry MJ, Jones SG et al. Effectiveness of an upper-gastrointestinal haemorrhage unit: a prospective analysis of 900 consecutive cases using the Rockall score as a method of risk standardisation. Eur J Gastroenterol Hepatol 2004; 16(5):487–94.

13. Stainsby D, MacLennan S, Thomas D et al. Guidelines on the management of massive blood loss. Br J Haematol 2006; 135(5):634–41.

14. Perel P, Roberts I. Colloids versus crystalloids for fluid resuscitation in critically ill patients. Cochrane Database Syst Rev 2007; 4.

15. Green FW, Kaplan MM, Curtis LE et al. Effect of acid and pepsin on blood-coagulation and platelet-aggregation – possible contributor to prolonged gastroduodenal mucosal hemorrhage. Gastroenterology 1978; 74(1):38–43.

16. Dorward S, Sreedharan A, Leontiadis GI et al. Proton pump inhibitor treatment initiated prior to endoscopic diagnosis in upper gastrointestinal bleeding. Cochrane Database Syst Rev 2007; 4.

   This systematic review of five randomised trials found no effect of pre-endoscopy PPI therapy on mortality but there was a significant reduction in active bleeding and the need for intervention at the time of endoscopy.

17. Lai KC, Hui WM, Wong BC et al. A retrospective and prospective study on the safety of discharging selected patients with duodenal ulcer bleeding on

the same day as endoscopy. Gastrointest Endosc 1997; 45(1):26–30.

18. Spiegel BMR, Vakil NB, Ofman JJ. Endoscopy for acute nonvariceal upper gastrointestinal tract hemorrhage: Is sooner better? A systematic review. Arch Intern Med 2001; 161(11):1393–404.

This systematic review of 23 studies concluded that early endoscopy improved outcome in patients with UGI bleeding in all risk categories.

19. Wong SK, Yu LM, Lau JY et al. Prediction of therapeutic failure after adrenaline injection plus heater probe treatment in patients with bleeding peptic ulcer [see comment]. Gut 2002; 50(3):322–5.

20. Park CH, Min SW, Sohn YH et al. A prospective, randomized trial of endoscopic band ligation vs. epinephrine injection for actively bleeding Mallory–Weiss syndrome. Gastrointest Endosc 2004; 60(1):22–7.

21. Huang SP, Wang HP, Lee YC et al. Endoscopic hemoclip placement and epinephrine injection for Mallory–Weiss syndrome with active bleeding. Gastrointest Endosc 2002; 55(7):842–6.

22. Park CH, Sohn YH, Lee WS et al. The usefulness of endoscopic hemoclipping for bleeding Dieulafoy lesions. Endoscopy 2003; 35(5):388–92.

23. Barkun A, Bardou M, Marshall JK, Nonvariceal Upper GI Bleeding Consensus Conference Group. Consensus recommendations for managing patients with nonvariceal upper gastrointestinal bleeding [see comment]. Ann Intern Med 2003; 139(10):843–57.

These are the most recently published comprehensive guidelines on the management of UGI bleeding based on studies published to date and include data from published and new meta-analyses as well as expert opinion.

24. Cook DJ, Guyatt GH, Salena BJ et al. Endoscopic therapy for acute nonvariceal upper gastrointestinal hemorrhage: a meta-analysis. Gastroenterology 1992; 102(1):139–48.

25. Sacks HS, Chalmers TC, Blum AL et al. Endoscopic hemostasis. An effective therapy for bleeding peptic ulcers. JAMA 1990; 264(4):494–9.

26. Forrest JA, Finlayson ND, Shearman DJ. Endoscopy in gastrointestinal bleeding. Lancet 1974; 2(7877):394–7.

27. Laine L, Peterson WL. Bleeding peptic ulcer. N Engl J Med 1994; 331(11):717–27.

28. Laine L, Freeman M, Cohen H. Lack of uniformity in evaluation of endoscopic prognostic features of bleeding ulcers. Gastrointest Endosc 1994; 40(4):411–17.

29. Consensus Conference. Therapeutic endoscopy and bleeding ulcers. JAMA 1989; 262(10):1369–72.

30. Bleau BL, Gostout CJ, Sherman KE et al. Recurrent bleeding from peptic ulcer associated with adherent clot: a randomized study comparing endoscopic treatment with medical therapy. Gastrointest Endosc 2002; 56(1):1–6.

31. Jensen DM, Kovacs TO, Jutabha R et al. Randomized trial of medical or endoscopic therapy to prevent recurrent ulcer hemorrhage in patients with adherent clots [see comment]. Gastroenterology 2002; 123(2):407–13.

32. Kahi CJ, Jensen DM, Sung JJ et al. Endoscopic therapy versus medical therapy for bleeding peptic ulcer with adherent clot: a meta-analysis [see comment; erratum appears in Gastroenterology 2006; 131(3):980–1]. Gastroenterology 2005; 129(3):855–62.

33. Kubba AK, Murphy W, Palmer KR. Endoscopic injection for bleeding peptic ulcer: a comparison of adrenaline alone with adrenaline plus human thrombin. Gastroenterology 1996; 111(3):623–8.

34. Rutgeerts P, Rauws E, Wara P et al. Randomised trial of single and repeated fibrin glue compared with injection of polidocanol in treatment of bleeding peptic ulcer [see comment]. Lancet 1997; 350(9079):692–6.

35. Johnston JH, Jensen DM, Mautner W. Comparison of endoscopic electrocoagulation and laser photocoagulation of bleeding canine gastric ulcers. Gastroenterology 1982; 82(5, Pt 1):904–10.

36. Havanond C, Havanond P. Argon plasma coagulation therapy for acute non-variceal upper gastrointestinal bleeding. Cochrane Database Syst Rev 2005; 2:CD003791.

37. Sung JJ, Tsoi KK, Lai LH et al. Endoscopic clipping versus injection and thermo-coagulation in the treatment of non-variceal upper gastrointestinal bleeding: a meta-analysis. Gut 2007; 56(10):1364–73.

38. Calvet X, Vergara M, Brullet E et al. Addition of a second endoscopic treatment following epinephrine injection improves outcome in high-risk bleeding ulcers. Gastroenterology 2004; 126(2):441–50.

39. Marmo R, Rotondano G, Piscopo R et al. Dual therapy versus monotherapy in the endoscopic treatment of high-risk bleeding ulcers: a meta-analysis of controlled trials [see comment]. Am J Gastroenterol 2007; 102(2):279–89.

These three meta-analyses provide compelling evidence that addition of a second endoscopic therapy is better than adrenaline alone.

40. Marmo R, Rotondano G, Bianco MA et al. Outcome of endoscopic treatment for peptic ulcer bleeding: is a second look necessary? A meta-analysis. Gastrointest Endosc 2003; 57(1):62–67.

41. Lau JY, Sung JJ, Lee KK et al. Effect of intravenous omeprazole on recurrent bleeding after endoscopic treatment of bleeding peptic ulcers [see comment]. N Engl J Med 2000; 343(5):310–16.

42. Leontiadis GI, Sharma VK, Howden CW. Proton pump inhibitor treatment for acute peptic ulcer bleeding [update of Cochrane Database Syst Rev 2004; 3:CD002094; PMID:15266462]. Cochrane Database Syst Rev 2006; 1:CD002094.

This Cochrane review of 24 randomised trials found that high-dose PPI therapy reduced re-bleeding, surgery and mortality rates following endotherapy for high-risk ulcers.

43. Poxon VA, Keighley MR, Dykes PW et al. Comparison of minimal and conventional surgery in patients with bleeding peptic ulcer: a multicentre trial. Br J Surg 1991; 78(11):1344–5.

44. Millat B, Hay JM, Valleur P et al. Emergency surgical treatment for bleeding duodenal ulcer: oversewing plus vagotomy versus gastric resection, a controlled randomized trial. French Association for Surgical Research. World J Surg 1993; 17(5):568–73.

45. Gilliam AD, Speake WJ, Lobo DN et al. Current practice of emergency vagotomy and *Helicobacter pylori* eradication for complicated peptic ulcer in the United Kingdom. Br J Surg 2003; 90(1): 88–90.

46. Lau JY, Sung JJ, Lam YH et al. Endoscopic retreatment compared with surgery in patients with recurrent bleeding after initial endoscopic control of bleeding ulcers [see comment]. N Engl J Med 1999; 340(10):751–6.

47. Shapiro N, Brandt L, Sprayregan S et al. Duodenal infarction after therapeutic Gelfoam embolization of a bleeding duodenal ulcer. Gastroenterology 1981; 80(1):176–80.

48. Trojanowski JQ, Harrist TJ, Athanasoulis CA et al. Hepatic and splenic infarctions: complications of therapeutic transcatheter embolization. Am J Surg 1980; 139(2):272–7.

49. De Wispelaere JF, De Ronde T, Trigaux JP et al. Duodenal ulcer hemorrhage treated by embolization: results in 28 patients. Acta Gastroenterol Belg 2002; 65(1):6–11.

50. Holme JB, Nielsen DT, Funch-Jensen P et al. Transcatheter arterial embolization in patients with bleeding duodenal ulcer: an alternative to surgery. Acta Radiol 2006; 47(3):244–7.

51. Lang EK. Transcatheter embolization in management of hemorrhage from duodenal ulcer: long-term results and complications. Radiology 1992; 182(3):703–7.

52. Ljungdahl M, Eriksson LG, Nyman R et al. Arterial embolisation in management of massive bleeding from gastric and duodenal ulcers. Eur J Surg 2002; 168(7):384–90.

53. Ripoll C, Banares R, Beceiro I et al. Comparison of transcatheter arterial embolization and surgery for treatment of bleeding peptic ulcer after endoscopic treatment failure. J Vasc Intervent Radiol 2004; 15(5):447–50.

54. Toyoda H, Nakano S, Takeda I et al. Transcatheter arterial embolization for massive bleeding from duodenal ulcers not controlled by endoscopic hemostasis. Endoscopy 1995; 27(4):304–7.

55. Toyoda H, Nakano S, Kumada T et al. Estimation of usefulness of N-butyl-2-cyanoacrylate–lipiodol mixture in transcatheter arterial embolization for urgent control of life-threatening massive bleeding from gastric or duodenal ulcer. J Gastroenterol Hepatol 1996; 11(3):252–8.

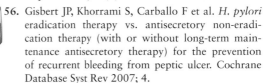

56. Gisbert JP, Khorrami S, Carballo F et al. *H. pylori* eradication therapy vs. antisecretory non-eradication therapy (with or without long-term maintenance antisecretory therapy) for the prevention of recurrent bleeding from peptic ulcer. Cochrane Database Syst Rev 2007; 4.

This Cochrane review included seven studies and a reduction in re-bleeding rates following *H. pylori* eradication compared with antisecretory therapy and no eradication.

8

Pancreaticobiliary emergencies

Rowan W. Parks

Introduction

Increasing specialisation in surgical practice has produced a trend towards concentration of elective pancreatic and complex biliary surgery in the hands of 'upper' gastrointestinal surgeons. However, the nature of surgical service provision often demands that pancreaticobiliary emergencies be treated by surgeons with principal specialist interests outwith the upper gastrointestinal tract. Thus the aim of this chapter is to provide an overview of current evidence guiding the treatment of the more commonly encountered pancreaticobiliary emergencies, including the management of acute cholecystitis, acute cholangitis and acute pancreatitis, for the emergency general surgeon.

Biliary colic and acute cholecystitis

The majority of acute gallbladder problems are the consequence of gallstones and have a range of clinical presentations.

Pathogenesis

Symptomatic cholelithiasis presents with a range of clinical syndromes. In the emergency setting the patient is most likely to present with either biliary colic or acute cholecystitis. It is often difficult at the initial assessment to distinguish between the two conditions because it is likely that biliary colic and acute cholecystitis form part of a spectrum. Biliary colic is thought to occur following the impaction of a gallstone within the cystic duct or gallbladder infundibulum, leading to gallbladder obstruction. In a functioning gallbladder, obstruction results in marked gallbladder contraction with the perception of pain. Following disimpaction of the stone, pain subsides. Disimpacted gallstones can either fall back into the gallbladder or pass into the common bile duct (CBD).

Continued gallbladder obstruction gives rise to an acute inflammatory process, although it should be borne in mind that there is often a poor correlation between the clinical presentation and the histopathological features of acute and chronic inflammation in the gallbladder wall. Initially in acute cholecystitis the inflammatory process within the gallbladder is sterile; however, bacterial colonisation of the obstructed bile and inflamed tissue occurs and may result in an empyema of the gallbladder. Further, if the inflammatory process is particularly severe, gallbladder ischaemia and necrosis can occur, with the consequent risk of gallbladder perforation and subsequent biliary peritonitis.

Clinical presentation

Biliary colic presents with severe upper abdominal pain in the epigastric and right upper quadrant regions, often radiating to the back or shoulders. Although termed 'colic', the pain is often constant but remits after a period of minutes to hours. It may be provoked by eating, and the patient may describe an association with ingestion of fatty foods. A history of previous similar episodes may be obtained. On examination during the acute episode the patient may be distressed because of the pain. Palpation of the abdomen may reveal epigastric/right upper quadrant tenderness but no evidence of peritoneal irritation. Blood investigations are usually normal.

In acute cholecystitis the pain is localised to the right upper quadrant, and may radiate through to the back or right shoulder tip. Because of peritoneal irritation the pain is exacerbated by movement and breathing. Commonly, the patient is nauseated and may have vomited. Systemic signs of inflammation including tachycardia and pyrexia would be expected and abdominal examination will typically reveal right upper quadrant tenderness with signs of localised peritonitis. Classically, Murphy's sign (pain on deep inspiration during palpation at the tip of the right ninth rib) can be elicited in patients with acute cholecystitis. A tender mass may be palpable in the right upper quadrant. Haematological investigations typically demonstrate a leucocytosis. Liver function tests may be deranged. An obstructive picture to the liver function tests may be a consequence of CBD stones but may also be a consequence of impacted gallstones in Hartmann's pouch pressing on or eroding into the common hepatic duct (Mirizzi's syndrome) or contiguous inflammation affecting the CBD or adjacent hepatic parenchyma.

Initial radiological imaging

Transabdominal ultrasonography is the initial investigation of choice in both biliary colic and acute cholecystitis. Standard grey-scale ultrasound has a sensitivity of greater than 95% for detecting gallstones. In addition, ultrasound can demonstrate signs of acute inflammation such as gallbladder wall thickening, pericholecystic fluid and a sonographic Murphy's sign (**Fig. 8.1**). Ultrasound is also able to visualise gas in the gallbladder wall in those patients with emphysematous cholecystitis. Newer techniques of colour velocity imaging and power Doppler sonography have greater accuracy than grey-scale ultrasonography in detecting acute cholecystitis, and may therefore be used to distinguish patients with true acute cholecystitis from those with upper abdominal pain and incidental chronic cholelithiasis. In addition, transabdominal ultrasound can detect the presence of biliary tree dilatation, suggesting choledocholithiasis.

Radionucleotide scans have been reported to have greater accuracy in diagnosing acute cholecystitis than standard ultrasound techniques. However, these techniques are time-consuming and involve the use of radiopharmaceuticals, and their use is now probably restricted to those individuals who are clinically suspected of having gall bladder disease in the presence of a normal ultrasound scan.

Figure 8.1 • Ultrasound of acute cholecystitis. Note the thickened gallbladder wall, the acoustic shadow produced by the gallstone in the neck and the surrounding pericystic fluid. This patient was also tender on pressing the transducer onto the gallbladder (sonographic Murphy's sign). With thanks to Dr Paul Allan, Consultant Radiologist, Royal Infirmary, Edinburgh.

Management of patients with acute gallbladder disease and suspected bile duct stones

Concomitant choledocholithiasis may be indicated by obstructive liver function tests or ultrasonographic evidence of biliary dilatation and/or evidence of ductal calculi. In the acute setting several additional factors complicate the decision-making process. Most importantly, if there are signs of generalised peritonitis then operative intervention cannot be deferred and investigation for CBD calculi becomes a secondary issue. In this situation, ductal stones can be dealt with if they are encountered at surgery. It is also important to bear in mind the clinical overlap between acute cholangitis and acute cholecystitis. Patients with sepsis secondary to impacted CBD calculi may have upper abdominal tenderness and guarding. Clearly, an appropriate index of suspicion together with findings on ultrasonography should result in such individuals being appropriately treated for their ductal calculi.

In the majority of patients with acute cholecystitis and deranged liver function tests there will be an opportunity to assess the CBD preoperatively. The management options include endoscopic retrograde cholangiopancreatography (ERCP) or magnetic resonance cholangiopancreatography (MRCP). MRCP has the advantage that it is a non-invasive modality that is as accurate as ERCP in detecting bile duct stones (**Fig. 8.2**);[1] however, therapeutic intervention can be undertaken at ERCP (**Fig. 8.3**).

Guidelines on the management of CBD stones published by the British Society of Gastroenterology recommend that where initial assessment, based on clinical features, liver function tests and ultrasound findings, suggest a high probability of CBD calculi, then it is reasonable to proceed directly to ERCP if this is considered the treatment of choice.[2] Where initial assessment suggests a low or uncertain index of suspicion for CBD calculi, then it is recommended that patients undergo MRCP or endoscopic ultrasound with ERCP reserved for those with abnormal or equivalent results.

An alternative management strategy is to undertake intraoperative cholangiography during cholecystectomy (**Fig. 8.4**). If a ductal stone is demonstrated on intraoperative cholangiography, the options are to undertake laparoscopic CBD exploration, convert to an open procedure with exploration of the CBD or to perform a postoperative ERCP. The potential risk with adoption of a postoperative ERCP strategy is failure to cannulate at endoscopy; however, in practice few patients require a second laparotomy.

Figure 8.2 • Magnetic resonance cholangiogram demonstrating a single calculus in the distal common bile duct.

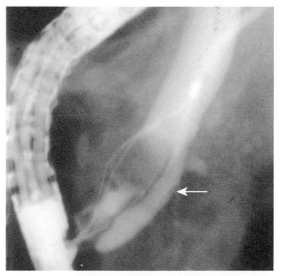

Figure 8.3 • Basket extraction of common bile duct calculi at endoscopic retrograde cholangiopancreatography. With thanks to Dr Kel Palmer, Consultant Gastro-enterologist, Western General Hospital, Edinburgh, UK.

Figure 8.4 • Operative cholangiograms obtained during laparoscopic cholecystectomy demonstrating a non-obstructing calculus in the cystic duct **(a)** and distal common bile duct **(b)**.

Given that many surgeons would no longer regard acute cholecystitis as a contraindication to the laparoscopic approach, a logical extension to the procedure is to combine laparoscopic cholecystectomy with laparoscopic exploration of the CBD for the treatment of ductal stones.

Systematic reviews of studies reporting the outcome of laparoscopic CBD exploration report morbidity rates of between 2% and 17% and mortality rates of 1–5%.[3] This is comparable to ERCP, with a recent Cochrane review of randomised controlled trials concluding that there was no clear difference in primary success rates, morbidity or mortality between the two approaches.[4]

A suggested algorithm for the management of patients with suspected biliary colic/acute cholecystitis and suspected CBD stones is described in **Fig. 8.5**.

Treatment

Biliary colic

The initial treatment for biliary colic consists of adequate analgesia and antiemetics. Although opiate analgesia is widely prescribed, non-steroidal anti-inflammatory drugs (NSAIDs) are also effective in relieving pain. Moreover, studies have suggested that NSAIDs can reduce the number of patients progressing from biliary colic to acute cholecystitis. Following symptom resolution, optimal definitive therapy in the form of laparoscopic cholecystectomy should be undertaken. Although it is preferable to undertake surgery during the index admission, patients may be discharged with plans for an interval procedure, but at the risk of recurrent symptoms.

Acute cholecystitis

Initial therapy in acute cholecystitis includes intravenous fluid resuscitation, analgesia, a nil-by-mouth regimen and administration of intravenous antibiotics. Although the initial inflammation is sterile, secondary infection with aerobic Gram-negative organisms, enterococci and anaerobes occurs. *Clostridium perfringens* infection of the necrotic gallbladder may be a particular complication in the diabetic patient. Few data exist to support the optimum antibiotic regimen, although a second- or third-generation cephalosporin combined with metronidazole is frequently prescribed.

Urgent surgical intervention is indicated in those patients with generalised peritonitis arising from a gallbladder perforation or in those with emphysematous cholecystitis (**Fig. 8.6**). Outwith these circumstances, the therapeutic options are to remove the gallbladder either during the index admission or

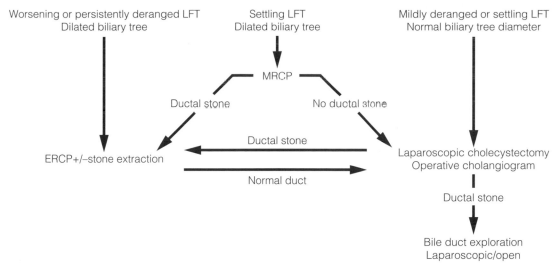

Worsening or persistently deranged LFT
Dilated biliary tree

Settling LFT
Dilated biliary tree

Mildly deranged or settling LFT
Normal biliary tree diameter

MRCP

Ductal stone

No ductal stone

ERCP+/–stone extraction

Ductal stone

Laparoscopic cholecystectomy
Operative cholangiogram

Normal duct

Ductal stone

Bile duct exploration
Laparoscopic/open

Figure 8.5 • Investigation and management of patients with biliary colic or acute cholecystitis and suspected bile duct stones. ERCP, endoscopic retrograde cholangiopancreatography; LFT, liver function tests; MRCP, magnetic resonance cholangiopancreatography.

Figure 8.6 • Computed tomography of emphysematous cholecystitis demonstrating gas in the gallbladder wall with extension into the hepatoduodenal ligament.

electively at a later admission. Early operation has the advantage of prompt definitive therapy but surgical intervention may be technically more difficult. The rationale for deferred surgery is to allow for resolution of inflammation, but the patient remains at risk of exacerbations during the 'waiting' period and subsequent 'delayed' surgery may still be very difficult.

Recent randomised controlled trials comparing early versus late laparoscopic cholecystectomy for acute cholecystitis have now confirmed that early laparoscopic cholecystectomy is both safe and has significant benefits for patients. Conversion rate, hospital stay and complications are all significantly lower in the early surgery group.[5–8]

The benefits of early laparoscopic cholecystectomy over early open cholecystectomy have also been assessed.[9] A total of 63 patients with acute cholecystitis were randomised to either early laparoscopic cholecystectomy ($n = 32$) or early open cholecystectomy ($n = 31$). Conversion to the open procedure was required in five patients randomised to laparoscopic cholecystectomy. Although there were no deaths or bile duct injuries in either group, the postoperative complication rate was significantly higher in the open group ($P = 0.0048$): seven patients (23%) had major and six (19%) had minor complications after open cholecystectomy, whereas only one (3%) minor complication occurred after the laparoscopic procedure. Both the postoperative hospital stay (median 4 days vs. 6 days; $P = 0.0063$) and duration of sick leave (mean 13.9 days vs. 30.1 days; $P < 0.0001$) were significantly shorter in the laparoscopic group.

As a result, early laparoscopic cholecystectomy should be attempted in all patients with acute cholecystitis who are fit for surgery, recognising that there will be some in whom the acute inflammation prevents adequate visualisation of the anatomy and conversion will be required.[5–9]

Antibiotic cover for urgent cholecystectomy

Antibiotic therapy following successful early cholecystectomy for acute non-gangrenous cholecystitis does not need to be continued beyond 12 hours.[10]

Non-surgical options for decompressing the gallbladder in acute cholecystitis

Although early laparoscopic cholecystectomy is optimal management in acute cholecystitis, surgery may not be feasible in some patients because of comorbid conditions. In these patients ultrasound-guided percutaneous cholecystostomy is a useful alternative (**Fig. 8.7**). If the diagnosis is in doubt, such as might be the case in the critically ill patient on the intensive care unit, percutaneous cholecystostomy can also be diagnostic,[11] with successful drainage of the gallbladder possible in up to 90% of patients.[12] Although cannulation of the gallbladder may be achieved through a transperitoneal approach, a transhepatic approach is to be preferred because of the lower risk of biliary peritonitis and the earlier maturation of the cholecystostomy tract. Following insertion of the drainage tube into the gallbladder, free drainage is established, although antibiotic instillation may also be carried out. On occasions, simple aspiration of the gallbladder may be effective; however, a recent randomised trial concluded that percutaneous cholecystostomy drainage was associated with a superior clinical response rate.[13] Signs of effective intervention usually occur within 24–48 hours; therefore in those in whom rapid improvement does not occur, a complication of either the acute cholecystitis (gallbladder necrosis, perforation) or of the insertion of the cholecystostomy tube (bile leak, visceral perforation) should be presumed and surgical intervention should be reconsidered. The cholecystostomy tube should be maintained until a mature fistula tract is achieved. Contrast radiology in the form of a 'tubogram' may be undertaken in order to confirm drain

Figure 8.7 • Ultrasound of a patient with acute cholecystitis. **(a)** Before treatment; note the microabscesses within the thickened gallbladder wall. **(b)** After successful percutaneous transhepatic drainage. With thanks to Dr Paul Allan, Consultant Radiologist, Royal Infirmary, Edinburgh.

position, cystic and common bile duct patency, as well as the presence and site of calculi.

To date there has only been one randomised clinical trial assessing the role of percutaneous cholecystostomy in patients with acute cholecystitis who are high-risk surgical candidates.[14] In this study, 123 patients with acute cholecystitis and an Acute Physiological and Chronic Health Evaluation (APACHE) II score of 12 or greater were randomised to either percutaneous cholecystostomy (PC; $n = 60$) or to conservative therapy (C; $n = 63$). Percutaneous cholecystostomy was associated with a number of major complications in the initial stages of the trial, although this appeared to be due to the use of non-locking drains inserted under computed tomography (CT) guidance. A change in technique to ultrasound-guided transhepatic placement of locking drains helped to lower procedure-related complications. Nevertheless, in this trial rates of clinical resolution (PC 86% vs. C 87%) and mortality (PC 17.5% vs. C 13%) were similar between the percutaneous cholecystostomy and conservative therapy groups.

As a result, percutaneous cholecystostomy should only be used in those patients not fit for surgery whose symptoms do not improve rapidly on standard conventional therapy.[14]

Following disease resolution, definitive therapy directed towards the gallbladder needs to be considered. Recurrent symptoms will occur in approximately one-third of patients who have previously had acute calculous cholecystitis and have not undergone definitive treatment.[15] Therefore interval cholecystectomy following optimisation of medical therapy treating comorbid disease should be considered. In those patients in whom surgical intervention is absolutely contraindicated, the cholecystostomy tube may be left in situ for a prolonged period. Cholelithiasis may also be treated by percutaneous extraction of the gallstone or direct dissolution with a solvent such as methyl-*tert*-butyl ether. However, recurrence of gallstones following these therapies is common, with studies suggesting that 10–20% of all patients treated by these methods develop further symptoms.[16–18]

Acute acalculous cholecystitis

Acute inflammation of the gallbladder can occur in the absence of gallstones and is termed acute acalculous cholecystitis (AAC). Although AAC may present as a complication of a number of clinical conditions, it occurs most frequently in the critically ill or postoperative patient. Despite the fact that AAC is an uncommon entity, it appears to be increasing in frequency.[19] Observational studies have suggested that AAC occurs in 0.004–0.05% of patients undergoing surgery.[20,21] However, although it is rarer than gallstone-induced acute cholecystitis, the mortality rate of AAC is significantly higher.[19]

The pathogenetic mechanisms in AAC are not clear. Most recent evidence suggests that AAC is a consequence of microvascular ischaemia resulting in gallbladder inflammation. Studies have demonstrated that the gallbladder arterial and capillary network is reduced and irregular in AAC compared with that in acute cholecystitis.[22] Further, in animal models the induction of a vasculitic process through the activation of factor XII causes AAC. As indirect evidence, AAC can occur as a consequence of systemic lupus erythematosus, polyarteritis nodosa and antiphospholipid syndrome. In critical illness states, gallbladder microvascular ischaemia probably occurs as a manifestation of the systemic inflammatory response syndrome.

The diagnosis of AAC is often difficult. Because it occurs principally in critically ill patients and in those who have recently had abdominal surgery, the symptoms and signs may be masked by co-existing problems. The critically ill patient may be sedated and/or ventilated, limiting history-taking, and abdominal signs may be masked by sedation or drug-induced paralysis. In the postoperative patient, abdominal signs may be limited by wound pain, and other more operation-specific complications may be considered as a cause for changes in the clinical condition.

Unfortunately, diagnostic imaging may also be unhelpful. Although ultrasonographic signs of AAC have been described (dilated gallbladder, gallbladder wall thickening, pericholecystic fluid and gallbladder sludge), these are not diagnostic. In a prospective series of 21 critically ill patients, all study subjects had gallbladder abnormalities on at least one occasion during serial ultrasound examinations; however, only four patients required intervention for AAC.[23] Similarly, although CT may demonstrate gallbladder abnormalities, these signs may again be non-diagnostic. Cholescintigraphy may be the most accurate method of identifying AAC. In a retrospective study of 27 patients with AAC, cholescintigraphy detected AAC in 9 of 10 patients (90%), whereas CT detected AAC in 8 of 12 (67%) and ultrasound detected AAC in 2 of 7 (29%).[24] However, these results must be viewed cautiously as every patient did not undergo all investigations. Moreover, other series have suggested a high incidence of false-positive cholescintigraphy scans in critically ill patients.[25] Because of the inaccuracy of imaging studies, the definitive diagnosis of AAC may only be made at laparotomy or diagnostic laparoscopy.[26] AAC must therefore be considered in all critically ill or postoperative patients with right upper quadrant pain, deranged liver function tests or unexplained sepsis. With the difficulty of diagnosis in mind, one prospective study assessed the benefit of percutaneous cholecystostomy in 82 critically ill patients with unexplained sepsis.[27] In 48 patients (59%) there was rapid improvement in the clinical condition within 48 hours but ultrasound did not predict which patients would respond to cholecystostomy.

 This study confirms the view that a low index of suspicion is required for the diagnosis of AAC in critically ill patients.[27]

The optimal therapeutic strategy in AAC is not clear. In all patients, broad-spectrum antibiotic therapy should be instituted as 65% of bile cultures will be positive, with *Escherichia coli* the most common organism. Therapeutic interventions include cholecystostomy with or without interval cholecystectomy, or early cholecystectomy. Several series have demonstrated that percutaneous cholecystostomy is not only an effective immediate intervention but may also constitute definitive treatment as the likelihood of recurrent episodes is small.[28,29] However, early cholecystectomy has been advocated because necrosis of the gallbladder may occur in up to 63% of cases,[24,30] with perforation occurring in approximately 15%. It would therefore appear reasonable to manage AAC in critically ill patients with initial percutaneous cholecystostomy, but in the absence of rapid clinical improvement a complication should be presumed and cholecystectomy carried out. In those patients managed successfully by percutaneous cholecystostomy there does not appear to be an absolute requirement for interval cholecystectomy.

Acute cholangitis

Acute cholangitis may be defined as an acute pyogenic infection within the biliary tree. Because of the possibility of rapid disease progression, acute cholangitis is a potentially life-threatening condition that requires urgent therapeutic intervention.

Pathogenesis

Acute cholangitis arises as a consequence of biliary stasis with subsequent bacterial infection. Although a number of pathological processes may lead to biliary stasis, the most common underlying causes of acute cholangitis are bile duct calculi, malignant bile duct obstruction and biliary stent occlusion. Biliary obstruction need not be complete as acute cholangitis can arise in a partially obstructed biliary system. Under normal conditions bile is sterile; however, in 58% of individuals with asymptomatic ductal calculi, bile cultures will be positive indicating bacterial colonisation.[31] In those progressing to acute cholangitis, cholangiovenous reflux of bacteria and bacterial products occurs because of increasing hydrostatic pressure within the biliary tree. This cholangiovenous reflux results in bacteraemia and the induction of a systemic inflammatory response, and it is this response, leading to organ dysfunction, that is responsible for the morbidity and mortality in acute cholangitis. Decompression of the biliary tree removes the inflammatory insult.

Aerobic Gram-negative bacilli (*E. coli*, *Klebsiella*, *Pseudomonas* species), enterococcus and anaerobes are the most common organisms cultured from the bile of patients with acute cholangitis.[31] In up to 50% of patients, anaerobic organisms may be associated with aerobic organisms. In the elderly, polymicrobial infection is more common than monomicrobial infection, and again concomitant anaerobic infection occurs in the majority. In approximately 35% of patients, blood cultures will be positive for the same organisms that are found in the bile.[32] The route of bacterial biliary colonisation is not clear; however, the types of bacteria involved suggest that they are derived from the intestinal tract.

Presentation

The presentation of acute cholangitis can be variable, ranging from mild symptoms and signs to overwhelming septic shock. Classically, patients with acute cholangitis present with the symptoms and signs that constitute Charcot's triad: upper abdominal pain, jaundice and pyrexia. However, the complete triad may be present in as few as 22% of patients.[33] Especially in the elderly patient, the presentation may be subtle, with signs of an acute confusional state being common, with deranged liver function tests being the only pointer to the diagnosis. Similarly, acute cholangitis must be included in the differential diagnosis for any patient presenting with rigors. It is not uncommon for patients who have previously had endoscopic biliary stents to present with a rigor as the major feature of an obstructed infected stent. At the other end of the spectrum, acute cholangitis can present with signs of septic shock and evidence of multiple organ dysfunction. Because the progression to septic shock can be rapid in patients with biliary obstruction, the diagnosis of acute cholangitis must be considered in any patient presenting with jaundice and signs of sepsis.

Investigation

Cholestatic liver function tests are found in the majority of patients with acute cholangitis, demonstrating elevated bilirubin, alkaline phosphatase and γ-glutamyl transferase. However, serum bilirubin may be normal in acute cholangitis arising in a partly obstructed biliary tree because the remaining unobstructed liver is able to compensate. A neutrophilia is typical and serum amylase may also be raised. Deranged coagulation tests can occur, either as a consequence of prolonged biliary obstruction resulting in vitamin K deficiency, or due to disseminated intravascular coagulation. It goes without saying that blood cultures must always be taken.

The initial radiological investigation of choice is transabdominal ultrasonography. This will demonstrate signs of bile duct obstruction, although false-negative scans can occur. Ultrasound may also determine the underlying pathology. CT can identify biliary dilatation in 78% of patients with acute cholangitis as well as the level of obstruction in 65% and the cause of the obstruction in 61%;[34] however, the initial information obtained is no greater than with ultrasonography.

Although the determination of the exact site and nature of the bile duct obstruction may require direct visualisation with either ERCP or percutaneous transhepatic cholangiography (PTC), the true value of these procedures is their potential for therapeutic intervention. For this reason, although MRCP has recently been reported to be accurate in identifying biliary obstruction and the underlying obstructing lesion, it does not have an early role in managing patients with acute cholangitis.

Management

Initial resuscitation aims to achieve adequate oxygen delivery, administration of an appropriate volume of intravenous fluid and appropriate analgesia. Efficacy of therapy is assessed by close monitoring of vital signs and, because of the potential for rapid decompensation, management of the patient in a high-dependency unit is usually required.

Aerobic Gram-negative bacilli are the most common organisms in acute cholangitis, and therefore empirical therapy with antibiotics covering these bacteria should be commenced. In addition, because anaerobic bacteria, although rarely cultured from blood, are frequently found in bile cultures in association with aerobic bacteria, antibiotic regimens should also have anaerobic activity. Piperacillin is an extended-spectrum penicillin with activity against aerobic Gram-negative bacilli, enterococcus and anaerobes. The addition of the β-lactamase inhibitor tazobactam increases the spectrum of activity.

In a randomised clinical trial involving 96 patients with acute cholangitis, piperacillin had similar efficacy to combination therapy with ampicillin and tobramycin, achieving clinical cure or significant improvement in 70% of patients.[35] Another randomised trial assessing single antibiotic therapy[32] demonstrated that intravenous ciprofloxacin alone improved the clinical condition in 85% of cases and had similar efficacy to a combination of ceftazidime, ampicillin and metronidazole.

Although appropriate antibiotic therapy is important, relief of biliary obstruction is crucial to successful disease resolution. Emergency operative intervention is associated with significant risk, with a reported mortality of 20% and a 50% complication rate for patients with severe acute cholangitis.[36] As a result, the mainstay of treatment now is endoscopic bile duct drainage, with improved results compared with surgical intervention.[37]

The benefits of endoscopic therapy over surgery in patients with acute cholangitis were confirmed several years ago in a randomised controlled trial, with significantly fewer complications and lower mortality in those undergoing endoscopic drainage.[38]

The method used to achieve non-surgical biliary drainage would appear to be less important than simply achieving adequate drainage. Within the confines of a randomised trial, one study[39] demonstrated that biliary decompression in acute cholangitis with a biliary stent inserted without a sphincterotomy was as efficacious as insertion of a nasobiliary drain. In patients in whom ERCP is unsuccessful, drainage by PTC should be undertaken in the acute situation, even in patients who do not have a dilated intrahepatic biliary tree.[40] Once external drainage has been achieved in the first instance, the placement of a biliary stent can be organised as a staged procedure.

In the case of gallstone-related acute cholangitis, following resolution of the episode of acute cholangitis, adequate clearance of the bile duct should be confirmed by direct cholangiography, ERCP, high-quality MRCP or operative cholangiography. Cholecystectomy should be undertaken if there are no contraindications in order to reduce the risk of further gallstone-related problems.[41,42]

In summary, based upon the studies mentioned above, effective management of patients with acute cholangitis requires both antibiotic therapy and relief of biliary obstruction. Endoscopic and percutaneous drainage techniques are effective in the early stages but may also provide definitive therapy in certain patients.

Acute pancreatitis

Acute pancreatitis is defined as an acute inflammatory process of the pancreas, with variable involvement of other regional or remote organ systems.[43] It is a common acute illness, with epidemiological data from the Health Service Statistics Division in Scotland reporting an annual incidence of 318 cases per million (365 cases per million in men, 275 cases per million for women).[44] Analysis of patterns of incidence in this particular population (which has remained relatively constant over the past decade) suggests an increase in the incidence of acute pancreatitis, particularly in those over 40 years of age. Similar increases in the incidence of acute pancreatitis have also been observed in Germany, Finland and Denmark. The factors giving rise to the observed increased incidences are not clear; however, at least in Finland, the increase in the incidence of acute pancreatitis is strongly correlated with an increase in alcohol consumption.

In practical terms the management of acute pancreatitis can be divided into two broad phases. The first phase includes the establishment of diagnosis, severity stratification, initial resuscitation and the choice of appropriate disease-specific initial therapy. The second phase relates to those with severe disease who will usually require further intervention for intra-abdominal complications or support for ongoing multiple organ failure. Recent guidelines[45–47] suggest that patients with complications arising from severe acute pancreatitis are most appropriately managed in a unit with specialist expertise and therefore this chapter only focuses on the initial phase of management.

Within this chapter the terminology used to describe patients with acute pancreatitis is in keeping with definitions agreed by the 1992 Atlanta consensus conference (Box 8.1).[43] The Atlanta classification attempted to introduce uniformity in the description of clinical severity and the various complications of the disease; however, with increasing understanding of the pathophysiology of pancreatitis, improved imaging techniques and newer therapeutic strategies, some authors have recently suggested that it may be time to consider revising the classification of acute pancreatitis.

Aetiology

Acute pancreatitis may be caused by a wide variety of aetiological agents (Box 8.2), although the majority of cases are due to either gallstones or alcohol excess. Recent epidemiological studies have

Box 8.1 • Terminology relating to acute pancreatitis as defined by the Atlanta consensus conference

Mild acute pancreatitis

Minimal organ dysfunction and an uneventful recovery

Severe acute pancreatitis

Associated with organ failure and/or local complications such as necrosis, abscess or pseudocyst

Acute fluid collections

Occur early in the course of acute pancreatitis, are situated in or near the pancreas, and always lack a wall of granulation or fibrous tissue

Pancreatic necrosis

Diffuse or focal areas of non-viable pancreatic parenchyma, typically associated with peripancreatic fat necrosis

Acute pseudocysts

Collection of pancreatic juice surrounded by a wall of fibrous or granulation tissue

Pancreatic abscess

Circumscribed intra-abdominal collection of pus arising in close proximity to the pancreas, but containing little or no pancreatic necrosis, which arises as a consequence of acute pancreatitis

demonstrated that alcohol excess is an increasingly frequent cause of acute pancreatitis. The prevalence of idiopathic acute pancreatitis varies between reported series and is probably a function of the degree of investigation undertaken to identify a cause. Recent UK guidelines state that no more than 20% of patients should be labelled as having idiopathic acute pancreatitis.[46]

Pathogenesis

The mechanisms through which each aetiological agent causes pancreatic acinar cell injury are not clear. However, after the initial pancreatic insult, it is believed that regardless of the aetiological agent the pathogenetic mechanisms of disease progression in acute pancreatitis are similar. Following pancreatic acinar cell injury, local pancreatic inflammation occurs. Although the inflammatory process may remain confined to the pancreas and peripancreatic tissues, a systemic inflammatory response may be triggered. This systemic inflammatory response is characterised by the systemic activation of leucocytes and endothelial cells and the secretion of proinflammatory cytokines, and is responsible for the development of the organ dysfunction that characterises severe acute pancreatitis. It is not clear why some patients develop severe acute pancreatitis

Box 8.2 • Aetiological agents in acute pancreatitis

Common

Gallstones
Alcohol

Uncommon

Trauma

Endoscopic retrograde cholangiopancreatography
Sphincterotomy
Biliary manometry
Pancreatic duct obstruction
Ampulla of Vater neoplasia

Drugs

Azathioprine

Metabolic

Hypercalcaemia
Hyperlipidaemia

Infection

Mumps
Coxsackie B
HIV

Vascular

Vasculitis
Cardiopulmonary bypass

Hereditary pancreatitis

Figure 8.8 • Grey Turner's sign in severe acute pancreatitis. Reproduced from Powell JJ, Parks RW. Diagnosis and early management of acute pancreatitis. Hosp Med 2003; 64:150–5. With permission from the BJHM.

whilst others with similar aetiological agents develop mild acute pancreatitis; however, there is evidence to implicate both excessive proinflammatory mediators and decreased anti-inflammatory mechanisms.

Clinical presentation

Presenting symptoms may range from mild discomfort to overwhelming abdominal pain. Typically, patients present with increasing epigastric/central abdominal pain radiating through to the back. This pain may be eased by sitting forward. Nausea is a predominant early symptom, with associated vomiting or retching. Before presenting with gallstone-induced acute pancreatitis, patients may have had symptoms consistent with biliary colic. Likewise, in alcohol-induced acute pancreatitis, patients will often have a long history of alcohol ingestion and/or recent binge drinking.

Signs of cardiovascular and respiratory dysfunction may be present. Examination may reveal abdominal signs ranging from localised epigastric tenderness to generalised peritonitis. More specific signs of severe acute pancreatitis include periumbilical bruising (Cullen's sign) and flank bruising (Grey Turner's sign; **Fig. 8.8**).

Diagnosis (see also Chapter 5)

Traditionally, the diagnosis of acute pancreatitis has depended on the detection of a serum amylase concentration more than three times the upper limit of normal. However, hyperamylasaemia may occur in several other conditions (Box 8.3), and a serum amylase concentration above the 'diagnostic' threshold does not definitely indicate acute pancreatitis. Conversely, acute pancreatitis may exist with serum amylase concentrations below this threshold. In those patients with a prolonged history prior to admission to hospital, serum amylase concentrations may have normalised. Amylase measurement therefore needs to be timely. Serum amylase levels do not provide prognostic information, nor can they be followed in order to monitor the early disease process. However, very high levels of serum amylase on admission are often suggestive of a gallstone aetiology.

Because of the limitations of the serum amylase test, other markers have been used to diagnose acute pancreatitis. Serum lipase is perhaps the most common and is more sensitive and specific than serum amylase. Moreover, because of its longer half-life, serum lipase is more accurate if there has been a delay in obtaining the initial sample.[45] However, as with serum amylase, serum lipase concentrations do not correlate with disease severity. In contrast, newer markers such as urinary trypsinogen activation peptide

Box 8.3 • Main differential diagnoses of hyperamylasaemia

Acute pancreatitis
Pancreatic pseudocyst
Mesenteric infarction
Perforated viscus
Acute cholecystitis
Diabetic ketoacidosis

and serum carboxy-peptide B activation peptide provide both diagnostic and prognostic information.

Although the vast majority of cases of acute pancreatitis can be diagnosed either clinically or biochemically, contrast-enhanced CT may be required in equivocal cases (**Fig. 8.9**).

Finally, in a few patients laparotomy may be required to confirm the diagnosis of acute pancreatitis while refuting other potential diagnoses such as acute mesenteric ischaemia or a perforated posterior duodenal ulcer. The decision to undertake diagnostic laparotomy is not made lightly as there is evidence that early operation has an adverse effect on outcome in acute pancreatitis.[48] In contrast, patients with acute intestinal ischaemia may present with abdominal pain and hyperamylasaemia and diagnostic delay may be critical. If the pancreas appears normal on CT, and in the absence of a firm diagnosis, laparoscopy or laparotomy should be considered if there are ongoing signs of peritonitis. Clearly, access to CT on a 24-hour basis is a prerequisite for this strategy.

Establishment of aetiology

Following diagnosis, usually confirmed biochemically, transabdominal ultrasound should be undertaken in all patients with acute pancreatitis to determine the presence or absence of gallstones. For those patients in whom alcohol is thought to be the causative agent, an accurate history must be taken, with collaborative information being obtained from other sources if necessary.

Management

General guidelines

Guidelines for the initial management of acute pancreatitis have been published by the 1997 Santorini consensus conference,[45] the British Society of Gastroenterology,[46] the American College of Gastroenterology,[47] the Japanese Society of Abdominal Emergency Medicine[49] and the International Association of Pancreatology.[50] Their recommendations are broadly similar and are described below.

Initial resuscitation

As in other acute abdominal emergencies, initial therapy is aimed at adequate resuscitation. Provision of oxygen to maintain arterial oxygen saturation, intravenous fluid therapy and adequate analgesia constitute the mainstays of therapy. In addition, the correction of metabolic abnormalities such as hyperglycaemia or hypocalcaemia may require administration of intravenous insulin or calcium. Patients with acute pancreatitis should be started on some form of thromboprophylaxis (see also Chapter 14). Antacid therapy with H$_2$ antagonists, proton-pump inhibitors

Figure 8.9 • Contrast-enhanced computed tomography of severe acute pancreatitis demonstrating a non-enhancing body of pancreas with an associated acute fluid collection.

or other gastroprotective agents may be commenced as prophylaxis against upper gastrointestinal haemorrhage in those patients with severe disease.

Severity stratification

Following resuscitation, patients should be categorised into either prognostically mild or severe disease, allowing decisions to be taken regarding the degree of monitoring, supportive care and intervention appropriate for each patient. Subjective clinical assessment of prognosis is inaccurate and a validated prognostic scoring system should be used. A number of systems currently exist and can be divided as follows:

- Multiple factor scoring systems – Glasgow,[51–53] Ranson[54] and APACHE II.[55]
- Biochemical scoring systems – C-reactive peptide (CRP)[56] and the Hong Kong system based on glucose and urea.[57]
- Immunological scoring – interleukin (IL)-6.[58]
- Radiological scoring – Balthazar[59] and Helsinki.[60]

It should be noted that the Ranson score is based on a North American population with alcohol as the predominant aetiological agent, whereas the Glasgow score is designed for use in a typical British population of gallstone-predominant disease. Further, practical confusion can result from the fact that there are at least three versions of the 'Glasgow' score: the original publication in 1978[51] and subsequent modifications in 1981[52] and 1984.[53] An APACHE II score of 9 or more has been validated for predicting prognostic severity in acute pancreatitis,[61] although a number of clinical trials have used lower cut-off points in order to predict severe disease, resulting in lower positive predictive values. Although an APACHE II score can be generated soon after admission, unlike the Ranson and Glasgow systems, it has the disadvantage of requiring collation of a sizeable number of variables. Comparative studies of the commonly used scoring systems have reported that no single system is superior to the others.[62] Accuracy to predict prognosis is typically 75–80%; however, a recent modification of the APACHE II system, which includes a clinical assessment of obesity (APACHE-O score), has been suggested to further improve predictive accuracy[63] and accuracy rates as high as 95% have been reported using computerised artificial neural networks.[64]

Finally, it should be noted that the currently used prognostic systems are a one-off or static assessment and serial or dynamic assessment may provide a more accurate determination of outcome. Indeed, it would appear that it is not the presence of organ dysfunction at presentation that is important in determining outcome, rather it is the response to initial resuscitation. Several authors have demonstrated that clinical outcome is worst in patients with persistent organ dysfunction, as manifested by worsening or static organ dysfunction scores following initial resuscitation, compared with patients whose organ dysfunction scores improve.[65–67]

Imaging in acute pancreatitis

As already mentioned, ultrasound should be performed in order to confirm or exclude the presence of gallstones. Following this, all patients with prognostically 'severe' acute pancreatitis should undergo contrast-enhanced CT between the third and tenth days of admission to determine the presence of pancreatic necrosis.[46]

Specific therapies for acute pancreatitis

The majority of patients recover from an episode of acute pancreatitis without complication and require little intervention. However, despite intense biomedical research activity there remains a dearth of effective specific therapies for severe acute pancreatitis. The importance of vigorous volume resuscitation and careful monitoring and treatment for metabolic, respiratory, renal and cardiac complications cannot be overemphasised. However, in addition to this supportive care, the therapeutic options are limited. Several randomised controlled trials have assessed the role of early ERCP and prophylactic antibiotics; however, controversy still persists regarding the relative values of both these therapeutic options. These treatments, together with other potential therapeutic options, are reviewed below.

Early ERCP

Early ERCP with endoscopic sphincterotomy (ES) in gallstone-induced acute pancreatitis aims to remove impacted ductal gallstones, thereby eliminating the initiating stimulus and hopefully reducing pancreatic inflammation. Three randomised trials assessing early ERCP have been published. They have produced some conflicting results and so it is worth discussing the results in some detail.

Neoptolemos et al.[68] randomised 121 patients with gallstone-induced acute pancreatitis, 53 of whom had prognostically severe disease, to either early ERCP (*n* = 59) or conventional therapy (*n* = 62). Although there was no difference in mortality between the two groups (1 for ERCP vs. 5 for conservative therapy; *P* = 0.23), there was a significant reduction in total complications (17% ERCP vs. 34% conservative; *P* = 0.03) and duration of hospital stay (median 9.5, range 6–36 days ERCP vs. 17.0, range 4–74 days; *P* = 0.035) in those patients with prognostically severe disease. Similarly,

Fan et al.[69] randomised 195 patients with acute pancreatitis, of whom 127 had gallstone-induced disease and 81 had prognostically severe disease, to either early ERCP ($n = 97$) or conventional therapy ($n = 98$). Again, there was no significant difference in mortality rates between the two groups (5 for ERCP vs. 9 for conservative therapy; $P = 0.276$). However, there was a significant reduction in the incidence of biliary sepsis following ERCP in those with prognostically severe acute pancreatitis (0% ERCP vs. 20% conservative; $P = 0.008$). Moreover, in those patients with gallstones a significant reduction in overall morbidity was observed (16% ERCP vs. 33% conservative; $P = 0.003$).

In contrast, a multicentre trial undertaken by Fölsch et al.[70] randomised 238 patients with gallstone-induced acute pancreatitis but without evidence of biliary obstruction to undergo either early ERCP ($n = 126$) or conservative management ($n = 112$). In total only 46 patients had prognostically severe disease. In contrast to the previous studies, the mortality rate was higher in the groups undergoing ERCP (10 for ERCP vs. 4 for conservative therapy; odds ratio 4.57, 95% CI 0.67–62.7, $P = 0.16$). Furthermore, ERCP was associated with an increased rate of respiratory failure (15 for ERCP vs. 5 for conservative; odds ratio 5.16, 95% CI 1.63–22.9, $P = 0.03$). Because of the trend towards increased mortality and the significantly increased rate of respiratory failure in those undergoing ERCP, the trial supervisory committee terminated the study early.

One further study exists that appears to support early ERCP/ES, although the results of this trial have to date only been published in abstract form. While the results suggest that early ERCP/ES is beneficial in patients with gallstone-induced acute pancreatitis, the conclusions that can be drawn must remain guarded as precise details regarding the study are limited.[71]

Rationalisation of the results of the three fully reported trials suggests that early ERCP/ES is of benefit in patients with prognostically severe gallstone-induced acute pancreatitis *with evidence* of cholangitis or biochemical evidence of obstructive liver function tests (serum bilirubin >90 μmol/L).[68–70]

Antibiotic therapy

The administration of prophylactic antibiotics in acute pancreatitis is based on the hypothesis that the prevention of infected pancreatic necrosis would improve outcome. Numerous studies have been undertaken to investigate the role of prophylactic antibiotics. Differing results have led to much debate. Early clinical studies did not show a benefit, possibly due to inclusion of patients with a low risk of infection or because antibiotics with poor pancreatic

penetration were used. However, more recent trials have now emerged and are worth considering further.

In a multicentre trial published in 1993, Pederzoli et al.[72] randomised 74 patients with CT-proven pancreatic necrosis to receive either imipenem or no initial antibiotic therapy. Pancreatic infection was significantly reduced in the antibiotic-treated group (30% vs. 12%; $P < 0.001$). Furthermore, rates of non-pancreatic infection were also significantly reduced; however, antibiotic therapy had no effect on the development of multiple organ failure, the need for operative intervention or on the mortality rate.

A Finnish study[73] randomised 60 patients with CT-proven pancreatic necrosis to receive either prophylactic intravenous cefuroxime or antibiotics only when there were clinical indications of infection. Although there was no difference in the rates of pancreatic infections between the two groups (30% cefuroxime vs. 40% control), prophylactic cefuroxime significantly reduced the mean number of infectious complications per patient (1.0 vs. 1.8; $P < 0.01$), mainly through a marked fall in the number of urinary tract infections. There was also a significant reduction in mortality in patients treated with cefuroxime (23.3% vs. 3.3%; $P = 0.028$), although this was not associated with any difference in local pancreatic infection.

Another study[74] randomised 23 patients with alcohol-induced severe acute pancreatitis to either standard medical therapy or standard medical therapy plus intravenous ceftazidime, amikacin and metronidazole. Antibiotic therapy resulted in a significant reduction in the number of patients with proven infections (0 vs. 7; $P < 0.03$), but there was no significant reduction in mortality rates. Schwarz et al.[75] reported a randomised controlled trial of 26 patients with CT-proven pancreatic necrosis in which the combination of ofloxacin and metronidazole lessened the physiological disturbance found in severe acute pancreatitis, but did not prevent or delay the development of infected pancreatic necrosis.

Subsequently two further studies were published that compared different antibiotics regimens in patients with necrotising pancreatitis. The first of these,[76] a multicentre, randomised, controlled trial involving 60 patients with pancreatic necrosis, observed that intravenous imipenum was more effective than perfloxacin at reducing rates of both infected pancreatic necrosis (34% vs. 10%; $P = 0.034$) and extrapancreatic infection (44% vs. 20%; $P = 0.059$), but had no effect on the mortality rate. The second of these studies again examined the effect of imipenem[77] in a randomised trial comparing the prophylactic use of imipenem with the therapeutic use of imipenem in patients with severe acute pancreatitis and CT-proven pancreatic necrosis. Patients enrolled in the prophylactic arm received imipenem from the time of admission, whereas patients in the therapeutic arm only commenced imipenem following the development of signs suggesting the development of infected pancreatic necrosis (pyrexia, leucocytosis, raised CRP, in the absence of another source of infection). There was no significant difference in the number of patients requiring necrosectomy or in the mortality rate between the two groups.

Recently the largest randomised placebo-controlled, double-blind trial on the use of prophylactic antibiotics has been published.[78] This multicentre study randomised 114 patients to receive either ciprofloxacin in combination with metronidazole or placebo. Only patients with a predicted severe attack were included, defined either by an elevated serum C-reactive protein above 150 mg/L or by pancreatic necrosis on CT scan. No beneficial effects with regard to reduction of pancreatic infection, systemic complications or hospital mortality were demonstrated; however, a shift to open antibiotic treatment was more frequent in patients receiving placebo, suggesting a subgroup of patients may warrant antibiotic treatment.

Using a different strategy aimed at eliminating the reservoir from which bacteria arise to colonise pancreatic necrosis, Luiten et al.[79] evaluated the role of selective gut decontamination. In a multicentre trial, 102 patients with prognostically severe acute pancreatitis were randomised to either conventional therapy or conventional therapy supplemented with selective gut decontamination using oral and rectal colistin, amphotericin and norfloxacin. In addition, patients in the selective gut decontamination group received intravenous cefotaxime until aerobic Gram-negative bacteria were eliminated from the oral cavity and rectum. Selective gut decontamination reduced rates of pancreatic infection compared with the control group (38% vs. 18%; $P = 0.03$). Although there was a reduction in mortality from 35% in the control group to 22% in the selective decontamination group, it did not reach significance ($P = 0.19$). However, when allowing for differences in disease severity, multivariate analysis suggested a significant survival benefit following gut decontamination ($P = 0.048$). Although the results of this trial appear promising, selective gut decontamination is not regarded as a standard for the prevention of pancreatic infection because of the difficulties of drug administration in the intensive care setting.

The inconsistencies among these trials may result from the relatively small number of patients per study and the limited statistical power to detect such differences. There is also considerable heterogeneity in patient selection and the antibiotics used. Other differences include variety in the non-antibiotic treatments, such as fluid resuscitation, enteral nutrition and timing of surgical intervention. Although many published guidelines recommend the use of antibiotics in patients with severe acute pancreatitis, none of the published randomised trials is in itself of sufficient power to mandate antibiotic prophylaxis.

In an attempt to strengthen the evidence regarding the use of antibiotic prophylaxis in acute pancreatitis, several meta-analyses have been performed. In 1998, Golub et al.[80] undertook a meta-analysis of all trials that had been published up to that point and reported that in patients with severe disease, the risk of death fell from 18.2% in patients not receiving antibiotic prophylaxis to 5.3% in those receiving prophylaxis (log odds ratio −0.32 to −2.44, $P = 0.008$). Similarly, Sharma and Howden[81] undertook a meta-analysis of three of the trials utilising broad-spectrum antibiotics in patients with severe disease. They suggested that antibiotic prophylaxis resulted in a 12.3% (95% CI 2.7–22%) absolute risk reduction in mortality rate, with eight (95% CI 5–37) patients needing treatment to prevent one death.

More recent meta-analyses, however, do not support the use of prophylactic antibiotics in patients with severe acute pancreatitis. In 2006, Mazaki et al.[82] analysed six trials and concluded that prophylactic antibiotics were not associated with a statistically significant reduction in infected necrosis (relative risk 0.77, CI 0.54–1.12, $P = 0.173$), non-pancreatic infections (relative risk 0.71, CI 0.32–1.58), surgical intervention (relative risk 0.78, CI 0.55–1.11) or mortality (relative risk 0.78, CI 0.44–1.39), but was associated with a significant reduction in hospital stay. In 2007, de Vries et al.[83] undertook a meta-analysis on six trials and reported that prophylactic antibiotics had no significant effect on infection of pancreatic necrosis (absolute risk reduction 0.055, CI −0.084 to 0.194) or mortality (absolute risk reduction 0.058, CI −0.017 to 0.134).

Furthermore, there is concern that the use of potent antibiotics may increase the rate of fungal-associated infected pancreatic necrosis and in turn adversely affect outcome. The use of antibiotic therapy has been shown to alter the organisms involved in the development of infected pancreatic necrosis,[84] and it has been suggested that higher rates of fungal infection have been reported in recent studies.[85] There is currently debate as to whether fungal-associated infected pancreatic necrosis is associated with increased mortality; however, a recent randomised trial of antifungal therapy in patients with severe acute pancreatitis showed a definite reduction in the incidence of fungal infection in the treatment group.[86]

In the light of all these conflicting studies, it is clear that further trials are needed to clarify the role of antibiotic and antifungal prophylaxis in acute pancreatitis. At present, a pragmatic approach may be that routine administration of prophylactic antibiotics to all patients with predicted severe acute pancreatitis is not indicated but should be considered in patients with evidence of pancreatic necrosis who appear septic (with leucocytosis, fever and/or organ failure). If blood and other cultures are subsequently found to be negative and no source of infection is identified, antibiotics should be discontinued. If positive microbiological cultures are obtained, appropriate antibiotics should be continued based on microbiological sensitivities.[80–83]

Early enteral nutrition

In those patients with severe acute pancreatitis the systemic inflammatory response may be maintained by intestinal dysfunction, leading to bacterial translocation from the intestinal lumen. Intestinal dysfunction may in part be a consequence of the nil-by-mouth regimen, leading to a loss of luminal nutrition in the intestine. The provision of enteral nutrition aims to ameliorate intestinal dysfunction, thereby reducing the systemic inflammatory response and improving outcome.

McClave et al.[87] randomised 32 patients with acute pancreatitis to receive either early enteral nutrition through an endoscopically placed feeding tube or parenteral nutrition following central or peripheral venous cannulation. Enteral nutrition appeared to be well tolerated, with no patients developing a significant complication from the study intervention. Importantly, enteral nutrition was able to supply a similar caloric intake to parenteral nutrition. However, the patients in the study had relatively mild disease and thus no significant differences in clinical outcome were observed, although enteral nutrition was associated with a significant reduction in the cost of patient care.

A similar study that randomised 34 patients with acute pancreatitis to receive, in addition to standard therapy, either early enteral nutrition or parenteral nutrition demonstrated that the introduction of early enteral nutrition was associated with a significant reduction in CRP and APACHE II scores.[88] Furthermore, in those receiving parenteral nutrition, serum anti-endotoxin IgM antibody levels increased whereas they remained unchanged in those receiving enteral nutrition.

In contrast to the previous two studies, all patients in the randomised controlled trial reported by Kalfarentzos et al.[89] had prognostically severe disease. In total, 38 patients were randomised to receive either enteral nutrition or parenteral nutrition. Enteral nutrition was delivered distal to the ligament of Treitz through a radiologically placed feeding tube. Even in this population of patients with severe disease, enteral nutrition was well tolerated, with the protein and caloric intake equalling that administered to the patients receiving parenteral nutrition. This ability to provide adequate nutrition via the enteral route appeared to translate into a clinical benefit. In those patients receiving enteral nutrition there were significantly fewer complications and a significant reduction in the number of infectious episodes. Further, the cost of nutritional support in the enteral feeding group was one-third of that in the parenteral nutrition group.

A slightly different study randomised 27 patients with prognostically acute pancreatitis to either enteral nutrition or standard care, where parenteral nutrition was not instituted from the outset.[90] Although no major complications arose from the provision of enteral nutrition, it was not possible to meet full nutritional requirements. In contrast to previous studies, enteral nutrition did not appear to affect markers of the inflammatory response (IL-6, tumour necrosis factor receptors, CRP). Moreover, the institution of enteral nutrition was associated with a significant deterioration in gut barrier function.

Recently, a large study from China randomised 96 patients with severe pancreatitis to parenteral nutrition versus nasojejunal feeding.[91] Measures of inflammation including CRP and IL-6 decreased earlier with enteral nutrition, as did APACHE II scores. Furthermore, mucosal permeability was improved, as inferred by urine endotoxin levels.

In an attempt to determine the efficacy of both enteral nutrition and antibiotic prophylaxis, Olah et al.[92] undertook a two-phase study. In the first phase, patients within 72 hours of the onset of prognostically severe acute pancreatitis were 'randomised' to either parenteral nutrition or enteral nutrition delivered by a nasojejunal feeding tube. In this phase of the study there was no significant difference in the rates of septic complications between the two treatment groups. The second phase of the study was a prospective cohort study, with all patients being given enteral nutrition and imipenem with prophylactic intent, with subsequent comparison of outcome measures obtained in phase 2 with those obtained in phase 1. Following their analysis, the authors of this study stated that the combination of enteral nutrition and antibiotic prophylaxis significantly reduced the rate of septic complications and the requirement for surgical intervention when compared with parenteral nutrition. However, the results of the study have to be interpreted with caution. The initial phase of the study was not truly 'randomised', with patients being allocated to treatment groups according to date of birth, whereas the second phase involved comparison of historical cohorts. Both of these flaws may result in bias.

Another small study randomised 17 patients with prognostically severe acute pancreatitis (APACHE II score = 6) to either enteral nutrition through a nasojejunal tube ($n = 8$) or parenteral nutrition ($n = 9$).[93] Not surprisingly, given the small numbers enrolled in the trial, there was no significant difference in morbidity between the two treatment groups, although the use of enteral nutrition was associated with an earlier institution of normal diet and resumption of normal bowel opening.

The interpretation of the results of all the published trials assessing the role of enteral nutrition and the subsequent translation of these into evidence-based clinical practice is difficult. Firstly, all the trials have insufficient power to determine the effects of enteral nutrition on the most relevant outcome measures of morbidity and mortality. The conclusions of two meta-analyses, one of which reported on six studies[94] and the other on two of the six studies,[95] were contradictory. In one, enteral nutrition was favoured;[95] in the other, the interpretation was that there were insufficient data upon which to make firm judgements.[94] Secondly, all the randomised trials to date have delivered enteral nutrition through a nasojejunal feeding tube requiring either radiological or endoscopic placement. However, a prospective observational study has reported that successful nasogastric feeding can be achieved in patients with severe acute pancreatitis.[96] Thirdly, other than the trial conducted by Powell et al.,[90] enteral nutrition was compared with early parenteral nutrition. In general, it is not standard practice to commence parenteral nutrition immediately following admission with acute pancreatitis. Furthermore, it is possible that the observed 'benefits' from the institution of enteral nutrition, as compared with parenteral nutrition, are in fact due to the induction of deleterious effects by parenteral nutrition. Fong et al.[97] have demonstrated that a nil-by-mouth regimen and the institution of parenteral nutrition in normal volunteers is associated with an increased inflammatory response following a stimulus and malnourished patients have an impairment of intestinal function and increased markers of the acute-phase response. Furthermore, the use of parenteral nutrition in acute pancreatitis is associated with a significant increase in line sepsis when compared with standard management.[98]

 Although there is no definitive evidence demonstrating that early enteral nutrition improves outcome in severe acute pancreatitis, all published studies demonstrate that enteral nutrition is feasible, safe and does not exacerbate the disease process. Further trials are required to determine the impact of early enteral nutrition in predicted severe acute pancreatitis on infectious complications and disease outcome.[94,95]

Other potential treatment strategies

Probiotic therapy

The use of probiotic therapy in acute pancreatitis is based on the hypothesis that colonisation of the proximal gastrointestinal tract by pathogenic bacteria is a precursor to the development of infected pancreatic necrosis. Probiotic therapy therefore aims to establish colonisation of the gastrointestinal tract by non-pathogenic bacteria, thereby reducing the risk of infective complications. This hypothesis was tested by randomising 45 patients with acute pancreatitis, 32 of whom had severe disease, to receive either live *Lactobacillus plantarum* ($n = 22$) or killed *Lactobacillus plantarum* ($n = 23$) delivered via a nasojejunal feeding tube, along with oat fibre as a bacterial substrate.[99] All patients received a standard enteral nutrition formula in addition to the live or killed *Lactobacillus plantarum*. Within this trial, probiotic therapy appeared to reduce the risk of developing either infected pancreatic necrosis or abscess. One patient who received live *Lactobacillus plantarum* developed pancreatic infection compared with seven patients in the control group ($P = 0.023$). Although these are encouraging results suggesting benefit from probiotic therapy, further trials are required.

Anticytokine therapy

With increased understanding of the pathogenetic mechanisms in acute pancreatitis, it is hoped that novel therapies will be developed that can perturb these mechanisms and improve outcome. Indeed, a large number of agents that either antagonise the proinflammatory response or augment the anti-inflammatory response have been demonstrated to ameliorate disease severity in animal models of acute pancreatitis. However, it should be noted that in these studies the agent is usually administered before or immediately after the induction of acute pancreatitis, a scenario that does not translate to the clinical situation. One such agent to undergo clinical trials was lexipafant, a high-affinity platelet-activating factor receptor antagonist which acts as a general down-regulator of the proinflammatory cytokine response. On the basis of encouraging results from initial trials, a large multicentre trial recruiting 1500 patients was undertaken. Although the trial results have not been formally reported, it is widely known that there was no improvement in mortality following the use of lexipafant, and that the manufacturers are now no longer pursuing this drug as a treatment for severe acute pancreatitis.

It is expected that further drugs perturbing the pathogenetic mechanisms of acute pancreatitis will be developed and will undergo clinical trials.

Prognosis

Current UK guidelines provide targets for mortality rates in acute pancreatitis.[46] These guidelines state that overall mortality should be less than 10% of patients admitted with acute pancreatitis, with a mortality rate less than 30% in those with prognostically severe acute pancreatitis. Encouragingly, recent epidemiological data have suggested that there has been a reduction in mortality rates over recent years.[44]

Treatment of gallstones in acute gallstone pancreatitis

In 1988, before laparoscopic surgery, Kelly and Wagner[100] randomised 165 patients with gallstone-induced acute pancreatitis to either early ($n = 83$) or late ($n = 82$) biliary surgery, with early surgery being undertaken within 48 hours of admission. In those with mild acute pancreatitis ($n = 125$) there was no significant difference in outcome between the two groups (morbidity: early 6.7% vs. late 3.3%,

$P > 0.10$; mortality: early 3.1% vs. late 0%, $P > 0.10$). However, in those with severe acute pancreatitis ($n = 40$) early biliary surgery resulted in a significant increase in morbidity and mortality (morbidity: early 82.6% vs. late 17.6%, $P < 0.001$; mortality: early 47.8% vs. late 11%, $P < 0.025$).

British Society of Gastroenterology guidelines recommend that patients with gallstone-induced mild acute pancreatitis should undergo cholecystectomy (laparoscopic) during the same hospital admission unless a clear plan for definitive treatment within the following 2 weeks has been made.[46] In patients with severe comorbid disease contraindicating cholecystectomy, definitive treatment may be provided by endoscopic sphincterotomy. In those with gallstone-induced severe disease, cholecystectomy should be delayed until disease resolution or undertaken as an additional procedure during surgery for a complication of the acute pancreatitis.

Key points

- Laparoscopic cholecystectomy is the gold standard intervention for the management of biliary colic and acute cholecystitis.
- Laparoscopic cholecystectomy during the index admission is both feasible and safe in patients with acute cholecystitis.
- Percutaneous cholecystostomy may be undertaken in those patients with acute cholecystitis who do not respond to conservative management and have significant comorbidity contraindicating emergency surgical intervention.
- Percutaneous cholecystostomy may be definitive therapy in patients with acute acalculous cholecystitis.
- Intravenous antibiotics and endoscopic drainage of the biliary tree form the basis of management for patients with acute cholangitis.
- Definitive management of acute cholangitis secondary to choledocholithiasis includes cholecystectomy in order to reduce the risk of further gallstone-related complications.
- Acute pancreatitis is an increasingly common life-threatening illness.
- Initial management of severe acute pancreatitis involves appropriate resuscitation and organ support.
- Prophylactic broad-spectrum antibiotics may reduce mortality and morbidity in severe acute pancreatitis.
- Early ERCP and ES should be undertaken in patients with gallstone-induced severe acute pancreatitis and evidence of either acute cholangitis or significant biliary obstruction (serum bilirubin >90 μmol/L).
- Surgery has little role in the initial management of severe acute pancreatitis.
- Cholecystectomy should be undertaken in patients with gallstone-induced acute pancreatitis.
- Complicated severe acute pancreatitis should be managed in a specialist unit.

References

1. Varghese JC, Farrell MA, Courtney G et al. A prospective comparison of magnetic resonance cholangiopancreatography with endoscopic retrograde cholangiopancreatography in the evaluation of patients with suspected biliary tract disease. Clin Radiol 1999; 54:513–20.

2. Williams E, Green J, Beckingham I et al. Guidelines on the management of common bile duct stones. Gut 2008; 57:1004–21.

3. Tranter SE, Thompson MH. Comparison of endoscopic sphincterotomy and laparoscopic exploration of the common bile duct. Br J Surg 2002; 89:1495–504.

4. Martin DJ, Vernon DR, Toouli J. Surgical versus endoscopic treatment of bile duct stones. Cochrane Database Syst Rev 2006; CD003327.

    No clear difference was found in primary success rates, morbidity or mortality between the two approaches in the above two studies.

5. Lo CM, Liu CL, Fan ST et al. Prospective randomized study of early versus delayed laparoscopic cholecystectomy for acute cholecystitis. Ann Surg 1998; 227:461–7.

    A randomised study of 99 patients to either early (within 72 hours) or delayed laparoscopic cholecystectomy. Early surgery was associated with a lower conversion rate (early 11% vs. delayed 23%; $P = 0.174$), lower complication rate (early 13% vs. delayed 29%; $P = 0.07$), shorter total hospital stay (early 6 days vs. delayed 11 days; $P < 0.001$) and shorter recuperation period (early 12 days vs. delayed 19 days; $P < 0.001$).

6. Lai PB, Kwong KH, Leung KL et al. Randomized trial of early versus delayed laparoscopic cholecystectomy for acute cholecystitis. Br J Surg 1998; 85:764–7.

    A randomised study of 104 patients to either early ($n = 53$) or delayed ($n = 51$) laparoscopic cholecystectomy. Surgery would appear to have been more difficult in the early group as manifested by significantly longer operating times (123 vs. 107 min; $P = 0.04$); however, this did not translate into a higher conversion rate (early 21% vs. delayed 24%; $P = 0.74$). Morbidity rates were similar between the two groups, with no bile duct injuries reported. Early surgery was associated with a significant reduction in overall hospital stay (7.6 vs. 11.6 days; $P < 0.001$).

7. Johansson M, Thune A, Blomqvist A et al. Management of acute cholecystitis in the laparoscopic era: results of a prospective, randomized clinical trial. J Gastrointest Surg 2003; 7:642–5.

    A study of 145 patients randomised to early laparoscopic cholecystectomy within the first 7 days (early; $n = 71$) or to interval cholecystectomy at 6–8 weeks (late; $n = 74$). In the late group, 26% failed conservative therapy and required urgent laparoscopic cholecystectomy. On an intention-to-treat basis, analysis demonstrated no significant difference in conversion rates (early 31% vs. delayed 29%; $P = 0.78$) or complications, although one major bile duct injury occurred in the delayed group. There was a reduction in overall hospital stay (early 5, range 3–63 days, vs. delayed 8, range 4–50 days; $P < 0.05$).

8. Kolla SB, Aggarwal S, Kumar A et al. Early vs delayed laparoscopic cholecystectomy for acute cholecystitis. Surg Endosc 2004; 18:1323–7.

    A study of 40 patients randomised to early (within 24 hours) or delayed (after 6–12 weeks) laparoscopic cholecystectomy. There was no significant difference in conversion rates, operative time, postoperative analgesia requirement or postoperative complications, but the early group had an increased intraoperative blood loss (228 mL vs. 114 mL) but shorter hospital stay (4.1 vs. 10.1 days).

9. Kiviluoto T, Siren J, Luukkonen P et al. Randomised trial of laparoscopic versus open cholecystectomy for acute and gangrenous cholecystitis. Lancet 1998; 351:321–5.

    There was a significantly lower complication rate in the laparoscopic group, with shorter hospital stay and quicker return to work.

10. Lau WY, Yuen WK, Chu KW et al. Systemic antibiotic regimens for acute cholecystitis treated by early cholecystectomy. Aust NZ J Surg 1990; 60:539–43.

    In a randomised trial of 203 patients, the continuation of cefamandole for 12 hours after surgery had equal efficacy with a prolonged dosage schedule of 7 days but was associated with less adverse drug reactions.

11. Lo LD, Vogelzang RL, Braun MA et al. Percutaneous cholecystostomy for the diagnosis and treatment of acute calculous and acalculous cholecystitis. J Vasc Intervent Radiol 1995; 6:629–34.

12. McGahan JP, Lindfors KK. Percutaneous cholecystostomy: an alternative to surgical cholecystostomy for acute cholecystitis? Radiology 1989; 173:481–5.

13. Ito K, Fujita N, Noda Y et al. Percutaneous cholecystostomy versus gallbladder aspiration for acute cholecystitis: a prospective randomized controlled trial. Am J Roentgenol 2004; 183:193–6.

14. Hatzidakis AA, Prassopoulos P, Petinarakis I et al. Acute cholecystitis in high-risk patients: percutaneous cholecystostomy vs conservative treatment. Eur Radiol 2002; 12:1778–84.

    A randomised trial of 123 patients with acute cholecystitis. Rates of clinical resolution and mortality were similar between the percutaneous cholecystostomy and conservative therapy groups.

15. Vetrhus M, Soreide O, Nesvik I et al. Acute cholecystitis: delayed surgery or observation. A randomized clinical trial. Scand J Gastroenterol 2003; 38:985–90.

16. McDermott VG, Arger P, Cope C. Gallstone recurrence and gallbladder function following percutaneous cholecystolithotomy. J Vasc Intervent Radiol 1994; 5:473–8.

17. Courtois CS, Picus DD, Hicks ME et al. Percutaneous gallstone removal: long-term follow-up. J Vasc Intervent Radiol 1996; 7:229–34.

18. Hellstern A, Leuschner U, Benjaminov A et al. Dissolution of gallbladder stones with methyl *tert*-butyl ether and stone recurrence: a European survey. Dig Dis Sci 1998; 43:911–20.

19. Glenn F, Becker CG. Acute acalculous cholecystitis. An increasing entity. Ann Surg 1982; 195:131–6.

20. Inoue T, Mishima Y. Postoperative acute cholecystitis: a collective review of 494 cases in Japan. Jpn J Surg 1988; 18:35–42.

21. Devine RM, Farnell MB, Mucha P Jr. Acute cholecystitis as a complication in surgical patients. Arch Surg 1984; 119:1389–93.

22. Hakala T, Nuutinen PJ, Ruokonen ET et al. Microangiopathy in acute acalculous cholecystitis. Br J Surg 1997; 84:1249–52.

23. Helbich TH, Mallek R, Madl C et al. Sonomorphology of the gallbladder in critically ill patients. Value of a scoring system and follow-up examinations. Acta Radiol 1997; 38:129–34.

24. Kalliafas S, Ziegler DW, Flancbaum L et al. Acute acalculous cholecystitis: incidence, risk factors, diagnosis, and outcome. Am Surg 1998; 64:471–5.

25. Kalff V, Froelich JW, Lloyd R et al. Predictive value of an abnormal hepatobiliary scan in patients with severe intercurrent illness. Radiology 1983; 146:191–4.

26. Almeida J, Sleeman D, Sosa JL et al. Acalculous cholecystitis: the use of diagnostic laparoscopy. J Laparoendosc Surg 1995; 5:227–31.

27. Boland GW, Lee MJ, Leung J et al. Percutaneous cholecystostomy in critically ill patients: early response and final outcome in 82 patients. Am J Roentgenol 1994; 163:339–42.

28. Shirai Y, Tsukada K, Kawaguchi H et al. Percutaneous transhepatic cholecystostomy for acute acalculous cholecystitis. Br J Surg 1993; 80:1440–2.

29. Sugiyama M, Tokuhara M, Atomi Y. Is percutaneous cholecystostomy the optimal treatment for acute cholecystitis in the very elderly? World J Surg 1998; 22:459–63.

30. Shapiro MJ, Luchtefeld WB, Kurzweil S et al. Acute acalculous cholecystitis in the critically ill. Am Surg 1994; 60:335–9.

31. Csendes A, Burdiles P, Maluenda F et al. Simultaneous bacteriologic assessment of bile from gallbladder and common bile duct in control subjects and patients with gallstones and common duct stones. Arch Surg 1996; 131:389–94.

32. Sung JJ, Lyon DJ, Suen R et al. Intravenous ciprofloxacin as treatment for patients with acute suppurative cholangitis: a randomized, controlled clinical trial. J Antimicrob Chemother 1995; 35:855–64.

A randomised trial assessing single antibiotic therapy demonstrated that intravenous ciprofloxacin alone improved the clinical condition in 85% of patients and had similar efficacy to a combination of ceftazidime, ampicillin and metronidazole.

33. Csendes A, Diaz JC, Burdiles P et al. Risk factors and classification of acute suppurative cholangitis. Br J Surg 1992; 79:655–8.

34. Balthazar EJ, Birnbaum BA, Naidich M. Acute cholangitis: CT evaluation. J Comput Assist Tomogr 1993; 17:283–9.

35. Thompson JE Jr, Pitt HA, Doty JE et al. Broad spectrum penicillin as an adequate therapy for acute cholangitis. Surg Gynecol Obstet 1990; 171:275–82.

A randomised clinical trial involving 96 patients with acute cholangitis in which piperacillin had similar efficacy to combination therapy with ampicillin and tobramycin, achieving clinical cure or significant improvement in 70% of patients.

36. Lai EC, Tam PC, Paterson IA et al. Emergency surgery for severe acute cholangitis. The high-risk patients. Ann Surg 1990; 211:55–9.

37. Tokyo guidelines for the management of acute cholangitis and cholecystitis. J Hepatobiliary Pancreat Surg 2007; 14:1–121.

38. Lai EC, Mok FP, Tan ES et al. Endoscopic biliary drainage for severe acute cholangitis. N Engl J Med 1992; 326:1582–6.

A randomised controlled trial comparing endoscopic biliary drainage with surgical decompression in 82 patients with severe acute cholangitis as manifested by signs of shock or progression of the disease despite appropriate antibiotics. In those undergoing endoscopic therapy there were fewer complications (34% vs. 66%; P > 0.05) but more importantly a significant reduction in mortality (10% vs. 32%; P < 0.03).

39. Lee DW, Chan AC, Lam YH et al. Biliary decompression by nasobiliary catheter or biliary stent in acute suppurative cholangitis: a prospective randomized trial. Gastrointest Endosc 2002; 56:361–5.

40. Pessa ME, Hawkins IF, Vogel SB. The treatment of acute cholangitis. Percutaneous transhepatic biliary drainage before definitive therapy. Ann Surg 1987; 205:389–92.

41. Boerma D, Rauws EA, Keulemans YC et al. Wait-and-see policy or laparoscopic cholecystectomy after endoscopic sphincterotomy for bile-duct stones: a randomised trial. Lancet 2002; 360:761–5.

42. Targarona EM, Ayuso RM, Bordas JM et al. Randomised trial of endoscopic sphincterotomy with gallbladder left in situ versus open surgery for common bile duct calculi in high-risk patients. Lancet 1996; 347:926–9.

43. Bradley EL. A clinically based classification system for acute pancreatitis. Summary of the International Symposium on Acute Pancreatitis, Atlanta, GA, 11–13 September 1992. Arch Surg 1993; 128:586–90.

44. McKay CJ, Evans S, Sinclair M et al. High early mortality rate from acute pancreatitis in Scotland, 1984–1995. Br J Surg 1999; 86:1302–5.

45. Dervenis C, Johnson CD, Bassi C et al. Diagnosis, objective assessment of severity, and management

of acute pancreatitis. Santorini consensus conference. Int J Pancreatol 1999; 25:195–210.

46. UK Working Party on Acute Pancreatitis. UK guidelines for the management of acute pancreatitis. Gut 2005; 54(Suppl. 3):iii1–9.

47. Banks PA. Practice guidelines in acute pancreatitis. Am J Gastroenterol 2006; 101:2379–400.

48. Mier J, Leon EL, Castillo A et al. Early versus late necrosectomy in severe necrotizing pancreatitis. Am J Surg 1997; 173:71–5.

49. Mayumi T, Ura H, Arata S et al. Evidence-based clinical practice guidelines for acute pancreatitis: proposals. J Hepatobiliary Pancreat Surg 2002; 9:413–22.

50. Uhl W, Warshaw A, Imrie C et al. IAP guidelines for the surgical management of acute pancreatitis. Pancreatology 2002; 2:565–73.

51. Imrie CW, Benjamin IS, Ferguson JC et al. A single-centre double-blind trial of Trasylol therapy in primary acute pancreatitis. Br J Surg 1978; 65:337–41.

52. Osborne DH, Imrie CW, Carter DC. Biliary surgery in the same admission for gallstone-associated acute pancreatitis. Br J Surg 1981; 68:758–61.

53. Blamey SL, Imrie CW, O'Neill J et al. Prognostic factors in acute pancreatitis. Gut 1984; 25:1340–6.

54. Ranson JH, Rifkind KM, Roses DF et al. Prognostic signs and the role of operative management in acute pancreatitis. Surg Gynecol Obstet 1974; 139:69–81.

55. Knaus WA, Draper EA, Wagner DP et al. APACHE II: a severity of disease classification system. Crit Care Med 1985; 13:818–29.

56. de Beaux A, Goldie AS, Ross JA et al. Serum concentrations of inflammatory mediators related to organ failure in patients with acute pancreatitis. Br J Surg 1996; 83:349–53.

57. Fan ST, Lai EC, Mok FP et al. Prediction of the severity of acute pancreatitis. Am J Surg 1993; 166:262–8; discussion 269.

58. Pezzilli R, Billi P, Miniero R et al. Serum interleukin-6, interleukin-8, and beta 2-microglobulin in early assessment of severity of acute pancreatitis. Comparison with serum C-reactive protein. Dig Dis Sci 1995; 40:2341–8.

59. Balthazar EJ, Robinson DL, Megibow AJ et al. Acute pancreatitis: value of CT in establishing prognosis. Radiology 1990; 174:331–6.

60. Schroder T, Kivisaari L, Somer K et al. Significance of extrapancreatic findings in computed tomography (CT) of acute pancreatitis. Eur J Radiol 1985; 5:273–5.

61. Larvin M, McMahon MJ. APACHE-II score for assessment and monitoring of acute pancreatitis. Lancet 1989; ii:201–5.

62. Wilson C, Heath DI, Imrie CW. Prediction of outcome in acute pancreatitis: a comparative study of APACHE II, clinical assessment and multiple factor scoring systems. Br J Surg 1990; 77:1260–4.

63. Triester SL, Kowdley KV. Prognostic factors in acute pancreatitis. J Clin Gastroenterol 2002; 34: 167–76.

64. Mofidi R, Duff MD, Madhavan KK et al. Identification of severe acute pancreatitis using an artificial neural network. Surgery 2007; 141:59–66.

65. Buter A, Imrie CW, Carter CR et al. Dynamic nature of early organ dysfunction determines outcome in acute pancreatitis. Br J Surg 2002; 89:298–302.

66. Johnson CD, Abu-Hilal M. Persistent organ failure during the first week as a marker of fatal outcome in acute pancreatitis. Gut 2004; 53:1340–4.

67. Mofidi R, Duff MD, Wigmore SJ et al. The association between early systemic inflammatory response, severity of multi-organ dysfunction and death in acute pancreatitis. Br J Surg 2006; 93:738–44.

68. Neoptolemos JP, Carr-Locke DL, London NJ et al. Controlled trial of urgent endoscopic retrograde cholangio-pancreatography and endoscopic sphincterotomy versus conservative treatment for acute pancreatitis due to gallstones. Lancet 1988; ii:979–83.

69. Fan ST, Lai EC, Mok FP et al. Early treatment of acute biliary pancreatitis by endoscopic papillotomy. N Engl J Med 1993; 328:228–32.

70. Fölsch UR, Nitsche R, Ludtke R et al. Early ERCP and papillotomy compared with conservative treatment for acute biliary pancreatitis. The German Study Group on Acute Biliary Pancreatitis. N Engl J Med 1997; 336:237–42.

71. Nowak A, Nowakowska Dulawa E, Marck T et al. Final results of the prospective, randomized, controlled study on endoscopic sphincterotomy versus conventional management in acute biliary pancreatitis [Abstract]. Gastroenterology 1995; 108:A380.

72. Pederzoli P, Bassi C, Vesentini S et al. A randomized multicenter clinical trial of antibiotic prophylaxis of septic complications in acute necrotizing pancreatitis with imipenem. Surg Gynecol Obstet 1993; 176:480–3.

73. Sainio V, Kemppainen E, Puolakkainen P et al. Early antibiotic treatment in acute necrotising pancreatitis. Lancet 1995; 346:663–7.

74. Delcenserie R, Yzet T, Ducroix JP. Prophylactic antibiotics in treatment of severe acute alcoholic pancreatitis. Pancreas 1996; 13:198–201.

75. Schwarz M, Isenmann R, Meyer H et al. Antibiotic use in necrotizing pancreatitis. Results of a controlled study [in German]. Dtsch Med Wochenschr 1997; 122:356–61.

76. Bassi C, Falconi M, Talamini G et al. Controlled clinical trial of pefloxacin versus imipenem in severe acute pancreatitis. Gastroenterology 1998; 115:1513–17.

77. Nordback I, Sand J, Saaristo R et al. Early treatment with antibiotics reduces the need for surgery

in acute necrotizing pancreatitis: a single-center randomized study. J Gastrointest Surg 2001; 5:113–18; discussion 118–20.

78. Isenmann R, Runzi M, Kron M et al. Prophylactic antibiotic treatment in patients with severe acute pancreatitis – A placebo-controlled double-blind trial. Gastroenterology 2004; 126:997–1004.

79. Luiten EJ, Hop WC, Lange JF et al. Controlled clinical trial of selective decontamination for the treatment of severe acute pancreatitis. Ann Surg 1995; 222:57–65.

80. Golub R, Siddiqi F, Pohl D. Role of antibiotics in acute pancreatitis: a meta-analysis. J Gastrointest Surg 1998; 2:496–503.

81. Sharma VK, Howden CW. Prophylactic antibiotic administration reduces sepsis and mortality in acute necrotizing pancreatitis: a meta-analysis. Pancreas 2001; 22:28–31.

82. Mazaki T, Ishii Y, Takayama T. Meta-analysis of prophylactic antibiotic use in acute necrotising pancreatitis. Br J Surg 2006; 93:674–84.

83. de Vries AC, Besselink MG, Buskens E et al. Randomised controlled trials of antibiotic prophylaxis in severe acute pancreatitis: relationship between methodological quality and outcome. Pancreatology 2007; 7:531–8.

84. Howard TJ, Temple MB. Prophylactic antibiotics alter the bacteriology of infected necrosis in severe acute pancreatitis. J Am Coll Surg 2002; 195: 759–67.

85. Beger HG, Rau B, Isenmann R et al. Antibiotic prophylaxis in severe acute pancreatitis. Pancreatology 2005; 5:10–19.

86. He YM, Lv XS, Ai ZL et al. Prevention and therapy of fungal infection in severe acute pancreatitis: a prospective clinical study. World J Gastroenterol 2003; 9:2619–21.

87. McClave SA, Greene LM, Snider HL et al. Comparison of the safety of early enteral vs parenteral nutrition in mild acute pancreatitis. J Parenter Enteral Nutr 1997; 21:14–20.

88. Windsor AC, Kanwar S, Li AG et al. Compared with parenteral nutrition, enteral feeding attenuates the acute phase response and improves disease severity in acute pancreatitis. Gut 1998; 42:431–5.

89. Kalfarentzos F, Kehagias J, Mead N et al. Enteral nutrition is superior to parenteral nutrition in severe acute pancreatitis: results of a randomized prospective trial. Br J Surg 1997; 84:1665–9.

90. Powell JJ, Murchison JT, Fearon KC et al. Randomized controlled trial of the effect of early enteral nutrition on markers of the inflammatory response in predicted severe acute pancreatitis. Br J Surg 2000; 87:1375–81.

91. Zhao G, Wang CY, Wang F et al. Clinical study on nutrition support in patients with severe acute pancreatitis. World J Gastroenterol 2003; 9:2105–8.

92. Olah A, Pardavi G, Belagyi T et al. Early nasojejunal feeding in acute pancreatitis is associated with a lower complication rate. Nutrition 2002; 18:259–62.

93. Gupta R, Patel K, Calder PC et al. A randomised clinical trial to assess the effect of total enteral and total parenteral nutritional support on metabolic, inflammatory and oxidative markers in patients with predicted severe acute pancreatitis (APACHE II = 6). Pancreatology 2003; 3:406–13.

94. Al-Omran M, Groof A, Wilke D. Enteral versus parenteral nutrition for acute pancreatitis. Cochrane Database Syst Rev 2003; CD002837.

95. Marik PE, Zaloga GP. Meta-analysis of parenteral nutrition versus enteral nutrition in patients with acute pancreatitis. Br Med J 2004; 328:1407.

96. Eatock FC, Brombacher GD, Steven A et al. Nasogastric feeding in severe acute pancreatitis may be practical and safe. Int J Pancreatol 2000; 28:25–31.

97. Fong YM, Marano MA, Barber A et al. Total parenteral nutrition and bowel rest modify the metabolic response to endotoxin in humans. Ann Surg 1989; 210:449–56; discussion 456–7.

98. Sax HC, Warner BW, Talamini MA et al. Early total parenteral nutrition in acute pancreatitis: lack of beneficial effects. Am J Surg 1987; 153: 117–24.

99. Olah A, Belagyi T, Issekutz A et al. Randomized clinical trial of specific *Lactobacillus* and fibre supplement to early enteral nutrition in patients with acute pancreatitis. Br J Surg 2002; 89:1103–7.

100. Kelly TR, Wagner DS. Gallstone pancreatitis: a prospective randomized trial of the timing of surgery. Surgery 1988; 104:600–5.

9

Acute conditions of the small bowel and appendix

Simon Paterson-Brown

Introduction

Acute disease of the small bowel, from which appendicitis is considered separately, contributes substantially to the workload of the general surgeon and many patients will present as emergencies. There are many causes of acute small-bowel disease and, because of the mobility and position of the bowel within the abdominal cavity, disease in any intraabdominal organ or any part of the investing layers of the abdominal cavity may involve the small bowel secondarily. The pattern of acute small-bowel disease varies with the age of the patient: some conditions are more common in young people, others in an older population. The incidence of acute surgical small-bowel pathology is difficult to estimate overall but is probably second to appendicitis as the site of disease requiring urgent surgical intervention. Acute small-bowel disease manifests itself in one of three main ways: (i) obstruction, (ii) peritonitis and (iii) haemorrhage. These categories are not mutually exclusive and more than one type of pathological process may exist in each clinical episode. Usually one category predominates but the clinical picture may change if the presentation or treatment is delayed.

Treatment of small-bowel disease may be operative or conservative, and the timing of any surgical intervention requires as much consideration as the causes and specific treatment of small-bowel disease.

Small-bowel obstruction

Although there are many causes of small-bowel obstruction (Box 9.1), the commonest cause in the developed world is adhesions secondary to previous surgery, followed by malignancy. By comparison, in the developing world the most common cause is hernia. A large retrospective study using the Scottish National Health Service medical linkage system estimated that 5.7% of all hospital readmissions following abdominal and pelvic surgery over a 10-year period were directly related to adhesions.[1] In order to avoid unnecessary surgery and to ensure the correct surgical approach is employed, an attempt should be made to diagnose the cause of the obstruction preoperatively where possible or at least to eliminate conditions that might require special treatment. In practice, however, the cause of the obstruction is often diagnosed at operation. A retrospective study of 102 patients undergoing surgery for adhesive small-bowel obstruction carried out between 1987 and 1992 and followed up for 14 years reported that a total of 273 further episodes of obstruction occurred, requiring 237 hospital admissions.[2] Nearly half of these further episodes resulted in more surgery.

Mechanism

The small bowel will respond to obstruction by the onset of vigorous peristalsis. This produces colicky abdominal pain usually in the central

Chapter 9

Box 9.1 • Causes of small-bowel obstruction

Within the lumen

Gallstone
Food bolus
Bezoars
Parasites (e.g. *Ascaris*)
Enterolith
Foreign body

Within the wall

Tumour
   Primary
      Small-bowel tumour
         Carcinoma
         Lymphoma
         Sarcoma
      Carcinoma of caecum
   Secondary
Inflammation
   Crohn's disease
   Radiation enteritis
   Postoperative stricture
   Potassium chloride stricture
   Vascultides (e.g. scleroderma)

Outside the wall

Adhesions
   Congenital
      Bands
   Acquired
      Postoperative
      Inflammatory
      Neoplastic
      Chemical (e.g. starch, talc)
      Pharmacological (e.g. practolol)
Hernia
   Primary
      Congenital (e.g. diaphragmatic)
      Acquired (e.g. inguinal, femoral, etc.)
   Secondary
      Incisional hernia
      Internal postoperative hernia (e.g. lateral space, mesenteric defect)

abdomen as the small bowel is of midgut embryological origin. As the obstruction develops, the proximal intestine dilates and fills with fluid, producing systemic hypovolaemia. Further fluid is lost through vomiting, which occurs early if the obstruction is proximal. As the process continues, the risk of complications increases. If the blood supply is compromised, infarction and perforation will occur. If the blood supply remains intact and the bowel is readily decompressed by vomiting and subsequent nasogastric suction, the peristalsis will eventually stop, leaving grossly dilated, non-functioning bowel; auscultation will reveal a silent abdomen. In the former scenario the pain, initially colicky, will

become continuous, whereas in the latter even the colicky pain may cease as peristalsis stops. The aim of management must be to identify possible strangulation before gangrene and perforation occurs, so that early surgery can be arranged. There is less urgency in the recognition of non-strangulating obstruction, and a period of decompression and intravenous fluid resuscitation may allow resolution to occur without surgery. However, failure of the obstruction to resolve after 24–48 hours is usually an indication for surgical intervention.

Presentation

The typical clinical presentation of small-bowel obstruction is central abdominal colicky pain, vomiting (which is often bile-stained), abdominal distension and a reduction or absence of flatus. Vomiting may be less of a feature and a greater degree of abdominal distension observed if the blockage is in the distal ileum – in which case the vomiting often becomes 'faeculant' as the stagnant small-bowel contents become degraded by bacterial colonisation. Bowel sounds increase and may be audible to the patient. Localised peritonitic pain and tenderness may develop and this suggests incipient strangulation. In some patients there may be an obvious causative feature such as an irreducible hernia. The presence of surgical scars is important, as is any history of previous intra-abdominal pathology.

Although small-bowel obstruction can occur without development of abdominal pain, the absence of this symptom should be viewed with caution. This is particularly the case in postoperative patients, where small-bowel obstruction and intestinal ileus can be difficult to differentiate. The history and examination of the patient should be sufficiently detailed to allow a diagnosis of small-bowel obstruction and to determine possible causes. Complicated small-bowel obstruction, with ischaemia or perforation, should be readily detectable by marked abdominal tenderness. It is essential to assess the patient's general state, particularly the degree of dehydration and its effect on the patient, so that adequate resuscitation is undertaken prior to any planned surgical treatment.

Investigation

The investigations undertaken in patients with small-bowel obstruction are aimed at:

1. assessing the general state of the patient;
2. confirming the diagnosis of small-bowel obstruction;
3. identifying, if possible, which patients should undergo early surgery (those with a high risk of strangulation) and those in whom a non-operative approach is appropriate.

Figure 9.1 • Small-bowel follow-through demonstrating a benign stricture in the proximal jejunum with gross proximal dilatation.

These investigations have been discussed in detail in Chapter 5 and, apart from emphasising the value of contrast studies (**Fig. 9.1**) and the increasing use of computed tomography (CT; **Fig. 9.2**), they will not be repeated here, except to reinforce the current view that to date identifying those patients with possible strangulation remains difficult, irrespective of which tests are used, and the surgeon must base most of his or her decision-making on clinical assessment.

Management

General management

As in all patients admitted to hospital with an abdominal emergency, the first step in management is fluid resuscitation. Patients usually need several litres of normal saline with potassium supplementation in the first few hours after admission. There remains controversy as to whether colloid or crystalloid fluid is most suitable and each unit will have its own protocols. As a rule of thumb, patients without significant clinical signs of hypovolaemia can usually be adequately resuscitated with normal saline. However, those who present with hypotension and tachycardia on admission will benefit from the addition of colloids as well as oxygen. Patients with a long history are likely to be severely dehydrated, with an alkalosis and associated hypokalaemia, the former due to loss of hydrogen ions in the vomit and the latter from renal compensation. Urinary catheterisation is essential to monitor response to resuscitation and measurement of central venous pressure can be very helpful in the elderly, particularly in

Figure 9.2 • Multislice CT scan with intravenous contrast demonstrating small-bowel obstruction. With thanks to Dr Dilip Patel, Consultant Radiologist, Royal Infirmary, Edinburgh.

those patients with coexisting morbidity. Adequate fluid replacement must be given before any surgical intervention is planned and can be given rapidly if required, even in the elderly, provided appropriate monitoring is used (see also Chapter 16).

Decompression of the stomach with a nasogastric tube will reduce vomiting in most patients, help to decompress the bowel and reduce the risk of airway contamination from aspiration. Fluid lost from the nasogastric tube should be replaced with additional intravenous crystalloids (normal saline) and potassium supplements. Analgesia should be given early and in adequate doses, with opiates the most commonly used. This will not mask signs of localised or generalised peritonitis and there is no justification for withholding adequate analgesia while waiting for further clinical assessment. However, the analgesia requirement needs to be reviewed regularly, especially in the early stages of management, as a persistent and recurrent requirement for increasing amounts of opiate analgesia is a strong sign that underlying strangulation is a possibility and surgery indicated. Again, as in all emergency patients, antithromboembolic prophylaxis should be commenced early and continued until resolution (see Chapter 14), particularly in elderly patients and those with malignancy.

Non-operative management

Intravenous fluids and nasogastric aspiration are the two components of the 'drip and suck' regimen, which is the first-line treatment for most patients with obstruction, particularly when the underlying cause is thought to be adhesions, as spontaneous resolution will occur in the majority. As mentioned earlier, this treatment plan should be abandoned at the first suggestion of underlying strangulation. Although non-operative management can be continued for several days in the absence of any suggestion of strangulation, surgical exploration is generally indicated if the obstruction fails to resolve after 24–48 hours. In some patients with known extensive adhesions from multiple previous explorations, it might be worth waiting longer and if so attention should be paid to nutritional support, sometimes necessitating insertion of a central line for parenteral feeding (see Chapter 17).

Surgical management

The particular circumstances of any given case determine the relative need for surgical intervention, but some of the commonest features in decision-making are listed in Box 9.2.

Operative principles

Once a decision to operate has been made, patients should be fully resuscitated, treatment of comorbidity optimised and the stomach emptied with a nasogastric tube. The wide range of possible surgical procedures should be explained to the patient. Prophylactic antibiotics and antithromboembolic prophylaxis (if not already started) should be administered.

Box 9.2 • Small-bowel obstruction: indications for surgery

Absolute indication (surgery as soon as patient resuscitated)

Generalised peritonitis
Visceral perforation
Irreducible hernia
Localised peritonitis

Relative indication (surgery within 24 hours)

Palpable mass lesion
'Virgin' abdomen
Failure to improve (continuing pain, high nasogastric aspirates)

Trial of conservatism (wait and see and/or investigate)

Incomplete obstruction
Previous surgery
Advanced malignancy
Diagnostic doubt (possible ileus)

Generally, a midline incision is the most flexible when the diagnosis is unknown. If the patient has a previous midline incision, this should be excised and extended cranially or caudally so that the peritoneal cavity can be entered through a virgin area rather than directly through the back of the old scar. In particular, loops of small bowel may be densely adherent to the back of the old scar and it can be difficult to recognise a change in tissue plane before the lumen of the bowel is entered. Although this is not a major problem if the small bowel is normal, it is clearly best avoided if the bowel wall is grossly distended, friable and diseased (such as from previous irradiation).

Having entered the abdominal cavity, the first step is to identify the point at which the dilated bowel proximal to the obstruction changes to collapsed distal bowel. It is important to demonstrate that such a change is present as this confirms the diagnosis of mechanical obstruction and identifies the obstructing point. The presence of uniformly dilated small bowel, or no definite point of change in diameter of the bowel, suggests that the clinical diagnosis of mechanical obstruction may be incorrect. Dilated bowel can be decompressed, usually by milking the contents proximally and aspirating via the nasogastric tube, which should be of a large size. If the small-bowel contents are thick and will not easily pass retrogradely to the stomach or if the bowel is so friable that retrograde decompression might produce a tear, then a suction catheter may be inserted through a small enterotomy. Decompression is particularly useful in a distal obstruction as a large number of dilated loops can be difficult to handle and make subsequent abdominal closure difficult. The large amount of fluid within the bowel makes it heavy and if it is removed from the abdominal cavity, it should be supported so that the mesentery is not stretched or damaged. The large surface area of dilated loops results in considerable insensible fluid loss and therefore if it is anticipated that the viscera will lie outside the abdominal cavity for a significant length of time, it should be placed in a waterproof 'bowel' bag or wrapped in moist swabs. The dilated bowel may be friable and should be handled with care.

Having identified the point of obstruction, the cause is dealt with. If it is due to adhesions, they should be divided as completely as possible, and although it is not necessary or helpful to divide every last adhesion within the abdomen (as these will inevitably re-form), enough should be divided to confirm that there remains no possible site of obstruction between the DJ flexure and the caecum. It is essential to recognise the patient in whom the clinical diagnosis of mechanical small-bowel obstruction is incorrect, and the presence of adhesions does not in itself confirm the diagnosis.

The small bowel should be resected if it is clearly ischaemic or there is disease or narrowing in the bowel at the point of obstruction and an anastomosis may be carried out if both ends of the bowel are healthy. However, even after removing the obstruction, exteriorisation of the bowel may be indicated if there is also generalised disease of the bowel and when an anastomotic dehiscence might be more likely. An ileostomy may be indicated in patients with Crohn's disease as part of their long-term management, and the possibility of such a step should be recognised, considered and discussed with the patient before undertaking the exploratory laparotomy.

Abdominal closure should always be carried out using a mass closure technique. Although continuous sutures are most popular, in those patients in whom closure is difficult or in whom healing might be reduced, interrupted mass closure should be considered. There are some patients with gross obstruction in whom, even after relief of obstruction, the swollen and oedematous bowel is clearly going to make closure very difficult and dehiscence a significant risk, irrespective of the method of closure. In these patients the use of a prosthetic mesh to allow temporary closure, with subsequent removal and formal closure a few days later, should be seriously considered. If at subsequent surgery it is still not possible to approximate the fascial edges, then the mesh can be left in situ and the wound edges mobilised and closed over the top. Further discussions on abdominal sepsis and dehiscence are covered in Chapter 18.

Special conditions

Radiation enteritis

Patients can present with an acute abdomen during radiotherapy due to radiation enteritis or with acute-on-chronic attacks many years later. Patients in the former scenario can present considerable diagnostic difficulties as they are often neutropenic or suffering other side-effects of their treatment. The possibility of a primary pathology, such as acute appendicitis, arising during the course of radiotherapy must also be borne in mind but, where possible, surgical exploration is best avoided.

A more common acute presentation is with adhesions due to previous radiotherapy and these patients normally have obstructive symptoms. Again, a non-operative management policy is the best course as laparotomy is fraught with difficulty. The adhesions are often dense and, if the small bowel is inadvertently injured during mobilisation, there is a significant risk that it might not heal whether it is repaired or anastomosed.

Malignant obstruction

Primary tumours of the small bowel are rare but can be the cause of acute small-bowel obstruction. A diagnosis in such situations is rarely made preoperatively and surgical management at laparotomy will depend on the exact nature of the disease.

A more common problem is the patient with advanced intra-abdominal malignancy, with or without a past history of surgical treatment for intra-abdominal malignancy, who presents with bowel obstruction. These patients usually respond to initial non-operative management and thus emergency laparotomy is less likely to be carried out. If the obstruction fails to settle or rapidly recurs, there is usually time to carry out appropriate investigations to determine the extent of the disease. Ascites can be a confusing clinical factor in such a patient and aspiration for cytology to confirm widespread malignancy can be helpful. Clearly, in the presence of advanced and disseminated malignancy laparotomy should be avoided at all costs. However, if the obstructive symptoms are difficult to manage non-operatively and the patient is otherwise in reasonable condition, a laparotomy may be useful in the short term. When surgery is necessary, the exact procedure will depend on the operative findings. The choice usually lies between resection or bypass.

However, it is important to recognise that not all patients have obstruction due to their malignant process. One study of patients who presented with obstruction following previous treatment of intra-abdominal malignancy, either by surgery or radiotherapy, reported that in around one-third of such patients the obstruction was due to a cause other than secondary malignancy.[3] In a study from Japan of 85 patients who had previously undergone surgery for gastric cancer and who were subsequently readmitted to hospital with intestinal obstruction, the cause was benign adhesions in 20%.[4]

The results of bypass entero-enterostomy for malignant adhesions are generally poor, with short periods of patient survival. For this reason there is growing expertise among palliative care physicians in the medical management of intestinal obstruction.[5] The principles involve the use of fluid diet, steroids and octreotide. The results of such management are variable but it does offer the opportunity to spare a patient the morbidity of laparotomy in the terminal phase of their disease. If in doubt, a CT may be helpful in demonstrating a single area of obstruction which might be amenable to surgery as compared to extensive intra-abdominal disease without a single area of obstruction.

A third option of surgical management, which is appropriate in a small minority of patients, is placement of a percutaneous gastrostomy tube. This is certainly highly effective at decompressing an obstructed stomach and is more acceptable than the use of a long-term nasogastric tube. On occasions after completion of a laparotomy, a feeding jejunostomy placed distal to the obstruction might be considered in order to maintain nutrition in a patient with proximal disease which is low volume but irresectable. Total parenteral nutrition may also be considered in patients with low volume but irresectable disease in whom the gastrointestinal (GI) tract cannot be accessed, but for it to be worthwhile facilities should exist to manage the patient at home.

Groin hernia

Any hernia can present with intestinal obstruction (**Fig. 9.3**) and if presentation is delayed, gangrene

Figure 9.3 • Supine abdominal radiograph demonstrating small-bowel obstruction in a patient with an irreducible femoral hernia.

may have occurred and a bowel resection may be necessary. A Richter hernia involves part of the circumference of the bowel wall and the lumen is not obstructed. Infarction of the trapped bowel wall segment can still occur and there will be exquisite localised tenderness over a potential hernia site; the indication for surgical intervention is usually clinically apparent.

Any patient with acute symptoms of a hernia that is irreducible should have urgent surgery, with repair carried out in the usual way. In the presence of obstruction necessitating bowel resection, it is probably best to avoid use of a prosthetic mesh. When there has been gross contamination of the surrounding area, the risk of complications is obviously increased and a full treatment course of antibiotics should be given. In most cases, direct approach to the hernia is appropriate. The incarcerated tissue may reduce under anaesthesia and it is unlikely, should this occur, that there will have been strangulation. However, the bowel loops must be inspected from within the hernia sac to ensure that a gangrenous loop of bowel or a strictured segment has not dropped back into the abdominal cavity.

A final consideration is the patient who has an asymptomatic hernia who develops acute intestinal obstruction and who then may demonstrate signs of an apparently irreducible swelling. The intestinal obstruction raises intra-abdominal pressure and this will, in turn, produce the irreducible hernia. The unwary may find the hernia difficult to reduce and, in their efforts to do so, elicit tenderness. This is likely to occur in patients with ascites and large-bowel obstruction due to colorectal cancer. Thus, it is worth obtaining a plain abdominal radiograph in all patients with an irreducible hernia and apparent bowel obstruction. The absence of dilated small-bowel loops, or the presence of a dilated colon, should suggest the possibility that the apparently 'incarcerated' hernia is a secondary effect of some other intra-abdominal pathology. If in doubt the groin hernia should be explored and, in the absence of conclusive evidence that this is the cause of obstruction, a full laparotomy carried out. A CT scan may help reach the correct diagnosis preoperatively.

Enterolith obstruction

Enterolith obstruction is rare: the commonest types are gallstone ileus and bezoars. Gallstone ileus typically occurs in the elderly female and is due to the development of a cholecystoduodenal fistula after an episode of acute cholecystitis. The gallstone may be visible on a plain abdominal radiograph and gas can often be seen within the biliary tree. At surgery the stone should be removed by proximal enterotomy and the intestine proximal to the obstruction carefully palpated to exclude the presence of a second large gallstone. In these circumstances the gallbladder should be left alone, as cholecystectomy can be difficult and hazardous but usually unnecessary.

Bezoars may arise in psychiatric patients, the normal population who have over-indulged in particular types of food (e.g. oranges and peanuts) and those who have ingested a foreign body. Rarely, they can occur with material that is collected within a jejunal diverticulum.

Intussusception

This form of obstruction is rarely diagnosed preoperatively in adults. In children, acute presentation is usually to the paediatric department and the main differential diagnosis is GI infection. This is discussed in more detail in Chapter 12. Intussusception in adults is usually caused by benign or malignant tumours of the bowel, which should be treated on their merits once detected at laparotomy.

Connective tissue disorders

There are several systemic connective tissue disorders that can affect the GI tract and result in a loss of peristaltic power. These patients generally present with chronic symptoms and the presence of the underlying disorder is established. Occasionally, symptoms suggesting acute GI obstruction are present and the differentiation between full mechanical obstruction and ileus can be difficult. Expectant management of these patients should be pursued whenever possible. The obstructed episode may progress to perforation of the bowel and the patient can present with free gas visible on erect chest radiographs.

Surgical intervention should be based on the clinical condition of the patient and a laparotomy is not always necessary. If peritonitis is present, the perforated bowel should be resected and consideration given to bringing the proximal bowel out as an ileostomy depending on the site and state of disease. In addition, postoperative ileus is common and the differentiation of a further episode of mechanical obstruction or continuing ileus presents a major diagnostic challenge.

Intestinal obstruction in the early postoperative period

GI ileus can occur after any intra-abdominal operation. The surgeon may also be asked to see patients who have undergone orthopaedic or gynaecological procedures who have apparent bowel obstruction. Each case must be judged on its merits but the differentiation between true mechanical obstruction and paralytic ileus can be difficult. In patients who genuinely have a mechanical obstruction, appropriate surgical intervention is frequently delayed as a result of this diagnostic dilemma. In these patients, the use of water-soluble contrast small-bowel studies and CT with both intravenous and oral contrast are often helpful and should be considered early.[6] Ultrasound is also useful as it may demonstrate lack of peristalsis, which would support the diagnosis of an ileus.[7]

Laparoscopy

Following the introduction and development of laparoscopic surgery, there have been a few reports regarding the use of laparoscopy and laparoscopic surgery in the treatment of small-bowel obstruction and the division of band adhesions.[8] It must be pointed out, however, that this is a risky procedure because of the distended loops of small bowel, and laparoscopy must be performed with great care and using an 'open' technique. It is probably most appropriate when the cause of the adhesive obstruction is likely to be a single band (**Fig. 9.4**), such as might occur in a patient who has previously had an appendicectomy but no other major abdominal surgery. Unless the surgeon has extensive experience in laparoscopic surgery, conventional open surgery should be the choice for the treatment of intestinal obstruction that requires operation.

Peritonitis

Small-bowel pathology may present as an acute abdomen, with either localised or generalised peritonitis. This may represent the end stage of any condition causing obstruction, but this section considers those conditions that present with primarily inflammatory signs.

Crohn's disease

Crohn's disease is a chronic relapsing inflammatory disease that can affect any part of the GI tract. A common presentation is inflammation of the terminal ileum and this occasionally presents as an acute abdomen. The small bowel alone is affected in approximately 30% of patients and the small

Figure 9.4 • Laparoscopic view of a band adhesion. With thanks to Luigi Sussman, Auckland, New Zealand.

bowel and colon together in 50%. The incidence of Crohn's disease is highest in the USA, the UK and Scandinavia and is rare in Asia and Africa, suggesting that dietary factors may be important. Similar to appendicitis, the disease can appear at any age but is most frequent in young adults and there may be a familial tendency. It is thought that the disease is most likely an immunological disorder, although the exact mechanism remains unclear. The final pathway is probably a microvasculitis in the bowel wall. Where possible, the management of patients with Crohn's disease should be undertaken by a surgeon with a special interest in this condition and the reader is referred to the much more detailed account of this disease in the *Colorectal Surgery* volume of the *Companion to Specialist Surgical Practice* series.[9] Only first principles for managing an acute episode are discussed in this chapter.

Presentation

A typical acute clinical episode presents with abdominal pain, diarrhoea and possible fever. These symptoms can be acute in onset in a patient who has previously been entirely well. An acute presentation is more likely in young adults, hence the differential diagnosis of Crohn's disease in patients with suspected appendicitis.

Two other clinical presentations occur, although they are less likely to be acute. First, resolving Crohn's disease will produce fibrosis in the ileum that can cause obstructive symptoms. These tend to be subacute or chronic and an acute presentation with small-bowel obstruction is rare. Second, entero-enteric or entero-cutaneous fistula occurs in Crohn's disease because of the transmural inflammation that is a characteristic histological finding.

Investigation

A patient who presents with right iliac fossa pain, but in whom the symptoms are more insidious than typical appendicitis, should give rise to clinical suspicion. Non-specific inflammatory markers may be markedly elevated (white cell count, platelet count, alkaline phosphatase, erythrocyte sedimentation rate). However, these markers can be raised in acute appendicitis and will not differentiate Crohn's disease. An ultrasound scan may show thickening of the bowel wall or a mass, and if these signs are present further investigation should be undertaken. A radiolabelled white cell scan, CT or small-bowel enema can suggest the diagnosis.

Surgery for acute Crohn's disease presenting de novo

If a patient with known Crohn's disease presents with an acute flare-up or during first presentation, and the diagnosis of Crohn's disease is established before surgery, the patient should be referred to a surgeon with a special interest in this condition. However, during the first presentation of this condition, the diagnosis is often only suspected at the time of laparotomy and the surgeon must proceed according to first principles. In the presence of a localised inflammatory mass or stricture, resection and primary anastomosis are appropriate. If surgery has been carried out for suspected appendicitis and a normal appendix with ileocaecal Crohn's disease is discovered, the appendix should be removed with careful repair of the caecum, so that the possible diagnosis of acute appendicitis is ruled out of any future attacks of pain. No further action needs to be taken at this time for the Crohn's disease and appropriate treatment can be started in the postoperative period. Fortunately, extensive Crohn's disease affecting the entire small bowel is an uncommon finding at laparotomy, but in this situation the bare minimum should be carried out once the diagnosis has been established and any acute pathology (such as stricture) dealt with. If a stricture is found it should be resected, both to treat the problem and to confirm the diagnosis. If multiple strictures are found, and this will be rare in the acute first presentation, resection of one and multiple stricturoplasties of the others should be carried out. The differential diagnosis of lymphoma should of course be considered and frozen section may help confirm the cause.

Mesenteric ischaemia

Mesenteric ischaemia can be due to embolism or thrombosis, arterial or venous, and may be acute or chronic. Chronic mesenteric ischaemia is also termed 'mesenteric claudication' and is usually caused by a stenosis in the proximal part of the superior mesenteric artery. Patients develop cramp-like abdominal pains after eating, caused by the increased oxygen requirements to the small intestine, which cannot be met by increased blood flow because of the stenosis. The disease is usually associated with atherosclerosis and the investigation of choice is mesenteric angiography. Further management should be transferred to a specialist vascular surgeon and is not discussed further here.

Acute mesenteric ischaemia can affect any part of the GI tract, but is most common in the small bowel and colon. Acute ischaemia to the small bowel will usually produce infarction, whereas ischaemia to the large bowel may present less dramatically with bloody diarrhoea and abdominal pain, which will usually settle over the course of a few days and is often termed 'ischaemic colitis'. Delayed strictures may occur.

Acute small-bowel ischaemia is caused by either thrombosis or embolus. Thrombosis may occur in the superior mesenteric artery or its branches, usually associated with underlying atherosclerosis.

Embolus is often associated with atrial fibrillation, when the patient may have mural thrombosis in the atrium that dislodges and impacts itself somewhere in the superior mesenteric artery distribution. Venous thrombosis in the distribution of the superior mesenteric vein is a less common cause of acute small-bowel ischaemia but may be related to increased blood coagulability, portal vein thrombosis, dehydration, infection, compression and vasoconstricting drugs.

Early detection of acute mesenteric ischaemia is difficult (see Chapter 5) and failure to detect this condition early continues to be one of the major causes of morbidity and mortality. The diagnosis is usually more common in the elderly patient who gives a history of vague abdominal pain getting worse, often colicky in nature. There may be a background history of atherosclerosis, but not invariably so. Examination findings are often unremarkable, lulling the clinician into a false sense of security. Detection of atrial fibrillation or decreased peripheral pulses should alert the clinician to an underlying vascular problem, but even then early diagnosis remains the exception rather than the rule.

The investigations for possible mesenteric ischaemia have been discussed in detail in Chapter 5 and are not repeated here. CT with intravenous contrast performed as a diagnostic test for the 'acute abdomen' may suggest the diagnosis, but angiography or CT angiography (**Fig. 9.5**) is more useful if the diagnosis is suspected. However, by this stage a more appropriate investigation is likely to be laparoscopy or laparotomy. Patients in whom a diagnosis is suspected should be resuscitated and prepared for

Figure 9.5 • Multislice CT scan with intravenous contrast demonstrating ischaemic bowel due to superior mesenteric vein thrombosis. With thanks to Dr Dilip Patel, Consultant Radiologist, Royal Infirmary, Edinburgh.

abdominal surgery. Once the diagnosis has been confirmed, a decision needs to be made as to whether the ischaemic bowel is salvageable by vascular reconstruction. If the underlying cause is thrombosis, then resection should be performed; however, if an embolus is present, then exploration of the superior mesenteric artery with removal of the embolus may save an extended small-bowel resection. This procedure is difficult and may require associated vascular reconstruction. Advice should be sought from a specialist vascular surgeon.

If surgical resection is carried out, primary anastomosis may be performed providing the blood supply to both proximal and distal margins is adequate. If embolectomy and reconstruction have been performed, then both distal and proximal ends should be brought out as stomas with repeat laparotomy performed in 48 hours. There is a tendency among some surgeons to staple off the proximal and distal ends of bowel, forcing the surgeon to re-explore the patient in 48 hours, rather than performing an anastomosis and basing further management on clinical condition. Following straightforward thrombosis, it is safe to perform primary anastomosis providing good pulses are evident in both proximal and distal resection margins. Attention must still be given in the postoperative period to the general condition of the patient in order that any possible secondary ischaemic event can be detected early.

Unfortunately, the majority of patients with mesenteric ischaemia only have the diagnosis made at laparotomy and the small intestine is invariably beyond salvage and requires resection. If the whole of the superior mesenteric artery has been affected, the majority of the small bowel and part of the proximal colon will often be involved and no resection should be performed. These patients should receive intravenous opiates and be kept well sedated, as death will occur shortly afterwards.

 Overall prognosis is better following acute mesenteric venous infarction as compared to acute mesenteric arterial ischaemia, and survival better following arterial embolism as compared to arterial thrombosis.[10]

Meckel's diverticulum

Meckel's diverticulum is a remnant of the omphalomesenteric or vitelline duct. It arises from the antimesenteric border of the distal ileum approximately 60 cm from the iliocaecal valve. It may contain ectopic tissue, usually gastric, and is estimated to be found in approximately 2% of patients. Meckel's diverticulum may remain completely asymptomatic throughout life, particularly if it has a broad base and does not contain ectopic gastric mucosa. Occasionally, a band may exist between Meckel's diverticulum and the umbilicus, which can cause small-bowel obstruction. This should be treated as for a congenital band adhesion, although resection of the diverticulum should accompany division of the band. Occasionally, the diverticulum may intussuscept, also causing obstruction. Again, this will require reduction and excision. The other two common complications of Meckel's diverticulum are inflammation, when the patient presents with signs and symptoms similar to acute appendicitis, and haemorrhage. Acute inflammation is rarely suspected before surgery and the patient is usually diagnosed on the operating table (**Fig. 9.6**) once a normal appendix has been found through a right iliac fossa incision or at laparoscopy. In the presence of inflammation Meckel's diverticulum should be excised and the small bowel repaired (**Fig. 9.7**). Occult GI bleeding may occur from a Meckel diverticulum that contains ectopic gastric mucosa and the diagnosis is usually established by isotope scan or CT angiogram. The treatment is surgical resection.

Figure 9.6 • Acutely inflamed Meckel's diverticulum identified at laparotomy.

Figure 9.7 • Operative view after resection of the Meckel's diverticulum shown in Fig. 9.6.

Haemorrhage

Disease of the small intestine is an occasional cause of acute GI haemorrhage. There are no specific clinical features that distinguish the small bowel as the source rather than the colon, except that the blood loss may be less 'fresh' and more like melaena. As discussed in Chapter 7, it is important to exclude bleeding from a gastroduodenal source at an early stage by upper GI endoscopy. The most commonly encountered causes are vascular malformation, peptic ulceration in a Meckel's diverticulum and small-bowel tumour. These are all treated by resection.

One of the major problems at operation is that a vascular abnormality may produce no external signs. The mobility and variable anatomical layout of the small bowel means that it can be difficult to identify a bleeding point that has been demonstrated by red cell scan or angiography. If a bleeding point is found during angiography, a catheter should be passed by the radiologist into the mesenteric branches as close as possible to the bleeding point to aid surgical localisation. If this has not been possible, intraoperative enteroscopy may be helpful. Occasionally, the only option is to place segmental soft bowel clamps throughout the small intestine, resecting the segment that fills up with blood after a period of waiting. However, blind resection is often unrewarding and the risks of rebleeding are high. If no bleeding point can be identified, the surgeon can either close and await events, hoping that further bleeding does not occur (and this can often be the case), or divide the small bowel around its midpoint, bringing out two stomas. Subsequent bleeding can then be identified to one or other side and enteroscopy used to localise it further.

Acute appendicitis

Acute appendicitis is the most common intra-abdominal surgical emergency that requires operation and has an incidence of 7–12% in the population of USA and Europe. Although frequently described as a childhood illness, the peak incidence is towards 30 years of age. It is slightly more common in males (1.3–1.6:1) but the operation of appendicectomy is more common in women because of other mimicking conditions (see below and also Chapter 5). The reader is referred to Chapter 5 for description of some of the general features and investigation of patients with acute abdominal pain, many of which relate directly to acute appendicitis.

Pathology

The aetiology of acute appendicitis is bacterial infection secondary to blockage of the lumen by faecoliths, parasitic worms, tumours of caecum or the appendix itself and enlargement of lymphoid aggregates within the appendix wall. In many cases, however, the cause of the obstruction is unknown. Barium contrast studies typically fail to demonstrate an appendiceal lumen in patients with acute appendicitis, and they are no longer used in the acute setting to make the diagnosis. There is little seasonal variation but there may be a familial tendency. The incidence has been falling since the 1930s, presumably because of improved living standards and general hygiene. Changes in dietary habits, such as an increase in dietary fibre, may also be a factor as appendicitis is less common in those countries with a high roughage diet (e.g. Central Africa).

The pathology of acute appendicitis is classically described as suppurative, gangrenous or perforated. Typically, there is full-thickness inflammation of the appendix wall; as the disease progresses, adjacent tissues, particularly the omentum, may also become inflamed. Haemorrhagic ulceration and necrosis in the wall indicate gangrenous appendicitis, and subsequent perforation may be associated with a localised periappendiceal mass/abscess or generalised peritonitis.

Clinical features

The presentation of acute appendicitis varies widely but the classical history is of central abdominal pain over 12–24 hours shifting to the right iliac fossa. Nausea and vomiting are common but diarrhoea less so. On examination, the patient usually exhibits a low-grade pyrexia and localised peritonism in the right lower quadrant. Rebound tenderness may be effectively demonstrated by percussion of the abdominal wall rather than the crude method of deep palpation and sudden release.

Appendicitis can occur at any age; although the main peak is in young adults, there is a second peak around the seventh decade. The condition is most difficult to diagnose at the extremes of age: in the very young because of the lack of history and frequent late presentation, and in the elderly because of a wider list of differential diagnoses and often less impressive physical signs. Acute appendicitis should be considered in the differential diagnosis of virtually any patient with an acute abdomen.

A further factor that may produce atypical signs is the variation in the position of the appendix. A retrocaecal appendix can give rise to tenderness in the right loin and/or right upper quadrant, whereas a pelvic appendix may be associated with very little abdominal discomfort but marked tenderness on rectal examination and a history of diarrhoea. Rectal examination tends to be of little value in the diagnosis of acute appendicitis unless the organ lies in the pelvis. If the diagnosis has been established

from abdominal examination, rectal examination contributes very little additional information in the male patient,[11] but obviously can be useful in the female to identify other possible pelvic conditions. Clearly, if a pelvic abscess is suspected a rectal examination is mandatory.

Acute appendicitis is one of a relatively dwindling number of conditions in which a decision to operate may be based solely on clinical findings. In this context, the description of classic history and/or the presence of localised peritonism are highly predictive of acute appendicitis. Features such as high fever, non-localising abdominal tenderness or prolonged history tend to make the diagnosis less likely. The risk of morbidity and mortality is significantly increased if the appendix perforates; thus, to err on the side of overdiagnosing acute appendicitis remains accepted best surgical practice. As discussed in Chapter 5, if in doubt, laparoscopy offers an alternative to what may turn out to be an unnecessary laparotomy.

Investigations

The majority of these investigations have been discussed at length in Chapter 5.

Urinalysis is helpful. Although pus cells and microscopic haematuria can occur in appendicitis, their absence may be useful in excluding significant urinary tract disease from a list of differential diagnoses. However, in the presence of signs of peritoneal irritation and pus cells without significant bacteria in the urine, urgent investigation of the renal tract is indicated to exclude pyelonephritis or pyonephrosis. If these diagnoses are excluded, an acutely inflamed retrocaecal appendix remains the most likely cause and appendicectomy is indicated.

Plain abdominal radiographs are virtually of no help in the diagnosis of acute appendicitis and are not routinely indicated. More recently, CT has been used to identify acute appendicitis,[12] but is probably best left for those patients in whom diagnostic doubt remains and laparoscopy is likely to be difficult (such as patients with multiple abdominal scars and those on the intensive care unit). As already mentioned, the reader is referred to Chapter 5 for a more detailed list of possible investigations and their usefulness.

Differential diagnosis

Just as appendicitis should be considered in any patient with abdominal pain, virtually every other abdominal emergency can be considered in the differential diagnosis of acute appendicitis. Some of the more common conditions that present in a similar fashion include gastroenteritis and mesenteric lymphadenitis, gynaecological diseases, right-sided urinary tract disease and disease of the distal small bowel. Gynaecological disorders are probably the most important group because the removal of a normal appendix is highest in young women. Acute salpingitis, Mittelschmerz pain and complications of ovarian cyst may all be difficult to differentiate. Torsion of an ovarian cyst usually presents with a notable acute onset of pain and may sometimes be distinguished on clinical grounds. It is important to recognise ruptured ectopic pregnancy, and females of childbearing age should routinely have a pregnancy test (although it must be remembered that appendicitis is not uncommon in the first trimester of pregnancy).

The continuing development of ultrasound techniques and laparoscopic surgery has prompted the view that the previous proportion of normal appendices removed in the 'open surgery' era (typically up to 20% of patients operated on) was unacceptably high. Although it is clearly advantageous to spare patients unnecessary surgery, the morbidity and mortality of failing to diagnose appendicitis until perforation has occurred is greater than that associated with the removal of a normal appendix. If the diagnostic tools discussed in Chapter 5 are not readily available, the best policy remains early surgery when there is clinical suspicion of acute appendicitis.

Management

A positive diagnosis of acute appendicitis requires urgent surgery as any further delay will result in a higher proportion of perforation.[13,14] Where the diagnosis is in doubt, in patients who are systemically well and/or have mild signs, early exploration in the middle of the night is not indicated and these patients can be safely observed with regular review or investigations as described in Chapter 5. The incidence of perforation in this subgroup of patients is no higher than if they are taken to theatre for early exploration.[15,16] All patients should be resuscitated with intravenous fluids and adequate analgesia.

Published data support the view that treatment with narcotic analgesia does not adversely affect the ability to diagnose appendicitis on clinical grounds and, indeed, may assist diagnosis by relieving the patient's anxiety.[17,18] Analgesia should therefore not be withheld pending clinical review.

Intravenous antibiotics may be given once a decision has been made to operate or to actively treat acute appendicitis non-operatively (see below).

Surgical treatment
Conventional appendicectomy
A classical appendicectomy incision is made over the point of maximum tenderness and this usually lies on a line between the anterior superior iliac spine and umbilicus in the right iliac fossa. The skin incision should be horizontal and placed in a skin crease if possible to achieve a satisfactory cosmetic result. The abdominal wall muscles may be separated in the traditional 'muscle splitting' fashion or the abdominal cavity may be entered at the lateral margin of the rectus muscle, with retraction of the muscle fibres medially. This lateral rectal approach may be associated with less postoperative discomfort. A right-sided Pfannenstiel incision is used by some surgeons in female patients because it allows ready access to the pelvis for the diagnosis and treatment of gynaecological conditions should these be present. This incision is inconvenient, however, if the caecum lies outside the pelvis or the appendix is retrocaecal. The need for such an approach has been replaced by the wider availability of diagnostic laparoscopy and this incision is no longer recommended.

Once the abdominal cavity has been entered, the appendix should be located by gentle palpation and it may be most easily mobilised from the inflammatory adhesions by finger dissection. If it is obviously inflamed, it should be removed, lavage performed and no further laparotomy carried out. If the appendix is macroscopically normal, examination should be undertaken of the terminal ileum (for at least 60 cm to exclude an inflamed Meckel diverticulum) and small-bowel mesentery and pelvis, both by palpation and direct visualisation with retraction of the abdominal wall. Any free peritoneal fluid should be examined and cultured. The presence of bile staining indicates bowel perforation at some point, such as perforated peptic ulcer, and faecal fluid indicates a colonic perforation. In both cases a full laparotomy is indicated. In the former situation, it is best to close the right iliac fossa incision in preference to an upper midline, but in the latter condition some surgeons advocate extending the right iliac fossa incision across to the left as a muscle-cutting lower abdominal transverse incision. If in doubt, a midline incision is best.

It used to be traditional to bury the appendix stump but there is now general recognition that simple ligation of the stump is adequate.[19] However, if the appendix has perforated at the base, formal repair of the caecal pole is advised. Leaving an excessively long stump should be avoided as this will inevitably become ischaemic and can produce symptoms postoperatively. Peritoneal lavage should always be carried out but surgical drains are unnecessary unless there is an established abscess cavity.

All patients should receive prophylactic antibiotics against the risk of wound infection, which is the commonest complication of appendicectomy. Regimens vary but the two most common are metronidazole alone or in combination with a broad-spectrum cephalosporin. A single dose is as effective as three doses for wound prophylaxis. In perforated appendicitis, however, a policy of instituting a full treatment course over 5 days is adopted by many surgeons, although there are no good data to support this view. Although the risk of deep vein thrombosis is relatively low in young patients, prophylaxis is best administered as a routine as not all patients will make a swift recovery and early postoperative mobilisation may be delayed. It goes without saying that it should be routinely employed in older patients.

Laparoscopic appendicectomy

The advantages of laparoscopic appendicectomy over the open approach have been extensively studied over the last 15 years, although many individual studies have produced conflicting results.[20–29]

 Two meta-analyses have confirmed the benefit of the laparoscopic approach in relation to less pain, faster recovery and a lower incidence of wound infections.[30,31] However, the Cochrane database systematic review of over 4000 patients suggested that there was a threefold increase in intra-abdominal abscesses and a longer operating time (16 minutes) in those patients undergoing the laparoscopic procedure.[32]

This may of course reflect either problems with surgical technique or poor patient selection. There is no rational reason why the laparoscopic approach should have a higher complication rate, if performed correctly, and indeed it brings with it the possibility of performing a better lavage than at open surgery.

As skill in laparoscopic techniques becomes increasingly more widespread, it is inevitable that laparoscopic appendicectomy will become more common.[33] It would therefore be reasonable to proceed with laparoscopic appendicectomy in any patient in whom an acutely inflamed appendix is discovered during diagnostic laparoscopy, providing the surgeon has the relevant skills. Likewise, in the other patients, and these will usually be men, offering the laparoscopic approach will depend on the surgical expertise available. Large and obese patients probably benefit more from the laparoscopic approach due to the larger wound required at open surgery.

Technique

The basic principles of laparoscopic appendicectomy mirror those of conventional open surgery. The appendix mesentery is usually divided first and may be cauterised with electrocoagulation at the level of the appendix, tied in continuity with ligatures or controlled by application of haemostatic clips. The appendix itself is usually ligated with a preformed loop ligature. An alternative, highly effective and rapid technique is to apply an endoscopic stapling device using vascular staples to the mesoappendix, which is divided as the first step. The appendix can then be removed after further application of the stapler or by using a pre-tied ligature. Unfortunately, the stapling device is expensive.

The inflamed appendix should be removed through an endoscopic port or, if it is excessively swollen, placed in a bag for retrieval as it is essential to remove the appendix through the abdominal wall without contaminating the soft tissues. This minimises the risk of wound infection, which appears to be significantly lower than after conventional surgery.[31] A very friable and perforated appendix should be handled very gently and care taken to remove all debris, including any loose faecolith. If manipulation of the swollen appendix is likely to result in perforation, conversion to an open operation should be considered. In this situation the laparoscope can be used to transilluminate the abdominal wall, allowing accurate placement of a conventional surgical incision, which it may be possible to keep to a smaller size than would otherwise have been used. A thorough lavage is essential in contaminated cases to prevent postoperative abscess formation. In patients with generalised peritonitis from a perforated appendix, it must be remembered that the advantages of the laparoscopic approach over the open approach are small, as even if the operation can be completed laparoscopically these patients rarely recover quickly due to the systemic nature of their disease.

There have been various descriptions of operative technique for laparoscopic appendicectomy and different positions for port placement are used. If ports are placed low in the abdominal wall, the cosmetic result may be improved, although some surgeons prefer to place one port in the right upper quadrant and one in the lower abdomen to allow the classical positioning of the long axis of laparoscopic instruments at right angles to each other. However, there is no evidence to suggest that one approach is better than another.

One of the reported complications of laparoscopic appendicectomy is leaving too long a stump and risking recurrent symptoms.[34] Care must be taken to ensure that the entire appendix has been fully mobilised to avoid this complication.

The normal appendix

Although the recognised complication rate associated with the open removal of a normal appendix lies somewhere between 17% and 21%, depending on whether other conditions have been found,[35,36] the longer-term sequelae of removing a normal appendix laparoscopically remains relatively unknown, but hopefully less. There is therefore the question as to what should be done if, at diagnostic laparoscopy, a normal appendix is seen but no other condition can be identified which could account for the patient's symptoms. Some surgeons might argue that in this case the appendix should be removed using the laparoscopic approach, because a normal-looking appendix can be found to have histological evidence of mucosal inflammation.[37] However, there have been other studies which have shown that even histologically normal appendices can subsequently be shown to contain inflammatory changes if more advanced analyses are used.[38] A study attempting to evaluate accurately the ability of laparoscopy to discriminate between a normal and an inflamed appendix demonstrated a sensitivity of 100% and a specificity of 85% only if an appendix with isolated mucosal inflammation was considered as normal. If an appendix with mucosal inflammation was considered to be inflamed, the sensitivity fell to 92% while the specificity remained at 85%.[39] As the significance of isolated mucosal inflammation in an otherwise normal-looking appendix is highly debatable, a pragmatic approach would be to remove the appendix when it looks inflamed at laparoscopy but do nothing further if it looks normal. The decision may differ in each patient and the final course of action has to be left to the operating surgeon. In a patient who has required repeated admissions to hospital with recurring right iliac fossa pain, it would make sense to remove the appendix, if normal, to at least exclude acute appendicitis from the differential diagnosis on any possible future admissions.

If a standard incision has been made for a planned open appendicectomy, conventional teaching dictates that the normal appendix should be removed to prevent confusion in the future should right iliac fossa pain recur. On the one hand, this hypothesis has never been fully tested and one would imagine that most patients are capable of understanding whether their appendix had been removed, provided they are given this information. On the other hand, removal of a normal appendix is associated with minimal morbidity, although the wound infection rate is the same for removal of a normal appendix as for a non-perforated inflamed appendix. In practice, a normal appendix should probably be removed in every patient, including those with Crohn's disease that affects the caecum at the base of the appendix, in order to prevent future diagnostic dilemma. The main longer-term complication of removing a normal appendix is small-bowel obstruction. This has been examined in a historical cohort study of 245–400 patients in Sweden with population-based matched controls.[40] This study calculated the cumulative risk of surgically treated small-bowel obstruction following open appendicectomy to be 1.3% after 30 years compared with 0.21% for non-operated controls. Higher risk was associated with those patients undergoing appendicectomy for other conditions, a perforated appendix and a normal appendix.

Removal of a normal appendix at diagnostic laparoscopy is not mandatory and should not be undertaken if a definitive diagnosis for the patient's symptoms, such as pelvic inflammatory disease, can be established. If no cause for symptoms is discovered, there are two arguments in favour of removing the appendix: (i) there is a small incidence of appendicitis on histological examination of a macroscopically normal appendix; and (ii) the removal of the appendix prevents the development of a diagnostic dilemma in a patient who continues to suffer from abdominal symptoms and signs following laparoscopy. It could also be argued that a major advantage of laparoscopy in suspected appendicitis is the ability to remove a normal appendix easily and with very low morbidity.

However, the counter-argument suggests that all operative interventions or procedures are associated with some form of risk and if the appendix is normal at laparoscopy there needs to be a good reason to remove it. Surgeons will no doubt have their own thoughts on this matter and decisions may vary between patients and the clinical presentation.

Non-surgical treatment

It has been suspected for many years that not only can acute appendicitis settle spontaneously, returning with recurrent symptoms at a later date, but that it can also be successfully treated with antibiotics, providing there are no signs of overt peritonitis. The former is supported by a study which reported that 71 of 1084 patients (6.5%) who underwent appendicectomy for acute appendicitis admitted to similar symptoms 3 weeks to 12 years previously.[41] The latter is supported by two randomised controlled studies comparing antibiotic treatment versus appendicectomy in patients with suspected appendicitis.[42,43] The more recent and larger of these two studies, carried out in 252 men, showed that although non-operative management was successful in 86% of patients, 14% of this group went on to develop recurrent symptoms within 1 year.[43] It therefore follows that when a diagnosis of acute appendicitis is suspected appendicectomy should be carried out. However, in the absence of overt peritonitis, it is reasonable to treat the patient with antibiotics if there are other factors that favour a non-operative approach. This decision is obviously made in the full knowledge that regular review is essential, that immediate operation is indicated if resolution does not take place within 12–24 hours or the patient's symptoms deteriorate and that there is a significant risk of recurrent symptoms during the course of the next 12 months.

Treatment of atypical presentation of acute appendicitis

Appendix mass

The natural history of acute appendicitis left untreated is that it will resolve, become gangrenous and perforate, or will become surrounded by a mass of omentum and small bowel that walls off the inflammatory process and prevents inflammation spreading to the abdominal cavity yet resolution of the condition is delayed. Such a patient usually presents with a longer history (1 week or more) of right lower quadrant abdominal pain, appears systemically well and has a tender palpable mass in the right iliac fossa. This condition is best managed conservatively as the risk of perforation has passed and removal of the appendix at this late stage can be difficult and is associated with a significant complication rate.[44] The differential diagnosis includes Crohn's disease in younger patients and carcinoma of the caecum in older patients. Confirmation is obtained from ultrasound or CT and it is not uncommon for these investigations to reveal an underlying abscess.[45] However, if the patient remains systemically well, non-operative treatment can still be pursued. Following resolution of the symptoms and mass, further investigations, which might include ultrasound, CT, barium enema and colonoscopy, must be used to exclude these other conditions.

In the past, routine interval appendicectomy (6 weeks to 3 months) was considered essential to prevent recurrent symptoms in the young and to exclude carcinoma in the elderly. However, providing carcinoma can be excluded by other means, routine interval appendicectomy is no longer considered essential. In the majority of cases the appendix has been destroyed and in one study only 9% of patients treated non-operatively for an appendix mass subsequently developed recurrent symptoms and all did so within 5 months.[45]

A recent systematic review has confirmed that non-operative management of an appendix mass will be successful in the majority of patients and recurrence of symptoms is low. As a result the routine use of interval appendicectomy is no longer justified.[46]

Appendix abscess

In some patients the appendix becomes walled off by omentum but has perforated and an abscess will develop localised to the periappendiceal region. This may be in the right paracolic gutter, the subcaecal area or the pelvis and can be visualised by either ultrasound (**Fig. 9.8**) or CT (**Fig. 9.9**). There may be a mass but, unlike a simple 'appendix mass',

Figure 9.8 • Ultrasound scan demonstrating an appendix abscess. With thanks to Dr Paul Allan, Consultant Radiologist, Royal Infirmary, Edinburgh.

Figure 9.9 • CT scan of the same patient as shown in Fig. 9.8, demonstrating the appendix abscess. With thanks to Dr Paul Allan, Consultant Radiologist, Royal Infirmary, Edinburgh.

the patient is systemically unwell with significant abdominal tenderness. As is the case in all abscesses, drainage is the best treatment, either under radiological control or surgically. The advantage of the latter is that through a standard right iliac fossa incision the residual necrotic appendix can be found and resected along with the inevitable faecolith, which if left contributes to a long and protracted recovery. There is no doubt, however, that surgical drainage can be associated with significant complications, not least because tissues and organs adjacent to the abscess will be friable and must be handled with great care. The alternative of non-operative management using radiologically guided drainage (**Fig. 9.10**) has been reported to produce significantly lower complications and equivalent early operation/reoperation rates.[47,48] It would therefore seem reasonable to use the non-operative approach in any patient who remains systemically well and in whom overt signs of peritonitis are absent.

Figure 9.10 • Radiograph of the same patient as shown in Figs 9.8 and 9.9, following percutaneous drainage of the appendix abscess, with drain in situ.

Chronic appendicitis

As mentioned above, there is certainly a group of patients who suffer from recurrent appendicitis[40] and who benefit from appendicectomy. Similarly, there are some patients who, having recovered from an acute attack of appendicitis, go on to suffer from recurrent less-acute episodes of abdominal pain. These also benefit from appendicectomy, usually as an elective procedure and increasingly carried out laparoscopically. In these patients, the macroscopic appearance of the appendix is abnormal; thus, when in doubt, laparoscopy is the best investigation, following which the appendix can be removed. Assessment in difficult cases can be helped by a

barium enema, which reveals a non-filling appendix lumen (**Fig. 9.11**), or even by CT (**Fig. 9.12**).

Postoperative complications and outcome

Hospital stay

The duration of hospital stay depends on local resources, policies, the patient's general condition and any coexisting disease. It is now fairly clear that laparoscopic appendicectomy is associated with a more rapid return to normal activities[30,31] than conventional surgery, but this does not necessarily relate to a shorter hospital stay. Much may depend on local factors and reports of routine early discharge (24–48 hours) after conventional appendicectomy[49] suggest that a full diet and early mobilisation are well tolerated by the majority of patients.

Wound infection

This is the commonest postoperative complication, occurring in around 15% of patients following a conventional right iliac fossa incision. In most patients there is superficial inflammation, which responds to antibiotics. In a smaller number there will be dehiscence of the wound and purulent discharge. Occasionally, surgical intervention may be required to drain a collection in the abdominal wall. The current practice of early discharge results in many wound infections developing once the patient is at home and the possibility of this complication should always be discussed with the patient. As already discussed, wound infection

Figure 9.11 • Barium enema in a patient with recurrent right-sided abdominal pain showing non-filling of the distal appendix lumen.

Figure 9.12 • CT scan of the same patient as in Fig. 9.11 showing an abnormal and thickened tip of appendix without contrast. These findings were confirmed at appendicectomy when a grossly abnormal distal half of appendix was found.

appears to be significantly less following laparoscopic appendicectomy.[30,31]

There is no clear evidence that injection of local anaesthetic into the wound is associated with any alteration in the incidence of wound infection but there is also minimal benefit in reducing postoperative wound pain.[50,51] The skin may be closed with interrupted stitches or a continuous suture and this does not appear to affect wound infection rates or subsequent management. Some surgeons prefer to leave the skin incision open if there has been gross contamination of the wound in perforated appendicitis. The subsequent cosmetic result of such a scar is usually entirely satisfactory but healing takes several weeks.

Other septic complications

Pericaecal fluid collections are relatively common and are usually indicated by the presence of abdominal discomfort and a low-grade pyrexia. They can be diagnosed by ultrasound and treated by antibiotics, especially in children,[52] or occasionally aspiration; formal drainage is rarely necessary. Pelvic abscess is an uncommon complication that presents with lower abdominal discomfort and swinging pyrexia. The symptoms may be delayed by 10 days or more and a soft tender mass may be palpable on rectal examination, but this is not always the case. Again, ultrasound or even CT diagnosis is required and, if pus is aspirated, a percutaneous drain should be placed if possible. Occasionally, a pelvic abscess may be difficult to drain percutaneously and in this situation the options are between antibiotics, drainage of the abscess into the rectum or to proceed to surgical drainage through the abdomen. The decision is influenced by the local circumstances and general condition of the patient. Prolonged use of antibiotics should be avoided and

further attempts made for drainage if the collection is not resolving on repeated ultrasound examinations.

In patients who have undergone laparoscopic appendicectomy for perforated appendicitis, signs of generalised peritonitis can develop in the first 48 hours. This may be due to dissemination of infected fluid through the abdominal cavity, possibly by circulation of the carbon dioxide used to create the pneumoperitoneum. The main differential diagnosis in this situation is iatrogenic injury to the intestine and, if in doubt, re-laparoscopy is indicated.

Prognosis

The mortality of appendicitis is associated with the age of the patient and delayed diagnosis (perforated appendix). The report from the Royal College of Surgeons of England showed a mortality of 0.24% and morbidity of 7.7% in 6596 patients undergoing open appendicectomy between 1990 and 1992.[53] A further prognostic consideration is the incidence of subsequent tubal infertility after appendicectomy. Although one report suggested that the increased risk of tubal infertility following perforated appendicitis was 4.8 in nulliparous women and 3.2 in multiparous women,[54] a more recent historical cohort study revealed no long-term consequence on fertility.[55] This latest study is another factor which opposes the view that it is better to carry out an unnecessary appendicectomy than risk delaying surgery, with the possible increased risk of perforation in particular, for acute appendicitis. As already discussed, a period of close observation with regular review in hospital is not associated with an increased risk of perforation, while the early and late complications of removing a normal appendix (using conventional surgery) range from 13% to 17%.[35,36]

Key points

- The main emergency conditions affecting the small bowel are obstruction, haemorrhage and ischaemia.
- Early management requires adequate clinical and radiological assessment, which might include contrast radiology and, increasingly, ultrasonography (see also Chapter 5).
- Early appendicectomy for acute appendicitis is better than non-operative treatment with antibiotics because of high recurrence rate.
- Laparoscopic appendicectomy results in less pain and faster return to normal activities than open appendicectomy but hospital stay remains similar and there is a higher risk of postoperative abscess formation.
- Non-operative approach is indicated in the majority of patients with appendix mass or abscess, with radiological drainage as required. Subsequent interval appendicectomy is only indicated in those patients with recurrent symptoms. However, care must be taken to ensure that underlying disease other than appendicitis has been excluded (e.g. caecal carcinoma and Crohn's disease).

References

1. Ellis H, Thompson JN, Parker MC et al. Adhesion-related hospital re-admissions after abdominal and pelvic surgery: a retrospective study. Lancet 1999; 353:1476–9.

2. Tingstedt B, Isaksson J, Andersson R. Long-term follow-up and cost analysis following surgery for small bowel obstruction caused by intra-abdominal adhesions. Br J Surg 2007; 94:743–8.

3. Walsh HPJ, Schofield PE. Is laparotomy for small bowel obstruction justified in patients with previously treated malignancy? Br J Surg 1984; 71:933–5.

4. Nakane Y, Okumura S, Akehira K et al. Management of intestinal obstruction after gastrectomy for carcinoma. Br J Surg 1996; 83:133.

5. Parker MC, Baines MJ. Intestinal obstruction in patients with advanced malignant disease. Br J Surg 1996; 83:12.

6. Sajja SBS, Schein M. Early post-operative small bowel obstruction. Br J Surg 2004; 91:683–91.

7. Ogata M, Mateer JR, Condon RE. Prospective evaluation of abdominal sonography for the diagnosis of bowel obstruction. Ann Surg 1996; 223:237–41.

8. Paterson-Brown S. Emergency laparoscopic surgery. Br J Surg 1993; 80:279–83.

9. Thompson-Fawcett MW, Mortensen NJMcC. Crohn's disease. In: Phillips RKS (ed.) Colorectal surgery, 4th edn. Edinburgh: Elsevier, 2009.

10. Schoots IG, Koffeman DA, Levi M et al. Systematic review of survival after acute mesenteric ischaemia according to disease aetiology. Br J Surg 2004; 91:17–27.

    Data from 45 observational studies including 3692 patients were reviewed. Prognosis after acute mesenteric venous thrombosis is better than for arterial ischaemia, and that for arterial embolism is better than that for arterial thrombosis.

11. Dixon JM, Elton RA, Rainey IB et al. Rectal examination in patients with pain in the right lower quadrant of the abdomen. Br Med J 1991; 302:386–8.

12. Rao PM, Rhea JT, Novelline RA et al. Effect of computed tomography of the appendix on treatment of patients and use of hospital resources. N Engl J Med 1998; 338:141–6.

13. Moss JG, Barrie JL, Gunn AA. Delay in surgery for acute appendicitis. J R Coll Surg Edinb 1985: 30:290–3.

14. Temple CL, Huchcroft SA, Temple WJ. The natural history of appendicitis in adults. A prospective study. Ann Surg 1995; 221:278–81.

15. McLean AD, Stonebridge PA, Bradbury AW et al. Time of presentation, time of operation, and unnecessary appendicectomy. Br Med J 1993; 306:307.

16. Surana R, Quinn F, Puri P. Is it necessary to perform appendicectomy in the middle of the night in children? Br Med J 1993; 306:1168.

17. Attard AR, Corlett MJ, Kidner NJ, Leslie AL, Fraser IA. Safety of early pain relief for acute abdominal pain. Br Med J 1992; 30:554–6.

    Assessment of patients with acute abdominal pain is not affected adversely by early analgesia.

18. Thomas SH, Cheema F, Reisner A et al. Effects of morphine analgesia on diagnostic accuracy in emergency department patients with abdominal pain: a prospective randomized trial. J Am Coll Surg 2003; 196:18–31.

    A randomised study of 74 patients who received either morphine or placebo. The diagnostic accuracy was not affected by morphine.

19. Engstrom L, Fenvo G. Appendicectomy: assessment of stump invagination: a prospective, randomised trial. Br J Surg 1985; 72:971–2.

20. Kum CK, Ngoi SS, Goh PMY et al. Randomized controlled trial comparing laparoscopic and open appendicectomy. Br J Surg 1993; 80:1599–600.

21. McAnena OJ, Austin O, O'Connell PR et al. Laparoscopic versus open appendicectomy: a prospective evaluation. Br J Surg 1992; 79:818–20.

22. Cox MR, McCall JL, Toouli J et al. Prospective randomized comparison of open versus laparoscopic appendectomy in men. World J Surg 1996; 20:263–6.

23. Tate JJT, Dawson IW, Chung SCS et al. Laparoscopic versus open appendicectomy: prospective randomised trial. Lancet 1993; 342:633–7.

24. Martin LC, Puente I, Sosa JL et al. Open versus laparoscopic appendectomy. Ann Surg 1995; 222:256–62.

25. Hansen JB, Smithers BM, Schache D et al. Laparoscopic versus open appendectomy: prospective randomised trial. World J Surg 1996; 20:17–21.

26. Minne L, Burnell A, Ratzer E et al. Laparoscopic vs open appendectomy. Arch Surg 1997; 132:708–12.

27. Reiertsen O, Larsen S, Trondsen E et al. Randomised controlled trial with sequential design of laparoscopic versus conventional appendicectomy. Br J Surg 1997; 84:842–7.

28. Hellberg A, Rudberg C, Kullman E et al. Prospective randomised multicentre study of laparoscopic versus open appendicectomy. Br J Surg 1999; 86:48–53.

29. Lintula H, Kokki H, Vanamo K. Single-blind randomised clinical trial of laparoscopic versus open appendicectomy in children. Br J Surg 2001; 88:510–14.

30. Sauerland S, Lefering R, Holthausen U et al. A meta-analysis of studies comparing laparoscopic with conventional appendectomy. In: Krahenbuhl L, Frei E, Klaiber Ch et al. (eds) Acute appendicitis: standard treatment or laparoscopic surgery? Basel: Karger, 1998; pp. 109–14.
   Less pain and earlier return to normal activity after the laparoscopic approach.

31. Golub R, Siddiqui F, Pohl D. Laparoscopic versus open appendectomy: a metaanalysis. J Am Coll Surg 1998; 186:545–53.
   Analysis of 1682 patients. Less postoperative pain, shorter hospital stay, faster return to normal activities and less wound infections following laparoscopic appendectomy.

32. Sauerland S, Lefering R, Neugebauer EAM. Laparoscopic versus open surgery for suspected appendicitis (Cochrane review). The Cochrane Library, 2004; Issue 4. www.cochrane.org/cochrane/revabstr/AB001546.htm

33. Paterson HM, Qadan M, de Luca SM et al. Changing trends in surgery for acute appendicitis. Br J Surg 2008; 95:363–8.

34. Milne AA, Bradbury AW. 'Residual' appendicitis following incomplete laparoscopic appendicectomy. Br J Surg 1996; 83:217.

35. Chang FC, Hogie HH, Welling DR. The fate of the negative appendix. Am J Surg 1973; 126:752–4.

36. Deutsch AA, Shani N, Reiss R. Are some appendicectomies unnecessary? J R Coll Surg Edinb 1983; 28:35–40.

37. Lau WY, Fan ST, Yiu TF et al. The clinical significance of routine histopathological study of the resected appendix and safety of appendiceal inversion. Surg Gynecol Obstet 1986; 162:256–8.

38. Wang Y, Reen DJ, Puri P. Is a histologically normal appendix following emergency appendicectomy always normal? Lancet 1996; 347:1076–9.

39. Champault G, Taffinder N, Ziol M et al. Recognition of a pathological appendix during laparoscopy: a prospective study of 81 cases. Br J Surg 1997; 84:671.

40. Andersson REB. Small bowel obstruction after appendicectomy. Br J Surg 2001; 88:1387–91.

41. Barber MD, McLaren J, Rainey JB. Recurrent appendicitis. Br J Surg 1997; 84:110–12.

42. Eriksson S, Granstrom L. Randomised controlled trial of appendicectomy versus antibiotic therapy for acute appendicitis. Br J Surg 1995; 82:166–9.

43. Styrud J, Eriksson S, Nilsson I et al. Appendectomy versus antibiotic treatment in acute appendicitis. A prospective multicentre randomized controlled trial. World J Surg 2006; 30:1033–7.

44. De U, Ghosh S. Acute appendicectomy for appendicular mass: a study of 87 patients. Ceylon Med J 2002; 47:117–18.

45. Bagi P, Dueholm S. Nonoperative management of the ultrasonically evaluated appendiceal mass. Surgery 1987; 101:602–5.

46. Deakin DE, Ahmed I. Interval appendicectomy after resolution of adult inflammatory appendix mass – is it necessary? Surgeon 2007; 5(1):45–50.
   A systematic review confirming that non-operative management will be successful in the majority of patients and recurrence of symptoms is low.

47. Hurme T, Nyalamo E. Conservative versus operative treatment of appendicular abscess. Ann Chir Gynaecol 1995; 84:33–6.

48. Oliak D, Yamini D, Udani VM et al. Initial nonoperative management for periappendiceal abscess. Dis Colon Rectum 2001; 44:936–41.

49. Salam IMA, Fallouji MA, El Ashaal YI et al. Early patient discharge following appendicectomy: safety and feasibility. J R Coll Surg Edinb 1995; 40:300–2.

50. Dahl IB, Moiniche S, Kehle H. Wound infiltration with local anaesthetics for post-operative pain relief. Acta Anaesthesiol Scand 1994; 38:7–14.

51. Turner GA, Chalkiadis G. Comparison of preoperative with postoperative lignocaine infiltration on postoperative analgesic requirements. Br J Anaesth 1994; 72:541–3.

52. Okoye BO, Rampersad B, Marantos A et al. Abscess after appendicectomy in children: the role of conservative management. Br J Surg 1998; 85:1111–13.

53. Baigrie RJ, Dehn TCB, Fowler SM et al. Analysis of 8651 appendicectomies in England and Wales during 1992. Br J Surg 1995; 82:933.

54. Mueller BA, Daling JR, Moore DE et al. Appendectomy and the risk of tubal infertility. N Engl J Med 1986; 315:1506–7.

55. Andersson R, Lambe M, Bergstrom R. Fertility patterns after appendicectomy: historical cohort study. Br Med J 1999; 318:963–7.

10

Colonic emergencies

David E. Beck
Charles B. Whitlow

Introduction

Emergency conditions of the large bowel are common and changes in their evaluation and management have occurred in recent years. Rather than rushing the patient to the operating room after a token resuscitation, current standards suggest that an initial appropriate period of resuscitation along with physiological and radiological evaluation should be undertaken. Many patients with colonic conditions can be managed non-operatively with bowel rest, antibiotics and blood components. Comorbid disease such as cardiac, pulmonary and metabolic conditions are optimised and critically ill patients are monitored in an intensive care setting. If adequate facilities and personnel are not readily available, transfer to a tertiary care facility should be considered if the patient can be readily stabilised.

The operative mortality for emergency colon resections is two to three times that associated with elective resection. As a result, surgeons have investigated ways of stabilising patients in order to convert emergency into more planned, elective procedures. Deciding if and when to operate can be difficult, and active observation and consultation with colleagues is often helpful in the decision-making process. Active participation of the attending/consultant surgeon in both the assessment and operative procedure is essential in this group of very challenging patients.

When emergency surgery is necessary, there has been a clear trend towards single rather than staged procedures for large bowel disorders. When feasible this approach reduces the length of hospital stay and avoids the risks of multiple operations. However, in some unfit or acutely septic patients, a staged approach may still be preferable.

Preparation for operation

Patients should be adequately informed of their likely diagnosis and management options. Alternatives and risks as well as the potential need for a stoma should be explained carefully. Patients requiring emergency large bowel surgery should be marked for potential stoma sites and if possible participation of a stoma therapist arranged.

The risk of postoperative deep vein thrombosis and pulmonary embolus is substantial in this group of patients, and prophylactic measures are essential. Options include intermittent pneumatic calf compression and subcutaneous low-molecular-weight heparin. Prophylactic antibiotic therapy is standard, with broad-spectrum single-dose therapy as effective as multiple-dose regimens. The duration of prophylactic antibiotics should be less than 24 hours. If significant infection or contamination is found intraoperatively, empirical therapeutic antibiotics may be indicated.

Disease process

Colonic emergencies can be divided into ischaemia, obstruction, perforation and bleeding. These categories will be discussed in turn, with attention to their pathophysiology, evaluation and management.

Colonic ischaemia

Although the colon has a generous overlapping blood supply, any interruption in blood flow produces ischaemia. Anatomical locations that have the potential to be vulnerable to ischaemic disease include: Griffith's point at the splenic flexure (junction of the superior mesenteric artery (SMA) and the inferior mesenteric artery (IMA)); Sudeck's critical point at the mid-sigmoid colon (junction of the IMA and hypogastric vasculature); and the caecum (distal distribution of the SMA).

Aetiological factors and pathophysiology

As outlined in Box 10.1, colonic ischaemia can result from a number of conditions.

Interruption of flow in large vessels following aortic surgery varies from 1–2% for elective cases to as high as 60% during emergency aneurysm repair.[1] Sudden occlusion of the IMA can also occur as a result of angiographic trauma with subintimal dissection or as a result of either blunt or penetrating abdominal trauma. Atheromatous narrowing or occlusion of the IMA is not unusual. However, in most cases this occurs gradually, and the collateral circulation from the superior mesenteric artery can compensate for the decrease in flow through collateral circulation via the marginal artery. If the IMA becomes acutely thrombosed or occluded with an embolus and the collateral circulation is inadequate, the clinical picture will be similar to that found after IMA ligation during aortic surgery.

Any of the connective tissue diseases that produce inflammation in the small intestinal arteries (intrinsic small-vessel disease) can also result in colonic ischaemia. This has been described in polyarteritis nodosa, systemic lupus erythematosus, rheumatoid arthritis, dermatomyositis, primary amyloidosis and Degos' disease. Colonic ischaemia resulting from small-vessel disease has also been described in patients with diabetes mellitus and chronic renal failure.

Ischaemic colitis has also been reported in approximately 1% of renal allograft recipients.[2] Another variant of ischaemic colitis occurs in patients who are severely ill with conditions that cause hypotension, decreased cardiac output or peripheral vasoconstriction, with a decreased flow to the end organ (low-flow states). This group of patients appears to have a higher incidence of full-thickness necrosis than do those with spontaneous ischaemic colitis who were previously well. Also noticed is the preponderance of patients with right-sided colonic involvement. The mortality associated with colonic infarction in these patients who are severely ill from another disease process is extremely high. In the group of 17 such patients reported by Sakai et al., the mortality rate was 57%.[3] One must therefore have a very high index of suspicion for full-thickness necrosis in this group of patients and be ready to intervene early.

Spontaneous ischaemic colitis occurs without any demonstrable vessel occlusion on angiography.[4] The pathological changes seen in the colon are identical to those reproduced in the laboratory with vessel occlusion; the presumption is that this entity is caused by a decreased flow to the colon. The spectrum of disease varies from mild submucosal oedema to frank full-thickness necrosis. Most cases are the milder self-limiting variety that are typically seen in middle-aged or elderly patients, often following episodes of dehydration. In younger patients, who are mostly women, there has been an association between ischaemic colitis and the use of oral contraceptives.[5]

Diagnosis

Colonic ischaemia usually presents in one of two ways. The milder cases are manifest by diffuse and/or bloody diarrhoea. Patients with frank colonic infarction frequently develop acidosis, glucose intolerance, renal failure, obvious sepsis, and abdominal distension or tenderness. The diagnosis of postoperative ischaemia can be made with flexible sigmoidoscopy performed at the bedside. If the symptoms are not explained by flexible sigmoidoscopy, a colonoscopy may occasionally be required to rule out more proximal disease. The endoscopic appearance of colonic ischaemia may range from submucosal oedema with haemorrhage and ulceration to the dusky blue mucosal colour of infarction. Frank gangrene mandates immediate surgery and resection; however, the colon with just mucosal oedema and haemorrhage may be watched closely.

The diagnosis can be made with endoscopy, barium enema or computed tomography (CT). Endoscopy

---

Box 10.1 • Classification of ischaemic colitis

I. Interruption of flow in large vessels
    A. Following ligation during aortic surgery
    B. Injury secondary to angiographic, blunt or penetrating trauma
    C. Spontaneous thrombosis of large vessels
II. Intrinsic small-vessel disease
III. Low-flow state in the critically ill
IV. Spontaneous ischaemic colitis without demonstrable vessel occlusion
    A. Self-limiting without sequelae
    B. With subsequent stricture formation
V. Miscellaneous
    A. Secondary to luminal obstruction
    B. Young adults
    C. Renal allograft recipients

Figure 10.1 • Endoscopic view of colonic ischaemia.

can be done in the office or at the bedside and the pathological state can be viewed directly (**Fig. 10.1**). A barium enema study performed soon after the onset of the pain will show a typical thumbprinting pattern that is the result of submucosal oedema and haemorrhage. However, a barium enema is contraindicated if the patient has peritoneal signs, is septic, there is a strong suspicion of bowel necrosis, or performance of an angiogram is contemplated. CT is rapidly becoming more common, and ischaemia presents as thickened bowel wall (**Fig. 10.2**).

There are three possible outcomes of ischaemic colitis:

1. **Resolution** of the process is the most common clinical course.

Figure 10.2 • CT scan of colonic ischaemia.

2. Progression to **full-thickness necrosis** is unusual, especially if there is no evidence of gangrenous bowel at the first examination.
3. The condition may evolve to an ulcerative stage, which may eventually result in **stricture** formation. During the ulcerative stage the endoscopic and radiographic findings may mimic Crohn's disease. Occasionally the early phases of this disease will go unnoticed or undiagnosed, and the patient will present with a stricture.

Ischaemic colitis may also be associated with a complete or partial bowel obstruction. In one reported series,[6] 10% of patients with colonic ischaemia had an associated carcinoma and another 10% had some other condition that potentially interfered with colonic motility. When ischaemic colitis occurs in association with tumour, the ischaemic area is usually proximal to the tumour and may or may not be associated with obstruction. The investigators in this study and others speculated that colonic blood flow could be decreased as a consequence of increased intraluminal pressure, hyperperistalsis with increased muscular spasm, and resultant diminution in blood flow in the colonic wall, or a decrease in aortic blood pressure and vena caval return with straining in obstructive lesions.[7] Knowledge of this association is of obvious importance to avoid using ischaemic bowel for an anastomosis.

Treatment

If the diagnosis of ischaemic colitis is made early, non-operative treatment is warranted in the first instance. Mild cases can be managed on an outpatient basis with a clear liquid diet, close observation and possibly antibiotic therapy. More serious cases require hospitalisation, bowel rest, nasogastric suction (if there are any signs of ileus), and optimisation of blood flow to the mucosa (intravenous hydration and optimisation of cardiac output). If the patient is receiving digitalis, a serum level should be checked because toxic digitalis levels can have a marked vasoconstrictive effect on visceral circulation. Parenteral antibiotics (such as a second- or third-generation cephalosporin) are used by some surgeons because of the suggestion that colonic ischaemia may allow colonic bacterial transmigration, although there are no strong data to support or refute their use. Patients with ischaemia resulting from arterities may respond to corticosteroid treatment.

Specific indications for surgery include peritonitis, perforation, sepsis and failure of non-operative therapy. At operation a wide resection of non-viable colon is performed. Primary anastomosis is usually unsafe because of the potential for postoperative progression of the ischaemia. A double-barrel stoma or end stoma and separate mucous fistula is safer and allows assessment of the bowel viability in the postoperative period. The mortality rate for ischaemic colitis among renal transplant patients is 70%.[2] Diagnostic manoeuvres should therefore be initiated at the first suspicion of ischaemia in these high-risk patients, and surgery should be aggressive once the diagnosis is made (resection of any compromised bowel with an end stoma). Primary anastomosis after resection is ill advised in these cases.

Colonic obstruction

Colonic volvulus

Volvulus can be defined as a twisting or torsion of bowel around its mesentery and occurs most commonly in the sigmoid colon (76%), but also in the caecum (22%) and the transverse colon (2%).[8] One report suggested that 40–60% of patients have had previous episodes of obstruction.[9] In the USA, volvulus represents a rare cause of intestinal obstruction, encompassing less than 5% of large bowel obstructions. However, worldwide it may represent more than 50% of the cases in some countries.[10]

Sigmoid volvulus

The sigmoid colon rotates through 180–720° in either a clockwise or anticlockwise direction to produce the volvulus.[11] A narrowed sigmoid mesocolon provides a pedicle for rotation. The condition is occasionally associated with Chagas' disease and Hirschsprung's disease, in which redundancy of the colon is a feature, in addition to non-specific motility disorders of the colon.[12]

A typical patient with a sigmoid volvulus presents with abdominal pain, constipation and feeling bloated. On examination there is marked distension, which is often asymmetrical. Severe pain and tenderness, associated with tachycardia and hypotension, may suggest colonic ischaemia. Patients who develop sigmoid volvulus in the industrialised world tend to be older, and one-third either have mental illness or are institutionalised.[12]

Findings on the plain abdominal radiograph are often characteristic. Massive distension of the sigmoid colon is visible; the bowel loses its haustration and extends in an inverted U from the pelvis to the right upper quadrant of the abdomen (**Fig. 10.3**). Fluid levels are seen in both limbs of the loop on the erect film, commonly at different levels ('pair of scales'). In one-third of patients, the appearances are atypical and a water-soluble contrast enema should be carried out. This may demonstrate narrowing of the contrast column at the point of twisting, which has been described as resembling the beak of a bird of prey.

Volvulus patients often present with significant fluid and electrolyte abnormalities, which require

Figure 10.3 • Radiograph of the abdomen demonstrates the characteristic massive dilation of the sigmoid colon arising from the pelvis and extending to the right diaphragm. The arrow points to three lines representing the twisted walls of the sigmoid colon which converge in the left lower quadrant.

careful correction. **Untwisting and decompression** are the initial treatments of choice as long as the patient lacks clinical features suggestive of colonic strangulation. Untwisting has been described using several techniques, including rigid or flexible sigmoidoscopy, colonoscopy, blind passage of a rectal tube, and instillation of rectal contrast during a barium enema examination.[13] Although the use of a rectal tube has been reported to be successful in more than 80% of patients,[14,15] there is the risk of reduction of gangrenous sigmoid colon and a small risk of perforation. This risk may be minimised by performing a laparotomy when the bowel content draining through the rectal catheter is bloodstained. The endoscopic method of decompression has the advantage that decompression can be done under vision, increasing the accuracy of insertion through the twisted segment in the sigmoid colon. In addition, the mucosa of the whole sigmoid loop can be visualised directly and the identification of gangrenous mucosal patches is an indication for operative management. The experience of colonoscopic reduction of sigmoid volvulus has also been encouraging.

If symptoms and signs suggest ischaemia of the colon, **laparotomy** should be undertaken after the patient has been adequately resuscitated. Likewise, the patient who has unsuccessful non-operative treatment and those who have clinical features suggestive of colonic ischaemia at colonoscopy should also undergo emergency laparotomy. Since it is likely that resection will be required, the patient should be placed in the lithotomy/Trendelenburg position on the operating table. If colonic distension makes it difficult to handle the colon, a needle inserted obliquely through a taenia coli attached to a suction apparatus aids decompression. If the colon is gangrenous, it should be resected with as little manipulation as possible; the most widely recommended procedure is a segmental colectomy with an end colostomy and closure of the rectal stump (Hartmann's operation). In a prospective randomised trial from West Africa, Bagarani et al. compared the operative treatment in 31 patients with or without gangrene.[16] When gangrene was present, the mortality for Hartmann's procedure was 12.5% compared with 33.3% when resection and anastomosis were performed.

A small number of surgeons have described resection and primary anastomosis with good results. A study from India reported 197 patients with acute sigmoid volvulus treated by single-stage resection and anastomosis, 23 of whom had gangrene of the bowel.[17] Only two patients had anastomotic leaks, both of which responded to non-operative management. The two mortalities occurred in elderly patients who presented with perforations. A study from Ghana reported 21 patients with acute sigmoid volvulus treated by single-stage resection and anastomosis, 15 of whom had gangrene of the bowel.[18] Only one patient had a minor anastomotic leak, which responded to conservative management. However, it is important to stress that the majority of the patients in these studies were young and these results may not be applicable to the typical Western patient. In contrast, a series from the USA with 228 patients reported a mortality rate of 24% for emergency operations and 6% for elective operations. This study found mortality to correlate with emergency surgery and necrotic colon.[14]

Intraoperative colonic irrigation may facilitate primary anastomosis in patients with sigmoid volvulus who require emergency operation, since faecal loading proximal to the volvulus may increase the risk of anastomotic dehiscence. However, it is still important that only patients who are generally fit and without systemic sepsis and peritoneal contamination are selected for this procedure.

Because the risk of recurrent volvulus after decompression and derotation has been reported to be between 40% and 60%,[9] **elective surgery** to prevent further volvulus should always be considered. The most widely accepted procedure is resection, which is now associated with an operative mortality of 2–3%. The operation may be performed as a laparoscopic-assisted procedure through a small incision under local anaesthesia if required.

A variety of fixation procedures have been described but have been associated with high recurrence rates. An exception to this poor outcome has been reported with mesosigmoplasty.[15] The technique consists of shortening and broadening the sigmoid mesocolon by making an incision in the peritoneum from root to apex; the peritoneum is then mobilised and closed in a transverse direction (**Fig. 10.4**). The same procedure is then performed on the opposite side of the mesocolon. Recurrence was seen in only 2 of 125 patients followed for a mean of 8.2 years.

Ileosigmoid knotting

Ileosigmoid knotting is a variant of sigmoid volvulus in which the ileum twists around the base of the mesocolon (**Fig. 10.5**). It is also known as double volvulus. Three factors are responsible for ileosigmoid knotting: (i) a long small bowel mesentery and freely mobile small bowel; (ii) a long sigmoid colon on a narrow pedicle; and (iii) ingestion of high-bulk diet in the presence of empty small bowel.[19] It has been suggested that when a large semi-liquid bulky meal empties into the proximal jejunum it increases the motility of the intestine and the heavy segment of the bowel falls into the left lower quadrant. The empty loops of ileum and jejunum are thereby forced into a clockwise rotation towards the right upper quadrant around the base of a narrow sigmoid mesocolon. Further peristalsis forms an ileosigmoid knot with two closed loops, one affecting the small bowel and the other in the sigmoid colon.[19]

The condition is characterised by very acute onset of agonising generalised abdominal pain and repeated vomiting. Gangrene of the ileum and sigmoid colon is common. Generalised peritonitis, sepsis and dehydration are recognised complications, with hypovolaemic shock occurring early. The erect plain abdominal radiograph shows a dilated sigmoid colon and fluid levels in the small bowel.

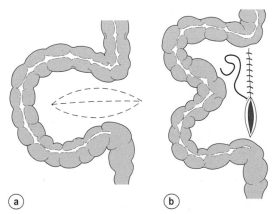

(a)   (b)

Figure 10.4 • The technique of mesosigmoidoplasty.

Figure 10.5 • Ileosigmoid knotting.

Initial management consists of resuscitation and administration of antibiotics followed by surgical intervention. Resection and anastomosis of the terminal ileum and a Hartmann procedure is the most commonly performed operation. Recent reports suggest that primary colonic anastomosis can be undertaken safely when there is a short history and the colon is clean and well vascularised. The condition unfortunately carries a very high mortality rate, ranging from 15% to 73%.[20]

Transverse colon volvulus

Volvulus affecting the transverse colon is less common than sigmoid volvulus, accounting for only 2.6% of all cases of colonic volvulus in one series.[21] Predisposing conditions include pregnancy, chronic constipation, distal colonic obstruction and previous gastric surgery. The plain abdominal radiograph usually shows gas-filled loops of large intestine with wide fluid levels. The condition is often mistaken for sigmoid volvulus and the diagnosis is rarely made preoperatively. After the operative diagnosis is confirmed and the transverse colon untwisted, evidence of distal obstruction should be sought. Operative choices include a transverse colectomy or an extended right hemicolectomy.

The rarity of the condition makes definitive statements difficult to support from the published literature but, in general, a primary anastomosis after resection is probably safe. An alternative method of treatment consists of suturing the right side of the transverse colon to the ascending colon with a similar procedure on the left side, thus shortening the unattached transverse colon.[22] In the presence of gangrenous bowel and significant peritoneal contamination, the safest approach may be to resect the affected colon and exteriorise both ends.

Caecal volvulus

Volvulus of the caecum is less common than volvulus of the sigmoid colon, representing 28% of all cases of colonic volvulus reported over a 10-year period in Edinburgh.[23] It is likely that incomplete rotation of the midgut leaves the caecum and ascending colon inadequately fixed to the posterior abdominal wall with a substantial length of mesentery. Conditions that alter the normal anatomy may predispose to caecal volvulus. There is an increased risk of caecal volvulus in pregnancy, and some patients are found to have adhesions from previous surgery. There is also an association with distal colonic obstruction. Volvulus usually takes place in a clockwise direction around the ileocolic vessels and, although the term 'caecal volvulus' is used, the condition also involves the ascending colon and ileum. As it twists, the caecum comes to occupy a position above and to the left of its original position. A similar condition, which is seen very occasionally, is 'caecal bascule'. In this condition, the caecum folds upwards on itself, producing a sharp kink in the ascending colon.

It is difficult to differentiate between caecal volvulus and other forms of proximal large bowel obstruction on clinical grounds. Some patients will have a previous history of episodes of obstruction that subsequently settled with non-operative treatment. The main presenting symptoms are colicky abdominal pain and vomiting. A tympanitic abdominal swelling will usually be present in the mid-abdomen.

On the supine abdominal radiograph, a comma-shaped caecal shadow in the mid-abdomen or left upper quadrant with a concavity to the right iliac fossa is diagnostic (**Fig. 10.6**) and there may be small bowel loops lying to the right side of the caecum. A single, long fluid level on the erect film is characteristic. If doubt persists, a contrast enema will show a beaked appearance in the ascending colon at the site of the volvulus (**Fig. 10.7**).

Management of caecal volvulus will depend to some extent on the clinical picture. The patient who is unfit for surgical treatment can be considered for colonoscopy since occasional successes have been reported using this method.[24] However, laparotomy is necessary in most patients. If the right colon is gangrenous at operation, the treatment of choice is a right hemicolectomy. A primary anastomosis should be possible in most cases even in the presence of contamination of the peritoneal cavity. It should be remembered that there is a markedly increased mortality in patients who have caecal gangrene. A report from the Mayo Clinic found a mortality rate of 12% in patients with caecal volvulus with a viable caecum, rising to 33% in the presence of colonic gangrene.[25]

There is more controversy about the procedure of choice in patients who have a viable caecum after reduction of the volvulus. On the one hand untwisting alone is associated with a high recurrence rate, but on the other hand resection, which avoids all risk of recurrence, carries a small risk of anastomotic leak. However, in one study of 22 patients there was no mortality and no anastomotic leaks. A 14% morbidity included one abdominal wall abscess, one intra-abdominal abscess and one medical complication.[26] The other two procedures commonly performed for caecal volvulus are caecostomy and caecopexy. Reports on the use of caecostomy demonstrate a wide variation in terms of both recurrence (0–25%) and mortality (0–33%). Some authors express concern over the morbidity of caecostomy and the occasional serious complication of abdominal wall sepsis and fasciitis, in addition to the potential for a persistent fistula.

Figure 10.6 • Abdominal radiograph demonstrates a massively dilated caecum folded over into the left upper quadrant with distended small bowel.

Figure 10.7 • Water-soluble contrast enema demonstrates a beak-like termination at the point of obstruction in the ascending colon with a markedly dilated caecum seen high in the abdomen.

The treatment of caecal volvulus has been reviewed in a large study comprising 561 published cases.[27] This review showed that caecopexy was associated with a mortality rate of 10% and a recurrence rate of 13%. If all circumstances are favourable, resection appears to be a justifiable procedure with minimal risk of recurrence, accepting that there may be a small number of patients who will have increased bowel frequency. In other circumstances, the minimum procedure compatible with survival becomes the goal.

Acute colonic pseudo-obstruction

Acute colonic pseudo-obstruction (ACPO) is the term used to describe the syndrome in which patients present with symptoms and signs of large bowel obstruction but in whom no mechanical cause can be demonstrated at contrast radiology. In more than 80% of patients with ACPO, an underlying precipitating condition exists, of which at least 50 have been described.[28] The most common of these associated conditions are metabolic disorders, trauma and cardiorespiratory disorders (Box 10.2). The term 'Ogilvie's syndrome' is loosely used in the literature as a synonym for ACPO, although it was actually used first to describe the pseudo-obstruction associated with retroperitoneal malignant infiltration. The mortality rate of ACPO is high, partly as a result of the underlying disorders but also related to failure to recognise the condition, leading to inappropriate operation. The true incidence is hard to ascertain since a number of unrecognised cases are likely to resolve spontaneously, but it has been estimated that some 200 deaths per annum in the UK may result from ACPO.[29]

Aetiology

The state of colonic motility at any point in time is determined by a balance of the inhibitory influence of the sympathetic nervous supply and the stimulatory effect of the parasympathetic system. It has been suggested that 'neuropraxia' of the sacral parasympathetic nerves may be a factor in the aetiology of

Box 10.2 • Predisposing conditions in acute colonic pseudo-obstruction

Chest infection
Myocardial infarction
Cerebrovascular accident
Renal failure
Puerperium
Retroperitoneal malignancy (Ogilvie's syndrome)
Orthopaedic trauma
Myxoedema
Electrolyte disturbance

ACPO, leading to a failure of propulsion in the left colon. This would also explain the 'cut-off' between dilated and collapsed bowel, which is located on the left side of the large bowel in 82% of patients.[30] Many of the conditions commonly associated with ACPO, such as sepsis, are likely to result from sympathetic overactivity.

Presentation

The clinical features of ACPO are almost identical to those of mechanical large bowel obstruction, making differentiation on clinical grounds alone almost impossible. Vanek and Al-Salti reviewed 400 patients and noted that the clinical features of ACPO are abdominal pain (83%), constipation (51%), diarrhoea (41%), fever (37%) and abdominal distension (100%).[30] On examination, the abdomen is generally very distended and tympanitic, but tenderness is often less than expected. The majority of patients will already have had operative procedures or have been hospitalised for some time because of some other disorder, and serum electrolytes are often abnormal.

Investigation (see also Chapter 5)

Plain radiographs of the abdomen in ACPO typically show gross distension of the large bowel with cut-off at the splenic flexure, rectosigmoid junction or, less commonly, the hepatic flexure (**Fig. 10.8**). Gas–fluid levels are less commonly seen on the plain radiograph in patients with ACPO compared with those presenting with mechanical obstruction.[31] It has been suggested that a prone lateral view of the rectum may be useful in making the diagnosis since gaseous filling of the rectum will tend to exclude mechanical obstruction. The caecal diameter should be measured on sequential abdominal radiographs since it is believed that the risk of caecal rupture increases greatly with increasing caecal diameter.[31]

There is overwhelming support for the use of a contrast enema in all patients with suspected ACPO in order to establish the diagnosis, since the differentiation from mechanical obstruction can be extremely difficult. This is well illustrated in a study reported by Koruth et al., who performed a contrast enema on 91 patients with suspected large bowel obstruction.[32] Of the 79 patients who were thought clinically to have mechanical obstruction, the diagnosis was confirmed in 50. There was free flow of contrast to the caecum in the remaining 29 patients. Of these 29, 11 had non-obstructing colonic pathology such as diverticular disease and ulcerative colitis and 18 patients had pseudo-obstruction. Of the 12 patients who were thought to have pseudo-obstruction before the water-soluble contrast enema, two were shown to have carcinoma of the colon.

Figure 10.8 • Plain abdominal radiograph of a patient with acute colonic pseudo-obstruction.

Management

The initial management of ACPO is non-operative and the underlying cause is treated if possible. Any medications that cause gut stasis should be discontinued, particularly analgesics. A nasogastric tube is routinely inserted to prevent swallowed air from entering the intestine and the use of enemas and flatus tubes is said to be of value in the treatment of early colonic pseudo-obstruction; in a number of patients even the water-soluble contrast enema used to establish the diagnosis may have a useful therapeutic effect. In most patients, the condition will resolve without intervention. One study found that it took an average of 6.5 days for complete resolution to take place in a group of 26 patients treated medically.[31] Progress should be checked by serial examination of the abdomen and by abdominal radiographs.

It is only when the risk of perforation increases substantially that more active intervention becomes necessary. The risk of perforation is approximately 3% and it has been shown that there is a correlation between perforation and the duration of distension.[33] The mean duration of distension was 6 days in the group of patients who went on to perforate compared with a mean duration of only 2 days in the group that did not progress to perforation.

In a randomised, double-blind, controlled trial of neostigmine only, 10 of 11 patients who were treated with intravenous neostigmine had prompt passage of flatus or stool, with reduced abdominal distension, compared with none of 10 patients who received placebo injection.[34]

These results were mirrored in a trial of 28 patients, with rapid resolution in 26. Time to pass flatus varied from 30 seconds to 10 minutes. In the two patients who failed to resolve, one was found to have a sigmoid cancer and the other died of multiorgan failure.[35] There is a risk of bradycardia with cholinergic agonists, and it has been suggested that patients with cardiac instability should not be treated with neostigmine. Interestingly, there is anecdotal evidence that the concomitant administration of glycopyrrolate with neostigmine seems to offset the risk of bradycardia and may be considered in patients with cardiac instability.[36] Epidural anaesthesia blocks sympathetic outflow, and improvement has been observed in a number of patients with ACPO who have had this form of treatment.[37]

The use of colonoscopy to decompress the colon in ACPO has become well established and it is successful in 73–90% of patients.[38] The procedure can be difficult and tedious, requiring a skilled colonoscopist, and air insufflation must be kept to a minimum. Frequent small-volume irrigation is required to ensure good visibility in the colon and maintain the patency of the colonoscope suction channel. A further advantage of colonoscopy is that necrotic patches can be identified on the colonic mucosa, allowing pre-emptive surgical treatment before perforation supervenes. The risk of perforation of the colon during colonoscopy for this condition has been estimated at around 3%,[39] and other complications are very unusual. It should be emphasised, however, that radiographs taken after successful clinical response often fail to show complete resolution of caecal distension, and one disadvantage of colonoscopic treatment is the tendency for the condition to recur. The overall rate of recurrence following initial colonoscopic decompression varies from 15% to 29%.[40] There is some difference of opinion about the best method of management of recurrent ACPO, but the safety and efficacy of repeat colonic decompression has now been reported.[28,38,40] A potential means of avoiding recurrence is intubation of the caecum with a long intestinal tube passed alongside the colonoscope.[41]

The indications for surgery include the following:

1. Caecal distension – the extent of distension varies between authors, from 9 to 12 cm,[42] the threshold rising with increasing availability of medical therapy.

2. Continuing caecal distension beyond 48–72 hours despite maximum medical therapy.
3. Pain over the right iliac fossa, i.e. the caecum.
4. Pneumoperitoneum.

There are doctors who recommend percutaneous caecostomies,[43] where a tube is inserted into the caecum using radiological guidance for the purpose of decompression. A trephine caecostomy may be performed under local anaesthesia. To avoid contamination, the caecum can be sutured to the incised external or internal oblique muscles and only opened when the peritoneal cavity is sealed off. Only when perforation of the caecum is suspected should a full laparotomy be performed. If a perforation or necrosis of the caecum has already occurred, a full laparotomy is necessary and a right hemicolectomy is the treatment of choice. When resection of the right colon is required, it is probably safest to bring out an ileostomy and mucous fistula and re-anastomose the two ends of bowel at a later date. Primary anastomosis may be feasible if contamination of the peritoneal cavity is not a feature and the remaining colon looks healthy.

Malignant large bowel obstruction

Approximately 85% of colonic emergencies are due to colon cancer and most of these occur in the elderly patient.[44] However, only 8–29% of colorectal cancer patients present with intestinal obstruction.[45] Approximately half of splenic flexure tumours present with obstruction, compared to 25% of those in the left colon, 6% of rectosigmoid lesions and 8–30% of right-sided carcinomas.[45] Both obstruction and perforation occur together in approximately 1% of all colon cancers, but in patients who have an obstruction caused by cancer, 12–19% will have a perforation.[46] The perforation may either be at the site of the tumour or in the caecum, caused by back pressure from the distal obstructing lesion.

The influence of obstruction on prognosis is controversial. Some studies suggest that the apparent adverse effect of obstruction on prognosis is a consequence of the stage of the disease rather than obstruction itself, as 27% have liver metastasis at the time of operation.[47] Other reports, however, suggest that obstruction is an independent predictor of poor prognosis.[48]

Presentation

Symptoms associated with large bowel obstruction frequently reflect the site of the tumour. In right-sided obstruction, particularly at the level of the ileocaecal valve, the onset of colicky central abdominal pain may be quite sudden and vomiting a relatively early feature. If the obstruction is at the rectosigmoid junction, there may be a history of a change in bowel habit and of rectal bleeding, with vomiting uncommon.

On examination, abdominal distension is the most notable feature. Peritoneal irritation suggests that perforation is either imminent or may have already occurred. Palpation of an irregular liver edge suggests that liver metastasis may be present and a palpable mass on rectal examination obviously suggests a carcinoma of the rectum.

Investigation

Plain abdominal radiography will usually provide the diagnosis of large bowel obstruction. The pattern of gas distribution in both the small and large bowel will depend on the site of obstruction and also on whether the ileocaecal valve is competent. However, as already mentioned differentiation from ACPO requires a contrast enema.

A water-soluble contrast enema (**Fig. 10.9**) should be carried out in all patients with suspected large bowel obstruction without evidence of perforation.[32]

A water-soluble contrast enema will exclude other conditions such as volvulus or pseudo-obstruction and, in addition, may go some way to cleansing the colon distal to the obstructing lesion. Sigmoidoscopy or colonoscopy can be useful, particularly if the suspected obstructing lesion is in the distal colon. In addition, either technique can be used to exclude synchronous carcinoma or adenoma below the level of obstruction.

Figure 10.9 • Water-soluble contrast enema demonstrating complete obstruction in the proximal sigmoid colon.

CT with intravenous and water-soluble rectal contrast is increasingly used in the emergency setting and this has the added advantage of providing information on the spread of disease preoperatively (**Fig. 10.10**).

Management

The morbidity and mortality rate associated with emergency procedures for obstruction of the colon is at least twice that for elective surgery. This has encouraged surgeons to develop methods such as the use of an expandable intraluminal stents. These can be used to palliate patients or to convert emergency operations into elective procedures. Several colonic stents are currently available and can be placed using radiological or endoscopic assistance. Various models can be deployed over guidewires or through an endoscope.

A review of 54 case series that included 1198 patients[49] found that, in 791 palliative patients, technical success was possible in 93% and clinical success (defined as decompression in less than 48 hours) in 91%. Stents also provided successful conversion to elective procedures in 92% of 407 patients. Intraluminal stenting was more successful in shorter, distal lesions and colonic primaries. Technical failure usually results from an inability to pass the guidewire or stent catheter across the lesion. Reported complications include perforation in 3.8%, stent migration in 12% and re-obstruction in 7%.

When surgery is undertaken, patients with right-sided obstruction should be positioned flat on the operating table. Those with left-sided large bowel obstruction are placed in the lithotomy/Trendelenburg position to allow access to the anus during the procedure for purposes of irrigation of the rectal stump or anal insertion of a surgical stapling instrument. It also allows the surgical assistant the option of standing between the patient's legs. The abdomen is opened through a midline incision. If the bowel is tense, it should be decompressed: first, to improve visualisation of the rest of the abdomen and, second, to prevent spillage of faecal content. The large bowel can be decompressed by inserting a 16G intravenous catheter or 18F nasogastric tube obliquely through the colonic wall, following which suction is applied. This is often enough to make it possible to handle the large bowel without fear of rupture as the distension is mainly gas. After localisation of the primary tumour, synchronous tumours should be excluded. The presence of direct spread to adjacent structures should also be assessed, in addition to any peritoneal seedlings and the presence of liver secondaries. Based on these observations, a decision can be made as to whether the operation is potentially curative or palliative.

When there is a prospect of curative resection, standard techniques of radical cancer therapy should be employed, including wide excision of the lesion en bloc with the appropriate blood vessels and mesentery. If the lesion is adherent to other structures, an attempt should be made to resect the affected part en bloc. High cure rates are possible with locally advanced tumours if a radical resection is performed and clear resection margins obtained. The presence of liver or peritoneal metastases does not preclude resection of the primary carcinoma and gastrointestinal continuity should be restored if at all possible.

If there is a closed loop obstruction because of competence of the ileocaecal valve, the caecum and right colon may be very tense. Decompression can be achieved as a preliminary to resection by making a small enterotomy in the terminal ileum and passing a Foley catheter through the ileocaecal valve into the caecum. This technique is particularly useful in situations where there is splitting of the taenia on the caecum, indicating impending rupture. The range of operations available for treatment of right-sided tumours causing obstruction includes right hemicolectomy with primary anastomosis, right hemicolectomy with exteriorisation of both ends of the large bowel, and ileo-transverse colon bypass. There is general agreement that a right hemicolectomy with primary anastomosis is the treatment of choice in most patients; however, this procedure is by no means free of complications. One report noted an operative mortality rate of 17% in 195 patients who had emergency right hemicolectomy with primary anastomosis for obstructing colonic carcinoma.[50] In addition, a leak rate of 10% was noted in 179 patients who had a right hemicolectomy and primary anastomosis for obstruction. This compares with a leak rate of 6% in 579 patients with right colon cancer who did not have an obstruction.[50] Other studies have shown similar mortality rates,

Figure 10.10 • Computed tomography scan of a patient with a perforated caecum (perforation indicated by arrow). The scan also revealed an obstructing splenic flexure tumour and extensive liver metastases.

and many of the deaths resulted from anastomotic failure. This suggests that instead of subjecting all patients with obstruction to right hemicolectomy with primary anastomosis, it may be wiser to use a policy of selection, subjecting patients with good risk status to primary anastomosis and managing patients with risk factors for anastomotic failure by resection and exteriorisation of the bowel ends.

The anastomotic technique used will depend on the surgeon's preference. If the obstructed bowel is very thickened and oedematous, care should be taken with the use of stapling instruments since there is a tendency for the instruments to cut through oedematous bowel. On these occasions a sutured anastomosis is preferable. Only on the relatively rare occasion when locally advanced disease is unresectable should the patient be subjected to an ileo-transverse colon bypass procedure. There is almost no place for caecostomy in the current management of right-sided large bowel obstruction; trephine ileostomy, which can usually be achieved under local anaesthesia, affords better palliation in very sick patients not fit for operation under general anaesthesia.

Most surgeons would advocate an extended right hemicolectomy for patients with transverse colon carcinoma, and decompression of the colon may be necessary to facilitate mobilisation. For the patient who has a large carcinoma obstructing the transverse colon, achieving clearance may be difficult because of involvement of the transverse mesocolon and adjacent organs. The splenic flexure is mobilised to assist with a primary anastomosis between ileum and upper descending colon. In the sick patient who already has a perforated caecum, resection and an ileostomy may be appropriate.

The two most frequent options are resection and either primary anastomosis or colostomy and rectal closure (Hartmann's procedure) for obstructing left-sided colonic tumours. A three-stage procedure (diverting colostomy, resection and colostomy closure) is now rarely used, and only in critically ill patients. Two-stage procedures became popular during the 1970s and remain the procedure of choice for most surgeons, with an overall mortality around 10%.[46] However, the main disadvantage of this approach, apart from the fact that a second operation is required for reconstruction, is that approximately 40% of patients will be left with a permanent stoma.

The second stage of the two-stage operation may be difficult because of adhesions, although it is facilitated if the rectal stump has been divided above the peritoneal reflection. The timing of the second stage is also important and most surgeons will wait 2–6 months. The second stage of the two-stage procedure is increasingly being performed using laparoscopic techniques. If successful the hospital stay is reduced, but conversion to open surgery may be necessary.

Primary resection and anastomosis is associated with a shorter hospital stay, reduced mortality and morbidity, and the avoidance of a stoma. It is increasingly becoming the operation of choice for colorectal surgeons, with the exact procedure depending on a number of factors. Subtotal colectomy followed by ileosigmoid or ileorectal anastomosis has been reported to have a low operative mortality of 3–11% and a hospital stay of around 15–20 days.[51] Segmental colectomy (left hemicolectomy, sigmoid colectomy or anterior resection of the rectosigmoid) with on-table irrigation followed by primary anastomosis has a reported operative mortality rate around 10%, anastomotic leakage around 4% and hospital stay of approximately 20 days.[52]

A retrospective study of 243 patients who underwent emergency operation for obstructing colorectal cancers showed that primary resection and anastomosis for left-sided malignant obstruction either by segmental resection with on-table lavage or by subtotal colectomy was not more hazardous than primary anastomosis for right-sided obstruction.[53] Single-stage resection with primary anastomosis was possible in 197 patients. Of the 101 patients with left-sided obstruction, segmental resection with on-table colonic lavage was performed in 75 patients and subtotal colectomy in 26. There were no differences in the mortality or leakage rates between patients with right-sided and left-sided lesions (mortality 7.3% vs. 8.9%; leakage 5.2% vs. 6.9% respectively).

More recent papers have described segmental resection and primary anastomosis without any attempt to clean the bowel. One study reported only one leak and one postoperative death in 58 consecutive patients with left-sided malignant colonic obstruction who underwent bowel decompression without irrigation, followed by resection and primary colocolic anastomosis.[54] The patients had a mean age of 63 (range 54–89) years, the leak occurring in a 61-year-old with a sigmoid carcinoma and the death in an 80-year-old due to myocardial infarction. None of the carcinomas described were rectosigmoid or rectal. A further study of left-sided obstruction in which 40 of 60 patients had carcinoma compared one-stage resection with Hartmann's procedure.[55] There was no significant difference in outcome or time taken to complete the operation, with the only death being in the Hartmann's group. Again, none of the tumours described was more distal than the sigmoid colon.

In certain circumstances one of these procedures may be more preferable. In the elderly segmental resection may be preferable to a more extensive resection, both in terms of operative morbidity and postoperative problems of incontinence. Subtotal colectomy is clearly the procedure of choice when there are synchronous tumours in the colon. When subtotal colectomy with ileorectal anastomosis is selected as the operation of choice, the whole colon is mobilised and the rectum washed out as for elective surgery. After resection of the colon, an ileorectal or ileosigmoid anastomosis is performed using either a sutured or stapled technique. The first randomised trial comparing subtotal versus segmental resection was reported in 1995.[56] This study involved 91 eligible patients recruited by 18 consultant surgeons in 12 centres; 47 were randomised to subtotal colectomy and 44 to on-table irrigation and segmental colectomy. There was no significant difference in operative mortality, hospital stay, anastomotic leakage or wound sepsis between the two groups. There was a significantly higher permanent stoma rate in the subtotal colectomy group compared with the segmental colectomy group (7 vs. 1). The high permanent stoma rate in the subtotal colectomy group was partly accounted for by four patients who were randomised to subtotal colectomy but who underwent Hartmann's procedure because this was thought clinically more appropriate by the operating surgeon. Two additional patients had the anastomosis taken down at a later date and a stoma formed. At follow-up 4 months after the operation, there was a significantly greater number of patients who had three or more bowel movements a day after subtotal colectomy than after segmental resection (14 of 35 vs. 4 of 35). One patient had 12 bowel movements per day after subtotal colectomy. Nearly one-third of patients randomised to subtotal colectomy had night-time bowel movements during the first few months after operation. In contrast, less than 10% of those who had segmental resection had this problem.

Segmental resection of the colon following intraoperative irrigation is the preferred treatment for left-sided malignant colonic obstruction.[56]

Although the study addressed the immediate and early results after these two procedures, it did not investigate the long-term implications of either procedure. It has been argued that there are advantages in performing a subtotal colectomy rather than segmental resection because synchronous tumours will be removed along with the obstructing lesion and, since the length of colon left is small, there should be less risk of developing a metachronous tumour. Clearly the operating surgeon needs to take all these factors into account when making the final decision on which procedure is most suitable for the individual patient.

Inflammation and infection

Acute colonic diverticulitis

Colonic diverticula are found with increasing age. It has been estimated that one-third of the population will have colonic diverticula by the age of 50 years and two-thirds after 80 years. Although the vast majority of individuals with colonic diverticula are asymptomatic, most patients who require surgical care do so because of an inflammatory complication. Acute diverticulitis can affect any part of the colon; in western Europe and North America, the left side is more commonly affected, whereas in Japan and China right-sided diverticulitis is more commonly seen. Symptomatic complications of diverticulitis occur in 10–30% of patients, but the need for surgery in acute diverticulitis is becoming less common.

Presentation

Diverticulitis is thought to result from inspissation of stool in the neck of a diverticulum, with consequent inflammation and possible microperforation. This results in local bacterial proliferation, leading to inflammation in the surrounding colonic wall and mesentery (acute phlegmonous diverticulitis). A collection of pus may form either in the mesentery of the colon or adjacent to the colonic wall. As the collection of pus enlarges, it becomes walled off by loops of small bowel or the peritoneum of the pelvis. Occasionally, free perforation into the peritoneal cavity occurs with consequent purulent or faecal peritonitis. The Hinchey grading system for acute diverticulitis has become fairly widely accepted, allowing more meaningful comparison between outcome studies (Table 10.1).[57]

From time to time other complications also arise. A fistula sometimes develops between bowel and another adjacent organ (ie. the bladder or vaginal cuff). Diverticular disease is responsible for around 10% of all cases of left-sided large bowel obstruction and is frequently difficult to differentiate from malignant left-sided large bowel obstruction on clinical grounds. Bleeding also occurs.

There has been controversy regarding the virulence of diverticular disease in younger patients and the possible increase in need for surgical intervention

Table 10.1 • Hinchey classification of peritoneal contamination in diverticulitis

Stage 1	Pericolic or mesenteric abscess
Stage 2	Walled-off pelvic abscess
Stage 3	Generalised purulent peritonitis
Stage 4	Generalised faecal peritonitis

in this group. Recently, Biondo et al. looked at 327 patients treated for acute left colonic diverticulitis and compared those aged 50 or less with those older than 50.[58] No difference was noted regarding severity or recurrence. Another study found that diverticulitis in the young does not follow a particularly aggressive course.[59] In general, there is a trend towards conservative management of acute diverticulitis, with early investigation and confirmation of the diagnosis being a fundamental part of this approach. The mortality and morbidity rates can be high if emergency surgery is necessary.

Investigation

Acute right-sided diverticulitis, a rare condition in the Western world, can be confused with appendicitis as it occurs in a somewhat younger age group than left-sided disease. In the more common left-sided disease, the plain abdominal radiograph may show non-specific abnormalities such as pneumoperitoneum, intestinal obstruction or a soft-tissue mass.

 CT is now the favoured modality for acute investigation of suspected acute colonic diverticultis.[60]

Features of acute diverticulitis include thickening of the bowel wall, increased soft-tissue density within the pericolic fat secondary to inflammation and a soft-tissue mass, which represents either a phlegmon or an abscess. Advantages of CT include the accurate assessment of the extent of pericolonic involvement and the diagnosis of abscess formation or perforation (**Fig. 10.11**). It is also useful for tracking the therapeutic percutaneous drainage of any abscess. When CT is compared with barium enema, CT is no more accurate in terms of diagnosis but

Figure 10.11 • Appearance of perforated sigmoid diverticular disease on computed tomography. The upper arrow shows a small pocket of free air and the lower arrow one of the diverticula.

undoubtedly provides better definition of the extent and severity of the inflammatory process, which is of prognostic value in the short and long term.[61] Ultrasonography has also been used for localised diverticulitis. The main disadvantages of ultrasonography are that assessment of bowel thickening is a non-specific finding and assessment is very operator dependent.

An alternative investigation is contrast enema. Despite the extensive literature on the use of contrast enema in acute diverticulitis, there is no consensus on either the best contrast agent or the optimal timing of the examination. There has been some interest with magnetic resonance imaging in the diagnosis of acute diverticulitis and prospective observational studies have been encouraging, but more formal evaluation is still required.[62]

Management

Right-sided disease may be encountered unexpectedly at surgery or be operated on for a complication diagnosed preoperatively. The treatment options are controversial, ranging from appendicectomy to hemicolectomy. A conservative approach with appendicectomy and antibiotics has resulted in a similar mortality, morbidity and recurrence as for resection of the diverticulum.[63] A right hemicolectomy is the correct operation when it is not possible to rule out the presence of a carcinoma.

A typical patient with localised left-sided diverticulitis will complain of pain in the left iliac fossa and will be febrile. Examination reveals tenderness and sometimes a mass is palpable per abdomen or on rectal examination. In women, a vaginal examination should also be performed to exclude gynaecological pathology. If sigmoidoscopy is performed, it should be done gently with minimal insufflation of air.

In the absence of generalised peritonitis, a nonoperative policy is adopted, with antibiotic therapy directed against Gram-negative and anaerobic bacteria. Most clinicians advocate bowel rest initially, and intravenous fluids and antibiotics. If the pain and fever settle within a few days, the patient can go home on oral antibiotics and a barium enema and sigmoidoscopy or colonoscopy can be performed as an outpatient several weeks later to exclude any malignancy.

If the patient continues with fever, pain or enlarging lower abdominal mass, a CT should be obtained. If there is an abscess, it can be drained percutaneously under radiological guidance. In the event of localised abdominal signs becoming more generalised or if there is a failure of the infective process to settle despite adequate conservative therapy, operation is indicated. In the small number of patients who require operation for localised diverticulitis, primary resection, with or without on-table irrigation and primary anastomosis, is becoming increasingly popular among specialist colorectal surgeons.

Pain from perforated sigmoid diverticulitis usually commences in the lower abdomen, mostly on the left side, and gradually spreads throughout the abdomen. In 25% of patients, however, signs and symptoms are predominantly right-sided.[64] On examination, there are signs of generalised peritonitis including guarding and rebound tenderness. About one-quarter of all patients will have free gas under the diaphragm on abdominal radiography, and at operation purulent peritonitis is more common than faecal peritonitis.[64] The majority of patients presenting in this way will clearly require operation following adequate resuscitation. Antibiotic therapy should be commenced early to cover both anaerobic organisms and Gram-negative bacteria. Some patients will improve so much with non-operative treatment that it may be appropriate to continue with this therapy for a longer period.

Operative management

The patient is placed in the lithotomy/Trendelenburg position and explored with a midline incision. Pus and faecal material should be removed from the peritoneal cavity and specimens sent for microscopy and both aerobic and anaerobic culture. Intraoperative irrigation of the peritoneal cavity with 6–10 L of warm saline solution is of value, while the addition of topical antibiotics to the solution (e.g. cephradine (cefradine) 1 g in 1 L of 0.9% saline), although logical, remains unproven.

In addition to treating the peritonitis, surgical treatment must minimise continued contamination of the peritoneal cavity. Krukowski and Matheson[65] analysed 57 reports on the treatment of acute diverticular disease and showed that the operative mortality rates from procedures that involve primary resection (10%) were less than half those from operations that did not include excision of the diseased colon (20%). A further reason for advocating primary resection is the difficulty experienced at the time of operation in deciding whether the lesion is a perforated carcinoma or an area of diverticulitis. At laparotomy, the appearance of both lesions may be similar when the colon is inflamed and oedematous. It has been estimated that as many as 25% of patients with a preoperative diagnosis of perforated diverticulitis may be found to have a perforated carcinoma. If there is reasonable suspicion of carcinoma, a radical resection of the lesion, together with the colonic mesentery, needs to be performed. Examination of the resected specimen at the earliest opportunity is recommended to aid further decision-making.

Failure to take the resection far enough distally beyond the sigmoid colon risks recurrence of diverticular disease. Therefore, Hartmann's resection with complete excision of the sigmoid and closure of the rectum, with formation of a left lower quadrant colostomy, has been the standard procedure advocated by most surgeons. If the operation is exceptionally difficult owing to the colon being very adherent to surrounding structures, making safe mobilisation impossible, it may be reasonable to create a proximal stoma, drain the area and transfer the patient to a tertiary referral centre.

There has been an increase in the use of primary anastomosis in selected patients who have operations for acute diverticulitis. The main reasons are: (i) that patients receive one operation rather than two; (ii) after a Hartmann operation many patients are left with a permanent stoma, either because of unwillingness or unfitness to have further surgery; and (iii) reversal operation after Hartmann's resection can be very difficult.

Biondo et al. used resection, intraoperative colonic lavage and primary anastomosis in 55 of 124 patients with complicated diverticular disease; 49 of the 55 had diverticulitis, 33 having localised and 16 generalised peritonitis.[66] Faecal peritonitis was considered a contraindication to a one-stage procedure. Four patients died, one from an anastomotic leak. Major complications included two anastomotic leaks (one of which was successfully treated with parenteral nutrition), four re-operations (three for abdominal wound dehiscence and one for anastomotic leak) and four deaths (three of those who died were over 70 years old). The study concluded that one-stage resection is feasible in selected patients.

 One-stage resection for acute complicated diverticultis without faecal peritonitis is feasible.[66]

A further study of primary anastomosis in emergency colorectal surgery showed no significant difference in the incidence of complications, even in patients with free peritonitis (21.9% perforation, 17.7% localised sepsis).[67] The necessity for intraoperative colonic lavage has also been challenged. Despite an increasing trend to perform primary anastomosis in patients who have perforated diverticulitis, the number of patients who are suitable for such a procedure will be small.

Neutropenic enterocolitis

Neutropenic enterocolitis, also known as typhlitis, is a potentially life-threatening condition characterised by an inflammatory process that usually involves the caecum and ascending colon. It occurs most often as a complication of chemotherapy and can progress to necrosis and perforation. Although it can affect any part of the small and large intestine, the cause of its predisposition for the right colon is unclear.

Clinical features include nausea, vomiting, abdominal pain, distension and diarrhoea, which can be bloody. Right iliac fossa tenderness and pyrexia are quite common and in later stages peritonitis may be present. CT is the diagnostic modality of choice and may reveal right-sided colon wall thickening, mesenteric stranding, pneumatosis and ascites (**Fig. 10.12**).

Management demands careful evaluation of the patient, with each case treated individually. An initial conservative approach includes fluid and electrolyte replacement, broad-spectrum antibiotics, correction of any attendant coagulopathy and complete bowel rest with parenteral nutrition. The use of recombinant granulocyte colony-stimulating factor to correct chemotherapy-induced neutropenia should be considered. Colonic perforation and generalised peritonitis are clear indications for surgery. The operative procedure of choice is a right hemicolectomy, with either exteriorisation of the bowel ends or a primary anastomosis depending on the extent of sepsis and peritoneal soiling. In general, most cases can be managed non-operatively.

Toxic colitis

Toxic colitis is a potentially fatal complication of inflammatory bowel disease, particularly if accompanied by megacolon. While several schemes exist to accurately identify toxic colitis, one reasonably simple system employs a definition that includes a disease flare-up accompanied by two of the following criteria: hypoalbuminaemia (<3.0 g/dL), leucocytosis (>10.5×10^9 cells/L), tachycardia (>100 beats/minute), temperature elevation (>38.6 °C).[68] Use of this relatively objective definition may aid in the diagnosis and care of these patients whose severe condition can be under-appreciated because of high dosages of steroids, immunomodulators or biological agents.

The initial management is directed at reversing physiological deficits with intravenous hydration, correction of electrolyte imbalances, and blood product transfusions. Free perforation, increasing colonic dilatation, massive haemorrhage, peritonitis and septic shock are indications for emergency operation after the patient has been adequately resuscitated. In the absence of these features, medical therapy is initiated with high dosages of intravenous corticosteroids, immunomodulators and/or biological agents. Broad-spectrum antibiotics directed against intestinal flora are prescribed to minimise the risk of sepsis secondary to transmural inflammation or microperforation. Anticholinergics, antidiarrhoeals and narcotics are avoided as they may worsen already impaired colonic motility or conceal ominous symptoms. Hyperalimentation may be started and the patient is closely observed with serial examinations and abdominal roentgenograms. Any worsening of the clinical course over the ensuing 24–72 hours mandates urgent laparotomy. If the patient improves minimally after 5–7 days of conventional therapy, the medical therapy should be altered or surgery should be advised. Experience with ciclosporin or infliximab in this setting is anecdotal, and should be weighed against operative therapy while understanding that surgery in this setting often relegates the patient to a lifelong ileostomy.[69]

The principal operative options in patients with toxic colitis are subtotal colectomy with end ileostomy or loop ileostomy with decompressive blowhole colostomy. The most difficult aspect of a subtotal colectomy is managing the distal bowel stump. The distal limb may be closed with sutures or staples and then delivered to the anterior abdominal wall, where it can lie without tension in the subcutaneous fat of the lower midline wound. If the bowel end is placed above the fascia, dehiscence of the rectal closure during the postoperative period results in a mucous fistula. If the closed stump is left within the peritoneal cavity, staple line dehiscence will produce a pelvic abscess. If the bowel wall is too friable to hold sutures or staples, creation of a mucous fistula is preferred.

The patient typically improves over the ensuing few days and can be typically discharged within a week of the operation. An appropriate elective procedure can be considered several months after the patient recovers.

Proctocolectomy with end ileostomy is rarely performed in the severely ill patient with toxic colitis because of the excessive rates of morbidity and mortality.[70] Proctectomy increases the difficulty of the procedure and risks pelvic bleeding as well as autonomic nerve damage. In rare instances of rectal perforation or profuse colorectal haemorrhage, proctocolectomy may be an option. The surgeon must be cautioned, however, that the macroscopic and microscopic differentiation of ulcerative colitis from Crohn's proctocolitis is especially difficult in severe colitis, and primary proctocolectomy would nullify the future option of a restorative procedure in a patient with ulcerative colitis.

Figure 10.12 • Computed tomography scan showing large retroperitoneal collection (indicated by arrows) secondary to acute necrotising enterocolitis with a delayed perforation of the posterior wall of the caecum and ascending colon.

The need for loop ileostomy combined with decompression blowhole colostomy has virtually disappeared with improved medical recognition and more sophisticated management of toxic colitis. The operation is still useful in extremely ill patients or those in whom colectomy would be especially hazardous (e.g. contained perforation, high-lying splenic flexure and pregnancy). Contraindications to the procedure include colorectal haemorrhage, free perforation and intra-abdominal abscess. The operation is considered only a temporising procedure, and a definitive operation is commonly performed approximately 6 months later.

Perforation

Stercoral perforation

The word *stercus* means dung or faeces. Perforation of the bowel caused by pressure necrosis from a faecal mass is a rare entity, first reported by Berry at the Pathological Society of London in 1894. Fewer than 100 cases have been reported in the literature, although this may reflect the poor outcome (with mortality rates approaching 50%), an increasing reluctance to publish case reports and ill-defined diagnostic criteria. There appears to be an equal incidence in men and women and the median age for these patients is said to be 60 years.[71]

Reported predisposing factors have included chronic constipation, megacolon, scleroderma, hypercalcaemia, renal failure and renal transplantation. Medications associated with stercoral perforation include narcotics, postoperative analgesia, antacids, calcium channel blockers and antidepressants. Only 11% of cases are accurately diagnosed prior to operation,[72] with investigations frequently non-contributory. Perforations usually occur on the antimesenteric border, with the majority occurring in the sigmoid colon and rectosigmoid region. Multiple perforations are found in about one-fifth of patients, with the remaining patients usually having ulceration extending away from the perforation.

The suggested clinicopathological diagnostic criteria are:

- A round or ovoid colonic perforation exceeding 1 cm in diameter.
- Faecolomas present within the colon.
- Microscopic evidence of pressure necrosis or ulcer and chronic inflammatory reaction around the perforation site.[73] This study, which constitutes one of the largest single-institution reports on stercoral perforation of the colon, defined strict clinical and pathological criteria for its diagnosis. Using these criteria stercoral

perforation of the colon would appear to occur more frequently than previously reported in the literature.

Management of these patients is surgical, with the resection margins sufficiently wide to encompass all areas of perforation or impending perforations. The bowel is universally loaded with stool and the tendency towards constipation is not removed by a limited resection. The operation should involve resection of the affected segment and exteriorisation of the bowel for left-sided perforations, with resection and primary anastomosis being reserved for those patients with a right-sided perforation. The risk of recurrent perforation in the proximal colon presents a further problem for those with a left-sided perforation. Milking the stool in an antegrade direction into the resected segment and orthograde colonic irrigation may combine to avoid early re-perforation. However, the fear of recurrent perforation from persistent constipation has led some surgeons to suggest a subtotal colectomy.

Anastomotic dehiscence

Breakdown of an anastomosis is one of the most significant complications after large bowel surgery. The presentation can be insidious but more commonly the patient becomes acutely ill, particularly if there is generalised peritonitis. If the diagnosis is not made and appropriate treatment undertaken, death is likely to follow. There is no doubt that the presence of anastomotic leakage significantly increases mortality. Fielding et al. noted a mortality rate of 22% in 191 patients who had leakage after large bowel anastomosis compared with only 7.2% in 1275 patients without a leak.[74] In the patients who survive this serious complication, morbidity and hospital stay are greatly increased.

Causes

A variety of general and local causative factors of anastomotic dehiscence have been described. General factors listed usually include poor nutritional state, anaemia, uraemia, diabetes, steroid administration and old age, while suggested local factors involved tension, ischaemia or infection of the anastomosis. The risk of anastomotic leakage in low colorectal anastomosis is several times higher than in either ileocolic or colocolic anastomosis. Watson et al. reported a clinical leak rate for ileocolic and colocolic anastomosis of 0.4%, whereas the leak rate after low colorectal anastomosis was 4.7%.[75] In a review of 477 large bowel anastomoses, which included 215 colorectal anastomoses, there were eight colorectal and one ileocolic leaks. All nine patients required laparotomy, and seven were salvaged with no mortality. Three colorectal leaks (small posterior defects in stapled anastomoses) were closed with interrupted endoanal sutures and a proximal loop stoma fashioned in two patients who did not already have one. The other two leaks (defect in suture line attributable to a single suture cutting through) were managed by creating a controlled external fistula. None of these patients had further complications and all the stomas were subsequently closed. It is therefore possible to salvage anastomotic leaks with a good outcome in selected patients with appropriate operative treatment.

Another important factor in dehiscence is the oxygen tension at the bowel ends used for the anastomosis. In an elegant study reported in 1987, it was shown that if tissue oxygen tension in the ends of bowel to be anastomosed fell to less than 20 mmHg (2.66 kPa), there was a high likelihood of anastomotic breakdown.[76] However, a significant factor in anastomotic failure is poor surgical technique, whether sutures or staples are used.

Presentation

In general, the clinical features of anastomotic dehiscence will depend on whether the leak is localised or more extensive, causing generalised peritonitis. At one end of the spectrum, when sepsis associated with the leak is localised, the patient may have minimal symptoms and only a few physical signs. There may be 'flu-like' symptoms of feeling vaguely unwell with shivering and nausea. If the anastomosis lies low in the pelvis, there may be some lower abdominal pain and tenderness and on rectal examination a defect can often be felt in the anastomosis. Tachycardia is a common general feature and is often associated with pyrexia. If a drain is still in situ, faecal material or pus may be seen.

At the other end of the spectrum is the scenario associated with a major leak, when faecal material or pus has leaked into the general peritoneal cavity. The effect on the patient is usually profound. Abdominal pain is difficult to control and tachycardia and tachypnoea are common. The temperature is raised and hypotension is often a feature. The patient is distressed and sweaty and on abdominal examination the abdomen is tender with abdominal guarding. Sometimes the features of even an extensive leak can be more insidious, with the patient not making progress as rapidly as expected and suffering abdominal pain that is vague rather than dramatic.

Delay in diagnosis of large bowel anastomotic leakage is still a major problem and leads to increased morbidity and mortality. It is crucial that surgeons are vigilant about deterioration of any patient who has a large bowel anastomosis and maintain a low threshold for ordering investigations to identify a leak. It should be remembered that the anastomosis may leak any time during the first 2–3 weeks after operation.

Investigations

Usually the white blood count is elevated, except in patients who have overwhelming sepsis, when it may be either normal or even low. However, the earliest derangement in the white blood count is an increase in the less mature polymorphic neutrophils (e.g. left shift). Erect chest radiograph or abdominal films will sometimes show gas under the diaphragm, but this sign is of debatable significance in the first few days after the original operation because of the presence of intra-abdominal air introduced at the time of operation. The absence of pneumoperitoneum should not discourage the clinician from pursuing investigations to check the integrity of the anastomosis.

Ultrasound examination can be helpful in the patient with a suspected collection of pus related to anastomotic leakage, but the value of this investigation is often impaired by the presence of dilated gas-filled loops of bowel, with dressings and drains on the abdomen further increasing technical difficulties. CT or contrast studies are the investigation of choice.

Water-soluble contrast enema is a simple investigation for assessing anastomotic leakage, particularly on the left side of the large bowel. In addition to demonstrating whether a leak has occurred, assessment of the extent of leakage is of value in deciding the overall management. It is important to be aware of two caveats, however; occasionally, when the contrast enema shows no leak, a later investigation will show one. The corollary of this is also rarely true. The enema may show a leak that is of no clinical consequence (radiological leak). It is therefore important to look at the overall clinical picture and attempt to assess all the clinical and radiological evidence before coming to a final conclusion about the presence of a clinically significant leak.

Management

Although the literature on colonic anastomotic leak rates is extensive, there is a paucity of information on how to treat the leakage. It is best to consider the management of localised leakage separate from those who present with generalised peritonitis. Most patients with **localised leakage** can be treated non-operatively with bowel rest and antibiotic therapy. If there is a large collection of pus around the anastomosis, it is usual to drain this percutaneously under ultrasound or CT guidance. Patients with **generalised peritonitis** from a large bowel anastomotic leak are usually dramatically ill and require resuscitation. Assuming that investigations have been performed and the diagnosis confirmed, the next step is to improve the patient's condition before surgical intervention.

Haemodynamic status needs to be assessed and treatment given to improve cardiac and respiratory function. Parenteral antibiotic administration is a priority and inotropic support may be necessary. Adequate pain control is important and these patients are best managed in a high-dependency unit or intensive therapy unit. Anaesthesia is alerted and only when the patient's condition is stabilised is operation undertaken.

The patient is usually placed in the lithotomy/Trendelenburg position. The previous midline incision is reopened and great care is taken not to damage adherent loops of small intestine. Bowel loops are dissected free and the area of anastomosis exposed. Faecal material and pus are removed from the peritoneal cavity and pelvis. Occlusion clamps are gently placed on bowel above and below the leaking anastomosis to limit further contamination. Extensive lavage of the peritoneal cavity is performed with saline or antibiotic solution.

The next steps depend on the size and location of the anastomotic defect. In the majority of cases, the anastomosis is taken apart and the proximal end of bowel is brought out as an end stoma and the distal end as a mucous fistula. If the distal stump is not long enough to be brought out on the abdominal wall, it should be closed carefully using a series of interrupted seromuscular sutures. Some surgeons will place a transanal drain to decompress the bowel. Surgeons must be aware that the more distal the leak, the lower the chances of bowel continuity being restored at a later date.

In selected patients (usually those with a small defect in a low colorectal anastomosis), the anastomosis may be salvaged. A defunctioning ileostomy can be constructed for diversion and the area of the leak can be drained. However, the faecal loading in the colon can lead to continued soiling unless it is removed with transanal irrigation. However, in a patient who has already had an anastomotic leak it is poor practice to risk a further leak and the patient's safety should be the prime objective.

Bowel damage at colonoscopy

The perforation rate at colonoscopy is now generally agreed to be about 1 in 500, varying with the level of intervention employed.

There are three proposed mechanisms for colonoscopic perforation:

1. mechanical perforation directly from the colonoscope or biopsy forceps;
2. barotrauma from overzealous air insufflation;
3. perforations occurring as a result of therapeutic procedures (use of energy sources).

Measurement of forces exerted during colonoscopy has only been reported in one paper from the Royal London Hospital,[77] where an electronic device was used in a research setting. The caecum and right colon are most susceptible to barotrauma, although diverticula can also be directly inflated. The use of carbon dioxide for insufflation may decrease perforation rates and increase levels of patient comfort. Therapeutic interventions, such as polyp removal with a hot biopsy or snare and balloon dilatation of strictures are, not surprisingly, associated with a higher risk of perforation.

The most common site of perforation is the sigmoid colon. Signs and symptoms of a perforation are not always obvious at the time of colonoscopy. In retrospective studies, the diagnosis of a perforation is delayed in about 50% of patients.[78] If the endoscopist is worried after an examination has been completed, an erect chest radiograph should be ordered as a screening test and the patient observed until symptoms have settled. In cases where there is a high index of suspicion, a water-soluble enema or CT can be used to confirm the diagnosis.

Non-operative treatment with close observation, intravenous fluids and antibiotics may be possible in selected patients.[79] The authors' approach is presented in **Fig. 10.13**. A large defect or symptoms of peritoneal contamination will usually require operative treatment. If the injury is operated upon early, a direct repair of the defect or small resection and a primary anastomosis is possible. It may also be possible to effect the repair laparoscopically. With delayed diagnosis or clinical deterioration during observation, patients will usually require a temporary defunctioning stoma.

Colonic bleeding

Although upper gastrointestinal and small bowel bleeding has been covered in Chapters 5 and 7, there remains the problem of patients who bleed from the colon. In approximately 20% of cases, the colon and rectum are the source of acute gastrointestinal haemorrhage. The most common aetiologies of this haemorrhage include diverticulosis, angiodysplasia, ischaemic colitis, inflammatory bowel disease, neoplasms, aorto-enteric fistulas and anorectal diseases such as haemorrhoids.[80] The general principles of management of many of these conditions has already been discussed, but each patient needs to be managed individually. Where possible, management of colonic bleeding is non-operative and usually stops spontaneously, permitting investigation to proceed at a leisurely pace. In some patients, however, the bleeding either does not spontaneously stop or is profuse and urgent investigation, followed occasionally by emergency surgery, is required.

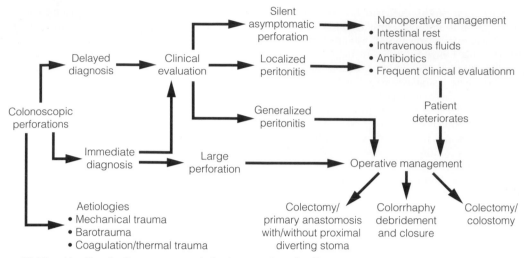

Figure 10.13 • Algorithm for the management of colonoscopic perforation.

In these patients, the source of bleeding is often difficult to identify.

Diagnosis and non-surgical management

Diagnostic tests utilised will vary according to institutional availability, patient characteristics, and the providers' experience and expertise. These investigations are used to localise the site of haemorrhage, cause it to stop or confirm its cessation. Options include radionuclide imaging, colonoscopy, CT angiography and selective angiography.

Radionuclide Imaging

Radionuclide imaging with 99mTc pertechnetate-tagged red cells detects the slowest bleeding rates (0.1 to 0.5 mL/min) but cannot reliably localise the site of baemorrhage.[81]

The timing of the radionucleotide blush is important. An immediately positive blush (within the first 2 minutes of scanning) is highly predictive of a positive angiogram (60%) and the need for surgery (24%), while a negative scan is highly predictive of a negative angiogram (93%) and the need for surgery falls to 7%.[82] A negative nuclear scan provides objective evidence that the patient is not actively bleeding and may be evaluated by colonoscopy.

Colonoscopy

Many authors believe that colonoscopy has the highest efficacy and should be the first study in patients with major bleeding that appears self-limited.[83] Whether colonoscopy should be undertaken 'emergently' depends on the patient's stability. In patients with hypotension and ongoing haemorrhage, it is difficult to safely cleanse the bowel with lavage

solutions, and the continued bleeding limits intraluminal visualisation and the ability to utilise therapeutic options. In general, these patients require prompt attention with angiography or surgery.

In stable patients with self-limited haemorrhage, colonoscopy is the preferred diagnostic study. The need for bowel preparation is controversial. Colonoscopy without preparation can be described as 'emergent' while administering a mechanical preparation and then performing colonoscopy within 24 hours of presentation is best termed 'urgent' colonoscopy. The rapid time preferred for mechanical cleansing usually mandates a lavage method.

Proponents of 'emergency colonoscopy' have demonstrated high caecal intubation rates (95%) and a diagnostic accuracy of 72–86%.[84] However, many of the reported series described atypical aetiologies for 'massive haemorrhage', including ischaemic colitis, inflammatory bowel disease and cancer. The usual rate of bleeding in these conditions is more amenable to urgent colonoscopy (within 24 hours) rather than emergent colonoscopy. Higher bleeding rates are more common with diverticular or angiodysplastic sources.

The benefit of colonoscopy depends on its ability to provide a definitive localisation of ongoing active bleeding and the potential for therapy. Many landmarks for colonoscopy may be obscured during haemorrhage. Even when pathology is identified, establishing the presence of stigmata of recent haemorrhage is more difficult than in the upper gastrointestinal tract. In addition, colonoscopy is associated with complications such as perforation. Inconclusive findings owing to technically unsatisfactory results are frequent and failure to achieve a firm diagnosis may reflect stricter diagnostic criteria rather than inferior diagnostic skill.

Because of the inability to appreciate all intraluminal landmarks and accurately locate the segment that is bleeding, once the enodoscopist highlights a source of bleeding, the region of the intestine is best marked with a tattoo of India ink. If the haemorrhage continues and the patient fails medical management, a tattoo greatly assists the surgeon in localising the site of bleeding. The endoscopist has many therapeutic options to control the bleeding, including thermal agents (heater probes and bipolar coagulation), monopolar or bipolar diathermy, topical or intramucosal epinephrine injection and endoscopically applied clips.

Angiography

Angiography aids as a diagnostic and therapeutic option in the treatment of intestinal haemorrhage. Acute, major haemorrhage with ongoing bleeding requires emergency angiography, while patients with an early blush during nuclear scintigraphy may benefit from therapeutic angiography. Angiograms may also define a potential source for haemorrhage in occult and recurrent gastrointestinal haemorrhage. In order to appreciate an angiographic blush of contrast, the study requires a bleeding rate of at least 1–1.5 mL/min. Appropriate patient selection increases yields and avoids excessive use of angiograms. Superselective catheterisation of branch arteries and multiple injections of contrast may be required to examine the entire territory. It is important to take late films in the venous phase as they may demonstrate abnormalities that may not be seen in the arterial phase. Major complications of diagnostic arteriography include arterial thrombosis, embolisation and renal failure caused by the contrast material.

The angiographic blush may suggest a specific aetiology, but this finding lacks the accuracy of colonoscopy. Highly accurate localisation also provides for focused therapy. The haemorrhagic site may receive highly selective, intra-arterial vasopressin infusion. This medication produces potent arterial contraction which may reduce or halt the haemorrhage. Infusion rates of vasopressin begin at concentrations of 0.2 U/min and may progress to 0.4 U/min. The systemic effects and cardiac impact of vasopressin may limit maximising the dosage. Vasopressin infusion controls bleeding in as many as 91% of patients, but unfortunately bleeding may recur in up to 50% of patients once the vasopressin is reduced. However, this has been reported as allowing surgery to be performed electively in 57% of patients.[85]

Angiographic technology also allows for arterial embolisation to control haemorrhage. Arterial embolisation of larger vessels produces intestinal ischaemia or infarction in approximately 20% of patients. Much safer superselective mesenteric angiography using microcatheters allows embolisation of the intestinal vasa recta or vessels as small as 1 mm.

The high re-bleeding rate with vasopressin has led to the suggestion that other, more definitive therapeutic manoeuvres should be undertaken during angiography such as superselective embolisation, which is effective in controlling colonic haemorrhage and is associated with a low rate of postembolisation colonic ischaemia. In a study of 27 patients, all were initially controlled with arterial embolisation although six re-bled, five of whom needed surgical intervention.[86]

Successful embolisation therapy provides immediate arrest of the bleeding. Embolisation agents include gelfoam pledgets, coils and polyvinyl alcohol particles. Success has been better in diverticular bleeds, which are usually fed by one vessel, than with angiodysplasias, which often have multiple feeding vessels.

CT angiography

Advanced CT angiography using thinly sliced, fast image acquisition combined with three-dimensional software packages has revolutionised the imaging of the vascular tree.[87] Vessels smaller than 'named' vessels can be visualised, and use of CT angiography has been reported in chronic conditions such as mesenteric ischaemia and inflammatory bowel disease. Case reports and animal modelling suggest feasibility for gastrointestinal haemorrhage. The sensitivity and specificity of CT angiography in patients with gastrointestinal haemorrhage are unknown and require further research.

Surgical management

Patients require surgical intervention if they continue to bleed profusely and medical, endoscopic and angiographic interventions have failed. Most sources of bleeding spontaneously resolve or are controlled with the therapeutic interventions described previously. Surgical therapy for intestinal bleeding is required infrequently and associated with significant mortality. Patients that are haemodynamically unresponsive to the initial resuscitation obviously require emergency surgery. In other patients the site of haemorrhage may be localised, yet the available therapeutic interventions fail to control the bleeding. Patient mortality increases with transfusion requirements. Bender et al. noted a reduced mortality (7%) for patients requiring less than 10 units of blood, while the mortality increased to 27% for patients receiving in excess of 10 units.[88] Therefore, patients with ongoing haemorrhage who require more than 6–7 units of blood during the resuscitation should undergo surgical intervention.

Surgeons should tailor their operative approach based on the preoperative diagnostic evaluations.

Surgery starts with a thorough examination of the entire intestine through a large midline open laparotomy incision. The first objective is location of intraluminal blood with the hope of segmentally isolating a possible source of bleeding.

If no source appears obvious after the exploration phase, the surgeon may consider intestinal enteroscopy. The enteroscope or colonoscope exposes the luminal surface and transilluminates the intestinal wall. Transillumination may identify vascular anomalies, small ulcers or tumours. Endoscopic access to the intestine may require a transoral, transgastric, transcolonic or transanal approach, or a combination of these. Intraoperative endoscopy is, however, a technically difficult endeavour. A team approach with two surgeons or the availability of an experienced endoscopist is important in order to identify the elusive lesions causing the haemorrhage.

Once the haemorrhage site is identified, an appropriate segmental resection can be performed. If no source of bleeding is confirmed, but appears to arise from the colon, the surgeon should perform a subtotal or total colectomy. Stable patients will tolerate a primary ileosigmoid or ileorectal anastomosis, while unstable patients are best served with an end ileostomy with closure of the rectal stump or a sigmoid mucous fistula.

Critical issues with operative management include delaying surgery until the haemorrhage reaches a critical point beyond 10 units of blood, with an associated mortality rate between 10% and 35%, and recurrence bleeding rates of 10% due to imprecise localisation of the bleeding.[89] Recurrence rates are higher (e.g. 20%) if a limited right or left colectomy is performed without precise localisation of the haemorrhage.[90] A total colectomy offers the same mortality but with a lower chance of recurrent or persistent bleeding. Therefore, a total colectomy is the preferred option if preoperative localisation is not possible, or a definite site of bleeding cannot be found at laparotomy.

Key points

- There has been a recent swing towards greater emphasis on preoperative investigations, especially CT, and daytime operating by specialist consultant surgeons for most urgent surgery. In cases of colonic emergencies where there is faecal contamination of the peritoneal cavity, emergency surgery may still be life-saving.

Ischaemia
- Mild cases are treated with bowel rest and optimisation of cardiovascular status. Severe cases usually require resection.

Colonic obstruction
- **Volvulus.** Emergency decompression using a proctoscope, a long soft tube such as a chest drain, or a colonoscope should, in most cases, be followed by elective definitive surgery.
- **Acute colonic pseudo-obstruction.** Some patients can be managed conservatively, employing regular review and frequent plain abdominal radiographs to check caecal diameter. As caecal diameter increases, decompression is required. Many patients will respond to a trial of neostigmine. If this treatment is not successful, the colon can be decompressed with the colonoscope. Failure may necessitate caecostomy or resection. If perforation or necrosis is suspected, a full laparotomy is necessary.
- **Malignant disease.** Right hemicolectomy with primary anastomosis is the treatment of choice for most patients with right-sided or transverse colonic obstruction. A subtotal colectomy may be the preferred option for patients who have a lesion at the splenic flexure. Most other patients who have an obstructing carcinoma in the left colon will be best treated by segmental colectomy with primary anastomosis where possible. Patients who are thought to be particularly at risk from lengthy emergency operations are best served by either segmental resection or colostomy.

Inflammation and/or infection
- **Diverticulits.** CT is now the investigation of choice for those patients presenting as emergencies. Abscesses can then be drained percutaneously and perforations requiring surgery diagnosed early.

One-stage surgery is ideal; however, in left-sided disease this is not appropriate for the unstable patient or in those with gross faecal contamination.

- **Typhlitis.** There should be a high index of suspicion for this condition in the neutropenic patient. The majority respond to conservative measures including antibiotics and complete bowel rest, but perforation should be actively excluded along the course of the disease, preferably with CT.

Perforation

- **Stercoral perforation.** This rare condition may be difficult to diagnose preoperatively. Awareness of the possibility of postoperative re-perforation, especially where limited resections have been performed, may be the key to a successful outcome.
- **Anastomotic leak.** Postoperative assessment of the abdomen is complex, with many signs being attributable to the surgery itself. In equivocal cases, further investigations should be instigated where there is uncertainty. Active observation should be employed by senior surgical staff. In some instances, transfer to a specialist colorectal unit needs to be considered after initial resuscitation and assessment.
- **Colonoscopic damage.** Signs and symptoms of perforation are not always obvious at the time of colonoscopy. A high index of suspicion, especially following interventional procedures, may allow conservative management or primary repair if surgery is performed early.

Haemorrhage

- The majority of colonic bleeding settles spontaneously, allowing subsequent investigation to take place 'electively'. However, ongoing bleeding should be investigated by CT angiography and then selective angiography, with or without embolisation. Surgery may be required and unless an obvious cause has been identified, subtotal colectomy with stoma formation is probably the safest procedure.

References

1. Hagihara PF, Ernst CB, Griffen WO Jr. Incidence of ischemic colitis following abdominal aortic reconstruction. Surg Gynecol Obstet 1979; 149:571–3.

2. Beck DE, Hicks TC. Other conditions: colonic volvulus, ischemia, radiation injury, and trauma. In: Beck DE (ed.) Handbook of colorectal surgery, 2nd edn. New York: Marcel Dekker, 2003; pp. 483–507.

3. Sakai L, Keltner R, Kaminski D. Spontaneous and shock-associated ischemic colitis. Am J Surg 1980; 140:755–60.

4. Marston A, Pheils M, Thomas ML et al. Ischaemic colitis. Gut 1966; 7:1–15.

5. Stamos MJ. Intestinal ischemia and infarction. In: Mazier WP, Levien DH, Luchtefeld MA et al. (eds) Surgery of the colon, rectum and anus. Philadelphia: WB Saunders, 1995; pp. 685–718.

6. Boley SJ, Schwartz S, Lash J et al. Reversible vascular occlusion of the colon. Surg Gynecol Obstet 1963; 116:53–60.

7. Boley SJ, Brandt LJ, Veith FJ. Ischemic disorders of the intestines. Curr Probl Surg 1978; 15:57–9.

8. Ballantyne GH. Review of sigmoid volvulus: clinical pattern and pathogenesis. Dis Colon Rectum 1982; 36:508.

9. Gibney EJ. Volvulus of the sigmoid colon. Surg Gynecol Obstet 1991; 173:243–55.

10. Hellinger MD, Steinhagen RM. Colonic volvulus. In: Wolff BG, Fleshman JW, Beck DE. (eds) ASCRS textbook of colorectal surgery. New York: Springer, 2007: pp. 286–98.

11. Sutcliffe MML. Volvulus of the sigmoid colon. Br J Surg 1968; 55:903–10.

12. Sonnenberg A, Tsou VT, Muller AD. The 'institutional colon': a frequent colonic dysmotility in psychiatric and neurologic disease. Am J Gastroenterol 1994; 89:62–6.

13. Mangiarte EC, Croce MA, Fabian TC et al. Sigmoid volvulus, a four decade experience. Am Surg 1989; 55:41–4.

14. Grossmann EM, Longo WE, Stratton MD et al. Sigmoid volvulus in Department of Veterans Affairs Medical Centers. Dis Colon Rectum 2000; 43:414–18.

15. Subrahmanyam M. Mesosigmoplasty as a definitive operation for sigmoid volvulus. Br J Surg 1992; 79:683–4.

16. Bagarani M, Conde AS, Longo R et al. Sigmoid volvulus in West Africa: a prospective study on surgical treatments. Dis Colon Rectum 1993; 36:186.

17. De U, Ghosh S. Single stage primary anastomosis without colonic lavage for left sided colonic obstruction due to acute sigmoid volvulus: a prospective study of one hundred and ninety seven cases. Aust NZ J Surg 2003; 73:390–2.

18. Naeeder SB, Archampong EQ. One-stage resection of acute sigmoid volvulus. Br J Surg 1995; 82:1635–6.

19. Akgun Y. Management of ileosigmoid knot. Br J Surg 1997; 84:672–3.

20. Miller BJ, Borrowdale RC. Ileosigmoid knotting: a case report and review. Aust NZ J Surg 1992; 62:402–4.

21. Anderson JR, Lee D, Taylor TV et al. Volvulus of the transverse colon. Br J Surg 1981; 7:12–18.

22. Mortensen NJMcC, Hoffman G. Volvulus of the transverse colon. Postgrad Med J 1979; 55:54–7.

23. Anderson JR, Lee D. Acute caecal volvulus. Br J Surg 1980; 67:39–41.

24. Anderson MJ, Okike N, Spencer RJ. The colonoscope in cecal volvulus: report of 3 cases. Dis Colon Rectum 1978; 21:71–4.

25. Ballantyne GH, Brandner MD, Beart RW et al. Volvulus of the colon. Ann Surg 1985; 202:83–92.

26. Tuech JJ, Pessaux P, Regenet N et al. Results of resection for volvulus of the right colon. Tech Coloproctol 2002; 6:97–9.

27. Rabanovici R, Simansky DA, Kaplan O et al. Cecal volvulus. Dis Colon Rectum 1990; 33:765–9.

28. Dorudi S, Berry AR, Kettewell MGW. Acute colonic pseudo-obstruction. Br J Surg 1992; 79:99–103.

29. Datta SN, Stephenson BM, Havard TJ et al. Acute colonic pseudo-obstruction. Lancet 1993; 341:690.

30. Vanek VW, Al-Salti M. Acute pseudo-obstruction of the colon (Ogilvie's syndrome): an analysis of 400 cases. Dis Colon Rectum 1986; 29:203–10.

31. Bachulis BL, Smith PE. Pseudo-obstruction of the colon. Am J Surg 1978; 136:66–72.

32. Koruth NM, Koruth A, Matheson NA. The place of contrast enema in the management of large bowel obstruction. J R Coll Surg Edinb 1985; 30:258–60.

33. Johnson CD, Rice RP, Kelvin FM et al. The radiological evaluation of gross cecal distension. Emphasis on cecal ileus. Am J Radiol 1985; 145:1211–17.

34. Ponec RJ, Saunders MD, Kimmey MB. Neostigmine for the treatment of acute colonic pseudo-obstruction. N Engl J Med 1999; 341:137–41.

    A randomised study of 21 patients with acute ACPO in which 11 patients were randomised to receive neostigmine and 10 patients received intravenous saline. The study showed that where the conservative treatment of ACPO fails, intravenous injection of 2.0 mg neostigmine results in rapid decompression of the colon.

35. Trevisani GT, Hyman NH, Church JM. Neostigmine. Safe and effective treatment for acute colonic pseudo-obstruction. Dis Colon Rectum 2000; 43:599–603.

36. Abbasakoor F, Evans A, Stephenson BM. Neostigmine for acute colonic pseudo-obstruction. N Engl J Med 1999; 341:1622–3.

37. Lee JT, Taylor BM, Singleton BC. Epidural anaesthesia for acute pseudo-obstruction of the colon. Dis Colon Rectum 1988; 31:686–91.

38. Strodel WE, Brothers T. Colonoscopic decompression of pseudo-obstruction and volvulus. Surg Clin North Am 1989; 69:1327–35.

39. Strodel WE, Norstrant TT, Eskhauser FE et al. Therapeutic and diagnostic colonoscopy in non obstructive colonic dilatation. Ann Surg 1983; 197:416–21.

40. Jetmore AB, Timmcke AE, Gathright JB et al. Ogilvie's syndrome: colonoscopic decompression and analysis of predisposing factors. Dis Colon Rectum 1992; 35:1135–42.

41. Stephenson KR, Rodriguez-Bigas MA. Decompression of the large intestine in Ogilvie's syndrome by a colonoscopically placed long intestinal tube. Surg Endosc 1994; 8:116–17.

42. Laine L. Management of acute colonic pseudo-obstruction. N Engl J Med 1999; 341:192–3.

43. Chevallier P, Marcy P, Francois E et al. Controlled transperitoneal percutaneous cecostomy as a therapy alternative to the endoscopic decompression for Ogilvie's syndrome. Am J Gastroenterol 2002; 97:471–4.

44. McKenzie S, Thomson SR, Baker LW. Management options in malignant obstruction of the left colon. Surg Gynecol Obstet 1992; 174:337–45.

45. Sjodahl R, Franzen T, Nystrom PO. Primary versus staged resection for acute obstructing colorectal carcinoma. Br J Surg 1992; 79:685–8.

46. Runkel NS, Schlag P, Schwarz V et al. Outcome after emergency surgery of the large intestine. Br J Surg 1991; 78:183–8.

47. Phillips RK, Hittinger R, Fry JS et al. Malignant large bowel obstruction. Br J Surg 1985; 72: 296–302.

48. Crucitti F, Sofo L, Doglietto GB et al. Prognostic factors in colorectal cancer: current status and new trends. J Surg Oncol 1991; 2(Suppl):76–82.

49. Sebastian S, Johnston S, Geoaghegan T et al. Pooled analysis of the efficacy and safety of self-expanding metal stenting in malignant colorectal obstruction. Am J Gastroenterol 2004; 9:2051–7.

50. Dudley H, Phillips R. Intraoperative techniques in large bowel obstruction: methods of management with bowel resection. In: Fielding LP, Welch J (eds) Intestinal obstruction. Edinburgh: Churchill Livingstone, 1987; pp. 139–52.

51. Deans GT, Krukowski ZH, Irvin ST. Malignant obstruction of the left colon. Br J Surg 1994; 81:1270–6.

52. Murray JJ, Schoetz DJ, Coller JA et al. Intra-operative colonic lavage and primary anastomosis in non-elective colon resection. Dis Colon Rectum 1991; 34:527–31.

53. Lee YM, Law WL, Chu KW et al. Emergency surgery for obstructing colorectal cancers: a comparison between right-sided and left-sided lesions. J Am Coll Surg 2001; 192:719–25.

54. Naraynsingh V, Rampaul R, Maharaj D et al. Prospective study of primary anastomosis without colonic lavage for patients with an obstructed left colon. Br J Surg 1999; 86:1341–3.

55. Turan M, Ok E, Sen M et al. A simplified operative technique for single-staged resection of left-sided colon obstructions: report of a 9-year experience. Surg Today 2002; 32:959–64.

56. The SCOTIA Study Group. Single stage treatment for malignant left sided colonic obstruction: a prospective randomised clinical trial comparing subtotal colectomy with segmental resection following intra-operative irrigation. Br J Surg 1995; 82:1622–7.

A multicentre, prospective, randomised trial comparing subtotal colectomy with segmental resection, intraoperative irrigation and primary anastomosis for left-sided malignant large bowel obstruction. Although postoperative mortality and length of stay in hospital were similar for both procedures, segmental resection with intraoperative colonic irrigation was superior to subtotal colectomy in terms of stoma rate and bowel function.

57. Hinchey EJ, Schaal PG, Richards GK. Treatment of perforated diverticular disease of the colon. Adv Surg 1978; 12:85–109.

58. Biondo S, Pares D, Marti Rague J et al. Acute colonic diverticulitis in patients under 50 years of age. Br J Surg 2002; 89:1137–41.

59. Reisman Y, Ziv Y, Kravrovitic D et al. Diverticulitis: the effect of age and location on the course of disease. Int J Colorectal Dis 1999; 14:250–4.

60. Ambrosetti P, Becker C, Terrier F. Colonic diverticulitis: impact of imaging on surgical management. A prospective study of 542 patients. Eur Radiol 2002; 12:1145–9.

This study prospectively evaluated 420 patients who underwent both CT and water-soluble contrast enema in the evaluation of acute diverticulitis. The performance of CT was significantly higher than contrast enema both in terms of sensitivity (98% vs. 92%) and in the evaluation of the severity of the inflammation (26% vs. 9%). Furthermore, contrast enema picked up an abscess in 20 patients compared with 69 patients using CT.

61. Hulnick DM, Megibow AJ, Balthazar EJ et al. Computed tomography in the evaluation of diverticulitis. Radiology 1984; 152:491–5.

62. Heverhagen JT, Zielke A, Ishaque N et al. Acute colonic diverticulitis: visualization in magnetic resonance imaging. Magn Reson Imaging 2001; 19:1275–7.

63. Chiu P, Lam C, Lam S et al. On-table cecoscopy. A novel diagnostic method in acute diverticulitis of the right colon. Dis Colon Rectum 2002; 45:611–14.

64. Dawson JL, Hanon I, Roxburgh RA. Diverticulitis coli complicated by diffuse peritonitis. Br J Surg 1965; 52:354.

65. Krukowski ZH, Matheson NA. Emergency surgery for diverticular disease complicated by generalised and faecal peritonitis: a review. Br J Surg 1984; 71:921–7.

66. Biondo S, Perea M, Ragué J et al. One-stage procedure in non-elective surgery for diverticular disease complications. Colorectal Dis 2001; 3:42–5.

67. Zorcolo L, Covotta L, Carlomagno N et al. Safety of primary anastomosis in emergency colorectal surgery. Colorectal Dis 2003; 5:262–9.

68. Scott SA. Surgery for Crohn's disease. In: Wolff BG, Fleshman JW, Beck DE et al. (eds) ASCRS textbook of colorectal surgery. New York: Springer, 2007; pp. 584–600.

69. Yamamoto T, Keighley MR. Long-term outcome of total colectomy and ileostomy for Crohn disease. Scand J Gastroenterol 1999; 34:280–6.

70. Binder SC, Miller HH, Deterling RA Jr. Emergency and urgent operations for ulcerative colitis; the procedure of choice. Arch Surg 1975; 110:284–9.

71. Dubinsky I. Stercoral perforation of the colon: case report and review of the literature. J Emerg Med 1996; 14:323–5.

72. Serpell JW, Nicholls RJ. Stercoral perforation of the colon. Br J Surg 1990; 77:1325–9.

73. Maurer CA, Renzulli P, Mazzucchelli L et al. Use of accurate diagnostic criteria may increase incidence of stercoral perforation of the colon. Dis Colon Rectum 2000; 43:991–8.

74. Fielding LP, Stewart Brown S, Blesovsky L et al. Anastomotic integrity after operation for large bowel cancer: a multicentre study. Br Med J 1980; 282:411–14.

75. Watson AJ, Krukoswski ZH, Munro A. Salvage of large bowel anastomotic leaks. Br J Surg 1999; 86:499–500.

76. Sheridan WG, Lowndes RH, Young HL. Tissue oxygen measurement as a predictor of colonic anastomotic healing. Dis Colon Rectum 1987; 30:867–71.

77. Anderson ML, Pasha TM, Leighton JA. Endoscopic perforation of the colon: lessons from a 10-year study. Am J Gastroenterol 2000; 95:3418–22.

78. Damore LJ, Rantis PC, Vernava AM et al. Colonoscopic perforations. Dis Colon Rectum 1996; 39:1308–14.

79. Araghizadeh F, Opelka FG, Hicks TC et al. Colonoscopic perforations. Dis Colon Rectum 2001; 44:713–16.

80. Abbaqsakoor F, Vaizey C. Colonic emergencies. In: Paterson-Brown S (ed.) A companion to

specialist surgical practice: Core topics in general and emergency surgery, 3rd edn. London: Elsevier; pp. 183–214.

81. Imbembo AL, Bailey RW. Diverticular disease of the colon. In: Sabiston D (ed.) Textbook of surgery. Philadelphia: WB Saunders, 1991; pp. 910–20.

82. Hammond KL, Beck DE, Hicks TC et al. Implications of negative technetium 99m-labeled red blood cell scintigraphy in patients presenting with lower gastrointestinal bleeding. Am J Surg 2007; 193:404–8.

83. Jensen DM, Machicado GA. Colonoscopy for diagnosis and treatment of severe lower gastrointestinal bleeding. Routine outcomes and cost analysis. Gastrointest Endosc Clin North Am 1997; 7(3):477–98.

84. Longstreth GF. Epidemiology and outcome of patients hospitalized with acute lower gastrointestinal hemorrhage: a population-based study. Am J Gastroenterol 1997; 92:419–24.

85. Browder W, Cerise EJ, Litwin MS. Impact of emergency angiography in massive lower gastrointestinal bleeding. Ann Surg 1986; 204:530–6.

86. DeBarros J, Rosas L, Cohen J et al. The changing paradigm for the treatment of colonic hemorrhage: superselective angiographic embolisation. Dis Colon Rectum 2002; 45:802–8.

87. Horton KM, Fishman EK. CT angiography of the GI tract. Gastrointest Endosc 2002; 55:S37–41.

88. Bender JS, Wiencek RG, Bouwman DL. Morbidity and mortality following total abdominal colectomy for massive lower gastrointestinal bleeding. Am Surg 1991; 57:536–40; discussion 540–1.

89. Corman ML. Vascular diseases. In: Corman ML (ed.) Colon and rectal surgery. Philadelphia: JB Lippincott, 1993; pp. 860–900.

90. Finne CO III. The aggressive management of serious lower gastrointestinal bleeding. Prob Gen Surg 1992; 9:597.

11

Anorectal emergencies

Hugh M. Paterson
B. James Mander

Introduction

Anorectal emergencies form a significant proportion of any general surgical emergency workload. Patients may present with anal pain, overt sepsis, rectal bleeding, anorectal trauma or retained foreign bodies. Acute anal pain may be caused by anorectal sepsis, anal fissures or thrombosed haemorrhoids.

Anorectal abscesses

Anorectal abscesses are among the commonest surgical emergencies. They predominantly occur in adults, may herald underlying disease and require prompt surgical drainage. The peak incidence is within the third and fourth decades and abscesses are three times more common in men than women. The annual incidence of acute anal abscess requiring operative drainage through the perineum in 2006/07 in Scotland was 1 in 5000 (Information Services Division, NHS Scotland).

An understanding of the anatomy of the anal canal is essential in order to understand the pathophysiology of abscess formation.

Anatomy

The anal canal is a 3–4 cm tube lined with epithelium that runs from the anorectal angle superiorly to the anal verge inferiorly (**Fig. 11.1**). It is surrounded by two funnels of muscle vital to the continence mechanism. The innermost ring is the internal anal sphincter, formed as a thickened extension of the circular muscle of the rectum. Beyond that is the external anal sphincter, formed from striated muscle, which becomes continuous superiorly with the levator plate. Between the two muscle layers is the intersphincteric space, which is the site of the anal glands. Ducts from these glands pass into the anal canal at the level of the dentate line. This marks the junction of the hindgut above, lined by columnar epithelium, and the proctodeum lined with squamous epithelium.

Aetiology

Primary anorectal abscesses arise as a result of anal gland infection (cryptoglandular), suppurating skin infections or pelvic pathology tracking through the levator plate. Cryptoglandular abscesses are believed to arise in anal glands found in the intersphincteric space,[1,2] which are connected to the anal epithelium at the dentate line. Support for the cryptoglandular theory comes from the observation that approximately 60% of patients will have an associated internal opening at the dentate line.[3] The suppuration can spread in a number of directions, resulting in abscesses in a variety of anatomical spaces (Fig. 11.1). The frequency with which abscesses are found in different locations is shown in Table 11.1.[4]

Suppurative skin conditions include furuncles, carbuncles and infected apocrine glands. They account for approximately 10–25% of all anorectal sepsis and are almost invariably staphylococcal in origin.[5] Because there is no communication with the anal mucosa, they are rarely associated with subsequent fistula formation.

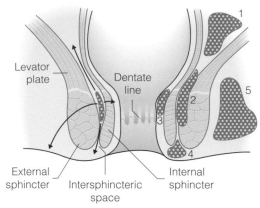

Levator
plate

Dentate
line

External
sphincter Intersphincteric
space

Internal
sphincter

Figure 11.1 • The spread of anal gland infection and common sites of anorectal sepsis. Infection of the anal gland within the intersphincteric space can spread in a variety of directions (see left side of diagram), resulting in abscess in a number of classical sites: 1, supralevator; 2, intersphincteric; 3, submucosal; 4, perianal; 5, ischiorectal. Note also the possibility of circumferential extension of sepsis ('horseshoeing') in the intersphincteric, ischiorectal and supralevator planes.

Table 11.1 • Location of anorectal sepsis by anatomical site

Anatomical site	Number	Percentage
Perianal abscess	437	42.7
Ischiorectal	233	22.8
Intersphincteric	219	21.4
Supralevator	75	7.3
Submucosal	59	5.8

Data from Ramunjam PS, Prasad MI, Abcarian H et al. Perianal abscesses and fistulae: a study of 1023 patients. Dis Colon Rectum 1984; 27:593–7. With kind permission from Springer Science and Business Media.

Secondary anorectal abscesses arise as a manifestation of other conditions and account for approximately 10% of patients.[6] Diseases such as inflammatory bowel disease (especially Crohn's disease), colorectal neoplasia, diabetes mellitus, AIDS and tuberculosis are commonly implicated. Other potential causes of sepsis include local trauma arising from foreign bodies inserted into the rectum or passing through the gut (such as bone fragments) and as a complication of the local treatment of haemorrhoids.

Clinical features

Patients with anorectal abscesses present with signs and symptoms of acute inflammation. While perianal and ischiorectal abscesses are usually associated with a visible painful swelling, the same is not true of intersphincteric abscesses. These are usually not visible, but characteristically patients have severe anal pain and fever. Not surprisingly, digital examination is frequently impossible without anaesthesia. Supralevator abscesses may be felt bimanually or diagnosed on further imaging modalities. In a few patients, particularly the immunocompromised and those with diabetes, the abscess may be associated with marked cellulitis that may progress to a life-threatening necrotising infection if not treated promptly.[7]

Investigation

Patients presenting with acute anorectal sepsis require appropriate work-up, with a full blood count and blood glucose assessment. All patients presenting with anorectal sepsis or severe anal pain warrant careful examination of the entire anorectum, including proctosigmoidoscopy. It is the authors' opinion that a full examination can only be conducted under general anaesthesia (EUA). Although it is acknowledged that in the USA anorectal abscesses are often treated under local anaesthesia in the 'office' (a situation almost certainly driven by financial pressures from insurance companies), formal EUA at the time of initial presentation is likely to be more cost-effective in the long term.[8] In the majority of cases of acute primary anorectal sepsis there is little difficulty in identifying the abscess clinically and therefore there is no value in routine radiological imaging. Further investigation should be reserved for recurrent sepsis or in primary cases where the source of sepsis is unclear.

Endoanal ultrasound

Endoanal ultrasound is undoubtedly an extremely sensitive method of identifying collections of pus close to the anal canal and associated fistulas.[9,10] In cases of complex anorectal suppurative disease (e.g. Crohn's disease) or in the management of severe anal pain the technique can be very useful for identifying pockets of pus (**Fig. 11.2**). As endoanal ultrasound may often not be available or familiar to the operating surgeon, its use in the emergency setting is unlikely to become routine in the immediate future.

Magnetic resonance imaging

Magnetic resonance imaging is very sensitive at delineating perianal sepsis and concomitant fistulas[11,12] and is extremely useful in cases of complex sepsis or when an abscess proves difficult to find.

Treatment

The principles of treatment of anorectal sepsis are to drain the abscess, minimise hospital stay and time off work, and preserve continence.

Figure 11.2 • Endoanal ultrasound examination carried out on a patient under general anaesthesia. This patient presented with severe anal pain and perianal induration but without any specific area of fluctuation. The ultrasound demonstrates an extensive ischiorectal abscess cavity (**c, d**) extending around the anal canal (**a**, internal sphincter; **b**, external sphincter). With thanks to Mr Mike Hulme-Moir, previous Clinical Fellow in Colorectal Surgery, Royal Infirmary, Edinburgh.

Abscess drainage

In the vast majority of patients, simple drainage of the abscess is achieved with an incision over the swelling, gentle breakdown of the loculi and subsequent dressing (for details of the management of specific abscesses, see the later section 'Technical tips'). Packing of the cavity makes subsequent dressing management painful, inhibits adequate drainage and should be discontinued.[13] Judgement needs to be exercised in tailoring the size of the incision to the size of the cavity to allow adequate drainage. Deroofing of the abscess cavity results in a larger than necessary wound, which increases the postoperative stay and the need for time off work for regular dressings. If the cavity is large, an alternative is to make a small skin incision and insert a de Pezzer- or Malecot-type drainage catheter. One study performed several years ago[14] compared a group of 91 patients who underwent this form of treatment with 54 patients who underwent more traditional incision and drainage. The use of a small incision and catheter drainage resulted in a shorter hospital stay (mean 1.4 vs. 4.5 days) and less community nursing than traditional incision and drainage. There was no increase in the rate of subsequent fistula formation or failure to adequately drain the abscess.

Primary closure

The rationale for primary closure after release of sepsis is that primary healing is common and further dressings are unnecessary. Early interest in the technique waned after studies showed little or no improvement in the time to healing or the incidence of recurrent sepsis.[15,16] Whatever benefit primary suture may hold in reducing time off work from repeated dressings is offset by the problems of failure to reduce the incidence of recurrent sepsis.

 This technique, along with the local anaesthetic management of abscesses in the accident and emergency setting, are therefore not recommended.

Role of antibiotics

There is no evidence supporting the use of antibiotics in the management of primary uncomplicated anorectal sepsis. However, they should be used during surgical drainage in patients at risk from bacteraemia (e.g. those with prosthetic heart valves) and in patients with florid cellulitis or necrotising infections. They also have a role in treating neutropenic patients in the absence of obvious fluctuation, though in this group an occult abscess must first be excluded by either further imaging or EUA.

Determining the likelihood of a concomitant fistula

Recent studies suggest that if actively sought, a fistula can be identified in at least 60% of patients with acute anorectal sepsis.[10,17] The chances of finding an internal opening are greater if there is an intersphincteric or supralevator abscess rather than a perianal or ischiorectal one.[4] However, although some patients undergoing simple incision and drainage of abscesses will represent with recurrent sepsis and an associated fistula, a significant proportion are adequately managed by simple drainage. In a follow-up study of 170 patients with perianal abscess treated by incision and drainage for an average of 90 months, 37% were found to develop a fistula and 10% recurrent abscess;[18] in another prospective study, 29% of patients developed recurrent sepsis after simple abscess drainage.[17] These figures are mirrored almost exactly by retrospective data,[19] demonstrating that although fistulas may be found in the acute setting, a significant proportion heal spontaneously after simple abscess drainage, and it is the epithelialisation of the tract that may be the crucial factor in preventing chronicity and recurrent sepsis.[20]

Although there is good evidence that at least 60% of acute primary anorectal abscesses are associated with a fistula, the majority of patients are adequately treated by simple incision and drainage.[17–19]

Gentle examination of the anal canal using a speculum while applying pressure to the abscess will sometimes reveal pus at the internal opening of a fistula, but if the opening is not immediately evident (as is often the case), what guidance exists to predict the subsequent development of a fistula? Although elegant studies have been performed to show that the culture of skin-derived organisms (usually *Staphylococcus aureus*) from pus drained from the acute abscess is useful in dismissing the likelihood of subsequent fistula, many surgeons consider the routine culture of such samples to be unhelpful. In patients in whom bowel-derived organisms are grown, the chance of identifying a fistula is only slightly better than 50%.[21] Furthermore, microbiological results are not immediately available and the patient would therefore require a second anaesthetic if no fistula is found initially and subsequent pus culture then suggests one is likely.

It has been suggested that if the cryptoglandular theory of acute anorectal sepsis was correct, the presence of intersphincteric sepsis at the time of presentation might be a more sensitive indicator of an underlying fistula than microbiological analysis of the pus.[22] In a study to test this hypothesis, a radial incision was made over the apex of the abscess in 22 patients. This was extended medially to allow dissection of the intersphincteric space to determine the presence of intersphincteric sepsis and a careful examination was made to determine if a fistula was present. Patients were followed up for a mean of 38 weeks. Demonstration of intersphincteric sepsis in association with an anorectal abscess was 100% sensitive and 100% specific for the presence of an underlying fistula in ano.[22] It should be acknowledged that two experienced colorectal surgeons performed this study

and, although highly sensitive and specific, there is no evidence that this technique can be safely utilised by surgeons without specialist training.

It is strongly recommended that a pus swab be sent for culture to determine the likelihood of a subsequent fistula. If skin organisms are cultured, no further follow-up is necessary. If bowel organisms are grown, a further outpatient appointment should be undertaken.

Role of synchronous fistulotomy

It is apparent that a proportion of patients with anorectal sepsis will have an associated fistula. If this can be dealt with simultaneously, then recurrence rates and patient inconvenience should be reduced. This potential benefit to the patient must be balanced against any risk of damage to the continence mechanism during definitive surgery. Furthermore, it may be difficult to delineate the anatomy of any fistulous track in the presence of gross oedema and inflammation, conditions which also risk the creation of false passages in inexperienced hands. As discussed above, one argument against concurrent fistulotomy is that only a minority of patients will suffer recurrent sepsis after simple drainage of an acute abscess.

There have been a number of randomised trials looking at the issue of the efficacy and safety of synchronous fistulotomy. One such study[23] studied 36 patients who underwent incision and drainage for anorectal abscesses accompanied by fistulectomy and 34 who underwent drainage alone. After a median follow-up of 42.5 months there was an impressive reduction in recurrence rates in the synchronous fistulectomy group compared with those treated simply by incision and drainage (2.9% vs. 40.6%). There was a trend towards increased disturbance of continence in the fistulotomy group at 1 year (39.4% vs. 21.4%) which did not reach statistical significance ($P < 0.106$), although the high rate of altered continence in the simple drainage group suggests that the assessment of incontinence lacked specificity. Another study randomised 38 patients to simple drainage versus drainage with fistulotomy. There was no difference in the rate of recurrent sepsis but a significantly higher rate of incontinence to flatus, delayed healing and longer hospitalisation in the fistulotomy group.[24] Two further randomised trails from Singapore have also looked into the issue of concomitant treatment of an underlying fistula.[25,26] In the first study, consecutive patients with a perianal or ischiorectal abscess and a demonstrable internal opening were randomised to either incision and drainage alone (21 patients) or incision and drainage with concurrent fistulotomy (24 patients). There were proportionally more low transphincteric fistulas in the fistulotomy group than in the patients treated with incision and drainage (58% vs. 33%). At 1-year follow-up there were three recurrences in the incision and drainage group and none in the synchronous fistulotomy group ($P = 0.09$).[25] There was no impaired continence in the fistulotomy group. The second study[26] included only perianal abscesses and randomised 52 consecutive patients to incision and drainage alone ($n = 28$) or incision and drainage with concomitant fistulotomy ($n = 24$). At a mean follow-up of 16 months there were seven (25%) recurrent fistulas in the group treated with incision and drainage alone compared with none in the fistulotomy patients ($P < 0.009$). All patients were fully continent after surgery.[26] Finally, using a policy of selective fistulotomy in 123 patients,[27] a fistula could not be found in 74% of patients and simple drainage was performed; the remainder underwent concurrent fistulotomy. Recurrent sepsis was seen in 11% and 13% respectively; altered continence was reported in 0% of the simple drainage group and two patients (6.5%) of the fistulotomy group ($P = 0.07$).

Available data on synchronous fistulotomy is conflicting. Although there seems to be a reduced incidence of recurrent sepsis, this is achieved at the cost of a higher rate of altered continence, and at present synchronous fistulotomy cannot be recommended.[23–26]

Technical tips

The management of specific abscesses is shown diagrammatically in **Fig. 11.3**. Simple perianal abscesses should be drained and the cavity gently curetted (Fig. 11.3a). With ischiorectal abscesses, the cavity is often huge (Fig. 11.3b). The cavity should be incised as near to the anal verge as possible. This is to bring the external opening of any subsequent fistula close to the anal verge to minimise the trauma of subsequent fistulotomy should it be required. A large horseshoe abscess in the ischiorectal space is better drained through multiple short incisions than one large circumferential incision. As mentioned earlier, the size of the drainage wound can be minimised if a drainage catheter is used. Intersphincteric abscesses require drainage into the anorectum, with excision of part of the internal sphincter (Fig. 11.3c). Submucosal abscesses, though rare, are drained into the anal canal. Supralevator or pelvic abscesses must be drained with care and ideally not through the perineum or a high fistula in ano will be created. In true pelvic abscesses unrelated to spread from the anal glands, drainage can be achieved into the rectum or vagina. If the abscess is related to pelvic pathology, the primary disease process will need to be excised along with drainage of the pus. Unless a fistula is obvious it should not be sought aggressively in tissues which are oedematous and swollen. Acute

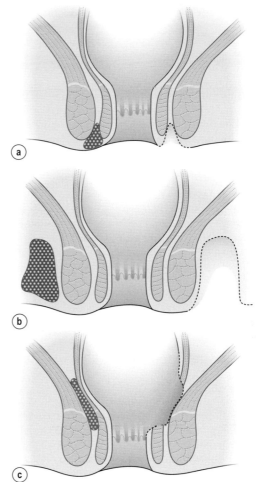

Figure 11.3 • Management of specific abscesses. **(a)** Perianal abscess is treated by excision of a small disc of skin and curettage of the cavity. **(b)** Ischiorectal abscess may require excision of a substantial amount of tissue to facilitate drainage. The alternative is to introduce a drainage catheter through a small stab incision. **(c)** Intersphincteric abscess is treated by excision of the mucosa and internal sphincter overlying the abscess. Such an abscess should not be drained through the perineal skin or a high fistula will result.

fistulotomy is only indicated if clearly superficial and only in the hands of experienced practitioners.

Management of secondary anal suppuration

Malignant disease

The abscess should be drained as per normal. It should be borne in mind that the presence of anorectal suppuration in these patients may well be caused by tumour extension beyond the bowel. This will have implications for the planning of definitive oncological treatment. If there is a significant malignant fistula, then the patient will require a defunctioning stoma.

Inflammatory bowel disease

Endoanal ultrasound is useful in identifying small collections in these patients. All collections of pus should be drained. In the majority of patients in the acute situation, setons should be placed across any fistulous openings.

Necrotising fasciitis

Treatment involves drainage of the pus and debridement of all non-viable tissue as well as high-dose antibiotics (best chosen with local microbiological advice). A second-look examination under anaesthetic may be required and a proximal stoma may be needed to facilitate wound healing.

Anorectal sepsis in children

Anorectal sepsis in children is rare. The largest series in the literature is from Edinburgh, which reported 69 patients in a catchment population of 1 million over a 10-year period.[21] The median age for development of the abscess was 3 years (range 1 month to 12 years), with the male to female ratio 9:1. In total, 24 patients (38%) presented with recurrent sepsis after simple incision and drainage but in only half of these was a fistula found. The study was unable to relate pus culture to the presence of a fistula. Recent data suggest that in this group, in whom anorectal sepsis is relatively uncommon, non-operative management may have a role. Needle aspiration and antibiotics were satisfactory in the management of 36 children over 2 years of age, only four requiring operative incision.[28]

Pilonidal sepsis

A pilonidal sinus is a chronic inflammatory condition associated with subcutaneous hair and is most commonly found in the natal cleft. Pilonidal abscesses are a common complication of the disease and usually present acutely with a tender, red, indurated swelling in, or adjacent to, the midline, close to the natal cleft. Midline pits are diagnostic of pilonidal disease and it is not uncommon for underlying abscesses to discharge spontaneously, leaving a secondary tract. The predominant organisms involved in pilonidal suppuration are staphylococci, but mixed anaerobes are also frequently cultured.[29]

As for all abscesses, the principles of treatment are drainage of the abscess and, if possible, eradication of the underlying disease while minimising the inconvenience to the patient. The surgical options include:

1. drainage of abscess and excision of disease at time of acute presentation;
2. drainage of abscess and staged definitive surgery;
3. drainage of abscess and staged definitive surgery only if required.

There are no good-quality randomised data on which approach is best. Attempts to excise the area surgically at the time of presentation are associated with high recurrence rates of up to 60%.[30] In addition, drainage alone may be a definitive treatment in itself. In a series of 73 patients treated with incision and drainage under local anaesthesia and followed for a median of 5 years, 42 patients (58%) healed primarily although nine (12%) subsequently developed a recurrence.[31] The likelihood of requiring a second procedure was increased if lateral tracts were present.

A comparative study from Israel assessed 58 patients with acute pilonidal abscess; 29 patients were treated with incision and drainage, the other 29 with wide excision (without closure). The results are displayed in Table 11.2. The risk of recurrent pilonidal suppuration was similar between patients undergoing incision and drainage with excision and those having incision and drainage alone, although those who underwent excision had a longer time off work.[32]

 There is enough evidence available to show that simple incision and drainage will cure approximately 50% of all pilonidal abscesses. It is therefore recommended that no excisional surgery is undertaken synchronously. Definitive surgery should be reserved for those who fail to heal or develop recurrence.[31,32]

Acute anal fissure

Anal fissures usually present as a chronic condition in the outpatient setting, although occasionally a patient will present as an emergency with acute intractable anal pain. A primary fissure is a benign superficial ulcer within the anal canal, with the patient characteristically presenting with severe pain after defecation and sometimes associated rectal bleeding. In the majority of patients it should be possible to diagnose the fissure simply by inspection. Gently parting the buttocks should reveal the lower edge of the fissure, usually in the midline posteriorly. It is often impossible to perform a digital rectal examination in these patients, although glyceryl trinitrate given sublingually has been shown to be helpful, allowing other pathology to be excluded in 13 of 16 patients presenting acutely.[33] If it is impossible to adequately assess for the presence of a fissure, or the patient has returned with worsening or

Table 11.2 • Results of treatment for acute pilonidal abscess

	Excision	Incision and drainage	P value
Number	29	29	
Recurrence	12 (41%)	16 (55%)	NS
Hospital stay (days)*	4 (2–8)	3 (0–12)	NS
Time off work (days)*	14 (3–60)	7 (3–30)	0.06
Time to healing (days)*	30 (15–70)	30 (10–60)	NS

Data from Matter I, Kunin J, Schein M et al. Total excision versus non-resectional methods in the treatment of acute and chronic pilonidal disease. Br J Surg 1995; 82:752–3. © British Journal of Surgery Society Ltd. Reproduced with permission. Permission is granted by John Wiley & Sonds Ltd on behalf of the BJSS Ltd.
* Values expressed as median (range); NS, non-significant.

intractable pain, then an EUA should be undertaken to exclude the presence of other pathology.

A large study (*n* = 308) comparing conservative therapy of acute anal fissure with surgical treatment at the time of acute presentation demonstrated that the fissures healed in 90% of patients without surgery, and the time to healing was not altered by early surgical intervention.[34]

The pain from an acute fissure arises from internal sphincter spasm. This can be alleviated by topical preparations such as glyceryl trinitrate or diltiazem, both of which have been shown to be efficacious in reducing sphincter pressure and healing chronic anal fissures,[35,36] although diltiazem has a lower side-effect profile.[37] Although surgery in the form of lateral sphincterotomy is undoubtedly effective in anal fissure, with recurrence rates less than 2%,[38] the technique has been associated with significant disturbances of continence in a proportion of patients and has therefore waned in popularity.[29] However, a recent meta-analysis suggests that the overall impact of medical treatments is only slightly better than placebo, with recurrence rates of approximately 50%,[39] while tailored surgical sphincterotomy in well-chosen patients can achieve superior results without incontinence.[40,41] Should a fissure be found acutely at EUA there is no place for acute sphincterotomy and local anaesthetic infiltration will provide good symptomatic relief.

It is strongly recommended that since the majority of acute fissures will heal spontaneously, pharmacological agents should be used as first-line treatment for symptomatic relief in the acute setting, with surgery being reserved for those who fail to heal or recur.[34,35,39]

Thrombosed haemorrhoids

Uncomplicated haemorrhoidal disease is usually painless and the presence of severe pain usually points to a complication or another diagnosis. Thrombosed prolapsed internal haemorrhoids are exquisitely tender and clinically obvious. Usually there is a history of a reducible prolapse prior to the onset of pain. The pain is so severe that the patient is often unable to sit, walk or defecate, and is caused by a combination of oedema of the perianal skin and thrombosis of the haemorrhoid. The condition, which is usually obvious on examination simply by parting the buttocks, may be further complicated by necrosis of the mucosa over the haemorrhoid.

The options for treatment are either non-operative or emergency haemorrhoidectomy. Non-operative measures consist of adequate analgesia combined with topical preparations such as nifedipine.[42] The rationale behind non-operative management is that, although intensely painful, the condition is usually self-limiting after 4–5 days and that haemorrhoidectomy itself is intensely painful for a similar period of time. However, the limitations of the non-operative approach are apparent from a study of 117 patients from St Mark's Hospital, London, in which 92 patients were followed up after discharge. Of 92 patients with thrombosed internal haemorrhoids treated non-operatively, 87% continued to have symptoms of prolapse and bleeding after discharge and 10% had a further admission to hospital with thrombosis.[43]

The concerns regarding emergency surgery are that the operative field may be infected and that the massive swelling and oedema distorts the anatomy so much that haemorrhoidectomy is extremely difficult. The sequelae of this is that too much tissue may be excised, with the attendant risk of anal stenosis and internal sphincter damage. Retrospective case series and case–control studies suggest that results in experienced hands can be favourable.[44,45] A case–control study from Singapore compared 204 patients who underwent acute haemorrhoidectomy with 500 treated electively over the same time period. The clinical end-points assessed were haemorrhage, anal stricture, recurrence of haemorrhoids, portal pyaemia and episodes of incontinence (Table 11.3). There was no difference in the profile or frequency of these complications between the two groups.[46]

Table 11.3 • Results from comparative study on emergency and elective haemorrhoidectomy

	Elective surgery (n = 500)	Emergency surgery (n = 204)	P value
Haemorrhage	27 (5.4)	10 (4.9)	NS
Blood transfusion	10 (2)	4 (2)	NS
Anal stenosis	15 (3)	12 (5.9)	NS
Disturbance of continence	26 (5.2)	9 (4.4)	NS
Sepsis	0	0	NS
Recurrence	38 (7.6)	14 (6.8)	NS

Numbers in parentheses are percentages. NS, non-significant.

Data from Eu KW, Seow Choen F, Goh HS. Comparison of emergency and elective haemorrhoidectomy. Br J Surg 1994; 81:308–10. © British Journal of Surgery Society Ltd. Reproduced with permission. Permission is granted by John Wiley & Sons Ltd on behalf of the BJSS Ltd.

In contrast to these results, the only prospective randomised study to compare non-operative treatment with haemorrhoidectomy in the acute setting found that the non-operative approach for prolapsed thrombosed internal haemorrhoids was associated with a shorter inpatient stay and less anal sphincter damage compared with operative treatment.[47]

Three studies have examined stapled versus conventional haemorrhoidectomy in the acute setting: all reported reduced pain, earlier discharge and faster return to work with the stapled procedure.[48–50]

Although there is good evidence to show that patients who present with acutely thrombosed haemorrhoids have a high risk of recurrent symptoms, there are not enough randomised data on non-operative versus operative treatment. Although emergency haemorrhoidectomy can be performed and in experienced hands appears to have a similar complication rate and profile to elective haemorrhoidectomy,[46,47] the case that all patients with thrombosed haemorrhoids should undergo definitive surgery in the acute setting remains unproven.

Anorectal haemorrhage

Massive per-rectal bleeding from an anorectal source is extremely rare. Nonetheless, proctosigmoidoscopy should always be undertaken to exclude bleeding from this area. In a series of 98 patients over the age of 65 presenting with major colonic haemorrhage, an anorectal source was found to be responsible in only four.[51] The pathologies implicated were rectal carcinoma, rectal prolapse, haemorrhoids and solitary rectal ulcer. Other anorectal pathologies occasionally reported as causes of major haemorrhage include cavernous haemangiomas of the rectum, anal fissures, rectal varices and proctitis.

Anorectal trauma

The rectum may be injured in its intraperitoneal or extraperitoneal parts by penetrating trauma, iatrogenic injuries or from inserted foreign bodies. Injuries to the intraperitoneal rectum can be primarily repaired.[52] However, where there are large injuries, significant contamination, devascularisation of the tissues or open fractures, resection and diversion should be considered. Injuries to the extraperitoneal rectum are treated by primary repair if possible or by proximal diversion, rectal washout and a presacral drain.[53] Sigmoidoscopy should be performed in all patients where blood is found in the rectal lumen or if an extraperitoneal haematoma is found adjacent to the rectum at laparotomy.

Anal injuries may complicate childbirth, with 0.4% of all vaginal deliveries associated with a third-degree (into the external sphincter) or fourth-degree (into the anal canal) tear.[54] However, prospective studies using endoanal ultrasound suggest that as many as 35% of women may have ultrasound evidence of internal or external anal sphincter damage following vaginal delivery.[55] Traditionally, obstetricians in the labour suite manage such tears by approximating the sphincter with interrupted sutures, but results following such repair are disappointing. Of 34 women with a third-degree tear who underwent primary repair, 16 had significant problems with incontinence and urgency and 85% still had a sphincter defect on endosonography.[56] A systematic review, albeit with limited data, concluded that early primary overlap repair was associated with less risks of faecal urgency and anal incontinence than end-to-end repair.[57]

Early primary overlap repair appears to be superior to end-to-end repair for third-degree obstetric injuries.[57]

Foreign bodies

The literature contains a large number of case reports of a vast array of foreign bodies inserted into the rectum for sexual gratification and there are a similarly large array of innovative techniques described to extract them safely.

The largest single series is from San Diego (but also including some patients from the Hammersmith Hospital in London).[58] Of 64 patients presenting with rectal foreign bodies, it was possible to remove the object in the emergency department under sedation in 31 (61%). Three patients with impacted bars of soap were successfully treated with admission and enemas, while 18 patients required EUA. Of these, five underwent laparotomy for rectal perforation, one required repair of a sphincter laceration and the other 12 underwent successful extraction. The authors of this study recommended that patients should undergo visualisation of the rectum after extraction to ensure there is no associated full-thickness injury. The likelihood of requiring an EUA was increased if the lesion was high up within the rectum on clinical examination or plain abdominal radiograph.

Key points

- Anorectal sepsis should be managed by prompt drainage of pus using sound anatomical principles.
- Synchronous fistulotomy is not recommended other than by an experienced coloproctologist.
- In the acute setting, pilonidal disease should be managed simply by incision and drainage.
- The first-line treatment of an acute anal fissure is pharmacological, with surgery being reserved for those that fail to heal.
- Thrombosed haemorrhoids should be managed non-operatively unless experienced colorectal assistance is available.
- The management of patients with anorectal trauma and retained foreign bodies is determined principally by the site of injury or impaction.

References

1. Eisenhammer S. The internal anal sphincter and the anorectal abscess. Surg Gynecol Obstet 1956; 103(4):501–6.

2. Parks AG. Pathogenesis and treatment of fistula in ano. Br Med J 1961; 1:63–9.

3. Buchan R, Grace RH. Anorectal suppuration: the results of treatment and the factors influencing the recurrence rate. Br J Surg 1973; 60(7):537–40.

4. Ramanujam PS, Prasad ML, Abcarian H et al. Perianal abscesses and fistulas. A study of 1023 patients. Dis Colon Rectum 1984; 27(9):593–7.

5. Eykyn SJ, Grace RH. The relevance of microbiology in the management of anorectal sepsis. Ann R Coll Surg Engl 1986; 68(5):237–9.

6. Winslett MC, Allan A, Ambrose NS. Anorectal sepsis as a presentation of occult rectal and systemic disease. Dis Colon Rectum 1988; 31(8):597–600.

7. Badrinath K, Jairam N, Ravi HR. Spreading extraperitoneal cellulitis following perirectal sepsis. Br J Surg 1994; 81(2):297–8.

8. Abcarian H. Editorial comment to Winslow et al. Dis Colon Rectum 1988; 31:601.

9. Law PJ, Talbot RW, Bartram CI et al. Anal endosonography in the evaluation of perianal sepsis and fistula in ano. Br J Surg 1989; 76(7):752–5.

10. Toyonaga T, Matsushima M, Tanaka Y et al. Microbiological analysis and endoanal ultrasonography for diagnosis of anal fistula in acute anorectal sepsis. Int J Colorectal Dis 2007; 22(2):209–13.

11. Sahni VA, Ahmad R, Burling D. Which method is best for imaging of perianal fistula? Abdom Imaging 2008; 33(1):26–30.

12. Lunniss PJ, Barker PG, Sultan AH et al. Magnetic resonance imaging of fistula-in-ano. Dis Colon Rectum 1994; 37(7):708–18.

13. Tonkin DM, Murphy E, Brooke-Smith M et al. Perianal abscess: a pilot study comparing packing with nonpacking of the abscess cavity. Dis Colon Rectum 2004; 47(9):1510–4.

14. Kyle S, Isbister WH. Management of anorectal abscesses: comparison between traditional incision and packing and de Pezzer catheter drainage. Aust NZ J Surg 1990; 60(2):129–31.

15. Mortensen J, Kraglund K, Klaerke M et al. Primary suture of anorectal abscess. A randomized study com-

paring treatment with clindamycin vs. clindamycin and Gentacoll. Dis Colon Rectum 1995; 38(4):398–401.

16. Leaper DJ, Page RE, Rosenberg IL et al. A controlled study comparing the conventional treatment of idiopathic anorectal abcess with that of incision, curettage and primary suture under systemic antibiotic cover. Dis Colon Rectum 1976; 19(1):46–50.

17. Oliver I, Lacueva FJ, Perez Vicente F et al. Randomized clinical trial comparing simple drainage of anorectal abscess with and without fistula track treatment. Int J Colorectal Dis 2003; 18(2):107–10.

18. Hamalainen KP, Sainio AP. Incidence of fistulas after drainage of acute anorectal abscesses. Dis Colon Rectum 1998; 41(11):1357–61; discussion 1361–2.

19. Vasilevsky CA, Gordon PH. The incidence of recurrent abscesses or fistula-in-ano following anorectal suppuration. Dis Colon Rectum 1984; 27(2):126–30.

These three studies indicate a rate of subsequent fistula or abscess of approximately 30% after simple drainage of primary anorectal sepsis without synchronous fistulotomy.

20. Lunniss PJ, Sheffield JP, Talbot IC et al. Persistence of idiopathic anal fistula may be related to epithelialization. Br J Surg 1995; 82(1):32–3.

21. Grace RH, Harper IA, Thompson RG. Anorectal sepsis: microbiology in relation to fistula-in-ano. Br J Surg 1982; 69(7):401–3.

22. Lunniss PJ, Phillips RK. Surgical assessment of acute anorectal sepsis is a better predictor of fistula than microbiological analysis. Br J Surg 1994; 81(3):368–9.

23. Schouten WR, van Vroonhoven TJ. Treatment of anorectal abscess with or without primary fistulectomy. Results of a prospective randomized trial. Dis Colon Rectum 1991; 34(1):60–3.

A study showing a drastically reduced rate of recurrence with synchronous fistulotomy, at a cost of higher rate of altered continence. The observation that 20% of the incision and drainage group were classified as exhibiting disturbed continence suggests that their assessment of incontinence lacked specificity.

24. Hebjorn M, Olsen O, Haakansson T et al. A randomized trial of fistulotomy in perianal abscess. Scand J Gastroenterol 1987; 22(2):174–6.

25. Tang CL, Chew SP, Seow-Choen F. Prospective randomized trial of drainage alone vs. drainage and fistulotomy for acute perianal abscesses with proven internal opening. Dis Colon Rectum 1996; 39(12):1415–17.

26. Ho YH, Tan M, Chui CH et al. Randomized controlled trial of primary fistulotomy with drainage alone for perianal abscesses. Dis Colon Rectum 1997; 40(12):1435–8.

Two randomised trials by experienced units showing markedly reduced rates of recurrence in abscesses treated by incision with synchronous fistulotomy without evidence of altered continence.

27. Seow-Choen F, Leong AF, Goh HS. Results of a policy of selective immediate fistulotomy for primary anal abscess. Aust NZ J Surg 1993; 63(6):485–9.

28. Serour F, Gorenstein A. Characteristics of perianal abscess and fistula-in-ano in healthy children. World J Surg 2006; 30(3):467–72.

29. Sondenaa K, Nesvik I, Andersen E et al. Bacteriology and complications of chronic pilonidal sinus treated with excision and primary suture. Int J Colorectal Dis 1995; 10(3):161–6.

30. Clothier PR, Haywood IR. The natural history of the post anal (pilonidal) sinus. Ann R Coll Surg Engl 1984; 66(3):201–3.

31. Jensen SL, Harling H. Prognosis after simple incision and drainage for a first-episode acute pilonidal abscess. Br J Surg 1988; 75(1):60–1.

32. Matter I, Kunin J, Schein M et al. Total excision versus non-resectional methods in the treatment of acute and chronic pilonidal disease. Br J Surg 1995; 82(6):752–3.

33. Larpent JL, Dussaud F, Gorce D et al. The use of glyceryl trinitrate in inexaminable patients with anal fissure. Int J Colorectal Dis 1996; 11(6):263.

34. Frezza EE, Sandei F, Leoni G et al. Conservative and surgical treatment in acute and chronic anal fissure. A study on 308 patients. Int J Colorectal Dis 1992; 7(4):188–91.

A large study concluding that the condition is self-limiting in the vast majority of patients.

35. Lund JN, Scholefield JH. A randomised, prospective, double-blind, placebo-controlled trial of glyceryl trinitrate ointment in treatment of anal fissure. Lancet 1997; 349(9044):11–14.

36. Knight JS, Birks M, Farouk R. Topical diltiazem ointment in the treatment of chronic anal fissure. Br J Surg 2001; 88(4):553–6.

37. Kocher HM, Steward M, Leather AJ et al. Randomized clinical trial assessing the side-effects of glyceryl trinitrate and diltiazem hydrochloride in the treatment of chronic anal fissure. Br J Surg 2002; 89(4):413–17.

38. Lewis TH, Corman ML, Prager ED et al. Long-term results of open and closed sphincterotomy for anal fissure. Dis Colon Rectum 1988; 31(5):368–71.

39. Nelson R. Non surgical therapy for anal fissure. Cochrane Database Syst Rev 2006; 4:CD003431.

40. Brown CJ, Dubreuil D, Santoro L et al. Lateral internal sphincterotomy is superior to topical nitroglycerin for healing chronic anal fissure and does not compromise long-term fecal continence: six-year follow-up of a multicenter, randomized, controlled trial. Dis Colon Rectum 2007; 50(4):442–8.

41. Ho KS, Ho YH. Randomized clinical trial comparing oral nifedipine with lateral anal sphincterotomy and tailored sphincterotomy in the treatment of chronic anal fissure. Br J Surg 2005; 92(4):403–8.

42. Perrotti P, Antropoli C, Molino D et al. Conservative treatment of acute thrombosed external hemorrhoids with topical nifedipine. Dis Colon Rectum 2001; 44(3):405–9.

43. Grace RH, Creed A. Prolapsing thrombosed haemorrhoids: outcome of conservative management. Br Med J 1975; 3(5979):354.

44. Mazier WP. Emergency hemorrhoidectomy – a worthwhile procedure. Dis Colon Rectum 1973; 16(3):200–5.

45. Greenspon J, Williams SB, Young HA et al. Thrombosed external hemorrhoids: outcome after conservative or surgical management. Dis Colon Rectum 2004; 47(9):1493–8.

46. Eu KW, Seow-Choen F, Goh HS. Comparison of emergency and elective haemorrhoidectomy. Br J Surg 1994; 81(2):308–10.

A large case–control study from an expert centre showing that almost identical results can be achieved in acute and elective settings. However, there is no suggestion that this technique should be undertaken without appropriate training in the emergency situation.

47. Allan A, Samad AJ, Mellon A et al. Prospective randomised study of urgent haemorrhoidectomy compared with non-operative treatment in the management of prolapsed thrombosed internal haemorrhoids. Colorectal Dis 2006; 8(1):41–5.

Randomised data on this question are lacking, but this study of 50 patients found that conservative treatment was associated with shorter admission duration and less anal sphincter damage as assessed by endoanal ultrasound, with no difference in the number of symptomatic patients at 24-month follow-up.

48. Wong JC, Chung CC, Yau KK et al. Stapled technique for acute thrombosed hemorrhoids: a randomized, controlled trial with long-term results. Dis Colon Rectum 2008; 51(4):397–403.

49. Lai HJ, Jao SW, Su CC et al. Stapled hemorrhoidectomy versus conventional excision hemorrhoidectomy for acute hemorrhoidal crisis. J Gastrointest Surg 2007; 11(12):1654–61.

50. Brown SR, Ballan K, Ho E et al. Stapled mucosectomy for acute thrombosed circumferentially prolapsed piles: a prospective randomized comparison with conventional haemorrhoidectomy. Colorectal Dis 2001; 3(3):175–8.

51. Boley SJ, DiBiase A, Brandt LJ et al. Lower intestinal bleeding in the elderly. Am J Surg 1979; 137(1):57–64.

52. McGrath V, Fabian TC, Croce MA et al. Rectal trauma: management based on anatomic distinctions. Am Surg 1998; 64(12):1136–41.

53. Weinberg JA, Fabian TC, Magnotti LJ et al. Penetrating rectal trauma: management by anatomic distinction improves outcome. J Trauma 2006; 60(3):508–13; discussion 513–14.

54. Sleep J, Grant A, Garcia J et al. West Berkshire perineal management trial. Br Med J (Clin Res Ed) 1984; 289(6445):587–90.

55. Sultan AH, Kamm MA, Hudson CN et al. Anal-sphincter disruption during vaginal delivery. N Engl J Med 1993; 329(26):1905–11.

56. Sultan AH, Kamm MA, Hudson CN et al. Third degree obstetric anal sphincter tears: risk factors and outcome of primary repair. Br Med J 1994; 308(6933):887–91.

57. Fernando R, Sultan AH, Kettle C et al. Methods of repair for obstetric anal sphincter injury. Cochrane Database Syst Rev 2006; 3:CD002866.

A systematic review suggesting that overlapping repair is superior to end-to-end repair, though the available data are limited.

58. Cohen JS, Sackier JM. Management of colorectal foreign bodies. J R Coll Surg Edinb 1996; 41(5):312–15.

12

Paediatric surgical emergencies

Dafydd A. Davies
Jacob C. Langer

Introduction

While paediatric surgery has increasingly become the domain of the subspecialist paediatric surgeon, adult general surgeons are still often faced with the challenges of assessing and managing children with surgical emergencies. The unique differences between adults and children must be taken into account when addressing every aspect of surgical management, including assessment, diagnosis, resuscitation and operative interventions. Children face a different spectrum of conditions, have different physiological responses to trauma, illness and surgical stress, and have different psychosocial needs.

This chapter will address the common abdominal paediatric surgical emergencies encountered by general surgeons. These will be categorised according to age: (i) neonates (up to 44 weeks postgestational age), (ii) infants (1 month to 2 years of age) and (iii) children (2 years of age and older).

Neonatal period

Prenatal diagnosis

Routine prenatal ultrasonography has become the standard of care in many parts of the developed world, and has resulted in the detection of many congenital anomalies before birth. Common detectable anomalies relevant to the general surgeon include: abdominal wall defects, congenital diaphragmatic hernia, intestinal obstruction and intra-abdominal masses.

Whenever possible these patients should be referred for prenatal consultation with obstetrics, neonatology and paediatric general surgery. In most cases, delivery should occur at a hospital with a neonatal intensive care unit and paediatric surgical service. If this is not possible they should be immediately transferred following delivery and resuscitation.

Intestinal obstruction

Intestinal obstruction is the most common abdominal emergency in the neonatal period, and is usually due to a congenital, developmental or genetic anomaly.

Assessment

Assessing neonatal patients for obstruction requires a thorough history, including the nature of any vomiting and the presence or absence of abdominal distension. Since neonates are unable to verbalise, surgeons must gather as many clues as possible from the prenatal, perinatal and family historical details (Table 12.1).

Examination of neonates with suspected intestinal obstruction should start with vital signs and an assessment of the level of resuscitation required. Certain forms of obstruction can cause severe dehydration or sepsis, which will need to be addressed early. Dysmorphic features may give clues to syndromes in which obstruction is common. The abdominal examination should make note of discoloration, distension and peritoneal signs such as guarding and rigidity. It is important to look for an incarcerated inguinal hernia as the

Table 12.1 • Important considerations in the neonatal history

Prenatal history	• Previous pregnancies (complications and outcomes) • Maternal gestational illnesses (e.g. gestational diabetes, pregnancy-induced hypertension) • Screening ultrasonography (dates and findings) • Other prenatal investigations and outcomes (e.g. maternal α-fetoprotein/β-human chorionic gonadotrophin/oestrogen levels, chorionic villous sampling, amniocentesis)
Perinatal history	• Weeks of gestation • Induced or spontaneous labour • Complications of delivery • APGAR scores
Neonatal history	• Complications • Infections • Feeding history (initiation, type, rate achieved) • Passage of meconium in the first 24 hours of life • Other anomalies identified
Family history	• Maternal and paternal health • Previous congenital anomalies • Cystic fibrosis • Cosanguinity

cause of obstruction. A thorough evaluation of the perineum must be done to ensure normal location and patency of the anus.

Routine blood work including electrolytes and complete blood count are helpful in assessing the level of dehydration as well as helping determine if electrolyte disturbances or sepsis are contributing to the presentation. It should be kept in mind that serum creatinine in the newborn reflects the mother's levels, and may not be helpful in assessing the neonate's renal function.

Abdominal radiography should be the initial imaging modality for neonates with possible intestinal obstruction. Typically, infants with duodenal obstruction have a 'double-bubble' appearance (**Fig. 12.1**), whereas those with distal intestinal obstruction will have multiple dilated bowel loops. It is impossible to differentiate distal small-bowel obstruction from colonic obstruction based on the plain abdominal radiograph in neonates, as the haustral markings seen in adults are not visible in this age group.

A contrast study is often required to definitively diagnose the aetiology of intestinal obstruction. If malrotation is suspected, an urgent upper gastrointestinal contrast study should be performed first. Once this has been excluded a contrast enema can be done to exclude distal pathology if this is indicated. For those infants with distal obstruction on plain radiograph, a contrast enema will help to differentiate the three most common causes of distal obstruction: meconium ileus, jejuno-ileal atresia and Hirschsprung's disease (**Fig. 12.2**). Water-soluble contrast should always be used instead of barium, to avoid the possibility of barium leaking into the

abdominal cavity should a perforation occur, and also because water-soluble contrast is more effective in relieving the obstruction in cases of meconium obstruction.

Neonates with suspected intestinal obstruction should be transferred in a temperature-controlled transport isolette to a specialised paediatric surgical unit for evaluation and definitive management. Resuscitation should begin as soon as the patient is assessed and should continue during transport. Nasogastric decompression with a large-calibre nasogastric tube (size 8–10 French) is important to improve ventilation, monitor resuscitation, and limit bowel distension and subsequent ischaemia.

Specific forms of intestinal obstruction

Oesophageal atresia

This anomaly is characterised by a gap in the oesophagus, resulting in a blind-ending proximal pouch. In 90% of cases, the distal oesophagus is connected to the back of the trachea as a tracheo-oesophageal fistula. Oesophageal atresia is usually first suspected when the baby has difficulty swallowing saliva and may have coughing or respiratory distress during the first feed.[1] Intubation may be needed if ventilation or respiration are significantly impaired. The diagnosis is confirmed by the inability to pass a 10–12 French nasogastric tube. This tube should be left in the proximal oesophageal pouch and placed on suction to prevent aspiration of secretions. Operative repair should only be performed by an experienced paediatric surgeon and involves division of the fistula and end-to-end anastamosis of the proximal and distal oesophagus.

Figure 12.1 • Abdominal radiograph of an infant showing the typical 'double-bubble' appearance resulting from duodenal obstruction.

Meconium ileus

Cystic fibrosis (CF) is the most common autosomal recessive disorder in Caucasian children.[2] The disease alters the regulation of chloride transport in epithelial cells resulting in a variety of clinical manifestations. Ten to fifteen percent of children born with CF will develop meconium ileus, in which the meconium becomes sticky and causes intraluminal obstruction. This can further lead to complications of volvulus, atresia or perforation. In addition, meconium ileus may occasionally occur in children without CF. A diagnostic work-up, including both sweat chloride determination and genetic studies, must be done on all children with meconium ileus.

Abdominal radiograph may show distal intestinal obstruction with a bubbly appearance in the right lower quadrant due to gas mixing with the viscous meconium (Fig. 12.2a).[2] There may also be intraperitoneal calcification if in-utero perforation has occurred.

Following resuscitation and nasogastric decompression, a water-soluble contrast enema will reveal a microcolon (small calibre) and multiple meconium plugs in the terminal ileum (Fig. 12.2a). In approximately 50% of cases, the contrast enema will relieve the obstruction. If progress is made, but the infant remains obstructed after the initial enema and is otherwise stable, the procedure can be repeated. If the contrast enema is unsuccessful in relieving the obstruction and/or no further progress has been made, a laparotomy must be done. If there is no volvulus or perforation, enterotomies are made and mechanical washout is performed. Complications of volvulus, acquired atresia or perforation are managed by intestinal resection with or without a stoma, depending on the condition of the bowel and of the patient.

Intestinal atresia/stenosis

Atresia and stenosis can occur at any point in the alimentary canal. The two prominent aetiological theories are failure of recanalisation of the intestine during fetal development, or an ischaemic event in utero.[3] Early resuscitative measures should be initiated and confirmatory diagnosis can usually be made with either upper or lower gastrointestinal contrast studies. The presence of a 'double-bubble' sign on abdominal radiograph is considered diagnostic for duodenal atresia (Fig. 12.1), although this finding associated with distal gas may also be due to stenosis, duodenal web or malrotation. Trisomy 21 is present in one-third of children with duodenal atresia. Patients with distal atresia will typically have multiple dilated loops of bowel on the plain abdominal radiograph. Although a diagnosis of proximal obstruction can be confidently made based on plain radiography, those with distal obstruction should always undergo water-soluble contrast enema to differentiate atresia from meconium ileus or Hirschsprung's disease.

Since most infants with intestinal atresia are stable once decompressed and resuscitated, we recommend transfer of such neonates to a facility with paediatric surgical expertise. Most of these anomalies are treated with a primary anastomosis. If there is significant dilatation of the proximal segment, tapering enteroplasty should be done, as the dilated bowel tends not to have effective peristalsis.

Hirschsprung's disease (HD)

HD is a congenital disorder characterised by lack of ganglion cells in the distal bowel. This results in failure of peristalsis and functional obstruction. The 'transition zone' is usually located in the recto-sigmoid region, but HD can affect the entire colon and in rare occurrences the small bowel. HD most often presents in the neonatal period with distal bowel obstruction and failure to pass meconium in the first 24 hours of life. Patients can present later in life with a history of severe constipation.

Figure 12.2 • Water-soluble contrast enemas of infants with distal bowel obstruction. **(a)** Meconium ileus, showing a microcolon, dilated proximal small bowel and a soap-bubble appearance in the right lower quadrant. **(b)** Ileal atresia, showing a microcolon, contrast entering the distal small bowel but dilated proximal small bowel without contrast. **(c)** Hirschsprung's disease: lateral film showing a contracted distal rectum with dilated bowel proximally.

Figure 12.2 • *(cont.)*

Early identification and management are important to prevent complications of HD such as enterocolitis and nutritional problems.

Water-soluble contrast enema has a sensitivity and specificity of 70% and 83% respectively, and may therefore be normal, particularly in the newborn.[4] The gold standard for the diagnosis of HD is rectal biopsy, either by a suction technique at the bedside or full-thickness biopsy.

Initial management, after resuscitation and nasogastric decompression, includes digital rectal stimulation and/or rectal irrigations (10 mL/kg normal saline).

 Although the historical teaching was routine diverting colostomy followed by a 'pull-through' operation several months later, the current standard of care is primary reconstructive surgery without a routine colostomy in most patients.[5] Preliminary colostomy should be reserved for infants presenting with severe enterocolitis or colonic perforation.

There are a number of options for surgical correction of HD, including the Swenson, Soave and Duhamel procedures. In recent years, laparoscopic and transanal approaches have been described, which have decreased morbidity and shortened hospital stay. All these operations should be done by an experienced paediatric surgeon.

Anorectal malformations

Anorectal malformations can be divided into low and high anomalies. Low anomalies are characterised by rectoperineal or rectovestibular fistulas in female patients. Most males with high malformations have a fistula from the rectum to the bladder neck or urethra. Females with high anomalies usually have a single channel (cloaca) formed by coalescence of the urethra, vagina and rectum. Less commonly, there may be rectal atresia without a fistula, and some infants present with an anal membrane or anal stenosis.

Infants with these malformations usually present in the first day of life with distal bowel obstruction. Low malformations in girls with large fistulas can permit adequate evacuation of stool and are occasionally missed. Careful examination of the perineum of all newborns for anal patency and position is important. Many of these patients will suffer from associated anomalies which need to be investigated prior to proceeding with anatomical repair of the anorectal malformation.

The next consideration is to determine if the defect is amenable to primary repair or whether faecal flow should be diverted with a colostomy followed by delayed secondary anatomical repair. Children with a rectoperineal fistula can usually be managed with a local procedure from below, without a colostomy. Children with high anomalies are usually managed with a preliminary colostomy.

Chapter 12

The use of a colostomy in females with a rectovestibular fistula is controversial. The colostomy can be made using either the transverse or the sigmoid colon, and can be a loop or divided stoma. We agree with Pena's recommendation for a divided colostomy in the proximal sigmoid colon.[6] Long-term continence in these patients is determined by the level of the rectal fistula, and the presence of an absent or hypoplastic sacrum. Depending on the nature of the anomaly, repair can be done using a posterior sagittal approach, a laparoscopic approach, or a combination of posterior and abdominal approaches. Technical expertise is crucial to success, and these procedures should only be performed by experienced paediatric surgeons.

Malrotation

The process of normal rotation and fixation occurs between the sixth and tenth weeks of development. If no rotation occurs, the patient is left in a position of non-rotation, which has a wide-based mesentery and does not require correction. Classic malrotation occurs when the process is interrupted part way through, leaving the caecum and the duodenal–jejunal junction (ligament of Treitz) close to each other (**Fig. 12.3**). Because this arrangement results in a narrow-based mesentery, the bowel is prone to midgut volvulus around the superior mesenteric vessels, which may lead to intestinal ischaemia. Malrotation with midgut volvulus is one of the true paediatric surgical emergencies. Failure to recognise

this condition early can be catastrophic, leading to loss of large portions of bowel and subsequent short-bowel syndrome or even death.

Rotation abnormalities are most often asymptomatic. While volvulus can occur at any time, it is most common in the first week of life.[7] The most common presentation of malrotation is bilious vomiting, which may occur for two reasons: midgut volvulus with kinking of the duodenum, or compression of the duodenum by Ladd's bands. Peritonitis and shock from midgut volvulus are late symptoms and are associated with a worse prognosis. Every attempt should be made to diagnose and correct malrotation before this occurs.[8] For this reason, every infant who presents with bilious vomiting should be considered to have malrotation with midgut volvulus until proven otherwise.

Any patient with suspected malrotation and volvulus needs urgent imaging and surgical consultation. Abdominal radiograph is often non-diagnostic but may show a dilated stomach, a 'double bubble' with distal gas, or a relatively gasless abdomen. Upper gastrointestinal contrast study is the preferred examination. A nasogastric tube placed prior to the examination aids not only decompression of the stomach, but also the administration of the water-soluble contrast. The chief radiographic signs of malrotation are: (1) abnormal position of the duodenojejunal junction, (2) spiral, corkscrew or Z-shaped course of the distal duodenum and proximal jejunum, and (3) location of the proximal jejunum in the right

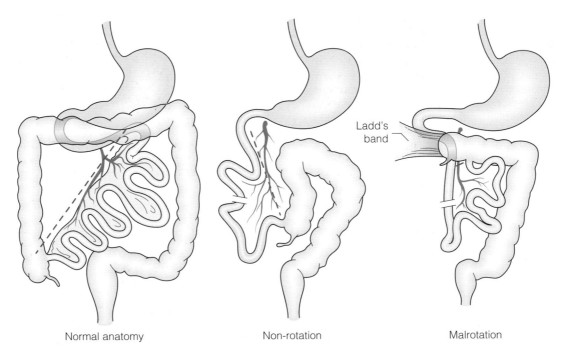

Normal anatomy   Non-rotation   Malrotation

Figure 12.3 • Schematic illustrations depicting normal intestinal rotation, non-rotation and malrotation. Bold dotted lines illustrate the width of the mesenteric base in each situation.

abdomen.[8] Abdominal ultrasound may show abnormal orientation of the superior mesenteric artery and vein, or a 'whirlpool sign'.[9]

The operation to correct malrotation involves a laparotomy (although a laparoscopic approach may be taken for children without evidence of volvulus).[10] If there is a volvulus, the bowel is untwisted and checked for viability. If there is ischaemia, the bowel is wrapped with warm towels and re-inspected. Grossly necrotic bowel is resected and the rest is left in situ, with a second-look laparotomy planned for 24–48 hours later. In children who have necrosis of the entire midgut, a palliative approach should be considered.

If the intestine is viable, a Ladd procedure should be done. This operation consists of five stages: (1) division of Ladd's bands, (2) mobilisation of the colon to the left side of the abdomen, (3) mobilisation and straightening of the duodenum, (4) dissection and widening of the small-bowel mesentery, and (5) appendicectomy.

Inflammatory conditions

Assessment

The diagnosis of peritonitis in the neonate is complicated by a number of factors, including the patient's inability to communicate with the surgeon, as well as several anatomical and physiological differences between neonates and older children/adults. The very thin abdominal wall may develop oedema and erythema as a result of underlying inflammation. Neonates breathe primarily with their diaphragms, so peritonitis results in rapid, shallow respiration, ultimately leading to elevation in pCO_2 and respiratory failure. Localised peritoneal signs can be elicited by palpation, but the examiner must be gentle, since the signs of involuntary guarding may be very subtle. In addition, the neonate does not have a well-developed omentum, so ability to localise inflammation may be impaired.

Neonates with peritonitis will often develop systemic sepsis, which may differ in its presentation compared to older children and adults. Signs of sepsis in neonates may include lethargy, temperature instability (either fever or hypothermia), increased ventilation requirements, thrombocytopenia, a high or low white blood cell count, and acidosis.

Specific forms of abdominal inflammation

Meconium peritonitis

This condition occurs when there has been prenatal intestinal perforation, resulting in chemical peritonitis. Prenatally there may be evidence of free fluid or calcification within the abdomen. In some cases, the fetus is able to localise and wall-off the perforation,

which may result in a meconium cyst. The aetiology of the perforation is often distal obstruction, usually from meconium ileus or intestinal atresia, but in some cases the perforation is idiopathic.

Management of meconium peritonitis involves fluid resuscitation, nasogastric drainage and antibiotics. If there is evidence of associated intestinal obstruction, a contrast enema may be helpful pre-operatively. Laparotomy should be carried out, with resection of the involved bowel and either stomas or primary anastomosis, depending on the condition of the child and the bowel.

Necrotising enterocolitis (NEC)

NEC is most commonly seen in low birth weight and small-for-gestational-age infants.[11] The aetiology of NEC is unknown, but a combination of bacterial colonisation, intraluminal substrate and intestinal ischaemia/hypoxia all appear to be important.[12]

NEC should be suspected in neonates with sepsis, increased abdominal girth, abdominal wall discoloration or bloody stools. Abdominal radiograph may show pneumatosis intestinalis, portal venous gas or free intra-abdominal air (**Fig. 12.4**). It is convenient to classify the severity of NEC using the Bell classification (Table 12.2), which helps to guide treatment and may assist the surgeon in decision-making about operative intervention.[13]

Initial management of NEC includes bowel rest, nasogastric decompression, broad-spectrum antibiotics, parenteral nutrition, and supportive measures to optimise perfusion and oxygenation of the bowel. Persistent clinical deterioration and signs of necrosis or perforation are generally considered indications for operative intervention. Options include bedside peritoneal drainage, or laparotomy with resection of grossly necrotic bowel and either primary anastomosis or stomas, depending on the status of the child and the bowel.[11,14]

A recent randomised control trial in neonates less than 1500 g with perforation found no significant difference in outcomes between peritoneal drainage and laparotomy.[15]

Prior to laparotomy parents should always be informed of the possibility of a long segment of necrosis requiring massive resection that would leave the child with short-bowel syndrome. Palliative management should be considered in these infants.

Isolated ileal perforation

This condition resembles NEC in that it primarily affects preterm and small-for-gestational-age infants. However, infants with isolated ileal perforation do not have any abnormalities of the intestine

Figure 12.4 • Abdominal radiographs of infants with necrotising enterocolitis. **(a)** Pneumatosis intestinalis. **(b)** 'Football sign' on supine film depicting intra-abdominal free air. **(c)** Free intra-abdominal air on lateral film.

other than localised perforation, usually in the distal ileum. It is unclear whether this represents a very localised form of NEC or a distinct entity. Clinically, these infants present with sudden deterioration, sepsis and free air without any evidence of pneumatosis seen on the abdominal radiograph. In general the same principles of treatment are applied to ileal perforation and NEC.

Other neonatal conditions

Incarcerated inguinal hernia

Inguinal hernias are very common throughout childhood and almost always arise from persistence of the processus vaginalis. If the processus contains only fluid, it is known as a hydrocoele; the hydrocoele is communicating if the processus remains

Table 12.2 • Bell stages of necrotising enterocolitis (NEC)

Stage 1 (suspect)	a. Any historical factors producing perinatal stress b. Systemic manifestations – temperature instability, lethargy, apnoea, bradycardia c. Gastrointestinal manifestations – poor feeding, increased nasogastric tube residuals, emesis (may be bilious or test positive for occult blood), mild abdominal distension, occult blood may be present in stool
Stage 2 (definite)	a. Any historical factors producing perinatal stress b. Above signs and symptoms plus persistent occult or gross gastrointestinal bleeding; marked abdominal distension c. Abdominal radiographs show significant intestinal distension with ileus; small-bowel separation (oedema in the bowel wall or peritoneal fluid), unchanging or persistent 'rigid' bowel loops, pneumatosis intestinalis, portal vein gas
Stage 3 (advanced)	a. Any historical factors producing perinatal stress b. Above signs and symptoms plus deterioration of vital signs, evidence of septic shock or marked gastrointestinal haemorrhage c. Abdominal radiographs may show pneumoperitoneum in addition to the others listed above

Reproduced from Bell MJ, Ternberg JL, Feigin RD et al. Neonatal necrotizing enterocolitis. Therapeutic decisions based upon clinical staging. Ann Surg 1978; 187(1):1–7. With permission from Lippincott, Williams & Wilkins.

open and non-communicating if the processus has become obliterated proximal to the fluid.

In most cases, inguinal hernias are asymptomatic and can be repaired electively. Incarceration of bowel may result in complete bowel obstruction and represents a surgical emergency, since both the bowel and the testis may become ischaemic. The risk of incarceration is greatest in newborns and is approximately 30% in the first 2 years of life. Premature infants are at highest risk.

Neonates and infants presenting with an incarcerated hernia should be resuscitated if necessary, following which an immediate attempt should be made to reduce the hernia. In contrast to the adult with an incarcerated hernia, testicular ischaemia is far more common than intestinal ischaemia, and it is appropriate to be aggressive about reducing the hernia. Multiple attempts and the use of sedation may be necessary. Ice should not be applied to the hernia, since it may induce hypothermia. Surgical repair of an incarcerated hernia in an infant is a formidable undertaking. The sac is often thin and oedematous, and the risks of injury to the cord structures and recurrence of the hernia are very high. Therefore, if a general surgeon is unable to reduce the hernia and a paediatric surgeon is available, the patient should be referred immediately.

 If the hernia is reduced, repair should be undertaken 24–48 hours later, to allow some of the oedema to settle, but before the risk of re-incarceration.[16]

Abdominal wall defects

Gastroschisis is characterised by an abdominal wall defect to the right of the umbilicus, through which most of the intestinal tract protrudes.[17] Omphalocele (also called exomphalos) is characterised by herniation of bowel with or without liver into the umbilical cord. Gastroschisis tends to be an isolated anomaly, whereas omphalocele is often associated with chromosomal, cardiac, renal, limb and facial anomalies.

If the diagnosis is made prenatally, delivery should occur at a centre with paediatric surgical support. Resuscitation and nasogastric decompression should begin in the delivery room. The bowel or sac should be wrapped in warm, saline-soaked, sterile gauze and covered with sterile plastic wrap to minimise heat and evaporative fluid loss.

Repair of both conditions should be done by an experienced paediatric surgeon. Options include primary closure, or staged closure using a Silastic® silo that allows the bowel to be reduced gradually into the abdomen over 1–6 days.[18]

Infancy

Hypertrophic pyloric stenosis (HPS)

HPS is an acquired condition in which the pylorus becomes abnormally thickened, causing gastric outlet obstruction. This occurs in infants during the first 2–12 weeks of life and is characterised by projectile, non-bilious vomiting usually occurring after feeds. HPS occurs in approximately 1 in 400 children, with a significant male predominance.[19]

Diagnosis is suspected based on a history of progressive, forceful, non-bilious vomiting in a child of the appropriate age. Physical examination usually reveals some level of dehydration and the presence of a palpable 'olive' in the epigastrium has a 99%

positive predictive value for the disease.[20] Vomiting of gastric contents leads to depletion of sodium, potassium and hydrochloric acid, resulting in the typical hypochloraemic, hypokalaemic, metabolic alkalosis. The kidneys attempt to conserve sodium at the expense of hydrogen ions, often leading to paradoxical aciduria.[21] The level of dehydration can be estimated by clinical examination, urine output, and serum chloride and bicarbonate levels. If the pyloric olive is not palpable, the diagnosis can be confirmed by ultrasound (pyloric length >16 mm and single wall thickness >3 mm). If an experienced sonographer is not available, the diagnosis can be made using a barium meal (**Fig. 12.5**).

Surgery should be deferred until the infant is fully resuscitated. This is accomplished by using normal saline or Ringer's lactate with potassium. Most children should receive a bolus of 20 mL/kg, and then an infusion consisting of 1.5 times the maintenance requirement (i.e. 6 mL/kg/h for this age group) until the urine output and electrolytes have been normalised.

Surgical management of HPS consists of extramucosal longitudinal splitting of the pyloric muscle. The original procedure described by Ramstedt in 1912 was done through a transverse right upper quadrant incision.[22] This technique has been modified in many institutions to utilise circumumbilical incisions or laparoscopic techniques. Following pyloromyotomy many infants will experience continued vomiting for 24–48 hours, although the majority will eventually tolerate feeds and be discharged. Postoperative complications are rare but include wound infection, duodenal or gastric perforation and incomplete pyloromyotomy.

Intussusception

Intussusception, or 'telescoping of the bowel', occurs when one portion of bowel invaginates into a more distant portion. This results in venous congestion, bowel wall oedema, intestinal obstruction and ultimately full-thickness necrosis of the intussusceptum. The peak incidence of intussusception is seen at 6–9 months of age.[23] The majority are ileocolic with hyperplastic lymphoid tissue in Peyer patches acting as a lead point.[24] Asymptomatic small-bowel to small-bowel intussusception may be seen incidentally on abdominal ultrasound, or sometimes may be associated with Henoch–Schonlein purpura or cystic fibrosis. Less than 5% of intussuceptions are due to a pathological lead point such as a Meckel diverticulum, polyp or small-bowel tumour such as lymphoma or leiomyoma. Intussusception occurring outside of the usual age range, or those that recur, should raise suspicion for a pathological lead point.

Few children with ileocolic intussusception will demonstrate the classic triad of intermittent severe abdominal pain with drawing up of the legs, palpable abdominal mass and 'red currant jelly' stool. Physicians must have a high index of suspicion due to the variability of symptoms. Patients may present with irritability, lethargy, abdominal pain, vomiting, diarrhoea or constipation, haematochezia, fever, dehydration or shock. Management should initially focus on diagnosis and resuscitation.

Following fluid resuscitation, imaging should be performed to confirm the diagnosis of intussusception. Abdominal radiograph may show air–fluid levels and distension of the small bowel. There may be a characteristic lack of air in the right lower quadrant. Ultrasonography has a high sensitivity and is currently the test of choice.[24]

 Traditionally, the treatment of intussusception has been barium enema. More recently, pneumatic reduction using air or CO_2 has been associated with an 80–95% success rate.[24]

If the intussusception is partially but not completely reduced it is worth trying again a few hours later, since some of the oedema may have been

Figure 12.5 • Images of hypertrophic pyloric stenosis. **(a)** Abdominal ultrasound. **(b)** Upper gastrointestinal contrast study.

eliminated by the first attempt and a second attempt may be associated with a 50% chance of success.[25]

Surgical intervention is reserved for those patients who fail hydrostatic or pneumatic reduction, or who have signs of infarcted or perforated bowel such as peritonitis or free air on abdominal radiograph at the time of presentation. At laparotomy, the intussusception is manually reduced if possible. If the intussusception is not reducible, the bowel appears necrotic or a pathological lead point is identified, a segmental resection should be performed with primary anastamosis. Recently some authors have documented excellent results using a laparoscopic approach to this condition.[26]

Children

Appendicitis

Appendicitis is the most frequent abdominal surgical emergency in children.[27] As in adults (see also Chapters 5 and 9), the classic presentation is mid-abdominal pain moving to the right lower quadrant, anorexia, vomiting, low-grade fever, and localised tenderness with peritoneal signs in the right lower quadrant. Presentation in children may be atypical, particularly in those under 5 years of age. Some authors have attempted to quantify the usefulness of specific findings in children using scoring systems. Clinical scoring systems such as the Alvarado Score and the Paediatric Appendicitis Score have been shown to be both sensitive and specific (Table 12.3).[28–30]

In the otherwise well, stable patient with an equivocal presentation, the diagnostic options include observation with serial examinations, or imaging with ultrasound or computed tomography (CT) (**Fig. 12.6**). There is a great deal of controversy as to which technique is more appropriate. Ultrasound is clearly more operator dependent, but recent

Table 12.3 • Paediatric Appendicitis Score: a score of 6 or more has been shown to be associated with a high likelihood of the child having acute appendicitis

Paediatric Appendicitis Score	Points
Percussion/hopping/coughing RLQ tenderness	2
Anorexia	1
Pyrexia	1
Nausea or vomiting	1
RLQ tenderness	2
Leucocytosis (WBC >10 000/μL)	1
Neutrophilia ('left shift')	1
Migration of pain to RLQ	1

RLQ, right lower quadrant; WBC, white blood cell count.
Reproduced from Samuel M. Pediatric appendicitis score.
J Pediatr Surg 2002; 37(6):877–81. © 2002, with permission from Elsevier.

analyses have suggested that CT in childhood may be associated with an increased risk of radiation-induced malignancy later in life.[31] Both have excellent accuracy.

Increasingly, surgeons are using a laparoscopic approach to appendicectomy in children. As in adults, the benefits of laparoscopic approach include reduced postoperative pain and length of stay, as well as a decrease in wound infection. There is some evidence that the rate of intra-abdominal abscess may be higher after laparoscopic appendicectomy in children with perforated appendicitis as compared to the open approach.[32] The laparoscopic approach may also be beneficial in children who are muscular or obese, and in adolescent females, where the incidence of ovarian pathology as a cause for the symptoms is higher.

Approximately 40% of children present with perforation, and the incidence is over 65% in those aged

Figure 12.6 • Ultrasound **(a)** and computed tomography **(b)** images of children with acute appendicitis. A faecolith (arrows) is visible at the base of the inflamed appendix in both images.

0–4 years.[27] In contrast to non-perforated appendicitis, these children usually present with prolonged symptoms, higher fever, higher white blood cell count and more diffuse peritoneal signs. Some children present with frank sepsis and diffuse peritoneal contamination; these children benefit from resuscitation, followed by immediate appendectomy and peritoneal washout. Many children with perforated appendicitis present with a prolonged history and a localised abscess or phlegmon on imaging. This condition can be managed either by early operation or by non-operative management consisting of broad-spectrum antibiotics and image-guided drainage of any purulent collections. The need for a subsequent interval appendectomy several months later is controversial. We reserve the use of interval appendicectomy for those with an appendicolith on imaging, since their risk of recurrent appendicitis is over 50%.[33]

Fluid resuscitation of the child with a surgical emergency

Fluid and electrolyte management in children are made challenging by differences in total body water and compensatory mechanisms, as well as changes in physiology throughout childhood. Total body water is as high as 80% of body weight in neonates, and decreases to the adult level of approximately 60% by 1 year. Degree of dehydration can be estimated from the history and physical examination. Children with mild dehydration (1–5% of body fluid volume) show few clinical signs but frequently have a history of 12–24 hours of vomiting or diarrhoea. Those with moderate dehydration (6–10%) are often lethargic, have low urine output (usually evident as fewer wet diapers), weight loss, loss of skin turgor, sunken eyes or fontanel, dry mucus membranes, and crying without tears. If severe dehydration (11–15%) is reached the child may develop cardiovascular or neurological instability. Children have very active peripheral vasoconstriction, so that the blood pressure will often be maintained until advanced intravascular volume depletion is reached with onset of hypotension, irritability or coma. However, tachycardia is an early sign that should be recognised and treated.[21]

The urgency of fluid replacement depends on the degree of dehydration and the cause of the fluid loss. The goals of treatment are the restoration and preservation of cardiovascular, neurological and renal perfusion. In the event of dehydration resulting from an inflammatory condition that will require urgent surgical intervention, such as appendicitis, isotonic fluid (normal saline or Ringer's lactate solution) should be given in 20 mL/kg boluses until signs of cardiovascular compromise subside. For situations in which there is no urgency to do an operation, such as pyloric stenosis, the fluid deficit can be replaced more slowly. This has the advantage of avoiding sudden fluid shifts, and the possibility of cerebral oedema and associated seizures, which are particularly likely in neonates and infants. The commonly used protocol is to calculate the fluid deficit and replace half over the first 8 hours and the other half over the subsequent 16 hours.

Paediatric trauma

The principles of trauma management are the same for children as they are for adults (see also Chapter 13). Securing the airway and ensuring adequate ventilation are paramount prior to treating bleeding and circulatory collapse. Fluid resuscitation is based on the patient's size, keeping in mind the differences in physiological response to hypovolaemia, as mentioned in the previous section. As with adults, two boluses of crystalloid (20 mL/kg) should be given through large-bore intravenous lines as quickly as possible. If there is still suspicion for ongoing bleeding, blood products are administered in 20 mL/kg boluses.

The principles of managing penetrating trauma in children are the same as in adults. However, children sustaining blunt abdominal trauma are more prone to solid-organ injury due to the low-lying nature of these organs with respect to the paediatric ribcage and the relative laxity of the abdominal wall. In general, injuries to the spleen, liver and kidney can and should all be managed non-operatively regardless of the grade of injury, with operations rare for blunt abdominal trauma in children. The indications for laparotomy in a child with blunt abdominal trauma include: evidence of peritonitis on abdominal examination, free intra-abdominal air on imaging, inability to normalise haemodynamic status despite resuscitation efforts, rapidly expanding abdominal girth associated with persistent hypotension, and need for transfusion of more than one-half of a blood volume over 24 hours.

Key points

- Neonatal and complex surgery in children should ideally take place in specialised paediatric surgical units, with subspecialised paediatric surgical, anaesthetic and intensive care unit support.
- Resuscitation is the first step in the management of all children with surgical problems.
- *Beware the child who vomits green!* Bilious vomiting in a neonate or child is usually associated with intestinal obstruction, and every child with bilious vomiting should be assumed to have life-threatening malrotation and midgut volvulus until proven otherwise.
- A high index of suspicion for intussusception should be maintained in children in the high-risk age group (3–12 months of age) presenting with intermittent abdominal pain, vomiting and/or bloody stools.
- Delayed passage of meconium (>24 hours of life) should arouse suspicion of Hirschsprung's disease.
- Incarcerated inguinal hernias should be reduced if possible and repaired within 48 hours of reduction.
- Tachycardia is an important sign of intravascular fluid depletion in children; hypotension is a late finding.

References

1. Spitz L. Oesophageal atresia. Orphanet J Rare Dis 2007; 2:24.

2. Chaudry G, Navarro OM, Levine DS et al. Abdominal manifestations of cystic fibrosis in children. Pediatr Radiol 2006; 36(3):233–40.

3. Dalla Vecchia LK, Grosfeld JL, West KW et al. Intestinal atresia and stenosis: a 25-year experience with 277 cases. Arch Surg 1998; 133(5):490–6; discussion 496–7.

4. de Lorijn F, Kremer LC, Reitsma JB et al. Diagnostic tests in Hirschsprung disease: a systematic review. J Pediatr Gastroenterol Nutr 2006; 42(5):496–505.

5. Nasr A, Langer JC. Evolution of the technique in the transanal pull-through for Hirschsprung's disease: effect on outcome. J Pediatr Surg 2007; 42(1):36–9; discussion 39–40.

6. Pena A, Hong A. Advances in the management of anorectal malformations. Am J Surg 2000; 180(5):370–6.

7. Torres AM, Ziegler MM. Malrotation of the intestine. World J Surg 1993; 17(3):326–31.

8. Strouse PJ. Disorders of intestinal rotation and fixation ("malrotation"). Pediatr Radiol 2004; 34(11):837–51.

9. Orzech N, Navarro OM, Langer JC. Is ultrasonography a good screening test for intestinal malrotation? J Pediatr Surg 2006; 41(5):1005–9.

10. Mazziotti MV, Strasberg SM, Langer JC. Intestinal rotation abnormalities without volvulus: the role of laparoscopy. J Am Coll Surg 1997; 185(2):172–6.

11. Lee JS, Polin RA. Treatment and prevention of necrotizing enterocolitis. Semin Neonatol 2003; 8(6):449–59.

12. Caplan MS, Jilling T. New concepts in necrotizing enterocolitis. Curr Opin Pediatr 2001; 13(2):111–15.

13. Bell MJ, Ternberg JL, Feigin RD et al. Neonatal necrotizing enterocolitis. Therapeutic decisions based upon clinical staging. Ann Surg 1978; 187(1):1–7.

14. Pierro A, Hall N. Surgical treatments of infants with necrotizing enterocolitis. Semin Neonatol 2003; 8(3):223–32.

15. Moss RL, Dimmitt RA, Barnhart DC et al. Laparotomy versus peritoneal drainage for necrotizing enterocolitis and perforation. N Engl J Med 2006; 354(21):2225–34.
   A randomised trial which showed no difference in outcomes between the two groups.

16. Baguley PE, Fitzgerald PG, Srinathan SK et al. Emergency room reduction of incarcerated inguinal hernia in infants: is routine hospital admission necessary? Pediatr Surg Int 1992; 7:366–7.

17. Langer JC. Abdominal wall defects. World J Surg 2003; 27(1):117–24.

18. Langer JC. Gastroschisis and omphalocele. Semin Pediatr Surg 1996; 5(2):124–8.

19. To T, Wajja A, Wales PW et al. Population demographic indicators associated with incidence of pyloric stenosis. Arch Pediatr Adolesc Med 2005; 159(6):520–5.

20. White MC, Langer JC, Don S et al. Sensitivity and cost minimization analysis of radiology versus olive palpation for the diagnosis of hypertrophic pyloric stenosis. J Pediatr Surg 1998; 33(6):913–17.

21. Rice HE, Caty MG, Glick PL. Fluid therapy for the pediatric surgical patient. Pediatr Clin North Am 1998; 45(4):719–27.

22. van der Bilt JD, Kramer WL, van der Zee DC et al. Laparoscopic pyloromyotomy for hypertrophic pyloric stenosis: impact of experience on the results in 182 cases. Surg Endosc 2004; 18(6):907–9.

23. Huppertz HI, Soriano-Gabarro M, Grimprel E et al. Intussusception among young children in Europe. Pediatr Infect Dis J 2006; 25(1, Suppl):S22–9.

24. Daneman A, Navarro O. Intussusception. Part 1: a review of diagnostic approaches. Pediatr Radiol 2003; 33(2):79–85.

25. Saxton V, Katz M, Phelan E et al. Intussusception: a repeat delayed gas enema increases the non-operative reduction rate. J Pediatr Surg 1994; 29(5):588–9.

26. Bailey KA, Wales PW, Gerstle JT. Laparoscopic versus open reduction of intussusception in children: a single-institution comparative experience. J Pediatr Surg 2007; 42(5):845–8.

27. Newman K, Ponsky T, Kittle K et al. Appendicitis 2000: variability in practice, outcomes, and resource utilization at thirty pediatric hospitals. J Pediatr Surg 2003; 38(3):372–9; discussion 372–9.

28. Owen TD, Williams H, Stiff G et al. Evaluation of the Alvarado score in acute appendicitis. J R Soc Med 1992; 85(2):87–8.

29. Samuel M. Pediatric appendicitis score. J Pediatr Surg 2002; 37(6):877–81.

30. Goldman RD, Crump S, Stephens D et al. Prospective validation of the pediatric appendicitis score. J Pediatr Surg 2008; 153:178–82.

31. Frush DP, Donnelly LF, Rosen NS. Computed tomography and radiation risks: what pediatric health care providers should know. Pediatrics 2003; 112(4):951–7.

32. Sauerland S, Lefering R, Neugebauer EA. Laparoscopic versus open surgery for suspected appendicitis. Cochrane Database Syst Rev 2004; 4(4):CD001546.

33. Ein SH, Langer JC, Daneman A. Nonoperative management of pediatric ruptured appendix with inflammatory mass or abscess: presence of an appendicolith predicts recurrent appendicitis. J Pediatr Surg 2005; 40(10):1612–15.

13

Abdominal trauma

Kenneth D. Boffard

Introduction

Without organised trauma care, some 20–35% of patients who reach hospital alive in the UK will die unnecessarily,[1] and almost 60% of patients in a recent study of the NHS received a standard of care that was less than good practice.[2] In the now classic study of trauma centres versus non-trauma centres in California published in 1979, West et al. demonstrated that the majority of preventable deaths resulted from unrecognised, and therefore untreated, intra-abdominal haemorrhage.[3]

Approximately 6% of all patients with blunt abdominal trauma will require laparotomy, primarily for haemorrhage from solid-organ injuries. Penetrating torso trauma poses its own decision-making problems, especially with regard to whether the peritoneal cavity has actually been penetrated, if so, whether intra-abdominal injury has occurred, and if so, how best to manage it.

Risk factors

One study which evaluated 3223 patients with blunt trauma found that the risk of abdominal injury was significantly increased in the presence of an arterial base deficit of 3 mmol/L or more, the presence of major chest trauma, the presence of pelvic fractures or the presence of hypotension.[4] In 482 paediatric patients haematuria and objective abdominal find-ings (distension, abrasions, contusions, blood in the gastrointestinal tract) were associated with abdominal injury.[5] Knudson et al. investigated the association between haematuria and blunt abdominal injuries in a group of patients that included adults and children.[6] In this study, the association between haematuria and significant intra-abdominal injuries not related to the kidney increased with the degree of haematuria. In patients with greater than 100 red blood cells per high-powered field, 17% had an intra-abdominal injury; this number increased to 24% in those with gross haematuria. When patients with a history of shock were evaluated, even microscopic haematuria (less than 100 red blood cells per high-powered field) was associated with a 29% incidence of abdominal injury.[6]

Criteria that identify patients at significant risk for abdominal injury, and therefore requiring objective evaluation, are:

- unexplained haemodynamic instability;
- unexplained hypovolaemic shock;
- associated major chest injury;
- presence of pelvic fracture;
- impaired sensorium;
- significant base deficit *or* significant rise in the serum lactate;
- presence of haematuria;
- objective physical findings (e.g. tenderness);
- major mechanism of injury.

Assessment in the emergency department

The entire philosophy of the abdominal injury can be summed up by answering the following questions:

- Is the abdomen involved in an injury process?
- Is a surgical procedure necessary to correct it?
- What additional support does the patient require?

In hypotensive patients, the goal is to stop the bleeding, and this includes the rapid determination of whether the abdomen is the cause of the hypotension. If intra-abdominal bleeding *is* the cause, then emergency measures will be needed to control that bleeding. These include emergency transfusion in order to 'buy time' or emergency thoracotomy in the emergency room to control the descending aorta and therefore bleeding distally. Transfusion alone is only a means to an end, and for hypotensive patients with penetrating torso injuries, delay in aggressive fluid resuscitation until rapid operative intervention has occurred improves outcome.[7] Haemodynamically stable patients without signs of abdominal irritation may undergo a more extended assessment in order to answer the above questions.

Most conventional texts emphasise the need for a careful history and physical examination of the abdomen. In trauma, it is extremely difficult to assess the abdomen, as the history may not be available and all the available physical signs are misleading. Fresh blood is not a peritoneal irritant. Positive findings may be relevant. Negative ones are not!

The mechanism of injury is critically important in assessing the potential for abdominal injury. This information may be obtained from the patient, relatives, police or emergency care personnel. When assessing the patient who has sustained a penetrating injury, pertinent historical information includes the time of injury, type of weapon, number and direction of (especially) bullet wounds (was it an entrance and an exit wound, or two entry wounds with the bullets retained?).

It is unacceptable to withhold analgesia. Judicious, properly titrated use of intravenous opiates will not significantly affect the clarity of the history, nor will it 'mask' pain, depress cerebration or respiration, or alter the blood pressure. What it will do is make the injury more comfortable for the patient and allow the clinician a much more accurate picture of both the history and the clinical presentation.

Diagnostic modalities in blunt abdominal trauma

The accuracy of physical examination of the abdomen in detecting intra-abdominal injuries is limited.

There are many patient factors that contribute to the difficult physical examination, including the presence of other painful distracting injuries, especially if they occur both above and below the abdomen, and an altered level of consciousness as a result of drugs, alcohol or head injury. Recognising these limitations, most trauma surgeons advocate a more objective evaluation of the abdomen in patients at risk for intra-abdominal injury.

Routine screening radiographs

As laid down by the Advanced Trauma Life Support (ATLS) Programme of the American College of Surgeons, routine radiographs include an anteroposterior chest film and a pelvic film.[8] Abdominal films are not usually useful. If possible (and it is safe to do so), an erect chest radiograph will provide more information than an erect abdominal film in looking for infradiaphragmatic air (see also Chapter 5).

In all cases of penetrating trauma, it is important to appreciate that the radiograph is unlikely to influence management in the *unstable* patient who requires an immediate laparotomy. However, in the stable patient, useful additional information regarding the track of the bullet can be obtained. It is essential in such a situation to make use of bullet markers to show the entry/exit wounds.[9] These can be simply paper-clips taped onto the skin. If there are wounds on both front and back, then one of the paper-clips can be unfolded. After the clips are applied to all torso wounds, the radiographs are taken and will give an indication of the track of the bullet, which wound is at the front and which at the back, and also the presence of other fragments.

Special diagnostic studies

The advantages and disadvantages of each of the objective methods of examining the abdomen for injuries are summarised in Table 13.1.

Computed tomography (CT)

With contrast-enhanced CT (CECT), it is possible both to recognise the organ that is injured and to grade the severity of the injury. There is only limited evidence that enteral (via stomach or rectum) contrast is helpful, and its use may delay the examination. Intravascular contrast is, however, essential. Both intraperitoneal and retroperitoneal injuries can be detected with CECT, and the amount of intra-abdominal blood loss can be estimated. Subsequent serial scanning can be used to follow the resolution (or progression) of an injury. The disadvantages of CECT include the need to move the patient to the radiology suite and the time required to perform the scan, although with the introduction of multi-slice spiral scanners, the latter factor has become less important. CT is also expensive and there is

Table 13.1 • Comparison of diagnostic methods for abdominal injury

Method	Advantages	Disadvantages
Clinical		
Clinical examination	Quick, non-invasive	Unreliable
Diagnostic		
Computed tomography 'Gold standard'	Organ-specific retroperitoneal information	Patient must be stable, expensive
Ultrasound	Quick, non-invasive	User dependent, unhelpful for hollow viscus injury
Diagnostic peritoneal lavage	Quick, inexpensive	Invasive, too sensitive, limited specificity
Laparoscopy	Organ specific	Painful, anaesthesia required, user dependent, patient must be stable
Laparotomy	Highly specific	Complications, expensive

the potential for allergic reactions to the injected contrast material, or for aspiration of oral contrast (a rare event).

Although CT is relatively insensitive in the detection of hollow viscus injuries, a bowel injury (and especially a duodenal injury) is suggested by finding a thickened bowel wall, extraluminal air and the presence of intraperitoneal fluid in the absence of a solid-organ injury.[10,11] CT may also miss a pancreatic injury early in its course. The accuracy of CT is generally poor in the detection of diaphragmatic, hollow-organ and mesenteric injuries, and there have been reports of a high incidence of false-negative results.[17] Despite these limitations, however, CT remains the method of choice for objective evaluation of the abdomen in *stable* trauma patients who are likely to have an intra-abdominal injury, and is currently the 'gold standard' investigation.

Diagnostic ultrasound

The sensitivity of ultrasound for the detection of free intraperitoneal fluid in the pericardial sac and in abdominal blunt trauma has been shown to be 81–99%.[13] The disadvantage of ultrasound is its lack of sensitivity for injuries that do not produce blood or peritoneal fluid and the fact that its accuracy is directly related to the experience of the ultrasonographer. Nonetheless, surgeons can be taught to perform and interpret ultrasound examinations

rapidly and accurately, with a sensitivity/specificity and accuracy each over 90%.[14–16] This diagnostic method has particular appeal in paediatric trauma patients and in the injured gravid patient.

In most centres, ultrasound has replaced diagnostic peritoneal lavage (DPL) for evaluation of the unstable patient following blunt trauma. However, the role of ultrasound in the diagnosis of penetrating abdominal trauma remains controversial, since the examination will miss small amounts of intraperitoneal fluid.

Diagnostic peritoneal lavage (DPL)

Root et al. introduced DPL as a method of evaluation of the abdomen,[17] and while it has frequently been superseded by more sophisticated (and potentially more expensive) techniques, it remains the standard against which all other diagnostic examinations are judged. The main advantage of DPL is that it can be performed quickly and with few complications by relatively inexperienced clinicians. DPL is also reproducible, and highly sensitive and specific for the detection of abdominal blood (>97%), but it does not identify the organ of injury. Injuries of the retroperitoneum will be missed by DPL, and the presence of pelvic fractures may lead to a false-positive result.

A DPL is generally considered as positive if:

- the red cell count is >100 000 cells/mm^3;
- the white cell count is >500/mm^3;
- there is amylase or bowel content in the lavage return.

In addition, if surgeons are committed to operating on all patients with a positive DPL, the ability to manage some patients non-operatively may be lost. The lavage is therefore regarded as an indicator of the presence of abdominal pathology, but not necessarily an indication for surgery (see section on non-operative management below).

Diagnostic laparoscopy

Laparoscopy has been found to be of little use in the evaluation of the patient with blunt abdominal trauma.[18] With few exceptions, laparoscopy requires general anaesthesia, is expensive, and in the patient with abdominal trauma has the potential to create a tension pneumothorax[19] or air embolus during insufflation. Isopneumonic (gasless) laparoscopy has been reported in an attempt to avoid the potential for air embolus by avoiding the pneumoperitoneum while maintaining the ability to use conventional surgical instruments.[20] The main disadvantage is the cost of the abdominal wall retraction system. Its use in penetrating injury has been reported in the successful repair of injuries of the diaphragm and stomach.[21]

An additional drawback of diagnostic laparoscopy is the current relative cost, compared with other modalities, especially those performed at the bedside, such as ultrasound. The technique can only be used on relatively stable patients, and laparoscopy is still limited in its ability to detect intestinal injury, especially in the hands of an operator unskilled in the specific techniques required to recognise intra-abdominal injury. Currently, laparoscopy is most useful in the patient with penetrating abdominal trauma when there is a question of peritoneal penetration or diaphragmatic injury.[22] The diaphragm is also an area where delay or missed diagnosis dramatically increases the morbidity.[23] Laparoscopy can identify not only clinically unsuspected diaphragm injuries, but also other injuries that have been 'missed' by other diagnostic tests.

Diagnostic laparoscopy does not confer any advantages or improvements over other techniques when it comes to investigation of retroperitoneal injuries to organs such as the duodenum and pancreas, and CT remains more accurate in this regard.

Laparotomy

Mandatory laparotomy

While laparotomy remains the most appropriate therapy for an unstable patient with obvious abdominal trauma, a non-therapeutic laparotomy is not necessarily benign. In a recent prospective study of unnecessary laparotomies performed in 254 trauma patients, complications occurred in 41% of patients, and included atalectasis, postoperative hypotension, pleural effusion, pneumothorax, prolonged ileus, pneumonia, surgical wound infection, small-bowel obstruction and urinary infection.[24]

Many centres still practice a policy of mandatory laparotomy for abdominal gunshot wounds because of the higher morbidity associated with delayed diagnosis.[25,26] However, a negative laparotomy rate (absence of injury) of 12% has been reported in gunshots, 23% in stab wounds and 6% in blunt trauma, suggesting that there is a more accurate investigation of the abdomen in blunt trauma.[27] Overall, negative laparotomies are associated with a morbidity of between 5% and 22%.[28]

Selective laparotomy (i.e. selective conservatism) in penetrating injury

Several studies have considered the possibilities of selectively treating certain patients by observation only, even when a laparotomy seems to be required. Two South African studies reviewed selective conservatism in the management of abdominal gunshot wounds. One reported no delayed laparotomies or morbidity, with only a 7% negative laparotomy rate,[26] and the other found a delayed laparotomy rate of 17%.[29]

It is obvious that the decision not to operate should be carefully considered and, if taken, meticulous and repeated re-examination of the patient for changing abdominal signs should be performed. A general dictum should be that the more uncertainty there is in the assessment, or the more inexperienced the assessor, the more aggressive should be the tendency towards laparotomy.

Operative management of abdominal trauma

Laparotomy for trauma

In patients who, by any of the diagnostic criteria above, are judged to need a laparotomy for control of their injuries, the timing of laparotomy in relationship to the detection and/or repair of concomitant injuries requires input from an experienced trauma surgeon. Although open to debate, the following scenarios are offered along with a suggested algorithm (**Fig. 13.1**).

The unstable patient with intra-abdominal bleeding

The unstable patient with obvious intra-abdominal haemorrhage should undergo immediate operative intervention. However, if other injuries are also pressing (e.g. severe closed head injury or associated pelvic haemorrhage), a 'damage control' procedure (abbreviated laparotomy) should be considered to allow management of the patient's physiology or of other life-threatening injuries.

During the laparotomy, however brief, if the patient had an initial Glasgow Coma Scale of less than 8/15, it is recommended that intracranial pressure monitoring should take place. The most lethal secondary brain injury is induced by hypotension or hypoxia.

If a widened mediastinum is present, the situation must be assessed and priorities of care selected. In the patient who is unstable because of intra-abdominal pathology, the diagnostic processes for the mediastinum may have to take place *after* the therapeutic laparotomy. Consideration should be given to the use of beta-blockade and hypotensive resuscitation, until the aorta/great vessels can be properly evaluated.

There are considerable data available to support medical treatment of contained thoracic aortic injuries and to delay repair or endovascular stenting until other injuries are stabilised.[30,31]

The unstable patient with intra-abdominal and pelvic haemorrhage

In a patient who is unstable with both intra-abdominal haemorrhage and pelvic bleeding, the surgeon must decide which injury is causing the hypotension. If the DPL is grossly positive, or an ultrasound demonstrates a large amount of fluid in Morrison's pouch, laparotomy should be performed promptly. As most fractures of the pelvis bleed extraperitoneally,

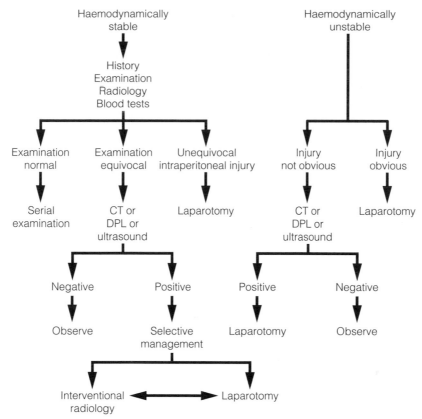

Figure 13.1 • Management of abdominal injury.

this bleeding is unlikely to originate in the pelvis. An unstable patient who has signs of bleeding from both pelvis and abdomen should have compression stabilisation of the pelvis first, either with a knotted sheet, a proprietary device or formal operative external fixation, followed by laparotomy, then angiography of the pelvis and embolisation of bleeding vessels. Ultrasound is unreliable for quantifying blood loss in such circumstances, and if the patient is stable enough, CT of both pelvis and abdomen should be carried out. Not only will CT provide significant information regarding the pelvic fractures, it will also give information as to possible injury to intra-abdominal organs. Furthermore it may exclude a diaphragmatic rupture, which has a significant association with pelvic fractures. Intrapelvic bleeding is best controlled by angio-embolisation (arterial) or external fixation (venous), sometimes in association with extraperitoneal pelvic packing.

The stable patient with combined head, chest and abdominal injuries

In stable patients with combined head/chest/abdominal injuries, CT with contrast can rapidly identify injuries that need operative intervention. In a study of 800 patients thought to have potentially correctable injuries to both the head and the abdomen,[32] of whom only 52 had a head injury requiring craniotomy, 40 required laparotomy, and only three needed both craniotomy and therapeutic laparotomy. The authors of this study lend support to the concept that if patients with combined head/abdominal trauma are *stable* and have a negative ultrasound (or DPL), they can undergo CT scanning of both the head and abdomen. Many patients with head trauma and stable liver/spleen injuries are now being treated non-operatively.[33]

The patient with abdominal injuries and limb fractures

With the exception of pelvic fractures, fracture/dislocations, and in the presence of vascular impairment, most fractures can be simply splinted during other surgical procedures. Open fractures should be irrigated and debrided within 6 hours of the injury and antibiotics administered. Although there is still considerable debate about the timing of fracture fixation in trauma patients with multiple priorities, those with head and/or pulmonary injuries still benefit from early fracture fixation, provided hypotension and hypoxia can be avoided during the surgery. There is a clear role for damage control orthopaedics as part of a damage control procedure.

Trauma laparotomy: a systematic approach

If it is decided that the injured patient would benefit from laparotomy, the operation should be approached in an orderly fashion. It is important to recognise the components of the 'trauma laparotomy'. The vital initial goals are to stop the bleeding and limit contamination.

Preparation

An adequately stocked *warm* operating theatre is essential. *Delay in surgery is the most common cause of unnecessary ongoing bleeding.* In addition to routine equipment, the following should be considered as mandatory equipment:

- rapid infusion devices with rapid warming capability (Alton Deane, Mallincrodt or Level One);
- patient warming blankets (e.g. Bair Hugger);
- autotransfusion if available.

Incision

A long midline abdominal incision is used, one that can be extended superiorly as a sternotomy. The ideal incision is always 'too big rather than too small' and should extend from the xiphisternum to the symphysis pubis.

Bleeding control

If, upon opening the abdomen, gross blood is encountered, as much as possible is scooped out, using a receiver, e.g. a kidney dish. Suction is ineffective as it is too slow, and the apparatus blocks with clots. The abdomen is packed using layered dry abdominal swabs:

- below the left hemidiaphragm;
- lateral to the descending colon;
- the pelvis;
- lateral to the ascending colon;
- below the liver;
- lateral to the liver;
- anterior to the dome of the liver, under the right subcostal margin;
- central abdomen.

Additional packs are used to isolate bleeding areas as required.

With blunt injuries, the most likely sources of bleeding are the liver, spleen and mesentery. The solid organs are packed and bleeders in the mesentery are clamped using mosquito forceps. No attempt is made to tie off individual vessels (which is time-consuming) until all major bleeding has been controlled with clamps. If necessary, a soft bowel clamp is used across the mesentery to control all mesenteric bleeding.

With penetrating injuries, the liver and retroperitoneal structures, vascular structures and mesentery are all examined.

If packing does not control the bleeding, the blood supply to the organ is isolated using proximal clamping or isolation techniques. If additional assistance is needed for blood pressure control, the abdominal aorta can be manually compressed at the hiatus. When the patient is reasonably stable, the packs are removed systematically, uncovering the most likely injury last. Any bleeding sites are then rapidly controlled by clamps, sutures or repacking as needed.

Contamination control

Gross contamination from the gastrointestinal tract is quickly controlled with sutures or staples.

Physiological control

No further surgery is performed until the anaesthesia team has the patient stabilised and the patient is warm (>35°C). This may require a period of resuscitation in the intensive care unit (see 'Damage control laparotomy' below).

Full inspection for injury

Once there is control of haemorrhage and contamination, a systematic inspection is performed.

In addition to inspecting the liver and spleen, a full trauma laparotomy includes exploration of the anterior/posterior stomach, the entire large and small bowel (including the duodenum), the diaphragm, the gastrohepatic ligament, the head, body and tail of the pancreas, and any central retroperitoneal haematomas. In order to achieve this, it will be necessary not only to perform a conventional reflection of the duodenum (the Kocher manoeuvre), but also to reflect the right and left hemicolon to view the great vessels (right and left medial visceral rotation manoeuvres).[34]

The abdomen is only closed when it is safe to do so (see 'Damage control laparotomy' and 'Abdominal compartment syndrome' below).

Damage control laparotomy

Since the mid-1980s, there has been a re-emergence of the concept of packing and closing, for abdominal injuries with profuse haemorrhage. Further experience with this technique has resulted in its extension to patients with other vascular/intestinal injuries, and new terms such as 'damage control' surgery, 'abbreviated laparotomy', 'staged laparotomy' or 'planned re-operation' have emerged.[35] The principle of damage control has been extended beyond the abdomen, to thoracic, extremity and orthopaedic damage control techniques.[36]

The concept of damage control has as its objective the delay in imposition of additional surgical stress at a moment of physiological frailty. The concept is not new – livers were not infrequently packed 100 years ago. However, the failure to understand the underlying rationale, or deal with the resulting disruption to physiological processes, led to disastrous results.

In 1979, analysis of fatal hepatic haemorrhage after trauma demonstrated that 82% of deaths following liver trauma were caused by uncontrollable haemorrhage and a progressive coagulopathy, seemingly exacerbated by hypothermia and acidosis.[37] The concept of packing was re-examined, and the technique of initial abortion of laparotomy, establishment of intra-abdominal pack tamponade and then completion of the procedure once coagulation has returned to an acceptable level proved to be life-saving. This approach was initially advocated for patients with severe liver injuries, especially those with retrohepatic venous injuries. When properly applied, packs above/below the liver can compress and control venous injuries long enough for the patient's coagulopathy, acidosis and temperature to be corrected.

Often, when the patient is returned to the operating room after packing for liver injuries, the bleeding has already stopped, and irrigation, debridement and formal closure are all that is required. The concept of staging applies both to routine and to emergency procedures, and it can apply equally well beyond the abdomen.

This approach has been used for patients with both penetrating and blunt injuries, and it generally includes clamping of major bleeding vessels, packing of bleeding solid-organ injuries and stapling/ dividing bowel injuries but *without* initial reconstruction. A variety of temporary methods of closure of the abdomen have been developed, including mesh and other synthetic material, plastic intravenous bags and towel clips. Currently, the 'vacuum sandwich' technique is the simplest method of choice. However, it must be remembered that the type of closure is much less important than the recognition of the need to terminate the operation and save the patient.

Patient selection for damage control

Patients are selected for a damage control approach if there is:

- inability to achieve haemostasis;
- inaccessible major venous injury, e.g. retrohepatic vena cava;
- anticipated need for a time-consuming procedure (>90 minutes);
- demand for non-operative control of other injuries, e.g. fractured pelvis;
- desire to reassess the intra-abdominal contents (directed relook).

Irrespective of setting, a coagulopathy in the presence of hypothermia is the single most common reason for abortion of a planned procedure or the curtailment of definitive surgery. It is important to abort the surgery *before* the coagulopathy becomes obvious.

Hirshberg and Mattox described three distinct indications for planned re-operation in severely injured patients:[38]

- avoidance of irreversible physiological insult in a hypothermic coagulopathic patient by rapid termination of the surgical procedure;
- inability to obtain direct haemostasis (by ligation, suture or vascular repair), necessitating indirect control of bleeding by packing or balloon tamponade;
- massive visceral oedema precluding formal closure of the abdomen or chest.

Garrison et al. described the following criteria which predicted the need to pack early for severe intra-abdominal haemorrhage:[39]

- Injury Severity Score (ISS) >35;
- coagulopathy with a prothrombin time >19 seconds;
- hypotension with a systolic blood pressure <70 mmHg for longer than 70 minutes;
- pH <7.2;
- serum lactate >5 mmol/L.
- temperature <34°C.

The cumulative experience with packing/damage control operations has resulted in a survival rate of 48%. In their study of 46 patients with penetrating abdominal injury who required >10 unit blood transfusion, Rotondo et al. identified a subset of patients they called their 'maximum injury' group, whose survival after damage control was markedly better than an equivalent group who underwent definitive laparotomy (10/13 survived, compared with 1/9).[35]

Damage control procedures can be considered under the following stages.

Stage 1: Damage control procedure

In damage control, the technical aspects of the surgery are dictated by the injury pattern, with the primary objectives as follows.

Arrest bleeding and the resulting (causative) coagulopathy

Procedures for haemorrhage control include:

- repair or ligation of accessible blood vessels;
- occlusion of inflow into the bleeding organ (e.g. Pringle's manoeuvre for bleeding liver);

- tamponade using wraps or packs;
- intravascular shunting;
- intraoperative or postoperative embolisation.

Limit contamination and the associated sequelae
This is achieved by:

- ligation or stapling of bowel;
- isolation of pancreatic injury;
- adequate suction drainage (e.g. with a Blake drain).

Temporary abdominal closure
The abdomen is only closed to limit heat and fluid loss and to protect viscera. Closure is usually achieved using the 'sandwich technique', which was first described by Schein et al. in 1986[40] and popularised by Rotondo et al.[35]

A sheet of self-adhesive incise drape (Opsite, Steridrape or Ioban) is placed flat and an abdominal swab placed upon it. The edges are folded over, to produce a sheet with membrane on one side and abdominal swab on the other. If extra firmness is required, a surgical drape can be used.

The membrane is utilised as an on-lay with the margins 'tucked in' under the edges of the open sheath, with the membrane in contact with the bowel.

The appreciable drainage of serosanguinous fluid which occurs is best dealt with by placing a pair of drainage tubes (e.g. sump-type nasogastric tubes or closed-system suction drains) through separate stab incisions onto the membrane and utilising continuous low-vacuum suction. This arrangement is covered by an occlusive incise drape applied to the skin, thus providing a closed system. Other techniques, such as the use of towel clips or the so-called 'Bogota bag', are now generally regarded as obsolete (see also Chapter 18).

Stage 2: Transfer to the intensive care unit for ongoing resuscitation

The timing of the transfer of the patient from the operating theatre to the intensive care unit is critical. Early transfer is cost-effective; premature transfer is counter-productive. In addition, once haemostasis has been properly achieved, it may not be necessary to abort the procedure and it may be possible to proceed to definitive surgery. Conversely, there are some patients with severe head injuries where the coagulopathy is induced by severe irreversible cerebral damage and further surgical energy is futile.

In the operating theatre, efforts must be started to reverse all the associated adjuncts, such as acidosis, hypothermia and hypoxia, and it may be possible to improve the coagulation status through these methods alone. Adequate time should still be allowed for this, following which reassessment of the abdominal injuries should take place, as it is not infrequent to discover further injuries or ongoing bleeding.

Stage 3: Resuscitation in the intensive care unit

Priorities on reaching intensive care are:

1. The restoration of body temperature using:
   (a) passive rewarming with warming blankets, warmed fluids, etc.
   (b) active rewarming using lavage of chest or abdomen.
2. Correction of clotting profiles by blood component repletion.
3. Optimisation of oxygen delivery:
   (a) volume loading to achieve optimum preload.
   (b) haemoglobin optimisation to a value of 9 g/dL.
   (c) temperature optimisation (>35°C).
4. Monitoring of intra-abdominal pressure to prevent abdominal compartment syndrome.

Stage 4: Return to the operating theatre for definitive surgery

The patient is returned to the operating theatre as soon as stage 3 is achieved. The timing is determined by:

- the indication for damage control in the first place.
- the injury pattern.
- the physiological response.

Patients with persistent bleeding despite correction of the other parameters merit early return to control the bleeding.

Every effort must be made to return *all* patients to the operating theatre within 24 hours (or, at most, 48 hours) of their initial surgery.

Stage 5: Definitive surgery and abdominal wall reconstruction if required

Once definitive surgery is complete and no further operations are contemplated, then the abdominal wall can be closed. This is often difficult and methods involved include:

- primary closure.
- closure of the sheath, leaving the skin open.
- grafts with Vicryl mesh, Gore-Tex sheets or other synthetic sheets.
- use of lateral relieving incisions to allow closure of sheath.

Abdominal compartment syndrome (see also Chapter 18)

There have been major developments in our under-standing of intra-abdominal pressure (IAP), intra-abdominal hypertension (IAH), and the far-reaching consequences of raised IAP for the physiology of the patient.[41] Clinically it is the cardiovascular, renal and pulmonary systems which are most affetced. Decreased cardiac output, increased periph-eral resistance, oliguria, anuria, increased airway pressures, decreased compliance and hypoxia may all occur. The syndrome which results is known as the abdominal compartment syndrome (ACS). Increasingly it is being recognised that ACS is not uncommon in trauma patients, and that failure to consider its prevention, detect it in a timely fashion and treat it aggressively results in a high mortality.

Definition

The first World Congress on ACS was held in 2005[42] and an internal consensus agreement relating to definitions is shown in Table 13.2.

 Specifically, ACS is defined as a sustained IAP ≥ 20 mmHg (with or without an abdominal perfusion pressure <60 mmHg) that is associated with new organ dysfunction/failure.

Pathology

The incidence of increased IAP may be 30% of post-operative general surgery patients in intensive care and after emergency surgery the incidence is even higher. The causes of acutely increased IAP are usu-ally multifactorial. The first clinical reports of postop-erative increased IAP were often after aortic surgery, with postoperative haemorrhage from the graft suture line. However, peritonitis and intra-abdominal sepsis, tissue oedema and ileus are the predominant causes of increased IAP. Raised IAP in trauma patients is often caused by a combination of blood loss and tis-sue oedema. Causes of increased IAP include:

* tissue oedema secondary to insults such as ischaemia, trauma and sepsis.
* paralytic ileus.
* intraperitoneal or retroperitoneal haematoma;
* ascites.

Table 13.2 • Consensus definitions related to IAP, IAH and ACS Reproduced with permission from the World Society of the Abdominal Compartment Syndrome.

Definition 1	IAP is the pressure concealed within the abdominal cavity
Definition 2	APP – MAP – IAP
Definition 3	FG = GFP – PTP = MAP – 2 × IAP FG, filtration gradient; GFP, glomerular filtration pressure; PTP, proximal tubular pressure
Definition 4	IAP should be expressed in mmHg and measured at end-expiration in the complete supine position after ensuring that abdominal muscle contractions are absent and with the transducer zeroed at the level of the mid-axillary line
Definition 5	The reference standard for intermittent IAP measurement is via the bladder with a maximal instillation volume of 25 mL of sterile saline
Definition 6	Normal IAP is approximately 5–7 mmHg in critically ill adults
Definition 7	IAH is defined by a sustained or repeated pathological elevation of IAP ≥12 mmHg
Definition 8	IAH is graded as follows: • Grade I: IAP 12–15 mmHg • Grade II: IAP 16–20 mmHg • Grade III: IAP 21–25 mmHg • Grade IV: IAP >25 mmHg
Definition 9	ACS is defined as a sustained IAP ≥20 mmHg (with or without an APP <60 mmHg) that is associated with new organ dysfunction/failure
Definition 10	Primary ACS is a condition associated with injury or disease in the abdomino-pelvic region that frequently requires early surgical or interventional radiological intervention
Definition 11	Secondary ACS refers to conditions that do not originate from the abdomino-pelvic region
Definition 12	Recurrent ACS refers to the condition in which ACS redevelops following previous surgical or medical treatment of primary or secondary ACS

- trauma with hypothermia, coagulopathy and acidosis, or as a consequence of over-resuscitation.[43]

Effect of raised IAP on organ function

Renal function

In 1945, Bradley demonstrated in a study of 17 volunteers that there was a reduction in renal plasma flow and glomerular filtration rate (GFR) in association with increased IAP. In 1982, Harman et al. showed that an increase in IAP from 0 to 20 mmHg in dogs resulted in a decrease in GFR of 25%.[44] When IAP reached 40 mmHg, the dogs were resuscitated and although their cardiac output returned to normal, their GFR and renal blood flow did not improve, indicating a local effect on renal blood flow. In a recent study, it was found that out of 20 patients with increased IAP and renal impairment, 13 already had impairment before the IAP increased.[45]

The most likely direct effect of increased IAP is an increase in the renal vascular resistance, coupled with a moderate reduction in cardiac output. The absolute value of IAP that is required to cause renal impairment is probably in the region of 20 mmHg. Furthermore maintaining adequate cardiovascular filling pressures in the presence of increased IAP also seems to be important.

Cardiac function

Increased IAP reduces cardiac output as well as increasing central venous pressure, systemic vascular resistance, pulmonary artery pressure and pulmonary artery wedge pressure. Cardiac output is affected mainly by a reduction in stroke volume, secondary to a reduction in preload and an increase in afterload. This is further aggravated by hypovolaemia. Paradoxically, in the presence of hypovolaemia, an increase in IAP can be temporarily associated with an increase in cardiac output. Venous stasis occurs in the legs of patients with IAP values above 12 mmHg. In addition, recent studies of patients undergoing laparoscopic cholecystectomy show up to a fourfold increase in renin and aldosterone levels.

Respiratory function

In association with increased IAP, there is diaphragmatic stenting, exerting a restrictive effect on the lungs with reduction in ventilation, decreased lung compliance, increase in airway pressures and reduction in tidal volumes. The mechanism by which increased IAP impairs pulmonary function appears to be purely mechanical. As IAP increases, the diaphragm is forced higher into the chest, thereby compressing the lungs. Adequate ventilation can still be achieved, but only at the cost of increased airway pressures.

In critically ill, ventilated patients the effect on the respiratory system can be significant, resulting in reduced lung volumes, impaired gas exchange and high ventilatory pressures. Hypercarbia can occur and the resulting acidosis can be exacerbated by simultaneous cardiovascular depression as a result of the raised IAP. The effects of raised IAP on the respiratory system in the intensive care setting can sometimes be life threatening, requiring urgent abdominal decompression. Patients with true ACS undergoing abdominal decompression demonstrate a remarkable change in their intraoperative vital signs.

Visceral perfusion

Interest in visceral perfusion has increased with increased awareness of gastric tonometry, and there is an association between IAP and visceral perfusion as measured by gastric pH. In a study of 73 patients after laparotomy, it was shown that IAP and pH are strongly associated, suggesting that early decreases in visceral perfusion are related to IAP at levels as low as 12 mmHg.[45] Visceral reperfusion injury is a major consideration after a period of raised IAP, and may of itself have fatal consequences.[45]

Intracranial contents

Raised IAP can have a marked effect on intracranial pathophysiology and cause severe rises in intracranial pressure.

Measurement of IAP

The most common method for measuring IAP uses a urinary catheter, as described by Kron et al.[46] (see also Chapter 18). The patient is positioned flat in the bed and a standard Foley catheter is used with a T-piece bladder pressure device attached between the urinary catheter and the drainage tubing. This piece is then connected to a pressure transducer. The pressure transducer is placed in the mid-axillary line and the urinary tubing is clamped. Approximately 50 mL isotonic saline is inserted into the bladder via a three-way stopcock. After zeroing, the pressure on the monitor is recorded.

Pitfalls of IAP measurement

The following factors are important in achieving effective IAP measurements:

- A strict protocol and staff education on the technique and interpretation of IAP is essential.
- Very high pressures (especially unexpected ones) are usually caused by a blocked urinary catheter.

- The size of the urinary catheter does not matter.
- The volume of saline instilled into the bladder is not critical, but it should be enough to overcome the resistance of the contracted bladder; usually, not more than 50 mL is adequate.
- A central venous pressure manometer system can be used but it is more cumbersome than online monitoring.
- Elevation of the urine catheter and measuring the urine column provides a rough guide and is simple to perform.
- If the patient is not lying flat, IAP can be measured from the pubic symphysis.
- IAP is not a static measurement and should be measured continuously. In addition, whether IAP is measured intermittently or continuously, consideration for abdominal perfusion measurement should be given.

Real-time continuous monitoring of IAP is effective and shows trends as well as actual pressures.

Abdominal perfusion pressure

Like the concept of cerebral perfusion pressure, calculation of the 'abdominal perfusion pressure' (APP), which is defined as mean arterial pressure (MAP) minus IAP, assesses not only the severity of IAP present, but also the adequacy of the patient's abdominal blood flow. APP has been studied as a resuscitation end-point in four clinical trials.[42] These demonstrated statistically significant differences in APP between survivors and non-survivors with IAH/ACS. Cheatham et al., in a retrospective trial of surgical and trauma patients with IAH (mean IAP 22 ± 8 mmHg), concluded that an APP >50 mmHg optimised survival based upon receiver operating characteristic curve analysis.[47] APP was also superior to global resuscitation end-points such as arterial pH, base deficit, arterial lactate and hourly urinary output in its ability to predict patient outcome. Three subsequent trials involving mixed medical–surgical patients (mean IAP 10 ± 4 mmHg) suggested that 60 mmHg represented an appropriate resuscitation goal.[48–50] Persistence of IAH and failure to maintain an APP ≥60 mmHg by day 3 following development of IAH-induced acute renal failure was found to discriminate between survivors and non-survivors.

Treatment of raised IAP

General support

In general, the best treatment is prevention, both by minimising the causative agents and early appreciation of the potential complications. There

are a number of key principles in the management of patients with potential ACS:

- regular (<8-hourly) monitoring of IAP;
- optimisation of systemic perfusion and organ function in the patient with IAH;
- institution of specific medical procedures to reduce IAP and the end-organ consequences of IAH/ACS;
- early surgical decompression for refractory IAH.

Reversible factors

The second aspect of management is to correct any reversible cause of ACS, such as intra-abdominal bleeding.[51] Massive retroperitoneal haemorrhage is often associated with a fractured pelvis and consideration should be given to measures that would control haemorrhage, such as pelvic fixation or vessel embolisation. In some cases, severe gaseous distension or acute colonic pseudo-obstruction can occur in patients in intensive care. This may respond to drugs such as neostigmine but if it is severe, surgical decompression may be necessary (see also Chapter 10). Ileus is a common cause of raised IAP in patients in intensive care. There is little that can be actively done in these circumstances apart from optimising the patient's cardiorespiratory status and serum electrolytes.

Abdominal evaluation for sepsis is a priority and surgery is obviously the mainstay of treatment in patients whose rise in IAP is caused by postoperative bleeding.

A report on secondary ACS, which can occur without abdominal injury, stated that, again, early recognition could improve outcome.[51]

Management

Management of IAH and ACS is summarised in **Fig. 13.2**.[42,50]

Surgery for raised IAP

As yet, there are few guidelines for exactly when surgical decompression is required in the presence of raised IAP. The indications for abdominal decompression are related to correcting pathophysiological abnormalities as much as achieving a precise and optimum IAP. The abdomen is decompressed and a temporary abdominal closure (TAC) is achieved. A large number of different techniques have been used to facilitate a TAC, including intravenous bags, Velcro, silicone and zips. Whatever technique, it is important that effective decompression be achieved with adequate incisions (see also Chapter 18).

Unfortunately, clinical infection is common in the open abdomen and the infection is usually polymicrobial. It is desirable to close the abdominal defect as soon as possible. This is often not possible because of persistent tissue oedema. The abdomen

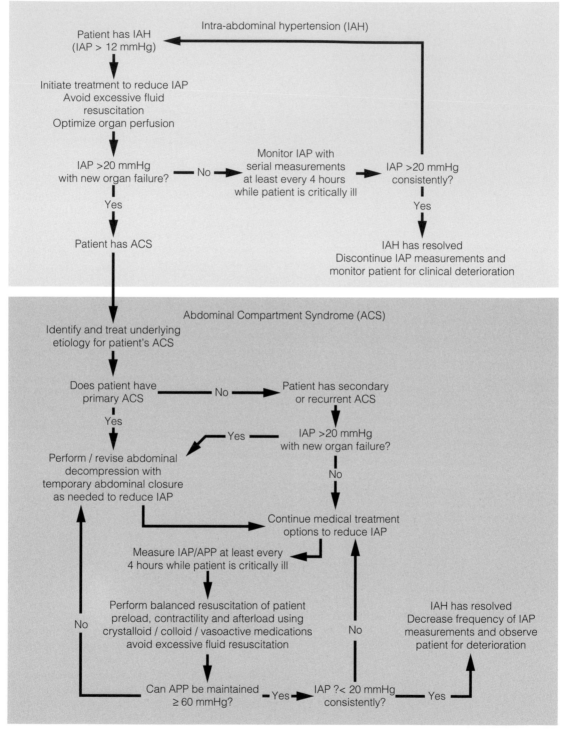

Figure 13.2 • Management algorithm for intra-abdominal hypertension (IAH)/abdominal compartment syndrome (ACS). Adapted from Malbrain ML, Cheatham ML, Kirkpatrick A et al. Results from the International Conference of Experts on intra-abdominal hypertension and abdominal compartment syndrome. I. Definitions. Intensive Care Med 2006; 32(11):1722–32. Cheatham ML, Malbrain ML, Kirkpatrick A et al. Results from the International Conference of Experts on intra-abdominal hypertension and abdominal compartment syndrome. II. Recommendations. Intensive Care Med 2007; 33(6):951–62. Reproduced with permission of the World Society of the Abdominal Compartment Syndrome. All rights reserved.

Medical treatment options to reduce IAP

1. Improve abdominal wall compliance
   Sedation and analgesia
   Neuromuscular blockade
   Avoid head of bed > 30 degrees

2. Evacuate intra-luminal contents
   Nasogastric decompression
   Rectal decompression
   Gastro/colo-prokinetic agents

3. Evacuate abdominal fluid collections
   Paracentesis
   Percutaneous drainage

4. Correct positive fluid balance
   Avoid excessive fluid resuscitation
   Diuretics
   Colloids / hypertonic fluids
   Hemodialysis / ultrafiltration

5. Organ support
   Maintain APP ≥ 60 mmHg with vasopressors
   Optimise ventilation, alveolar recruitment
   Use transmural (tm) airway pressures
   $Pplat_{tm} = Pplat - IAP$
   Consider using volumetric preload indices
   If using PAOP/CVP, use transmural pressures
   $PAOPtm = PAOP - 0.5 * IAP$
   $CVPtm = CVP - 0.5 * IAP$

Definitions

IAH – Intra-abdominal hypertension

ACS – Abdominal compartment syndrome

IAP – Intra-abdominal pressure

APP – Abdominal perfusion pressure (MAP-IAP)
Primary ACS – A condition associated with injury or disease in the abdomino-pelvic region that frequently requires early surgical or interventional radiological intervention

Secondary ACS – ACS due to conditions that do not originate from the abdomino-pelvic region

Recurrent ACS – The condition in which ACS redevelops following previous surgical or medical treatment of primary or secondary ACS

Figure 13.2 • (cont.)

should be closed, preferably using a sandwich technique or a silo.[52] There is no indication for prophylactic antibiotics.

Summary

Patients with raised IAP require close and careful monitoring, aggressive resuscitation and a low index of suspicion for requirement of surgical abdominal decompression. The formation of the World Society on ACS has been a major advance, with production of consensus definitions, formation of a research policy, with multicentre trials, and the publishing of the consensus guidelines on ACS.[42]

Scoring systems for injuries

Penetrating Abdominal Trauma Index

Moore et al. facilitated identification of the high-risk patient when they developed the Penetrating Abdominal Trauma Index (PATI) scoring system (Tables 13.3 and 13.4).[53] In a group of 114 patients with gunshot wounds to the abdomen, they showed that a PATI score >25 dramatically increased the risk of postoperative complications (46% of patients with a PATI score of >25 developed serious postoperative complications compared with 7% of those with a PATI of <25). Subsequent reports have confirmed the accuracy of a high PATI score in predicting postoperative complications and have also identified multiple blood transfusions and the presence of underlying medical illness as a further predictor of postoperative complications.[54]

Organ Injury Scaling systems

The American Association for the Surgery of Trauma (AAST) has developed an Organ Injury Scaling system for all major injuries in the body.[54–61] The scores not only allow a clear anatomical language when dealing with organ injury but also, since surgical policies are often dictated by the injuries sustained, a degree of consistency in both treatment and prognosis. The scaling system is outlined in the Appendix to this chapter and can be accessed at http://www.aast.org on the Internet.

Surgical decision-making in abdominal trauma

Experience in dealing with injury clearly leads to a better outcome: good judgement comes from experience. Unfortunately, experience comes from bad judgement!

There is limited evidence-based decision-making in trauma, although certain practice guidelines have been developed.[62]

Antibiotic prophylaxis in abdominal trauma[63,64]

Guidelines for patient selection and specific antimicrobial regimens are based on good evidence (Box 13.1), those regarding high-risk patients and duration of therapy less so (Box 13.2). The trauma surgery setting is fundamentally different to that of elective surgery, especially with regard to prophylactic antibiotics. Antibiotics are given after the peritoneal insult and possible contamination has occurred (Boxes 13.3 and 13.4).

Hepatic injury

Repair and resection for treatment of hepatic trauma demand a working knowledge of the anatomy of the liver. Segmental anatomical resection has been well documented but usually is not applicable to injury. The three main hepatic veins divide the liver into four sections: right posterior lateral, right anterior medial, left anterior and left posterior. Each of these sectors receives a portal pedicle. The liver is practically divided into eight Couinaud's segments (Fig. 13.3).

Understanding the anatomy also helps to explain some of the patterns of injury following blunt trauma. There are also differences in tissue elasticity, which determine injury patterns. The forces from blunt injury are usually direct compressive forces or shear forces. The elastic tissue within arterial blood vessels makes them less susceptible to tearing than any other structures within the liver. Venous and biliary ductal tissues are moderately resistant to shear forces, whereas the liver parenchyma is the least resistant of all. Therefore, fractures within the liver parenchyma tend to occur along segmental fissures or directly into the parenchyma. This causes shearing of lateral branches to the major hepatic and portal veins. With severe deceleration injury, the origin of the hepatic veins may be ripped from the inferior vena cava, causing devastating haemorrhage. Similarly, the small branches from the caudate lobe entering directly into the cava are at high risk of shearing with linear tears on the caval surface.

Direct compressive forces usually cause tearing between segmental fissures in an anterior posterior sagittal orientation. Horizontal fracture lines into the parenchyma give the characteristic burst pattern to such liver injuries. If the fracture lines are parallel, these have been dubbed 'bear claw'-type injuries and probably represent where the

Table 13.3 • Calculation of the Penetrating Abdominal Trauma Index (PATI)

Organ injured	Risk factor	Score value	Injury
Duodenum	5	1	Single wall
		2	<25% wall
		3	>25% wall
		4	Duodenal wall and blood supply
		5	Requiring pancreatico-duodenectomy
Pancreas	5	1	Tangential
		2	Through-and-through (duct intact)
		3	Requiring major debridement or distal duct injury
		4	Proximal duct injury
		5	Requiring pancreaticoduodenectomy
Liver	4	1	Non-bleeding: peripheral
		2	Bleeding, central or requiring minor debridement
		3	Requiring major debridement or hepatic vessels artery ligation
		4	Requiring lobectomy
		5	Requiring lobectomy with caval repair or extensive bilobar debridement
Large bowel	4	1	Serosa
		2	Single wall
		3	<25% wall
		4	>25% wall
		5	Colon wall and blood supply
Major vascular	4	1	<25% wall transected
		2	>25% wall transected
		3	Complete transection: primary repair
		4	Requiring interposition grafting or bypass
		5	Requiring ligation
Spleen	3	1	Non-bleeding
		2	Requiring cautery or haemostatic agent
		3	Requiring minor debridement or suturing
		4	Requiring partial resection
		5	Requiring splenectomy
Kidney	3	1	Non-bleeding
		2	Requiring minor debridement or suturing
		3	Requiring major debridement
		4	Pedicle or major caliceal injury
		5	Requiring nephrectomy
Extrahepatic biliary	3	1	Contusion
		2	Requiring cholecystectomy
		3	<25% common duct wall
		4	>25% common duct wall
		5	Requiring biliary enteric reconstruction

(Continued)

Table 13.3 • Calculation of the Penetrating Abdominal Trauma Index (PATI)—Cont'd

Organ injured	Risk factor	Score value	Injury
Small bowel	2	1	Single wall
		2	Through-and-through
		3	<25% wall or two to three injuries
		4	25% wall or four to five injuries
		5	Wall or blood supply or more than five injuries
Stomach	2	1	Single wall
		2	Through-and-through
		3	Requiring minor debridement
		4	Requiring wedge resection
		5	Requiring >35% resection
Ureter	2	1	Contusion
		2	Laceration
		3	Requiring minor debridement
		4	Requiring segmental resection
		5	Requiring reconstruction
Bladder	1	1	Single wall
		2	Through-and-through
		3	Requiring debridement
		4	Requiring wedge resection
		5	Requiring reconstruction
Bone	1	1	Periosteum
		2	Cortex
		3	Through-and-through
		4	Intra-articular
		5	Major bone loss
Minor vascular	1	1	Non-bleeding small haematoma
		2	Non-bleeding large haematoma
		3	Requiring suturing
		4	Requiring ligation of isolated vessels
		5	Requiring ligation of named vessels

The PATI score is obtained for each organ by multiplying its risk factor by the injury estimate score (e.g. duodenum >25% wall injured would be 5 × 3 and liver non-bleeding peripheral injury would be 4 × 1). The final PATI score is the sum of the individual organs (e.g. in this case 15 + 4 = 19).

Reproduced from Moore EE, Dunn EL, Moore JB et al. Penetrating Abdominal Trauma Index. J Trauma 1981; 21:439–45.[53] With permission from Lippincott, Williams & Wilkins.

ribs have been compressed directly into the parenchyma. Occasionally, there will be a single fracture line across the horizontal plane of the liver, usually between the anterior and posterior segments. This can cause massive haemorrhage if there is direct extension or continuity with the peritoneal cavity.

The liver is at risk in any penetrating trauma to the right upper quadrant of the abdomen. CECT has enhanced the diagnosis of significant liver injury in the stable patient. Virtually all penetrating injuries to the abdomen should be explored promptly, especially when they occur in conjunction with hypotension. The surgeon should be aware that penetrating injuries to the right lower chest, presenting with haemothorax, may have penetrated the diaphragm, with the bleeding originating from the liver.

The treatment of severe liver injuries begins with temporary control of haemorrhage. Most catastrophic bleeding from hepatic injury is venous

Table 13.4 • Use of the Penetrating Abdominal Trauma Index (PATI) to assess the likelihood of postoperative complications

PATI score	Percentage of patients developing complications
1–5	0
6–15	6
16–25	12
26–35	44
36–45	47
46–55	50
>55	50

Reproduced from Moore EE, Dunn EL, Moore JB et al. Penetrating Abdominal Trauma Index. J Trauma 1981; 21:439–45.[53] With permission from Lippincott, Williams & Wilkins.

Box 13.1 • Evidence-based guidelines for prophylactic antibiotic administration: summary of recommendations

1. Patients with peritoneal contamination due to traumatic bowel injury repaired within 12 hours are not considered to have established intra-abdominal infections, and should be treated with prophylactic antimicrobials for 24 hours or less (**Evidence level I**)
2. Systemic antibiotics should be administered as soon as possible after injury for patients with penetrating trauma requiring surgical intervention (**Evidence level II**)
3. A single broad-spectrum agent is at least as safe and effective as a double or triple antibiotic therapeutic regimen (**Evidence level II**)
4. Patients with a fully removable focus of inflammation (e.g. bowel necrosis) should be treated with prophylactic antimicrobials for 24 hours or less (**Evidence level II**)
5. Patients with more extensive conditions should be treated as having more extensive infections, and given *therapeutic* antimicrobials for greater than 24 hours (**Evidence level III**)

From Mazuski JE, Sawyer RG, Nathens AB et al. The Surgical Infection Society Guidelines on antimicrobial therapy for intra-abdominal infections: an executive summary. Surg Infect 2002; 3(3):161–73.[63] With permission from Mary Ann Liebert, Inc.

Box 13.2 • Evidence-based guidelines for duration of antibiotic therapy: summary of recommendations

1. High postoperative septic complications can be expected in patients with gunshot injuries to the colon, high PATI scores, major blood loss and common need for postoperative care. There is no evidence to date that extending prophylactic antibiotic therapy beyond 24 hours decreases that high risk (**Evidence level II**)
2. Antimicrobial therapy of most established intra-abdominal infections should be limited to no more than 5 days (**Evidence level II**)
3. Antimicrobial therapy can be discontinued in patients when they have no clinical evidence of infection such as fever or leucocytosis (**Evidence level II**)
4. Continued clinical evidence of infection at the end of the time period designated for antimicrobial therapy should prompt appropriate diagnostic investigations rather than prolongation of antimicrobial treatment (**Evidence level III**)
5. If adequate source control cannot be achieved, a longer duration of antimicrobial therapy may be warranted (**Evidence level III**)

Box 13.3 • Evidence-based guidelines for antimicrobial regimens: summary of recommendations

1. Antimicrobial regimens for abdominal infections should cover common aerobic and anaerobic enteric flora. No regimen has been demonstrated to be superior to another (**Evidence level I**)
2. Once-daily administration of aminoglycoside is the preferred dosing regimen for patients receiving these agents for intra-abdominal infections (**Evidence level II**)
3. Aminoglycosides should be avoided in the acute trauma patient due to difficulty in reaching adequate minimum inhibitory concentrations without toxicity (**Evidence level III**)
4. For less severely ill patients with community-acquired infections, antimicrobial agents having a narrower spectrum of activity, such as antianaerobic cephalosporins, are preferable to more costly agents having broader coverage of Gram-negative organisms and/or a greater risk of toxicity (**Evidence level III**)
5. The routine use of intraoperative cultures is controversial, and there is no evidence that altering the antimicrobial regimen on the basis of intraoperative culture results improves outcome (**Evidence level III**)

in nature and can therefore be controlled by liver packs. If there is bright red blood pouring from the parenchyma, it is then appropriate to apply a vascular clamp to the porta hepatis (Pringle's manoeuvre), via the gastrohepatic ligament. If this controls the

bleeding, the surgeon should be suspicious of hepatic arterial or possible portal venous injury. While control is being obtained, it is important to establish more intravenous access lines and other monitoring devices as needed. (The treatment of bleeding is to

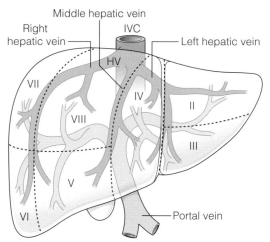

Figure 13.3 • Couinaud's segments of the liver. IVC, inferior vena cava; PV, portal vein. Reproduced from Garden OJ, Bismuth H. Anatomy of the liver. In: Carter DC, Russell RCG, Pitt HA et al. (eds) Operative surgery: hepatobiliary and pancreatic surgery. London: Chapman & Hall, 1996; pp. 1–4. With kind permission from Springer Science and Business Media.

stop the bleeding!) Hypothermia should be anticipated and corrective measures taken.

After haemostasis and haemodynamic resuscitation has been achieved, any packs in the two lower abdominal quadrants are removed. If there is

abdominal contamination, it is appropriate to control this as rapidly as possible. The packs in the left upper quadrant are then removed. If there is an associated spleen injury a decision must be made either to remove it promptly or to clamp the hilum of the spleen temporarily with a vascular clamp to reduce further bleeding. Finally, the packs are removed in the right upper quadrant and the injury to the liver rapidly assessed.

If there is bleeding from the porta hepatis, careful exploration for a portal vein injury should be carried out, with repair or shunting. Traction on the dome of the liver which produces a sudden gush of retrohepatic blood should make the surgeon suspicious of injury to the posterior hepatic veins or inferior vena. The options for hepatic vein and cava injuries include direct compression (packing), extension of the laceration, atrial–caval shunt, non-shunt isolation (Heaney technique) and veno-venous bypass. Liver packs can also be definitive treatment, particularly when there is bilobar injury, or they can simply buy time if the patient develops a coagulopathy, hypothermia or there are no blood resources. (The reader is also referred to Chapter 17 of *Hepatobiliary and Pancreatic Surgery* in this Companion to Specialist Surgical Practice series.)

Pancreatic injury

Penetrating pancreatic trauma should be obvious since the patient will almost invariably have been explored for an obvious injury.[65] Once the retroperitoneum has been violated it is imperative for the surgeon to do a thorough exploration in the central region. This includes:

- an extended Kocher manoeuvre to examine the entire duodenum;
- a right medial visceral rotation to examine the back of the head of the pancreas;
- division of the ligament of Treitz to examine the front of the pancreas;
- division of the gastrocolic omentum to examine the top of the pancreas;
- a left medial visceral rotation to examine the anterior and posterior surfaces of the tail of the pancreas as it extends towards the splenic hilum.

Any parenchymal haematoma of the pancreatic head should be thoroughly explored and should include irrigation of the haematoma and adequate drainage with a low suction drain (e.g. a Blake drain).

Blunt pancreatic trauma is much more of a problem since the pancreas is a retroperitoneal organ and there may be no anterior peritoneal signs.[56] History can be helpful – for example, if there is a history of epigastric trauma. The physical examination is often misleading. Amylase and blood count are non-specific; CT is 85% accurate and endoscopic retrograde cholangiopancreatography can be helpful in selected stable patients.

Injuries to the tail and body of the pancreas can usually either be drained or, if a strong suspicion for major ductal injury is present, resection can be carried out. The injuries that vex the surgeon most, however, are those to the head of the gland, particularly those with juxtaposed injuries and/or involving the duodenum. Resection (Whipple procedure) is usually reserved for those patients who have destructive injuries or those in whom the blood supply to the duodenum and pancreatic head has been embarrassed. This procedure should only be embarked upon as a planned procedure in the stable patient, with consideration being given to appropriate damage control procedures in all others. The remainder are usually treated with variations of drainage and pyloric exclusion. This would include tube duodenostomy and extensive closed drainage around the injury site. Common duct drainage is not indicated. (As for hepatic trauma, the reader is referred to Chapter 17 of *Hepatobiliary and Pancreatic Surgery* in this Companion to Specialist Surgical Practice series.)

Aorta and inferior vena cava injury

Aortic and caval injuries are primarily a problem of access (rapid) and control of haemorrhage. If the surgeon opens the abdomen and there is extensive retroperitoneal bleeding centrally, there are two options. If the bleeding is primarily venous in nature, the right colon should be mobilised to the midline, including the duodenum and head of the pancreas using a right medial visceral rotation. This will expose the infrarenal cava and infrarenal aorta. It will also facilitate access to the portal vein.

If the bleeding is primarily arterial in nature, it is best to approach the injury from the left. Initial control can be obtained by direct pressure at the oesophageal hiatus, or via the lesser sac. Additional exposure can be obtained by simply dividing the left crus of the diaphragm. Exposure includes reflecting the left colon medially and mobilising the pancreas, kidney and spleen to the midline. By approaching the aorta from the left lateral position it is possible to identify the plane of Leriche more rapidly than by approaching it through the lesser sac. The problem is the coeliac and superior mesenteric ganglia, both of which can be quite dense and hinder dissection around the origins of the coeliac and superior mesenteric arteries.

Treatment of aortic or caval injuries is usually straightforward, either by direct suture or occasion-

ally grafting. Caval injuries below the renal vein, if extensive, can be ligated, although repair is preferred. Injuries above the renal veins in the cava should be repaired if at all possible. If there is injury to the posterior wall of the vein, it is preferable to isolate the segment and repair it from within the vein using an anterior approach. (The reader is also referred to Chapter 9 of *Vascular and Endovascular Surgery* in this Companion to Specialist Surgical Practice series.)

Colonic injury

The significant morbidity and financial costs associated with creation and reversal of colostomy, and the destructive effect of colostomy on a patient's quality of life, have been cited as evidence to support the primary repair of colonic wounds.[64,66–68]

Many studies have shown primary repair of colonic injuries to be safe in patients at low risk of postoperative complications; however, identification of the high-risk patient in whom avoidance of an intraperitoneal colonic suture line may be beneficial is still controversial. Some authors suggest the exclusion of patients from primary repair in the presence of shock, major blood loss, more than two organs injured, faecal contamination more than 'minimal', delay to repair of more than 8 hours and wounds of the colon or abdominal wall so destructive as to require resection.[69] In a review of 140 patients with colonic injuries that required resection,[70] it is suggested that the majority of patients can safely undergo colonic resection with primary colo-colonic anastomosis, even for severe injuries. However, there is a subgroup of critically injured patients at higher risk of anastomotic leakage (indicated by a high PATI score and preoperative hypotension) who may be best treated by colostomy.[71] There is a group of critically injured patients (reliably identified by high PATI scores, high blood transfusion requirements and/or premorbid cardiovascular compromise) in whom suboptimal gut perfusion and postoperative acidosis is likely to be prolonged and for whom colonic repair or anastomosis is unsafe.[72]

In the 'physiologically challenged' patient, hypoperfusion of splanchnic tissues leads to local tissue hypoxia, and repair or anastomosis under those circumstances is more likely to fail. This high-risk group should be treated by damage control techniques with restoration of continuity of the bowel once the physiological insult has been corrected. Patients should be selected for damage control by the recognition of a severe injury pattern (i.e. high PATI score) plus a combination of physiological variables, the most important of which are hypothermia, lactic acidosis, hypotension and blood transfusion requirements.[54] These factors reflect the physiological status of the patient, for us the critical determinant of the choice and extent of surgery.[64]

Outcome is determined by the patient's physiological envelope and not by anatomical integrity[54,64,72,73] (Box 13.5).

Complex pelvic fracture

Complex pelvic fractures can be some of the most difficult injuries to treat. Initially, they can cause devastating haemorrhage and subsequently may be associated with overwhelming pelvic sepsis and distant multiple organ failure.

For those patients who present with complex pelvic fractures and who are haemodynamically stable, diagnostic studies should be carried out as rapidly as possible, including plain films of the pelvis, CECT and arteriogram. All haemodynamically unstable patients with such pelvic fractures should be taken to the operating theatre as soon as possible, to allow continuing resuscitation, including packing.[74]

The priorities facing the surgeon are to control the pelvic haemorrhage and rule out other intra-abdominal organ injuries with associated haemorrhage.

Sometimes it is prudent to perform a rapid laparotomy to rule out additional haemorrhage, but if there is not a strong suspicion of abdominal bleeding, it is best to avoid laparotomy until the pelvic bleeding has been arrested (Box 13.6). Extrapelvic packing should be considered.

Stabilisation of the pelvis is initially by compression (using a knotted sheet or external fixation). External fixation is used for stabilisation of the anterior pelvis but will fail if the posterior pelvis is unstable. These patients may require plating of the sacroiliac joint and are best managed by temporary stabilisation using a pelvic binder, and then assessed by CT and arteriography. Based on location of the injury, colostomy may be required in order to prevent contamination of a perineal wound in the post-injury period. In general, all compound injuries involving the perineum and perianal area should have a diverting colostomy.

In patients with associated major perineal injuries, after the initial fixation of the pelvis has been obtained, daily wound examination, debridement and gradual removal of packs should take place. A caveat of pack removal is that the longer they are left in, the greater the risk of pelvic sepsis.

Box 13.5 • Evidence-based guidelines for management of colon injuries: summary of recommendations

1. Primary repair is supported for *non-destructive* (involvement of <50% of the bowel wall without devascularisation) colon wounds in the absence of peritonitis. The risk is not obviated by colostomy, and intra-abdominal sepsis frequently occurs in the absence of suture line disruption. Accordingly, the majority of colon injuries in civilian practice may be managed by primary repair (**Evidence level I**)

2. Patients with penetrating colon wounds which are *destructive* can undergo resection and primary anastomosis if they are:
   (a) haemodynamically stable without evidence of shock
   (b) have no significant underlying disease
   (c) have minimal associated injuries (PATI <25, ISS <25)
   (d) have no peritonitis

   (**Evidence level II**)

3. Given the small number of patients in high-risk categories with destructive colon injuries requiring resection who were randomised to primary repair, there is still room to consider colostomy in the management of these patients (**Evidence level II**)

4. Patients with shock, underlying disease, significant associated injuries or peritonitis should have destructive wounds managed by resection and colostomy (**Evidence level II**)

5. Colostomies performed following colon and rectal trauma can be closed within 2 weeks if contrast enema is performed to confirm distal healing. This recommendation pertains to patients who do not have non-healing bowel injury, unresolved wound sepsis or are unstable (**Evidence level II**)

6. A barium enema should not be performed to rule out colon cancer or polyps prior to colostomy closure for trauma in patients who otherwise have no indications for being at risk (**Evidence level II**)

7. Multiple blood transfusions, shock and a high PATI reliably identify patients at high risk for septic complications following penetrating colon injuries (**Evidence level II**)

From Stewart RM, Fabian TC, Croce MA et al. Is resection with primary anastomosis following destructive colon wounds always safe? Am J Surg 1994; 168:316–19.[54] Cornwell EE IIIrd, Campbell KA. Trauma. In: Gordon TA, Cameron JL (eds) Evidence-based surgery. Hamilton, Ontario: BC Decker, 2000; pp. 415–28.[64] Cayten CG, Fabian TC, Garcia VF et al. Patient Management Guidelines for penetrating intraperitoneal injuries. EAST Practice Parameter Working Group, 1998. Available at www.east.org.[73]

Non-operative approach to abdominal solid-organ injuries[75] (Box 13.7)

Liver

In 1990, it was suggested that a number of patients with blunt liver injuries might be candidates for expectant management.[76] In a multicentre study, it was found that, in the hands of experienced trauma surgeons, the success with the non-operative approach to liver injuries was greater than 98%.[77]

Currently, all patients with liver injuries following blunt trauma should be considered candidates for non-operative management, if haemodynamic stability can be assured. Unlike the spleen, delayed haemorrhage from the liver is rare. The complications in those patients managed expectantly are frequently related to the biliary system and can usually be managed by endoscopic or interventional techniques. While non-operative management has most frequently been applied to patients with blunt injuries, a few stable patients with liver injuries as the result of penetrating trauma have also been managed expectantly.[78]

Box 13.6 • Evidence-based guidelines for management of haemorrhage in pelvic fracture: summary of recommendations

1. Patients with evidence of unstable fractures of the pelvis associated with hypotension should be considered for some form or pelvic stabilisation (**Evidence level II**)
2. Patients with evidence of unstable pelvic fractures who warrant laparotomy should receive external pelvic stabilisation prior to laparotomy incision (**Evidence level II**)
3. Patients with a major pelvic fracture who have signs of ongoing bleeding after non-pelvic sources of blood loss have been ruled out should be considered for pelvic angiography and possible embolisation (**Evidence level II**)
4. Patients with major pelvic fractures who are found to have bleeding in the pelvis, which cannot be adequately controlled at laparotomy, should be considered for pelvic angiography and possible embolisation (**Evidence level II**)
5. Patients with evidence of arterial extravasation of intravenous contrast in the pelvis by computed tomography should be considered for pelvic angiography and possible embolisation (**Evidence level II**)
6. Patients with hypotension and gross blood in the abdomen of evidence of intestinal perforation warrant emergency laparotomy (**Evidence level II**)
7. The diagnostic peritoneal tap appears to be the most reliable diagnostic test for this purpose. Urgent laparotomy is warranted for patients who demonstrate signs of continued intra-abdominal bleeding after adequate resuscitation, or evidence of intestinal perforation (**Evidence level II**)
8. Patients with evidence of unstable fractures of the pelvis not associated with hypotension but who do require a steady and ongoing resuscitation should be considered for some form of external pelvic stabilisation (**Evidence level III**)

From DiGiacomo JC, Bonadies JA, Cole FJ et al. Practice Management Guidelines for haemorrhage in pelvic fracture. EAST Practice Management Guidelines Work Group, 2001. Available at www.east.org.[74]

Box 13.7 • Evidence-based guidelines for the non-operative management of abdominal injury: summary of recommendations

1. Non-operative management of blunt hepatic and/or splenic injuries in a haemodynamically stable patient is reasonable (**Evidence level II**)
2. The severity of hepatic or splenic injury (as suggested by CT grade or degree of haemoperitoneum), neurological status and/or the presence of associated injuries are not contraindications to non-operative management (**Evidence level II**)
3. Abdominal CT is the most reliable method to identify and assess the severity of injury to the spleen or liver (**Evidence level II**)
4. The clinical status of the patient should dictate the frequency of follow-up scans (**Evidence level III**)
5. Initial CT of the abdomen should be performed with oral and intravenous contrast to facilitate the diagnosis of hollow viscus injuries (**Evidence level III**)
6. Medical clearance to resume normal activity status should be based on evidence of healing (**Evidence level III**)
7. Angiographic embolisation is an adjunct in the non-operative management of the haemodynamically stable patient with hepatic and splenic injuries and evidence of ongoing bleeding (**Evidence level III**)

From Alonso M, Brathwaite C, Garcia V et al. Practice Management Guidelines for the nonoperative management of blunt injury to the liver and spleen. EAST Practice Management Guidelines Work Group, 2003. Available at http://www.east.org.[75]

Spleen

In children, the success of non-operative management of the spleen is over 90%, but this has not been the experience in adults. Currently, most surgeons will attempt to manage non-operatively the injured adult spleen with an AAST grade I–III injury; the management of grade IV or V injuries remains controversial. In a recent report of 190 consecutive patients with splenic injuries managed at a single institution,[79] 102 (54%) were initially treated without surgery, including 15 patients with intrinsic splenic pathology and six patients with isolated stab wounds. Only two of these patients failed non-operative management and both survived.

It was suggested that 65% of all blunt splenic injuries and selected stab wounds can be managed non-operatively, with minimal transfusions, morbidity or mortality, with a success rate of 98%. In contrast, splenectomy, when necessary, is associated with an excessive transfusion and an inordinately high postoperative sepsis rate.

Interventional radiology

In a significant number of patients, interventional radiology, with arterial embolisation (AE), stent or stent-graft placement, has become either the first line of treatment or an important adjunct to non-operative management of abdominal and other injuries.[80] Clinical evaluation, however, determines the course of treatment. Patients who are haemodynamically stable should be evaluated with CECT.

Pelvic fractures

Severe pelvic fractures, particularly with disruption of the sacroiliac joints, are associated with a high risk of severe arterial and venous bleeding. The application of a sheet or external fixation may control the venous bleeding, which constitutes about 85% of all pelvic bleeding. However, arterial bleeding often requires AE, which has become the first line of treatment in patients stable enough to reach angiography.[81] Established indications are CT evidence of ongoing bleeding such as contrast extravasation and pelvic haematoma with bladder compression and ongoing transfusion requirements without evidence of other extrapelvic bleeding sources.

There is also a possibility in this subgroup of patients for severe venous bleeding. The patient in shock refractory to resuscitation should be considered for damage control with (extraperitoneal) pelvic packing before AE.

AE is carried out after performing an abdominal aortography followed by selective catheterisation of the internal iliac arteries. When contrast extravasation is demonstrated, the bleeding vessels are catheterised superselectively and embolised with coils, or a combination of coils and gelfoam particles.

Blunt splenic injuries

Indications for AE include CT evidence of ongoing bleeding with contrast extravasation outside or within the spleen, a drop in haemoglobin, tachycardia and haemoperitoneum as well as formation of pseudoaneurysm. Selective catheterisation of the splenic artery is performed, followed by superselective catheterisation of the bleeding arteries or feeders to the pseudoaneurysm.[82,83]

Liver injuries

Non-operative management of blunt liver injuries in haemodynamically stable or stabilised patients has become standard practice. The introduction of AE has been reported to increase the success rate of non-operative management to well above 80%.[84]

Operative treatment of liver injuries, even in experienced hands, still carries a high mortality and morbidity risk. AE seems to be a valuable adjunct to operative management since most patients are haemodynamically abnormal at the end of a damage control laparotomy, and ongoing arterial bleeding is difficult to rule out clinically.

The indications for AE should include CT evidence of ongoing bleeding with contrast extravasation outside or within the liver, a drop in haemoglobin, tachycardia and haemoperitoneum as well as formation of pseudoaneurysm. The risk of bleeding with non-operative management in Organ Injury Scaling grade IV and V liver injuries is significant, and operative intervention, with packing, followed by AE is preferable.[85]

Key points

- In order to avoid missed injuries and preventable deaths, trauma patients who have any of the risk factors for abdominal injury should undergo objective evaluation of the abdomen.
- Delay in surgery is the most common cause of unnecessary ongoing bleeding.
- In patients who are unstable, the preferred objective study is a bedside ultrasound. If an ultrasound examination is unavailable or equivocal, a DPL should be performed.

- In stable patients, abdominal CT with oral and intravenous contrast is the preferred method of objective examination of the abdomen.
- When laparotomy is required, it should be approached in a systematic fashion and the treatment of injuries prioritised.
- In patients who are cold, coagulopathic and acidotic, a damage control operation should be accomplished promptly.

Web references

ICD-10 Codes. World Health Organisation; http://www.who.int/classifications/apps/icd/icd10online/2007.

Organ Injury Scaling of the American Association for the Surgery of Trauma; http://www.aast.org 2008.

References

1. Anderson ID, Woodford M, de Dombal T et al. A retrospective study of 1000 deaths from injury in England and Wales. Br Med J 1988; 296:1305–8.

2. National Confidential Enquiry into Patient Outcome and Death (NCEPOD). Trauma: who cares? www.ncepod.org/2007b.htm, accessed January 2008.

3. West JC, Trunkey DD, Lim RC. System of trauma care: a study of two counties. Arch Surg 1979; 114:455–60.

4. Mackersie RC, Tiwary AD, Shackford SR et al. Intra-abdominal injury following blunt trauma: identifying the high-risk factors. Arch Surg 1989; 124:809–13.

5. Taylor GA, Eichelberger MR. Abdominal CT in children with neurologic impairment following blunt trauma. Ann Surg 1989; 210:229–33.

6. Knudson MM, McAninch JA, Gomez R et al. Haematuria as a predictor of abdominal injury after blunt trauma. Am J Surg 1992; 164:482–6.

7. Bickell WH, Wall MJ, Pepe PE et al. Immediate versus delayed fluid resuscitation for hypotensive patients with penetrating torso injuries. N Engl J Med 1994; 331:1105–9.

8. American College of Surgeons. Advanced Trauma Life Support Programme: abdominal trauma. Washington, DC: American College of Surgeons, 1997.

9. Brooks A, Bowley DM, Boffard KD. Bullet markers – a simple technique to assist in the evaluation of penetrating trauma. J R Army Med Corps 2002; 148(3):259–61.

10. Donohue JH, Federle MP, Griffiths BG et al. Computed tomography in the diagnosis of blunt intestinal and mesenteric injuries. J Trauma 1987; 27:11–17.

11. Brasel KJ, Olson CH, Stafford R et al. Incidence and significance of free fluid on abdominal computed tomographic scan in blunt trauma. J Trauma 1998; 44:889–92.

12. Sherck JP, Oakes DD. Intestinal injuries missed by computed tomography. J Trauma 1990; 30:1–7.

13. McKenney MG, Martin L, Lopez C. 1000 consecutive ultrasounds for blunt abdominal trauma. J Trauma 1996; 40:607–12.

14. Rozycki GS, Ochsner MG, Schmidt JA et al. A prospective study of surgeon-performed ultrasound as the primary adjuvant modality for injured patient assessment. J Trauma 1995; 39:492–7.

15. Shackford SR. Focused ultrasound examinations by surgeons: the time is now [Editorial]. J Trauma 1993; 35:181–2.

16. Rozycki GS, Ballard RB, Feliciano DV et al. Surgeon performed ultrasound for the assessment of truncal injuries: lessons learned from 1540 patients. Ann Surg 1998; 229:557–67.

17. Root HD, Hauser CW, McKinley CR et al. Diagnostic peritoneal lavage. Surgery 1965; 57:633–7.

18. Brooks AJ, Boffard KD. Current technology: laparoscopic surgery in trauma. Trauma 1999; 1:53–60.

19. Fabian TC, McCord S. Therapeutic laparoscopy in trauma. Trauma Quart 1993; 34:313–15.

20. Smith RS, Fry WR, Tsoi EKM. Gasless laparoscopy and conventional instruments. Arch Surg 1993; 70:632–7.

21. Zantut LF, Ivatury RR, Smith S. Diagnostic and therapeutic laparoscopy for penetrating abdominal trauma: a multicentre experience. J Trauma 1997; 42:825–31.

22. Fabian TC, Croce MA, Steward RM et al. A prospective analysis of diagnostic laparoscopy in trauma. Ann Surg 1993; 217:557.

23. Degiannis E, Levy R, Sofianos C et al. Diaphragmatic herniation after penetrating trauma. Br J Surg 1996; 83:88–91.

24. Renz BM, Feliciano DV. Unnecessary laparotomies for trauma: a prospective study of morbidity. J Trauma 1995; 38:350–6.

25. Moore EE, Moore JB, van Duzer-Moore S et al. Mandatory laparotomy for gunshot wounds penetrating the abdomen. Am J Surg 1980; 140: 847–51.

26. Muckart DJ, Abdool-Carim AT, King B. Selective conservative management of abdominal gunshot wounds: a prospective study. Br J Surg 1990; 77:652–5.

27. Ross SE, Dragon GM, O'Malley KF et al. Morbidity of negative celiotomy in trauma. Injury 1995; 26: 393–4.

28. Weigelt JA, Kingman RG. Complications of negative laparotomy for trauma. Am J Surg 1988; 156:544–7.

29. Demetriades D, Charalambides D, Lakhoo M et al. Gunshot wound of the abdomen: role of selective conservative management. Br J Surg 1991; 78:220–2.

30. Maggisano R, Nathens A, Alexandrova NA et al. Traumatic rupture of the thoracic aorta: should one always operate immediately? Ann Vasc Surg 1995; 9:44–6.

31. Camp PC, Shackford SR, Knudson MM et al. Outcome following blunt traumatic thoracic aortic laceration: identification of a high risk cohort. J Trauma 1997; 43:413–22.

32. Wisner DH, Victor NS, Holcroft JW. The priorities in the management of multiple trauma: intracranial versus intra-abdominal injury. J Trauma 1993; 35:271–8.

33. Archer LP, Rogers RB, Shackford SR. Selective non-operative management of liver and splenic injuries in neurologically impaired adult patients. Arch Surg 1996; 131:309–15.

34. Cattel RB, Braasch JW. A technique for the exposure of the third and fourth parts of the duodenum. Surg Gynecol Obstet 1960; 111:379–83.

35. Rotondo MF, Schwab CW, McGonigal MD et al. 'Damage control': an approach for improved survival in exsanguinating penetrating abdominal injury. J Trauma 1993; 35:375–82.

36. Loveland JA, Boffard KD. Damage control in the abdomen and beyond. Br J Surg 2004; 91(9): 1095–101.

37. Elerding SC, Aragon GE, Moore EE. Fatal hepatic haemorrhage after trauma. Am J Surg 1979; 138:883–8.

38. Hirshberg A, Mattox KL. Planned re-operation for severe trauma. Ann Surg 1995; 222:3–8.

39. Garrison JR, Richardson JD, Hilakos A et al. Predicting the need to pack early for severe intra-abdominal haemorrhage. J Trauma 1996; 40:923–9.

40. Schein M, Saadia R. Jamieson JR. The "sandwich technique" in the management of the open abdomen. Br J Surg 1986; 73(5):369–70.

41. Burch J, Moore E, Moore F et al. The abdominal compartment syndrome. Surg Clin North Am 1996; 76:833–42.

42 World Society for Abdominal Compartment Syndrome. www.wsacs.org, accessed online January 2008.

43. Balogh Z, McKinley BA, Cocanour CS et al. Supranormal trauma resuscitation causes more cases of abdominal compartment syndrome. Arch Surg 2003; 138:637–42.

44. Harman PK, Kron IL, McLachlan HD. Elevated intra-abdominal pressure and renal function. Ann Surg 1982; 196:594–7.

45. Sugrue M, Buist MD, Hourihan F et al. Prospective study of intra-abdominal hypertension and renal function after laparotomy. Br J Surg 1995; 82:235–8.

46. Kron IL, Harman PK, Nolan SP. The measurement of intra-abdominal pressure as a criterion for abdominal re-exploration. Ann Surg 1984; 199:28–30.

47. Cheatham ML, White MW, Sagraves SG et al. Abdominal perfusion pressure: a superior parameter in the assessment of intra-abdominal hypertension. J Trauma 2000; 49:621–6.

48. Malbrain ML, Chiumello D, Pelosi P et al. Incidence and prognosis of intraabdominal hypertension in a mixed population of critically ill patients: a multiple-centre epidemiological study. Crit Care Med 2005; 33:315–22.

49. Malbrain ML, Chiumello D, Pelosi P et al. Prevalence of intra-abdominal hypertension in critically ill patients: a multicentre epidemiological study. Intensive Care Med 2004; 30:822–9.

50. Malbrain ML, Cheatham ML, Kirkpatrick A et al. Results from the International Conference of Experts on Intra-abdominal Hypertension and Abdominal Compartment Syndrome. I. Definitions. Intensive Care Med 2006; 32:1722–32.

51. Maxwell RA, Fabian TC, Croce MA et al. Secondary abdominal compartment syndrome: an underappreciated manifestation of severe haemorrhagic shock. J Trauma 2000; 47:995–9.

52. Sugrue M, Jones F, Janjua J et al. Temporary abdominal closure. J Trauma 1998; 45:914–21.

53. Moore EE, Dunn EL, Moore JB et al. Penetrating Abdominal Trauma Index. J Trauma 1981; 21:439–45.

54. Stewart RM, Fabian TC, Croce MA et al. Is resection with primary anastomosis following destructive colon wounds always safe? Am J Surg 1994; 168:316–19.

55. Moore EE, Shackford SR, Pachter HL et al. Organ Injury Scaling: spleen, liver and kidney. J Trauma 1989; 29:1664–6.

56. Moore EE, Cogbill TH, Malangoni MA et al. Organ Injury Scaling: pancreas, duodenum, small bowel, colon and rectum. J Trauma 1990; 30:1427–9.

57. Moore EE, Cogbill TH, Jurkovich GJ. Organ Injury Scaling III: chest wall, abdominal vascular, ureter, bladder and urethra. J Trauma 1992; 33:337–8.

58. Moore EE, Malangoni MA, Cogbill TH et al. Organ Injury Scaling IV: thoracic, vascular, lung, cardiac and diaphragm. J Trauma 1994; 36:299–300.

59. Moore EE, Cogbill TH, Jurkovich GJ et al. Organ Injury Scaling: spleen and liver (1994 revision). J Trauma 1995; 38:323–4.

60. Moore EE, Jurkovich GJ, Knudson MM et al. Organ Injury Scaling VI: extrahepatic biliary, oesophagus, stomach, vulva, vagina, uterus (nonpregnant), uterus (pregnant), fallopian tube, and ovary. J Trauma 1995; 39:1069–70.

61. Moore EE, Malangoni MA, Cogbill TH et al. Organ Injury Scaling VII: cervical vascular, peripheral vascular, adrenal, penis, testis and scrotum. J Trauma 1996; 41:523–4.

62. Hoff WS, Holevar M, Nagy KK et al. Practice Management Guidelines for the evaluation of blunt abdominal trauma. EAST Practice Management Guidelines Work Group, 2001. Available at http://www.east.org.

63. Mazuski JE, Sawyer RG, Nathens AB. The Surgical Infection Society Guidelines on antimicrobial therapy for intra-abdominal infections: an executive summary. Surg Infect 2002; 3(3):161–73.

64. Cornwell EE IIIrd, Campbell KA. Trauma. In: Gordon TA, Cameron JL (eds) Evidence-based surgery. Hamilton, Ontario: BC Decker, 2000; pp. 415–28.

65. Boffard KD, Brooks AJ. Pancreatic trauma. Eur J Surg 2000; 166:4–12.

66. Brasel KJ, Borgstrom DC, Weigelt JA. Management of penetrating colon trauma: a cost utility analysis. Surgery 1999; 125:471–9.

67. Bern JD, Velmahos GC, Chan LS et al. The high morbidity of colostomy closure after trauma: further support for the primary repair of colon injuries. Surgery 1998; 123:157–64.

68. Pachter HL, Hoballah JJ, Corcoran TA et al. The morbidity and financial impact of colostomy closure in trauma patients. J Trauma 1990; 30:1510–14.

69. Stone HH, Fabian TC. Management of perforating colon trauma: randomisation between primary colon closure and exteriorisation. Ann Surg 1979; 190:430–6.

70. Murray JA, Demetriades D, Colson M et al. Colonic resection in trauma, colostomy versus anastomosis. J Trauma 1999; 46:250–4.

71. Cornwell EE, Velmahos GC, Berne TV et al. The fate of colonic suture lines in high risk patients: a prospective analysis. J Am Coll Surg 1998; 187:58–63.

72. Hirschberg A, Walden R. Damage control for abdominal trauma. Surg Clin North Am 1997; 77:813–21.

73. Cayten CG, Fabian TC, Garcia VF et al. Patient Management Guidelines for penetrating intraperitoneal injuries. EAST Practice Parameter Working Group, 1998. Available at http://www.east.org.

74. DiGiacomo JC, Bonadies JA, Cole FJ et al. Practice Management Guidelines for haemorrhage in pelvic fracture. EAST Practice Management Guidelines Work Group, 2001. Available at http://www.east.org.

75. Alonso M, Brathwaite C, Garcia V et al. Practice Management Guidelines for the nonoperative management of blunt injury to the liver and spleen. EAST Practice Management Guidelines Work Group, 2003. Available at http://www.east.org.

76. Knudson MM, Lim RC, Oakes DD et al. Nonoperative management of blunt liver injuries in adults: the need for continued surveillance. J Trauma 1990; 30:1494–500.

77. Pachter HL, Knudson MM, Esrig B et al. Status of nonoperative management of blunt hepatic injuries in 1995: a multicenter experience with 404 patients. J Trauma 1996; 40:31–8.

78. Renz BM, Feliciano DV. Gunshot wounds to the right thoracoabdomen: a prospective study of nonoperative management. J Trauma 1994; 37:737–44.

79. Pachter HL, Guth AA, Hofstetter SR et al. Changing patterns in the management of splenic trauma: the impact of nonoperative management. Ann Surg 1998; 227:708–19.

80. Dondelinger RF, Trotteur G, Ghaye B et al. Traumatic injuries: radiological hemostatic intervention at admission. Eur Radiol 2002; 12(5):979–93.

81. Velmahos GC, Toutouzas KG, Vassiliu P et al. A prospective study on the safety and efficacy of angiographic embolization for pelvic and visceral injuries. J Trauma 2002; 53(2):303–8.

82. Dent D, Alsabrook G, Erickson BA et al. Blunt splenic injuries: high nonoperative management rate can be achieved with selective embolization. J Trauma 2004; 56(5):1063–7.

83. Haan JM, Biffl W, Knudson MM et al. Western Trauma Association Multi-institutional Trials Committee. Splenic embolization revisited: a multicenter review. J Trauma 2004; 56(3):542–7.

84. Johnson JW, Gracias VH, Gupta R et al. Hepatic angiography in patients undergoing damage control laparotomy. J Trauma 2002; 52:1102–6.

85. Asensio JA, Roldan G, Petrone P et al. Operative management and outcomes in 103 AAST-OIS grades IV and V complex hepatic injuries: trauma surgeons still need to operate, but angioembolization helps. J Trauma 2003; 54:647–53.

Appendix: Scaling system for organ-specific injuries

Scaling system for organ-specific injuries

Table A1

Cervical vascular organ injury scale

Grade*	Description of injury	ICD-9	ICD-10	AIS-2005
I	Thyroid vein	900.8	S15.8	
	Common facial vein	900.8	S15.8	
	External jugular vein	900.81	S15.2	1–3
	Non-named arterial/venous branches	900.9	S15.9	
II	External carotid arterial branches (ascending pharyngeal, superior thyroid, lingual, facial, maxillary, occipital, posterior auricular)	900.8	S15.0	1–3
	Thyrocervical trunk or primary branches	900.8	S15.8	1–3
	Internal jugular vein	900.1	S15.3	1–3
III	External carotid artery	900.02	S15.0	2–3
	Subclavian vein	901.3	S25.3	3–4
	Vertebral artery	900.8	S15.1	2–4
IV	Common carotid artery	900.01	S15.0	3–5
	Subclavian artery	901.1	S25.1	3–4
V	Internal carotid artery (extracranial)	900.03	S15.0	3–5

*Increase one grade for multiple grade III or IV injuries involving more than 50% vessel circumference. Decrease one grade for less than 25% vessel circumference disruption for grade IV or V.

Reproduced from Moore EE, Malangoni MA, Cogbill TH et al. Organ Injury Scaling VII: cervical vascular, peripheral vascular, adrenal, penis, testis and scrotum. J Trauma 1996; 41(3):523–4.[61] With permission from Lippincott, Williams & Wilkins.

Table A2

Chest wall injury scale

Grade*	Injury type	Description of injury	ICD-9	ICD-10	AIS-2005
I	Contusion	Any size	911.0/922.1	S20.2	1
	Laceration	Skin and subcutaneous	875.0	S20.4	1
	Fracture	<3 ribs, closed	807.01/807.02	S22.3	1–2
		Non-displaced clavicle, closed	810.00/810.03	S42.0	2
II	Laceration	Skin, subcutaneous and muscle	875.1	S20.4	2
	Fracture	≥3 adjacent ribs, closed	807.03/807.08	S22.4	1
		Open or displaced clavicle	810.10/810.13	S42.0	2–3
		Non-displaced sternum closed	807.2	S22.2	2
		Scapular body, open or closed	811.00/811.18	S42.1	2
III	Laceration	Full thickness including pleural penetration	862.29	S21.9	2
	Fracture	Open or displaced sternum	807.2	S22.2	2
		Flail sternum	807.3	S22.2	2
		Unilateral flail segment (<3 ribs)	807.4	S22.5	3–4
IV	Laceration	Avulsion of chest wall tissues with underlying rib fractures	807.10/807.18	S22.8	4
	Fracture	Unilateral flail chest (≥3 ribs)	807.4	S22.5	3–4
V	Fracture	Bilateral flail chest (≥3 ribs on both sides)	807.4	S22.5	5

*This scale is confined to the chest wall alone and does not reflect associated internal or abdominal injuries. Therefore, further delineation of upper versus lower or anterior versus posterior chest wall was not considered, and a grade VI was not warranted. Specifically, thoracic crush was not used as a descriptive term; instead, the geography and extent of fractures and soft tissue injury were used to define the grade. Upgrade by one grade for bilateral injuries.

Reproduced from Moore EE, Cogbill TH, Jurkovich GJ. Organ Injury Scaling III: chest wall, abdominal vascular, ureter, bladder and urethra. J Trauma 1992; 33:337–8.[57] With permission from Lippincott, Williams & Wilkins.

Table A3

Heart injury scale

Grade*	Description of injury	ICD-9	ICD-10†	AIS-2005
I	Blunt cardiac injury with minor ECG abnormality (non-specific ST or T wave changes, premature arterial or ventricular contraction or persistent sinus tachycardia)	861.01	S26.0	3
	Blunt or penetrating pericardial wound without cardiac injury, cardiac tamponade or cardiac herniation	861.01	S26.0	3
II	Blunt cardiac injury with heart block (right or left bundle branch, left anterior fascicular or atrioventricular) or ischaemic changes (ST depression or T wave inversion) without cardiac failure	861.12	S26.0	3
	Penetrating tangential myocardial wound up to, but not extending through endocardium, without tamponade	861.01	S26.0	3–4
III	Blunt cardiac injury with sustained (≥6 beats/min) or multifocal ventricular contractions	861.01	S26.0	3–4
	Blunt or penetrating cardiac injury with septal rupture, pulmonary or tricuspid valvular incompetence, papillary muscle dysfunction, or distal coronary arterial occlusion without cardiac failure	861.01	S26.0	3–4
	Blunt pericardial laceration with cardiac herniation	861.12	S26.0	3
	Blunt cardiac injury with cardiac failure	861.12	S26.0	3
	Penetrating tangential myocardial wound up to, but extending through, endocardium, with tamponade			

(Continued)

Table A3

Heart injury scale—Cont'd				
Grade*	Description of injury	ICD-9	ICD-10†	AIS-2005
IV	Blunt or penetrating cardiac injury with septal rupture, pulmonary or tricuspid valvular incompetence, papillary muscle dysfunction, or distal coronary arterial occlusion producing cardiac failure	861.03	S26.0	5
	Blunt or penetrating cardiac injury with aortic mitral valve incompetence	861.03	S26.0	5
	Blunt or penetrating cardiac injury of the right ventricle, right atrium, or left atrium	861.03	S26.0	5
V	Blunt or penetrating cardiac injury with proximal coronary arterial occlusion	861.03	S26.0	5
	Blunt or penetrating left ventricular perforation	861.13	S26.0	5
	Stellate wound with <50% tissue loss of the right ventricle, right atrium, or of left atrium	861.03	S26.0	5
VI	Blunt avulsion of the heart; penetrating wound producing >50% tissue loss of a chamber	861.13	S26.0	6

*Advance one grade for multiple wounds to a single chamber or multiple chamber involvement.
†With ICD-10 use supplementary character: 0 without open wound into thoracic cavity; 1 with open wound into thoracic cavity.
Reproduced from Moore EE, Malangoni MA, Cogbill TH et al. Organ Injury Scaling IV: thoracic, vascular, lung, cardiac and diaphragm. J Trauma 1994; 36(3):299–300.[58] With permission from Lippincott, Williams & Wilkins.

Table A4

Lung injury scale					
Grade*	Injury type	Description of injury	ICD-9	ICD-10†	AIS-2005
I	Contusion	Unilateral, <1 lobe	861.12/861.31	S27.3	3
II	Contusion	Unilateral, single lobe	861.20/861.30	S27.3	3
	Laceration	Simple pneumothorax	860.0/1/4/5	S27.0	3
III	Contusion	Unilateral, >1 lobe	861.20/861.30	S27.3	3
	Laceration	Persistent (>72 h) air leak from distal airway	860.0/1/4/5	S27.3	3–4
	Haematoma	Non-expanding intraparenchymal	862.0/861.30	S27.3	
IV	Laceration	Major (segmental or lobar) air leak	862.21/861.31	S27.4	4–5
	Haematoma	Expanding intraparenchymal		S25.4	
	Vascular	Primary branch intrapulmonary vessel disruption	901.40	S25.4	3–5
V	Vascular	Hilar vessel disruption	901.41/901.42	S25.4	4
vi	Vascular	Total uncontained transection of pulmonary hilum	901.41/901.42	S25.4	4

*Advance one grade for bilateral injuries up to grade III. Haemothorax is scored under thoracic vascular injury scale.
†With ICD-10 use supplementary character: 0 without open wound into thoracic cavity; 1 with open wound into thoracic cavity.
Reproduced from Moore EE, Malangoni MA, Cogbill TH et al. Organ Injury Scaling IV: thoracic, vascular, lung, cardiac and diaphragm. J Trauma 1994; 36(3):299–300.[58] With permission from Lippincott, Williams & Wilkins.

Table A5

Thoracic vascular injury scale

Grade*	Description of injury	ICD-9	ICD-10	AIS-2005
I	Intercostal artery/vein	901.81	S25.5	2–3
	Internal mammary artery/vein	901.82	S25.8	2–3
	Bronchial artery/vein	901.89	S25.4	2–3
	Oesophageal artery/vein	901.9	S25.8	2–3
	Hemiazygos vein	901.89	S25.8	2–3
	Unnamed artery/vein	901.9	S25.9	2–3
II	Azygos vein	901.89	S25.8	2–3
	Internal jugular vein	900.1	S15.3	2–3
	Subclavian vein	901.3	S25.3	3–4
	Innominate vein	901.3	S25.3	3–4
III	Carotid artery	900.01	S15.0	3–5
	Innominate artery	901.1	S25.1	3–4
	Subclavian artery	901.1	S25.1	3–4
IV	Thoracic aorta, descending	901.0	S25.0	4–5
	Inferior vena cava (intrathoracic)	902.10	S35.1	3–4
	Pulmonary artery, primary intraparenchymal branch	901.41	S5.4	3
	Pulmonary vein, primary intraparenchymal branch	901.42	S25.4	3
V	Thoracic aorta, ascending and arch	901.0	S25.0	5
	Superior vena cava	901.2	S25.2	3–4
	Pulmonary artery, main trunk	901.41	S25.4	4
	Pulmonary vein, main trunk	901.42	S25.4	4
VI	Uncontained total transection of thoracic aorta or pulmonary hilum	901.0	S25.0	5
	Uncontained total transection of pulmonary hilum	901.41/ 901.42	S25.4	5

*Increase one grade for multiple grade III or IV injuries if more than 50% circumference. Decrease one grade for grade IV injuries if less than 25% circumference.
Reproduced from Moore EE, Malangoni MA, Cogbill TH et al. Organ Injury Scaling IV: thoracic, vascular, lung, cardiac and diaphragm. J Trauma 1994; 36(3):299–300.[58] With permission from Lippincott, Williams & Wilkins.

Table A6

Diaphragm injury scale

Grade*	Description of injury	ICD-9	ICD-10	AIS-2005
I	Contusion	862.0	S27.8	2
II	Laceration <2 cm	862.1	S27.8	3
III	Laceration 2–10 cm	862.1	S27.8	3
IV	Laceration >10 cm with tissue loss ≤25 cm^2	862.1	S27.8	3
V	Laceration with tissue loss >25 cm^2	862.1	S27.8	3

* Advance one grade for bilateral injuries up to grade III.
Reproduced from Moore EE, Malangoni MA, Cogbill TH et al. Organ Injury Scaling IV: thoracic, vascular, lung, cardiac and diaphragm. J Trauma 1994; 36(3):299–300.[58] With permission from Lippincott, Williams & Wilkins.

Table A7

Spleen injury scale (1994 revision)					
Grade*	Injury type	Description of injury	ICD-9	ICD-10†	AIS-2005
I	Haematoma	Subcapsular, <10% surface area	865.01/865.11	S36.0	2
	Laceration	Capsular tear, <1 cm parenchymal depth	865.02/865.12	S36.0	2
II	Haematoma	Subcapsular, 10–50% surface area; intraparenchymal, <5 cm in diameter	865.01/865.11	S36.0	2
	Laceration	Capsular tear, 1–3 cm parenchymal depth that does not involve a trabecular vessel	865.02/865.12	S36.0	2
III	Haematoma	Subcapsular, >50% surface area or expanding; ruptured subcapsular or parenchymal haematoma; intraparenchymal haematoma ≥5 cm or expanding	865.03	S36.0	3
	Laceration	>3 cm parenchymal depth or involving trabecular vessels	865.03	S36.0	3
IV	Laceration	Laceration involving segmental or hilar vessels producing major devascularisation (>25% of spleen)	865.13	S36.0	4
V	Laceration	Completely shattered spleen	865.04	S36.0	5
	Vascular	Hilar vascular injury with devascularised spleen	865.14	S36.0	5

*Advance one grade for multiple injuries up to grade III.
†With ICD-10 use supplementary character: 0 without open wound into abdominal cavity; 1 with open wound into abdominal cavity.
Reproduced from Moore EE, Cogbill TH, Jurkovich GJ et al. Organ Injury Scaling: spleen and liver (1994 revision). J Trauma 1995; 38(3):323–4.[59] With permission from Lippincott, Williams & Wilkins.

Table A8

Liver injury scale (1994 revision)					
Grade*	Type of injury	Description of injury	ICD-9	ICD-10†	AIS-2005
I	Haematoma	Subcapsular, <10% surface area	864.01/864.11	S36.1	2
	Laceration	Capsular tear, <1 cm parenchymal depth	864.02/864.12	S36.1	2
II	Haematoma	Subcapsular, 10–50% surface area; intraparenchymal <10 cm in diameter	864.01/864.11	S36.1	2
	Laceration	Capsular tear 1–3 parenchymal depth, <10 cm in length	864.03/864.13	S36.1	2
III	Haematoma	Subcapsular, >50% surface area of ruptured subcapsular or parenchymal haematoma; intraparenchymal haematoma >10 cm or expanding	864.04/864.14	S36.1	3
	Laceration	3 cm parenchymal depth	864.04/864.14	S36.1	3
IV	Laceration	Parenchymal disruption involving 25–75% hepatic lobe or 1–3 Couinaud's segments within a single lobe	864.04/864.14	S36.1	4
V	Laceration	Parenchymal disruption involving >75% of hepatic lobe or >3 Couinaud's segments within a single lobe	864.04/864.14	S36.1	5
	Vascular	Juxtahepatic venous injuries, i.e. retrohepatic vena cava/central major hepatic veins	864.04/864.14	S36.1	5
VI	Vascular	Hepatic avulsion	864.04/864.14	S36.1	5

*Advance one grade for multiple injuries up to grade III.
†With ICD-10 use supplementary character: 0 without open wound into abdominal cavity; 1 with open wound into abdominal cavity.
Reproduced from Moore EE, Cogbill TH, Jurkovich GJ et al. Organ Injury Scaling: spleen and liver (1994 revision). J Trauma 1995; 38(3):323–4.[59] With permission from Lippincott, Williams & Wilkins.

Table A9

Extrahepatic biliary tree injury scale				
Grade*	Description of injury	ICD-9	ICD-10†	AIS-2005
I	Gallbladder contusion/haematoma	868.02	S36.1	2
	Portal triad contusion	868.02	S36.1	2
II	Partial gallbladder avulsion from liver bed; cystic duct intact	868.02	S36.1	2
	Laceration or perforation of the gallbladder	868.12	S36.1	2
III	Complete gallbladder avulsion from liver bed	868.02	S36.1	3
	Cystic duct laceration	868.12	S36.1	3
IV	Partial or complete right hepatic duct laceration	868.12	S36.1	3
	Partial or complete left hepatic duct laceration	868.12	S36.1	3
	Partial common hepatic duct laceration (<50%)	868.12	S36.1	3
	Partial common bile duct laceration (<50%)	868.12	S36.1	3
V	>50% transection of common hepatic duct	868.12	S36.1	3–4
	>50% transection of common bile duct	868.12	S36.1	3–4
	Combined right and left hepatic duct injuries	868.12	S36.1	3–4
	Intraduodenal or intrapancreatic bile duct injuries	868.12	S36.1	3–4

*Advance one grade for multiple injuries up to grade III.
†With ICD-10 use supplementary character: 0 without open wound into abdominal cavity; 1 with open wound into abdominal cavity.
Reproduced from Moore EE, Jurkovich GJ, Knudson MM et al. Organ Injury Scaling VI: extrahepatic biliary, oesophagus, stomach, vulva, vagina, uterus (non-pregnant), uterus (pregnant), fallopian tube, and ovary. J Trauma 1995; 39(6):1069–70.[60] With permission from Lippincott, Williams & Wilkins.

Table A10

Pancreas injury scale					
Grade*	Type of injury	Description of injury	ICD-9	ICD-10†	AIS-2005
I	Haematoma	Minor contusion without duct injury	863.81/863.84	S36.1	2
	Laceration	Superficial laceration without duct injury		S36.1	2
II	Haematoma	Major contusion without duct injury or tissue loss	863.81/863.84	S36.1	2
	Laceration	Major laceration without duct injury or tissue loss		S36.1	3
III	Laceration	Distal transection or parenchymal injury with duct injury	863.92/863.94	S36.1	3
IV	Laceration	Proximal transection or parenchymal injury involving ampulla	863.91	S36.1	4
V	Laceration	Massive disruption of pancreatic head	863.91	S36.1	5

*Advance one grade for multiple injuries up to grade III. 863.51, 863.91 – head; 863.99, 862.92 – body; 863.83, 863.93 – tail. Proximal pancreas is to the patient's right of the superior mesenteric vein.
†With ICD-10 use supplementary character: 0 without open wound into abdominal cavity; 1 with open wound into abdominal cavity.
Reproduced from Moore EE, Cogbill TH, Malangoni MA et al. Organ Injury Scaling: pancreas, duodenum, small bowel, colon and rectum. J Trauma 1990; 30(11):1427–9.[56] With permission from Lippincott, Williams & Wilkins.

Chapter 13

Table A11

Oesophagus injury scale

Grade*	Type of injury	Description of injury	ICD-9	ICD-10†	AIS-2005
I	Contusion	Contusion/haematoma	862.22/826.32	S10.0/S27.8/S36.8	2
	Laceration	Partial thickness laceration	862.22/826.32	S10.0/S27.8/S36.8	3
II	Laceration	Laceration <50% circumference	862.22/826.32	S10.0/S27.8/S36.8	4
III	Laceration	Laceration >50% circumference	862.22/826.32	S10.0/S27.8/S36.8	4
IV	Tissue loss	Segmental loss or devascularisation <2 cm	862.22/826.32	S10.0/S27.8/S36.8	5
V	Tissue loss	Segmental loss or devascularisation >2 cm	862.22/826.32	S10.0/S27.8/S36.8	5

* Advance one grade for multiple lesions up to grade III.
† With ICD-10: cervical oesophagus, S10.0; thoracic oesophagus, S27.8; abdominal oesophagus, S36.8. With ICD-10 use supplementary character: 0 without open wound into abdominal or thoracic cavity; 1 with open wound into abdominal or thoracic cavity. Reproduced from Moore EE, Jurkovich GJ, Knudson MM et al. Organ Injury Scaling VI: extrahepatic biliary, oesophagus, stomach, vulva, vagina, uterus (non-pregnant), uterus (pregnant), fallopian tube, and ovary. J Trauma 1995; 39(6):1069–70.[60] With permission from Lippincott, Williams & Wilkins.

Table A12

Stomach injury scale

Grade*	Type of injury	Description of injury	ICD-9	ICD-10†	AIS-2005
I	Contusion	Contusion/haematoma	863.0/863.1	S36.3	2
	Laceration	Partial thickness laceration	863.0/863.1	S36.3	2
II	Laceration	<2 cm in gastro-oesophageal junction or pylorus	863.0/863.1	S36.3	3
		<5 cm in proximal {1/3} stomach	863.0/863.1	S36.3	3
		<10 cm in distal {2/3} stomach	863.0/863.1	S36.3	3
III	Laceration	>2 cm in gastro-oesophageal junction or pylorus	863.0/863.1	S36.3	3
		>5 cm in proximal {1/3} stomach	863.0/863.1	S36.3	3
		>10 cm in distal {2/3} stomach	863.0/863.1	S36.3	3
IV	Tissue loss	Tissue loss or devascularisation <{2/3} stomach	863.0/863.1	S36.3	4
V	Tissue loss	Tissue loss or devascularisation >{2/3} stomach	863.0/863.1	S36.3	4

* Advance one grade for multiple lesions up to grade III.
† With ICD-10 use supplementary character: 0 without open wound into abdominal cavity; 1 with open wound into abdominal cavity. Reproduced from Moore EE, Jurkovich GJ, Knudson MM et al. Organ Injury Scaling VI: extrahepatic biliary, oesophagus, stomach, vulva, vagina, uterus (non-pregnant), uterus (pregnant), fallopian tube, and ovary. J Trauma 1995; 39(6):1069–70.[60] With permission from Lippincott, Williams & Wilkins.

Table A13

Duodenum injury scale					
Grade*	Type of injury	Description of injury†	ICD-9	ICD-10‡	AIS-2005
I	Haematoma	Involving single portion of duodenum	863.21	S36.4	2
	Laceration	Partial thickness, no perforation	863.21	S36.4	3
II	Haematoma	Involving more than one portion	863.21	S36.4	2
	Laceration	Disruption <50% of circumference	863.31	S36.4	4
III	Laceration	Disruption 50–75% of circumference of D2	863.31	S36.4	4
		Disruption 50–100% of circumference of D1, D3, D4	863.31	S36.4	4
IV	Laceration	Disruption >75% of circumference of D2	863.31	S36.4	5
		Involving ampulla or distal common bile duct	863.31	S36.4	5
V	Laceration	Massive disruption of duodenopancreatic complex	863.31	S36.4	5
	Vascular	Devascularisation of duodenum	863.31	S36.4	5

*Advance one grade for multiple injuries up to grade III.
†D1, first position of duodenum; D2, second portion of duodenum; D3, third portion of duodenum; D4, fourth portion of duodenum.
‡With ICD-10 use supplementary character: 0 without open wound into abdominal cavity; 1 with open wound into abdominal cavity.
Reproduced from Moore EE, Cogbill TH, Malangoni MA et al. Organ Injury Scaling: pancreas, duodenum, small bowel, colon and rectum. J Trauma 1990; 30(11):1427–9.[56] With permission from Lippincott, Williams & Wilkins.

Table A14

Small-bowel injury scale					
Grade*	Type of injury	Description of injury	ICD-9	ICD-10†	AIS-2005
I	Haematoma	Contusion or haematoma without devascularisation	863.20	S36.4	2
	Laceration	Partial thickness, no perforation	863.20	S36.4	2
II	Laceration	Laceration <50% of circumference	863.30	S36.4	3
III	Laceration	Laceration ≥50% of circumference without transection	863.30	S36.4	3
IV	Laceration	Transection of the small bowel	863.30	S36.4	4
V	Laceration	Transection of the small bowel with segmental tissue loss	863.30	S36.4	4
	Vascular	Devascularised segment	863.30	S36.4	4

*Advance one grade for multiple injuries up to grade III.
†With ICD-10 use supplementary character: 0 without open wound into abdominal cavity; 1 with open wound into abdominal cavity.
Reproduced from Moore EE, Cogbill TH, Malangoni MA et al. Organ Injury Scaling: pancreas, duodenum, small bowel, colon and rectum. J Trauma 1990; 30(11):1427–9.[56] With permission from Lippincott, Williams & Wilkins.

Table A15

Colon injury scale					
Grade*	Type of injury	Description of injury	ICD-9†	ICD-10‡	AIS-2005
I	Haematoma	Contusion or haematoma without devascularisation	863.40–863.44	S36.5	2
	Laceration	Partial thickness, no perforation	863.40–863.44	S36.5	2
II	Laceration	Laceration <50% of circumference	863.50–863.54	S36.5	3
III	Laceration	Laceration ≥50% of circumference without transection	863.50–863.54	S36.5	3
IV	Laceration	Transection of the colon	863.50–863.54	S36.5	4
V	Laceration	Transection of the colon with segmental tissue loss	863.50–863.54	S36.5	4

*Advance one grade for multiple injuries up to grade III.
†With ICD-9: 863.40/863.50, non-specific site in colon; 863.41/863.51, ascending; 863.42/863.52, transverse; 863.43/863.53, descending; 863.44/863.54, sigmoid.
‡With ICD-10 use supplementary character: 0 without open wound into abdominal cavity; 1 with open wound into abdominal cavity.
Reproduced from Moore EE, Cogbill TH, Malangoni MA et al. Organ Injury Scaling: pancreas, duodenum, small bowel, colon and rectum. J Trauma 1990; 30(11):1427–9.[56] With permission from Lippincott, Williams & Wilkins.

Table A16

Rectum injury scale					
Grade*	Type of injury	Description of injury	ICD-9	ICD-10†	AIS-2005
I	Haematoma	Contusion or haematoma without devascularisation	863.45	S36.6	2
	Laceration	Partial-thickness laceration	863.45	S36.6	2
II	Laceration	Laceration < 50% of circumference	863.55	S36.6	3
III	Laceration	Laceration ≥50% of circumference	863.55	S36.6	4
IV	Laceration	Full-thickness laceration with extension into the perineum	863.55	S36.6	5
V	Vascular	Devascularised segment	863.55	S36.6	5

*Advance one grade for multiple injuries up to grade III.
†With ICD-10 use supplementary character: 0 without open wound into abdominal cavity; 1 with open wound into abdominal cavity.
Reproduced from Moore EE, Cogbill TH, Malangoni MA et al. Organ Injury Scaling: pancreas, duodenum, small bowel, colon and rectum. J Trauma 1990; 30(11):1427–9.[56] With permission from Lippincott, Williams & Wilkins.

Table A17

Abdominal vascular injury scale				
Grade*	Description of injury	ICD-9	ICD-10†	AIS-2005
I	Non-named superior mesenteric artery or superior mesenteric vein branches	902.20/902.39	S35.2	NS‡
	Non-named inferior mesenteric artery or inferior mesenteric vein branches	902.27/902.32	S35.2	NS
	Phrenic artery or vein	902.89	S35.8	NS
	Lumbar artery or vein	902.89	S35.8	NS
	Gonadal artery or vein	902.89	S35.8	NS
	Ovarian artery or vein	902.81/902.82	S35.8	NS
	Other non-named small arterial or venous structures requiring ligation	902.80	S35.9	NS
II	Right, left, or common hepatic artery	902.22	S35.2	3
	Splenic artery or vein	902.23/902.34	S35.2	3
	Right or left gastric arteries	902.21	S35.2	3
	Gastroduodenal artery	902.24	S35.2	3
	Inferior mesenteric artery/trunk, or inferior mesenteric vein/trunk	902.27/902.32	S35.2	3
	Primary named branches of mesenteric artery (e.g. ileocolic artery) or mesenteric vein	902.26/902.31	S35.2	3
	Other named abdominal vessels requiring ligation or repair	902.89	S35.8	3
III	Superior mesenteric vein, trunk and primary subdivisions	902.31	S35.3	3
	Renal artery or vein	902.41/902.42	S35.4	3
	Iliac artery or vein	902.53/902.54	S35.5	3
	Hypogastric artery or vein	902.51/902.52	S35.5	3
	Vena cava, infrarenal	902.10	S35.1	4
IV	Superior mesenteric artery, trunk	902.25	S35.2	3
	Coeliac axis proper	902.24	S35.2	3
	Vena cava, suprarenal and infrahepatic	902.10	S35.1	3
	Aorta, infrarenal	902.00	S35.0	4
V	Portal vein	902.33	S35.3	3
	Extraparenchymal hepatic vein only	902.11	S35.1	3

(Continued)

Table A17

Abdominal vascular injury scale—Cont'd				
Grade*	Description of injury	ICD-9	ICD-10†	AIS-2005
	Extraparenchymal hepatic veins + liver	902.11	S35.1	5
	Vena cava, retrohepatic or suprahepatic	902.19	S35.1	5
	Aorta suprarenal, subdiaphragmatic	902.00	S35.0	4

*This classification system is applicable to extraparenchymal vascular injuries. If the vessel injury is within 2 cm of the organ parenchyma, refer to the specific organ injury scale. Increase one grade for multiple grade III or IV injuries involving >50% vessel circumference. Downgrade one grade if <25% vessel circumference laceration for grades IV or V.
†With ICD-10 use supplementary character: 0 without open wound into abdominal cavity; 1 with open wound into abdominal cavity.
‡NS, not scored.
Reproduced from Moore EE, Cogbill TH, Jurkovich GJ. Organ Injury Scaling III: chest wall, abdominal vascular, ureter, bladder and urethra. J Trauma 1992; 33:337–8.[57] With permission from Lippincott, Williams & Wilkins.

Table A18

Adrenal organ injury scale				
Grade*	Description of injury	ICD-9	ICD-10†	AIS-2005
I	Contusion	868.01/868.11	S37.9	1
II	Laceration involving only cortex (<2 cm)	868.01/868.11	S37.8	1
III	Laceration extending into medulla (≥2 cm)	868.01/868.11	S37.8	2
IV	>50% parenchymal destruction	868.01/868.11	S37.8	2
V	Total parenchymal destruction (including massive intraparenchymal haemorrhage) Avulsion from blood supply	868.01/868.11	S37.8	3

*Advance one grade for bilateral lesions up to grade V.
†With ICD-10 use supplementary character: 0 without open wound into abdominal cavity; 1 with open wound into abdominal cavity.
Reproduced from Moore EE, Malangoni MA, Cogbill TH et al. Organ Injury Scaling VII: cervical vascular, peripheral vascular, adrenal, penis, testis and scrotum. J Trauma 1996; 41(3):523–4.[61] With permission from Lippincott, Williams & Wilkins.

Table A19

Kidney injury scale					
Grade*	Type of injury	Description of injury	ICD-9	ICD-10†	AIS-2005
I	Contusion	Microscopic or gross haematuria, urological studies normal	866.01	S37.0	2
	Haematoma	Subcapsular, nonexpanding without parenchymal laceration	866.01	S37.0	2
II	Haematoma	Non-expanding perirenal haematoma confined to renal retroperitoneum	866.01	S37.0	2
	Laceration	<1.0 cm parenchymal depth of renal cortex without urinary extravagation	866.11	S37.0	2
III	Laceration	>1.0 cm parenchymal depth of renal cortex without collecting system rupture or urinary extravasation	866.11	S37.0	3
IV	Laceration	Parenchymal laceration extending through renal cortex, medulla and collecting system	866.02/866.12	S37.0	4
	Vascular	Main renal artery or vein injury with contained haemorrhage	866.03/866.13	S37.0	4
V	Laceration	Completely shattered kidney	866.04/866.14	S37.0	5
	Vascular	Avulsion of renal hilum which devascularises kidney	866.13	S37.0	5

*Advance one grade for bilateral injuries up to grade III.
†With ICD-10 use supplementary character: 0 without open wound into abdominal cavity; 1 with open wound into abdominal cavity.
Reproduced from Moore EE, Shackford SR, Pachter HL et al. Organ Injury Scaling: spleen, liver and kidney. J Trauma 1989; 29(12):1664–6.[55] With permission from Lippincott, Williams & Wilkins.

Table A20

Ureter injury scale

Grade*	Type of injury	Description of injury	ICD-9	ICD-10†	AIS-2005
I	Haematoma	Contusion or haematoma without devascularisation	867.2/867.3	S37.1	2
II	Laceration	<50% transection	867.2/867.3	S37.1	2
III	Laceration	≥50% transection	867.2/867.3	S37.1	3
IV	Laceration	Complete transection with <2 cm devascularisation	867.2/867.3	S37.1	3
V	Laceration	Avulsion with >2 cm of devascularisation	867.2/867.3	S37.1	3

*Advance one grade for bilateral up to grade III.

†With ICD-10 use supplementary character: 0 without open wound into abdominal cavity; 1 with open wound into abdominal cavity.
Reproduced from Moore EE, Cogbill TH, Jurkovich GJ. Organ Injury Scaling III: chest wall, abdominal vascular, ureter, bladder and urethra. J Trauma 1992; 33:337–8.[57] With permission from Lippincott, Williams & Wilkins.

Table A21

Bladder injury scale

Grade*	Injury type	Description of injury	ICD-9	ICD-10†	AIS-2005
I	Haematoma	Contusion, intramural haematoma	867.0/867.1	S37.2	2
	Laceration	Partial thickness	867.0/867.1	S37.2	3
II	Laceration	Extraperitoneal bladder wall laceration <2 cm	867.0/867.1	S37.2	4
III	Laceration	Extraperitoneal (≥2 cm) or intraperitoneal (<2 cm) bladder wall laceration	867.0/867.1	S37.2	4
IV	Laceration	Intraperitoneal bladder wall laceration ≥2 cm	867.0/867.1	S37.2	4
V	Laceration	Intraperitoneal or extraperitoneal bladder wall laceration extending into the bladder neck or ureteral orifice (trigone)	867.0/867.1	S37.2	4

*Advance one grade for multiple lesions up to grade III.

†With ICD-10 use supplementary character: 0 without open wound into pelvic cavity; 1 with open wound into pelvic cavity.
Reproduced from Moore EE, Cogbill TH, Jurkovich GJ. Organ Injury Scaling III: chest wall, abdominal vascular, ureter, bladder and urethra. J Trauma 1992; 33:337–8.[57] With permission from Lippincott, Williams & Wilkins.

Table A22

Urethra injury scale

Grade*	Injury type	Description of injury	ICD-9	ICD-10†	AIS-2005
I	Contusion	Blood at urethral meatus; urethrography normal	867.0/867.1	S37.3	2
II	Stretch injury	Elongation of urethra without extravasation on urethrography	867.0/867.1	S37.3	2
III	Partial disruption	Extravasation of urethrography contrast at injury site with visualisation in the bladder	867.0/867.1	S37.3	2
IV	Complete disruption	Extravasation of urethrography contrast at injury site without visualisation in the bladder; <2 cm of urethra separation	867.0/867.1	S37.3	3
V	Complete disruption	Complete transaction with ≥2 cm urethral separation, or extension into the prostate or vagina	867.0/867.1	S37.3	4

*Advance one grade for bilateral injuries up to grade III.

†With ICD-10 use supplementary character: 0 without open wound into pelvic cavity; 1 with open wound into pelvic cavity.
Reproduced from Moore EE, Cogbill TH, Jurkovich GJ. Organ Injury Scaling III: chest wall, abdominal vascular, ureter, bladder and urethra. J Trauma 1992; 33:337–8.[57] With permission from Lippincott, Williams & Wilkins.

Table A23

Uterus (non-pregnant) injury scale				
Grade*	Description of injury	ICD-9	ICD-10†	AIS-2005
I	Contusion/haematoma	867.4/867.5	S37.6	2
II	Superficial laceration (<1 cm)	867.4/867.5	S37.6	2
III	Deep laceration (≥1 cm)	867.4/867.5	S37.6	3
IV	Laceration involving uterine artery	902.55	S37.6	3
V	Avulsion/devascularisation	867.4/867.5	S37.6	3

* Advance one grade for multiple injuries up to grade III.
† With ICD-10 use supplementary character: 0 without open wound into pelvic cavity; 1 with open wound into pelvic cavity.
Reproduced from Moore EE, Jurkovich GJ, Knudson MM et al. Organ Injury Scaling VI: extrahepatic biliary, oesophagus, stomach, vulva, vagina, uterus (non-pregnant), uterus (pregnant), fallopian tube, and ovary. J Trauma 1995; 39(6):1069–70.[60] With permission from Lippincott, Williams & Wilkins.

Table A24

Uterus (pregnant) injury scale				
Grade*	Description of injury	ICD-9	ICD-10†	AIS-2005
I	Contusion or haematoma (without placental abruption)	867.4/867.5	S37.6	2
II	Superficial laceration (<1 cm) or partial placental abruption <25%	867.4/867.5	S37.6	3
III	Deep laceration (≥1 cm) occurring in second trimester or placental abruption >25% but <50%	867.4/867.5	S37.6	3
	Deep laceration (≥1 cm) in third trimester	867.4/867.5	S37.6	4
IV	Laceration involving uterine artery	902.55	S37.6	4
	Deep laceration (≥1 cm) with >50% placental abruption	867.4/867.5	S37.6	4
V	Uterine rupture			
	Second trimester	867.4/867.5	S37.6	4
	Third trimester	867.4/867.5	S37.6	5
	Complete placental abruption	867.4/867.5	S37.6	4–5

* Advance one grade for multiple injuries up to grade III.
† With ICD-10 use supplementary character: 0 without open wound into pelvic cavity; 1 with open wound into pelvic cavity.
Reproduced from Moore EE, Jurkovich GJ, Knudson MM et al. Organ Injury Scaling VI: extrahepatic biliary, oesophagus, stomach, vulva, vagina, uterus (non-pregnant), uterus (pregnant), fallopian tube, and ovary. J Trauma 1995; 39(6):1069–70.[60] With permission from Lippincott, Williams & Wilkins.

Table A25

Fallopian tube injury scale				
Grade*	Description of injury	ICD-9	ICD-10†	AIS-2005
I	Haematoma or contusion	867.6/867.7	S37.5	2
II	Laceration <50% circumference	867.6/867.7	S37.5	2
III	Laceration ≥50% circumference	867.6/867.7	S37.5	2
IV	Transection	867.6/867.7	S37.5	2
V	Vascular injury; devascularised segment	902.89	S37.5	2

* Advance one grade for bilateral injuries up to grade III.
† With ICD-10 use supplementary character: 0 without open wound into abdominal or pelvic cavity; 1 with open wound into abdominal or pelvic cavity.
Reproduced from Moore EE, Jurkovich GJ, Knudson MM et al. Organ Injury Scaling VI: extrahepatic biliary, oesophagus, stomach, vulva, vagina, uterus (non-pregnant), uterus (pregnant), fallopian tube, and ovary. J Trauma 1995; 39(6):1069–70.[60] With permission from Lippincott, Williams & Wilkins.

Table A26

Ovary injury scale				
Grade*	Description of injury	ICD-9	ICD-10†	AIS-2005
I	Contusion or haematoma	867.6/867.7	S37.4	1
II	Superficial laceration (depth <0.5 cm)	867.6/867.7	S37.4	2
III	Deep laceration (depth ≥0.5 cm)	867.6/867.7	S37.4	3
IV	Partial disruption or blood supply	902.81	S37.4	3
V	Avulsion or complete parenchymal destruction	902.81	S37.4	3

*Advance one grade for bilateral injuries up to grade III.
†With ICD-10 use supplementary character: 0 without open wound into abdominal or pelvic cavity; 1 with open wound into abdominal or pelvic cavity.
Reproduced from Moore EE, Jurkovich GJ, Knudson MM et al. Organ Injury Scaling VI: extrahepatic biliary, oesophagus, stomach, vulva, vagina, uterus (non-pregnant), uterus (pregnant), fallopian tube, and ovary. J Trauma 1995; 39(6):1069–70.[60] With permission from Lippincott, Williams & Wilkins.

Table A27

Vagina injury scale				
Grade*	Description of injury	ICD-9	ICD-10†	AIS-2005
I	Contusion or haematoma	922.4	S30.2	1
II	Laceration, superficial (mucosa only)	878.6	S31.4	1
III	Laceration, deep into fat or muscle	878.6	S31.4	2
IV	Laceration, complex, into cervix or peritoneum	868.7	S31.4	3
V	Injury into adjacent organs (anus, rectum, urethra, bladder)	878.7	S39.7	3

*Advance one grade for multiple injuries up to grade III.
†With ICD-10 use supplementary character: 0 without open wound into abdominal or pelvic cavity; 1 with open wound into abdominal or pelvic cavity.
Reproduced from Moore EE, Jurkovich GJ, Knudson MM et al. Organ Injury Scaling VI: extrahepatic biliary, oesophagus, stomach, vulva, vagina, uterus (non-pregnant), uterus (pregnant), fallopian tube, and ovary. J Trauma 1995; 39(6):1069–70.[60] With permission from Lippincott, Williams & Wilkins.

Table A28

Vulva injury scale				
Grade*	Description of injury	ICD-9	ICD-10	AIS-2005
I	Contusion or haematoma	922.4	S30.2	1
II	Laceration, superficial (skin only)	878.4	S31.4	1
III	Laceration, deep (into fat or muscle)	878.4	S31.4	2
IV	Avulsion; skin, fat or muscle	878.5	S38.2	3
V	Injury into adjacent organs (anus, rectum, urethra, bladder)	878.5	S39.7	3

*Advance one grade for multiple injuries up to grade III.
Reproduced from Moore EE, Jurkovich GJ, Knudson MM et al. Organ Injury Scaling VI: extrahepatic biliary, oesophagus, stomach, vulva, vagina, uterus (non-pregnant), uterus (pregnant), fallopian tube, and ovary. J Trauma 1995; 39(6):1069–70.[60] With permission from Lippincott, Williams & Wilkins.

Table A29

Testis injury scale				
Grade*	Description of injury	ICD-9	ICD-10	AIS-2005
I	Contusion/haematoma	911.0–922.4	S30.2	1
II	Subclinical laceration of tunica albuginea	922.4	S31.3	1
III	Laceration of tunica albuginea with <50% parenchymal loss	878.2	S31.3	2
IV	Major laceration of tunica albuginea with ≥50% parenchymal loss	878.3	S31.3	2
V	Total testicular destruction or avulsion	878.3	S38.2	2

*Advance one grade for bilateral lesions up to grade V.
Reproduced from Moore EE, Malangoni MA, Cogbill TH et al. Organ Injury Scaling VII: cervical vascular, peripheral vascular, adrenal, penis, testis and scrotum. J Trauma 1996; 41(3):523–4.[61] With permission from Lippincott, Williams & Wilkins.

Table A30

Scrotum injury scale				
Grade	Description of injury	ICD-9	ICD-10	AIS-2005
I	Contusion	922.4	S30.2	1
II	Laceration <25% of scrotal diameter	878.2	S31.2	1
III	Laceration ≥25% of scrotal diameter	878.3	S31.3	2
IV	Avulsion <50%	878.3	S38.2	2
V	Avulsion ≥50%	878.3	S38.2	2

Reproduced from Moore EE, Malangoni MA, Cogbill TH et al. Organ Injury Scaling VII: cervical vascular, peripheral vascular, adrenal, penis, testis and scrotum. J Trauma 1996; 41(3):523–4.[61] With permission from Lippincott, Williams & Wilkins.

Table A31

Penis injury scale				
Grade*	Description of injury	ICD-9	ICD-10	AIS-2005
I	Cutaneous laceration/contusion	911.0/922.4	S30.2/31/2	1
II	Buck's fascia (cavernosum) laceration without tissue loss	878.0	S37.8	1
III	Cutaneous avulsion Laceration through glans/meatus Cavernosal or urethral defect <2 cm	878.1	S38.2	3
IV	Partial penectomy Cavernosal or urethral defect ≥2 cm	878.1	S38.2	3
V	Total penectomy	876.1	S38.2	3

*Advance one grade for multiple injuries up to grade III.
Reproduced from Moore EE, Malangoni MA, Cogbill TH et al. Organ Injury Scaling VII: cervical vascular, peripheral vascular, adrenal, penis, testis and scrotum. J Trauma 1996; 41(3):523–4.[61] With permission from Lippincott, Williams & Wilkins.

Table A32

Peripheral vascular organ injury scale

Grade*	Description of injury	ICD-9	ICD-10	AIS-2005
I	Digital artery/vein	903.5	S65.5	1–3
	Palmar artery/vein	903.4	S65.3	1–3
	Deep palmar artery/vein	904.6	S65.3	1–3
	Dorsalis pedis artery	904.7	S95.0	1–3
	Plantar artery/vein	904.5	S95.1	1–3
	Non-named arterial/venous branches	903.8/904.7	S55.9/S85.9	1–3
II	Basilic/cephalic vein	903.8	S45.8/S55.8	1–3
	Saphenous vein	904.3	S75.2	1–3
	Radial artery	903.2	S55.1	1–3
	Ulnar artery	903.3	S55.0	1–3
III	Axillary vein	903.02	S45.1	2–3
	Superficial/deep femoral vein	903.02	S75.1	2–3
	Popliteal vein	904.42	S85.5	2–3
	Brachial artery	903.1	S45.1	2–3
	Anterior tibial artery	904.51/904.52	S85.1	1–3
	Posterior tibial artery	904.53/904.54	S85.1	1–3
	Peroneal artery	904.7	S85.2	1–3
	Tibioperoneal trunk	904.7	S85.2	2–3
IV	Superficial/deep femoral artery	904.1/904.7	S75.0	3–4
	Popliteal artery	904.41	S85.0	2–3
V	Axillary artery	903.01	S45.0	2–3
	Common femoral artery	904.0	S75.0	3–4

*Increase one grade for multiple grade III or IV injuries involving >50% vessel circumference. Decrease one grade for <25% vessel circumference disruption for grades IV or V.
Reproduced from Moore EE, Malangoni MA, Cogbill TH et al. Organ Injury Scaling VII: cervical vascular, peripheral vascular, adrenal, penis, testis and scrotum. J Trauma 1996; 41(3):523–4.[61] With permission from Lippincott, Williams & Wilkins.

14

Venous thromboembolism: prevention, diagnosis and treatment

Rhona M. Maclean

Introduction

Venous thromboembolism (VTE) is a common and increasing cause of cardiovascular disease in the Western world, associated with significant morbidity and mortality. It is now believed that deep vein thrombosis (DVT) and pulmonary embolism (PE) are two manifestations of that same disease process: VTE. The two major complications of DVT of the lower leg are the post-thrombotic syndrome, with its sequelae of leg pain, swelling, venous insufficiency and ulceration, and PE, which is potentially life-threatening. VTE is a multifactorial disease, involving both genetic and environmental interactions; these environmental factors include both hospitalisation and surgical intervention. It is therefore important not only to recognise and treat VTE in a timely and appropriate manner, but also to institute evidence-based thromboprophylaxis strategies to hospitalised patients in order to reduce the risk of its development.

Epidemiology

The estimated incidence of a first episode of VTE is approximately 1–2 per 1000 person-years in white Caucasians, with a lower incidence in Hispanics and Asians.[1,2] A high prevalence of silent DVTs and PEs, particularly in the severely ill, and a low rate of post-mortem examinations will likely make the true incidence much higher. The risk of developing VTE increases steadily with age, with an incidence of >5.0 per 1000 person-years in those over 80 years of age.[2] In the absence of risk factors such as central

venous access, sepsis or malignancy, VTE is vanishingly rare in childhood with an overall incidence of 0.05–0.07 per 10 000.[3] The incidence of VTE is approximately equal in men and women; however, the incidence rates are higher in women than men in the childbearing years, likely due to the recognised risk factors of the combined oral contraceptive pill, hormone replacement therapy and pregnancy, whereas after the age of 45 incidence rates are generally higher in men. Clinical studies excluding autopsy data have consistently shown that the incidence of DVT is approximately twice that of PE.[1,2] It has been estimated that there are over 130 000 cases of VTE in the UK each year, at a cost (direct and indirect) of around £640 million per year.[4]

It is now generally agreed that DVT and PE are the result of the same disease process, VTE; of patients presenting with symptomatic PE, up to 80% will have asymptomatic DVT, and in those presenting with symptomatic DVT, 50–80% can be shown by imaging to have PE.[5]

Approximately 40–50% of episodes of VTE are idiopathic in nature (defined as having had no recent surgery, trauma, cancer, pregnancy or immobilisation), the remainder presenting with a thrombosis after an obvious precipitating event.[1,2] Of patients diagnosed with VTE, the majority (73.7%) present as outpatients and of these a significant proportion have either undergone surgery (23.1%) or been hospitalised (36.8%) in the preceding 3 months.[6]

The mortality associated with VTE is surprisingly high; in a retrospective epidemiological study, Naess et al. reported a 30-day fatality rate of 4.6% with DVT and 9.7% following PE.[2] Cancer was associated with a worse outcome, with a 30-day fatality rate of 19.1%. Mortality rates associated with PE are high, with approximately 25% of patients dying after a year, many due to malignancy, others from cardiopulmonary disease or recurrent VTE.[7] Overall, pulmonary emboli are thought to be responsible for 10% of deaths of hospital inpatients.[8]

Many PEs are diagnosed for the first time at post-mortem examination and in only 30–45% of hospital inpatients who die as a result of major PE was that diagnosis considered before death.[9]

Thrombosis in the deep veins damages the deep venous valves, causes post-thrombotic scarring and stiffening of the vessel wall. This frequently results in venous insufficiency, reflux and venous hypertension, which in turn can result in swelling, pain and heaviness in the affected leg – the post-thrombotic syndrome. In its severe form, it causes marked skin changes: lipodermatosclerosis (varicose eczema and atrophy of the subcutaneous tissues), hyperpigmentation and ulceration, and can be a major cause of morbidity. The incidence of the post-thrombotic syndrome has been reported at approximately 28% after 5 years, with 9% having severe post-thrombotic syndrome.[7] Up to 5% of patients with PE will develop pulmonary hypertension.[7]

Following cessation of oral anticoagulation after a first episode of VTE, the risk of recurrence is 7–12.9% after 1 year and 21.5–22.8% after 5 years.[10,11]

A prospective study of patients in Cambridge, UK, followed 570 patients with a first episode of VTE for 2 years after the cessation of oral anticoagulant therapy.[12] The risk of recurrence at 2 years in those who had presented with VTE within 6 weeks of surgery or in pregnancy or postpartum was 0%, in contrast to those who had had idiopathic events (19.4%) and those who had had a non-surgical risk factor for VTE (8.8%). In this cohort, the presence or absence of a detectable inherited thrombophilia did not significantly influence the risk of recurrence of VTE. Patients with clear precipitants to VTE are at low risk of recurrence once stopping anticoagulation if the underlying risk factor has resolved.

Pathophysiology of venous thromboembolism

The results of Virchow's classic pathological studies of fatal postpartum thrombosis were presented in the 1860s. He described a triad of factors: slowing of venous blood flow (stasis), changes in the blood which increase the propensity to develop thrombosis (hypercoagulability), and damage to the blood vessel wall (venous injury). These are now widely know as Virchow's triad.

This model remains a valid concept today (Table 14.1). Stasis (or paralysis) is associated with an increased risk of VTE. There is an increased risk of VTE in stroke patients in the paralysed limb;[13] however, paralysis may have other effects on the venous system in addition to slowing venous blood flow. It has been demonstrated that intraoperative paralysis causes 'microtears' in the venous endothelium, exposing circulating blood to procoagulant components in the subendothelium (e.g. collagen, von Willebrand factor, tissue factor).[14] Stasis, in and of itself, is likely to be insufficient to cause VTE, and most patients with significant immobility are likely to have a systemic illness, increasing the risk of VTE by other mechanisms.

It is obvious that surgery (especially in orthopaedic arthroplasty) or trauma can cause venous injury, thus increasing the risk of thrombosis. Inflammatory cytokines can also cause venous injury, down-regulating thrombomodulin, stimulating tissue factor expression on monocytes or endothelial cells, or inducing apoptosis of the endothelium, rendering them thrombogenic.[15]

It has become increasingly apparent that blood hypercoagulability is the component of Virchow's triad with the largest role in the development of VTE with both inherited and acquired forms (see below). The acquired forms are associated with an inflammatory response with increased levels of cytokines such as tumour necrosis factor and interleukin-1. These cytokines can stimulate endothelial cells and monocytes to express tissue factor, impair fibrinolysis by increasing levels of plasminogen activator inhibitor-1 (PAI-1), and in some circumstances reducing levels of tissue plasminogen activator. There is some evidence that fibrinolysis is reduced in patients with VTE (reduced PAI-1 levels in patients with VTE).[16]

As a thrombus forms, close to the vein wall the valve pocket thrombus is rich in red blood cells caught within a fibrin mesh, and is described as red thrombus. Extending away from the vein wall, the thrombus becomes white with the accumulation of platelets and fibrin into the clot.[17] The thrombus then either propagates proximally to form a free-floating non-occlusive clot or extends to attach to the vein's wall just beyond the valve pocket, often occluding the vein[18] (**Fig. 14.1**).

These DVTs usually start in the calf veins; the thrombi developing after surgery often originate in the valve cusps of the soleal veins. Venographic and leg scanning studies undertaken as early as the 1960s show that many such thrombi start to develop intraoperatively; of these half will resolve spontaneously within 72 hours, 18% will extend proximally and 50% of these proximal thromboses will embolise. Some thromboses, however, begin postoperatively; 20–34% of patients diagnosed as having DVT by screening tests in hospital had been shown to have

Table 14.1 • Interpretation of Virchow's triad using modern understanding of the physiological mechanisms of thrombosis

Virchow's triad	Modern interpretation
Stasis	Immobility • Of minor importance except that it may indicate underlying disease activity • Paralysis induces 'microtears' in the endothelium
Blood coagulability	Impaired inhibition of coagulation • Deficiencies of antithrombin, protein C, protein S, factor V Leiden prothrombin G20210A Effects of inflammatory cytokines • Increased monocyte tissue factor • Increased plasminogen activator inhibitor
Venous injury	Direct trauma • Torsion during surgery • Hydrodynamic trauma from tourniquet use Effects of inflammatory cytokines • Endothelial cell apoptosis • Increased endothelial cell tissue factor • Decreased thrombomodulin expression

Reproduced from Zwicker J, Bauer KA. Thrombophilia. In: Kitchens CS, Alving BA, Kessler CM (eds) Consultative hemostasis and thrombosis. Elsevier Science, 2002; p. 198.[29] With permission from Elsevier.

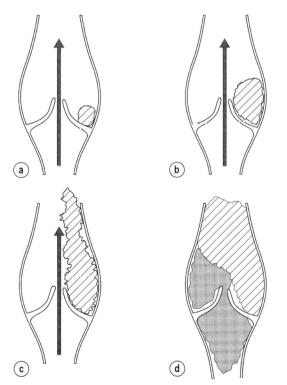

Figure 14.1 • Clot formation and propagation: **(a)** nidus of clot forming in recess of the valve pocket; **(b)** propagation of clot to fill the pocket; **(c)** propagation of free-floating thrombus without vein occlusion; **(d)** thrombus extension and attachment to opposite vein wall causing occlusion and secondary thrombus propagation both proximal and distal. Reproduced from Hamilton G, Platt SA. Deep vein thrombosis. In: Beard JD, Gaines PA (eds) Vascular and endovascular surgery. London: WB Saunders, 1998; pp. 351–96. With permission from Elsevier.

legs free of thrombosis postoperatively. It has been estimated that 10% of symptomatic PEs cause death within 1 hour of onset (Box 14.1). There is an ongoing debate as to the significance of calf vein thrombosis and whether, if detected, it should be treated. A recent study of isolated symptomatic muscular calf vein thromboses suggested that they are not as innocuous as originally thought; 7% of patients had symptomatic PEs at presentation, and after completing 1–3 months of anticoagulation, 18% had recurrent episodes of VTE within 3 years.[19]

Hypercoagulability

Inherited predispositions to venous thromboembolism

There are four predominant anticoagulant mechanisms which maintain the fluidity of blood and limit the production of thrombin and fibrin clot at the site of venous injury: antithrombin, proteins C and S, the tissue factor pathway inhibitor system, and the fibrinolytic system (**Fig. 14.2**). Deficiencies of the components of these pathways can cause a thrombotic state (although a defect in the tissue factor pathway inhibitor system has not yet been described). In addition to these inherited coagulopathies, a number of acquired hypercoagulable states can increase the propensity of developing VTE (Box 14.2). The inherited thrombophilias most clearly linked with predispositions to VTE are antithrombin, protein C and S deficiencies, activated protein C resistance (factor V Leiden), the prothrombin gene variant, hyperhomocysteinaemia and elevated levels of coagulation factor VIII.

Most deep vein thrombosis (DVT) starts in the calf veins

About half the episodes of DVT associated with surgery start intraoperatively and about half resolve spontaneously within 72 hours

The risk of progression of postoperative DVT is greatest in the presence of continuing risk factors and where the initial thrombosis is large

After orthopaedic surgery, 75% of episodes of DVT occur in the operated leg

Symptomatic risk of venous thromboembolic disease is highest within 2 weeks of surgery but is maintained for 2–3 months

Isolated calf DVT is rarely symptomatic and rarely results in clinically significant pulmonary embolism

Approximately 25% of episodes of untreated symptomatic calf DVT extend to the proximal veins within 1 week of presentation

Approximately 70% of patients with symptomatic pulmonary embolism have a DVT (approximately two-thirds involve the proximal veins)

Without treatment approximately 50% of patients with symptomatic proximal DVT or pulmonary embolism will have a recurrent thrombosis in 3 months. The greatest risk of fatal postoperative pulmonary embolism occurs 3–7 days after surgery and 10% of symptomatic DVTs are fatal within 1 hour of first symptoms

Between 5% and 10% of patients with pulmonary embolism present with shock

Isolated calf DVT is associated with half the risk of recurrence of proximal DVT or pulmonary embolism

The risk of recurrence is similar following proximal DVT and pulmonary embolism

Recurrent DVT in the same leg predisposes to post-thrombotic syndrome

Approximately 50% resolution of perfusion defects occurs after 2–4 weeks of treatment for pulmonary embolism, with complete resolution in two-thirds of patients thereafter

Pulmonary hypertension will develop in approximately 5% of patients with pulmonary embolism

Adapted from Kearon C. Natural history of venous thromboembolism. Circulation 2003; 107:I22–30.[7] With permission from Lippincott, Williams & Wilkins/American Heart Association.

Antithrombin deficiency

Antithrombin is a critical regulator of the haemostatic system: it irreversibly inactivates thrombin (factor IIa), activated factor X (factor Xa) and, to a lesser extent, factors IXa, XIa and XIIa, limiting the ongoing propagation of thrombosis. Its activity is accelerated by the presence of endothelial glycosaminoglycans as well as unfractionated heparin (UFH), low-molecular-weight heparin (LMWH)

and fondaparinux. Deficiency of antithrombin was first reported by Egeberg,[20] who found reduced antithrombin levels (40–50% of normal) in members of a Norwegian family with a strong predisposition to venous thrombosis. Antithrombin deficiency has been found to have a prevalence of between 0.2 and 0.02 per 1000 of the population,[21] and can be found in approximately 1% of consecutive patients presenting with VTE.[22] Antithrombin deficiency is classified as type I deficiency (reduced quantity of a normally functioning protein), type II deficiency (abnormally functioning protein) and type III deficiency (absence of functional antithrombin). Homozygosity for type I deficiency is thought to be fatal in utero. Type I deficiency and those type II deficiencies affecting the antithrombin reactive site have a higher risk of VTE than type II deficiencies affecting the antithrombin heparin-binding site. Studies have reported antithrombin deficiency to confer a 5–50-fold increased risk of VTE. Acquired deficiency of antithrombin can occur in a number of different clinical situations, including pregnancy, liver disease, sepsis, acute thrombosis, disseminated intravascular coagulation (DIC) and nephrotic syndrome. Levels of antithrombin are reduced in patients who are receiving treatment with heparin, L-asparaginase or estrogens.

Protein C and S deficiencies

Proteins C is synthesised by the liver and protein S by hepatocytes, megakaryocytes, endothelial and brain cells. Proteins C and S are both vitamin K-dependent proteins, therefore their activity is reduced by coumarin anticoagulation. Protein C is cleaved by thrombin to its active state, activated protein C (APC); thrombomodulin and the endothelial protein C receptor are both required for its activation, and bind its cofactor protein S. This APC–protein S complex then inactivates coagulation factors Va and VIIIa.

Thrombosis associated with protein C deficiency was first described in 1981[21] and subsequently 1 in 500 of the general population has been shown to have reduced levels of protein C.[23] Protein C deficiency has been reported to confer a relative risk of developing VTE of 6.5–15, and will be found in 1–3% of patients presenting with VTE.[21]

Protein S deficiency was first described in 1984. Reduced levels of protein S have been described in 1–3% of patients with VTE and approximately 1.3% of controls; the relative risk of VTE with protein S deficiency is 2. There appears to be a significantly increased risk of VTE in thrombophilic families with protein S deficiency compared to unselected patients with protein S deficiency; this is thought to be due to the additive effect of other thrombophilic defects (such as factor V Leiden) in those kindreds. Protein S deficiency accounts for approximately 1% of patients presenting with VTE.[21]

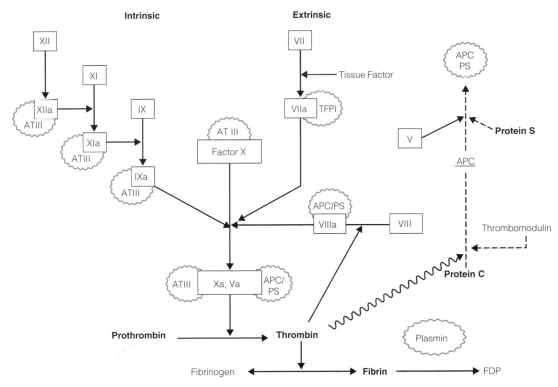

Figure 14.2 • Outline of the clotting cascade demonstrating the points of action of the four main anticoagulant mechanisms: antithrombin III (ATIII), plasmin, proteins C and S (APC/PS) and tissue factor pathway inhibitor (TFPI). FDP, fibrin degradation products. Reproduced from Hamilton G, Platt SA. Deep vein thrombosis. In: Beard JD, Gaines PA (eds) Vascular and endovascular surgery. London: WB Saunders, 1998; pp. 351–96. With permission from Elsevier.

Box 14.2 • Risk factors for venous thromboembolism

Inherited	Selective estrogen receptor modulators
Antithrombin deficiency	Infection/sepsis
Protein C deficiency	Immobility/paresis
Protein S deficiency	Heart or respiratory failure
Factor V Leiden	Inflammatory bowel disease
Prothrombin G20210A	Nephrotic syndrome
Elevated factor VIII levels	Haemoglobinopathies
Dysfibrinogenaemia	Myeloproliferative disease
	Paroxysmal nocturnal haemoglobinuria
Acquired	Paraproteinaemia
Surgery	Obesity
Trauma	Smoking
Acute medical illness	Varicose veins
Malignancy	Central venous lines
Cancer therapies (hormonal, chemotherapy or radiotherapy)	
Previous VTE	
Antiphospholipid syndrome	
Increasing age	
Pregnancy and puerperium	
Estrogen-containing oral contraceptives or hormone replacement therapy	

Neonates are deficient in proteins C and S (levels not normalising until adulthood). As with antithrombin deficiency, liver disease, sepsis, DIC and acute thrombosis all reduce protein C and S levels, as of course can coumarin anticoagulation. Protein S (but not protein C) levels are also reduced in pregnancy and with estrogens.

Factor V Leiden and APC resistance

Activated factor V is inactivated by APC; Dahlback et al. described a family who were relatively resistant to APC using a coagulation-based assay.[24] This APC resisitance was subsequently shown to be due to factor V Leiden. In Caucasian populations, factor V Leiden (factor V R506Q) is the most prevalent genetic risk factor for VTE (2–18% of the general population), whereas it is present in <1% of Africans/South-East Asians. Factor V Leiden is relatively resistant to inactivation by APC/protein S (causing APC resistance). Heterozygosity for factor V Leiden increases the risk of VTE three- to eightfold; those who are homozygous for the mutation have an 80-fold increased risk, and present with VTE at a younger age. In most Caucasian populations, it is found in >20% of unselected patients presenting with VTE.[21]

Prothrombin G20210A

Prothrombin is a vitamin K-dependent coagulation factor synthesised in the liver. First described in 1996, the prothrombin G20210A mutation is in the 3′-untranslated region of the prothrombin gene, and has been reported to improve the stability of prothrombin mRNA, increasing plasma prothrombin activity. The prothrombin G20210A mutation is found in approximately 2–3% of the Caucasian population and confers a threefold increased risk of VTE. It is found in 2–6% of unselected patients presenting with VTE.[21]

Hyperhomocysteinaemia

Classical homocystinuria, which causes extremely high levels of plasma homocysteine, is associated with both venous and arterial thrombosis. The association between mild and moderate increases in plasma homocysteine and VTE is not as clear-cut. Although retrospective studies suggested that mild elevations in plasma homocysteine (>18.5 μmol/L) were associated with venous thrombosis, homozygosity for the methylene tetrahydrofolate reductase gene variant (MTHFR C677T), which causes mildly elevated homocysteine levels, was shown not to be associated with VTE,[21] casting doubt on the hypothesis.

Prospective studies of folate and vitamin B supplementation to reduce homocysteine levels failed to show an improved outcome in patients with previous thrombosis. A recent publication has clearly demonstrated that mild elevations in homocysteine levels are not associated with venous or arterial thrombosis, but are associated with increased factor VIII levels.[25]

Elevated factor VIII levels

High plasma factor VIII (FVIII) levels have been demonstrated to increase the risk of VTE and the risk of recurrence after a first episode.[21,26] When compared to those with FVIII levels less than 100 IU/dL, those with levels above 150 IU/dL have a six-fold increased risk of VTE. FVIII is an acute-phase reactant protein; however, the association with thrombosis persists on adjustment for C-reactive protein levels, suggesting that elevated FVIII levels are causally associated with VTE. It is well recognised that individuals with blood group O have not only reduced von Willebrand factor levels (and FVIII levels) compared with those with a non-O blood group, but also a reduced risk of VTE. It is largely thought that this is due to the lower levels of FVIII in group O individuals.[21,27]

Other inherited thrombophilias

Fibrinogen is a large protein, made up of three different polypeptide chains (alpha, beta and gamma). There are more than 300 reported abnormal fibrinogens, of which a minority have been reported to be associated with thrombosis.[28]

Elevations in levels of coagulation factors IX and XI are lesser risk factors for VTE. Defects of fibrinolysis have also been reported to increase thrombosis risk: increased levels of thrombin-activatable fibrinolysis inhibitor or PAI-1 and plasminogen deficiency have been reported to increase the risk of VTE, but the clinical relevance of these findings is uncertain.[29]

Acquired or secondary causes of hypercoagulability

The antiphospholipid syndrome (APLS)

A diagnosis of the APLS requires the presence of both clinical features (most commonly venous or arterial thrombosis or adverse pregnancy outcome) and the presence of persistent (on two occasions more than 12 weeks apart) lupus anticoagulant or moderate- or high-titre antiphospholipid antibodies (anti-cardiolipin IgG/IgM or anti-β$_2$-glycoprotein-1 IgG/IgM antibodies). Lupus anticoagulants interfere in phospholipid-dependent coagulation investigations, and therefore can cause prolongation of the activated partial thromboplastin time (APTT) assay. The mechanism of these antibodies in the development of thrombosis has not been established; however, a number of hypotheses have been suggested: antibodies interfering with endogenous anticoagulant mechanisms, triggering procoagulant changes in leucocytes, platelets or endothelial cells; or activation of complement triggering an inflammatory reaction.[30]

The APLS can be either secondary (usually associated with systemic lupus erythematosus (SLE) or systemic sclerosis) or primary (no underlying autoimmune disease). Approximately half of patients with SLE have demonstrable antiphospholipid antibodies; however, as SLE is rare, these patients will account for only a small number of those presenting with VTE.

Antiphospholipid antibodies themselves, however, are not infrequent, being described in 1–5% of the general population, and are found in 5–15% of those presenting with VTE. They are more prevalent in those with acute infection and malignant disease, and are associated with a number of different medications (including antipsychotic drugs). It is thought that lupus anticoagulants are most strongly associated with venous thrombosis (5–10-fold increased risk), with up to a fourfold increased risk with anticardiolipin IgG antibodies.[31]

 Patients with the APLS and venous thrombosis should be anticoagulated with warfarin with a target international normalised ratio (INR) of 2.5, and this anticoagulation should be continued long term.[30]

Heparin-induced thrombocytopenia (HIT)

HIT is an adverse effect of heparin with a high risk of thrombosis (thrombosis risk 30–75%; **Fig. 14.3**) and is associated with a significant morbidity and mortality. It occurs more frequently in patients receiving UFH compared to LMWH, following therapeutic rather than prophylactic treatment, and in surgical rather than medical patients, although is very rare in pregnancy. Typically in HIT, the platelet count from a patient receiving UFH or LMWH falls by ≥50% from baseline (rarely below 20×10^9/L) between days 5 and 10 of heparin therapy. Less often, if a patient has received heparin within the last 100 days, HIT can present acutely after heparin administration with systemic symptoms (rigors, cardiorespiratory distress). Skin lesions at the site of heparin injection sites have also been shown to be associated with HIT.[32] Half of patients with HIT will develop thrombosis, and unless heparin is stopped and alternative anticoagulation commenced, there is a considerable risk of further thrombosis developing.[33]

The thrombocytopenia is due to the production of IgG antibodies directed at heparin–platelet factor 4 (PF4) complexes, which form on the surface of platelets and endothelial cells. It is thought that these antibody–heparin–PF4 complexes bind to the platelet (and possibly endothelial) surface, causing platelet activation, thrombocytopenia and venous and/or arterial thrombosis. Rarely thrombosis can present before the onset of thrombocytopenia.

 With the exception of prophylactic LMWH in pregnancy, all patients receiving heparin should have a platelet count checked on the day treatment is started, after 24 hours of therapy (if exposed to heparin within the previous 100 days) and thereafter every 2–4 days until day 14. If the platelet count falls by ≥50% of baseline or the patient develops new venous or arterial thrombosis or skin allergy, then a diagnosis of HIT should be considered and a clinical assessment made (Table 14.2). If the diagnosis of HIT is likely, heparin should be stopped (including heparin flushes) and due to the high risk of thrombosis, an alternative anticoagulant (e.g. danaparoid, lepirudin or fondaparinux – discuss with haematologist) should be commenced pending the results of further investigations. Warfarin should not be started until the platelet count has fully recovered, and care should be taken to continue an additional anticoagulant until the INR is >2.0 for 2 days.

Figure 14.3 • Skin necrosis caused by heparin-induced thrombocytopenia. Reproduced from Hamilton G, Platt SA. Deep vein thrombosis. In: Beard JD, Gaines PA (eds) Vascular and endovascular surgery. London: WB Saunders, 1998; pp. 351–96. With permission from Elsevier.

HIT is rarely associated with bleeding and so platelet transfusions should not be given due to the risk of thrombosis,[33] unless there is active bleeding.

Hormone replacement therapy (HRT) and combined oral contraceptive pill (cOCP)

Venous thrombosis in young women is rare; the absolute risk of developing a VTE is <1 per 10 000 per year in women of reproductive age. In users of the cOCP, this risk increases to 2 or 3 per 10 000 per year. The risk is highest in the first year of use, diminishes thereafter, and is reduced by the use of the lower dose estrogen preparations (twofold reduction in VTE with 30 µg ethinylestradiol compared with 50 µg ethinylestradiol preparations).

> Third-generation pills (containing the progestogens desogestrel or gestodene) are associated with a twofold higher risk of venous thrombosis when compared to the second-generation preparations (containing norgestrel or levonorgestrel).[34]

As well as the differences between the contraceptive preparations, there are differences between women. Obese women (body mass index >30) have a twofold increased risk of VTE, but a 10-fold increased risk if taking the cOCP. Women with thrombophilia (antithrombin, protein C or S deficiencies, factor V Leiden of the prothrombin gene variant) who take the cOCP are at particularly high risk of VTE. Heterozygous carriers of factor V Leiden are at significantly increased risk of VTE (20–30-fold), with homozygous carriers at even greater risk. Those who are heterozygous for the prothrombin gene variant have a 16-fold increased risk of VTE.[35] More recently, transdermal contraceptive patches have been introduced containing both estrogen and progestogen, but the risk of VTE with these preparations appears to be similar to the oral preparations.[36]

HRT was initially thought to be of significant benefit to postmenopausal women, not only reducing vasomotor symptoms but also reducing the risk of osteoporosis, cardiovascular disease and gynaecological malignancies. While it is clearly effective at reducing vasomotor symptoms, it does not reduce cardiovascular risk, prevents osteoporotic fractures only while being taken, with the benefit declining soon after stopping, and increases the risk of breast cancer. As a result it is no longer recommended as treatment for osteoporosis.

> Although HRT was thought to confer a lower risk of thrombosis compared to the cOCP, three studies published in 1996 demonstrated a two- to fourfold increased risk of VTE in women using HRT compared with non-users.[37–39]

As with the cOCP, the risk is highest in the first year of HRT, and there is a synergistic effect with the inherited thrombophilias.[34] Unlike the cOCP, there appears to be a lower risk of VTE when the transdermal route is used compared with oral preparations.[40]

Travel- and flight-related thrombosis

The first report of VTE associated with air travel was in 1954. The term 'economy-class syndrome' was first used in 1977 in a report of eight patients presenting with VTE shortly after flying in economy class.[41] It has since been shown that travel in relatively cramped conditions, whether plane, train or car, increases the risk of developing VTE. Prolonged sitting in cramped conditions, dehydration and

Table 14.2 • Estimating the pretest probability of HIT: the four Ts

	Points (0, 1 or 2 for each of four categories: maximum possible score = 8)*		
	2	**1**	**0**
Thrombocytopenia	>50% fall or platelet nadir 20–100 × 10⁹/L	30–50% fall or platelet nadir 10–19 × 10⁹/L	Fall <30% or platelet nadir <10 × 10⁹/L
Timing of platelet count fall or other sequelae	Onset between days 5 and 10, or less than 1 day if exposure to heparin within last 100 days	Consistent with immunisation but not clear or thrombocytopenia >10 days	Platelet count falls too early (without recent heparin exposure)
Thrombosis or other sequelae	New thrombosis, skin necrosis, systemic reaction after heparin	Progressive or recurrent thrombosis, erythematous skin lesions, suspected thrombosis not proven	None
Other causes for thrombocytopenia?	No other cause evident	Possible other cause	Definite other cause

* Score 6–8 = high; 4–5 = intermediate; 0–3 = low.
Adapted from Warkentin TE et al. Laboratory diagnosis of immune heparin induced thrombocytopenia. Curr Haematol Rep 2003; 2:148–57.[32] © Current Medicine.

hypobaric hypoxia induce a number of physiological changes (increase in haematocrit, reduction in lower limb venous velocity, coagulation activation) which could, plausibly, increase the risk of VTE.[42] Eight studies prospectively identified travellers, excluded the presence of active VTE (duplex ultrasound or D-dimer measurement), then reassessed them on their return for the presence of VTE. The studies varied in their inclusion/exclusion criteria and by intervention during the flight (low/moderate or high risk ± aspirin/exercise/elastic stockings during the flights) and by duration of flight. Incidences of VTE of between 0% and 10% were reported, with symptomatic thromboses in <1%.[42] Two of these studies reported that the majority of passengers presenting with VTE had additional risk factors present.

A cohort study of employees of multinational corporations undertaking flights of >4 hours showed a threefold increased risk in the development of symptomatic VTE in the 8 weeks after the flight. The risk increased with exposure to more flights within a short period of time and with increased flight duration. The risk was found to be higher in those under the age of 30, in women taking the cOCP and in individuals who were particularly tall, short or overweight.[43]

A further study (MEGA study) which investigated the effect of travelling (different modes and duration) on the risk of VTE found that travel of >4 hours increased the risk of venous thrombosis twofold, with the risk of flying being similar to the risk of travelling by car, train or bus.[44]

The risk of symptomatic PE associated with travel is low (<0.5 per million passengers) and the risk of fatality lower still.[42] Therefore, although travel is a weak risk factor for VTE, it appears to be largely confined to those with additional risk factors for VTE who are undertaking long flights.

There is no evidence for the use of aspirin for thromboprophylaxis for flying, and if thromboprophylaxis is to be considered (i.e. those with additional risk factors) it should consist of below-knee elastic compression hosiery (15–30 mmHg at the ankle) or LMWH (although there is little evidence for its use for this indication, it has been shown to be effective for thromboprophylaxis in surgical and medical patients).[42]

Medical illness and malignancy

VTE is an all too frequent cause of morbidity and mortality in hospitalised medical patients. Hospitalisation itself is associated with an eightfold

increased risk of VTE, with specific patient groups being at particularly high risk. It has therefore been proposed that hospitalised medical patients are risk-assessed for their level of risk of developing VTE. Congestive cardiac failure, acute infection, central venous line, paralytic stroke, pregnancy/postpartum, previous VTE, thrombophilia, nephrotic syndrome, HRT, cancer and chemotherapy are all moderate risk factors for VTE (odds ratio 2–9).[45]

Cancer is clearly associated with VTE; 15% of patients with VTE have malignancy and 2–3% of patients with VTE are found to have malignancy at time of presentation. The risk of developing cancer is particularly high in the 6 months after diagnosis of VTE; therefore a careful clinical history and examination should be taken in all patients presenting with a new thrombotic event. Patients with certain cancers (stomach, lung, breast, pancreas, gynaecological, lymphoma) are at particularly high risk of thrombosis, thought to be caused by tissue factor-like substances and microparticles activating the coagulation cascade. Surgery and immobilisation further increase this patient group's risk of thrombosis.

Cancer patients with thrombosis are at high risk of both recurrent thrombosis and of the bleeding complications of anticoagulant therapy. A randomised prospective trial involving patients with cancer, demonstrated that patients treated with LMWH for 6 months had approximately 50% fewer recurrent thromboses when compared with those receiving oral anticoagulant therapy with a target INR of 2.5. Bleeding rates and mortality were similar in both groups.[46]

Surgery

Major surgery is one of the greatest risk factors for VTE, the risk being greatest with certain orthopaedic surgical procedures (hip arthroplasty, hip fracture, knee arthroplasty), neurosurgery, and abdominal and pelvic surgery (especially if associated with malignancy). Major trauma is also associated with a very high risk of VTE. It has been recognised that in addition to the surgical procedure itself, a number of other factors increase the risk of thrombosis in the surgical patient (Box 14.2). It is also now understood that the risk of VTE does not end at the time of discharge; 56% of all VTE episodes within 91 days of surgery occur after discharge.[47]

Age is an important risk factor for VTE, many studies showing an increased risk in patients over 40 years of age, the risk considerably greater in those >70 years. Major illness, trauma or surgical intervention further increase this risk. VTE is therefore a disease predominantly of the middle-aged and elderly (THRIFT study group).[48] Of the secondary risk factors for VTE, obesity, congestive cardiac failure, prolonged immobilisation, previous VTE, malignancy or lower limb orthopaedic surgery are the most important.

Without thromboprophylaxis, there is a high risk of DVT in hospitalised patients (up to 60–80% in those with major trauma/high-risk orthopaedic surgery). These figures are largely taken from studies in the 1970s and 1980s. Mechanical and chemical thromboprophylaxis are now routinely employed to minimise the risk of VTE, which has been further reduced by improvements in surgical and anaesthetic techniques over recent years.

Summary of pathophysiology

Our understanding of the pathophysiology of VTE has advanced significantly in recent years, and is now understood to be a multifactorial process. An individual's risk of developing a venous thrombosis is clearly linked to the number of risk factors present. Thromboembolic disease will develop in the patient already primed with an underlying risk factor (whether inherited, such as factor V Leiden, or acquired, such as cancer) in whom other prothrombotic events or conditions, such as major surgery, are superimposed.

Diagnosis of venous thromboembolic disease

Many patients present with leg pain or swelling, chest pain or breathlessness, in whom it is not possible to exclude VTE on the basis of clinical history and examination alone. Only approximately 25% of patients with symptoms thought to be due to a DVT or PE will have those diagnoses subsequently confirmed; therefore many could be unnecessarily exposed to imaging investigations with their associated risks. As a result, over the last 5–10 years, diagnostic strategies have been developed which utilise both clinical pretest probability scoring tools (for DVT and PE) and D-dimer estimation.

Clinical features of DVT

The symptoms and signs of VTE (whether DVT or PE) tend to be non-specific. The most common symptoms and signs of DVT are pain, swelling, mild erythema, tenderness along the thigh or calf, muscle induration and mild pyrexia, although many patients with DVT will have none of these clinical features. Unilateral pitting oedema is the most significant clinical sign, indicating thrombosis in 70% of patients. Homan's sign (pain or discomfort on

foot dorsiflexion) is unreliable. In practice, any patient presenting with new-onset limb pain, irrespective of clinical features on examination, should be investigated for DVT.

Uncertain clinical presentations are more common in those with distal thromboses. Patients with distal iliac or femoral vein thromboses can present with a very painful, swollen, white leg (phlegmasia caerulea alba). The pallor is thought to be due to skin capillary compression by oedema, which, as it also makes it difficult to palpate the pedal pulses, is not infrequently mistaken for acute arterial insufficiency. A less frequent but dramatic presentation is that of 'phlegmasia caerulea dolens', which occurs when the whole iliac system is thrombosed. The entire leg is swollen, acutely painful, dusky blue in colour and patchy areas of venous gangrene can develop. The cyanosis and swelling distinguishes this from arterial ischaemia (in which the limb is white and rarely is there any swelling). The venous gangrene is a result of the venous congestion caused by the extent of the iliac vein thrombosis and also by extension of the thrombosis into the venules and capillaries. There also tends to be a significant thrombophilia (often acquired, such as heparin-induced thrombocytopenia) in such patients.

It is important to remember that venous thrombosis is not the only cause of a painful and/or swollen leg. Rupture of a Baker's cyst presents with sudden-onset lower leg pain, swelling and cellulites, with a painful and erythematous lower limb. Muscular tears and bleeding into a muscle in a patient already on anticoagulant therapy can also be difficult to differentiate from a DVT. It is also important to remember that (rarely) malignancies such as sarcoma can present with a unilateral swollen leg.[49]

Pretest probability in DVT

A major advance in the management of patients with possible DVT has been the development of clinical prediction tools. These incorporate clinical symptoms, signs and risk factors, and categorise patients as being at low (score <1), moderate (score 1–2) or high (score >2) probability for DVT. More recently the rule has been adapted to categorise patients as 'DVT likely' or 'DVT unlikely' (Table 14.3).

 A recent systematic review reported the incidence of DVT in the low-, moderate- and high-risk groups to be 5%, 17% and 53% respectively.[50]

The pretest probability score has allowed the development of improved diagnostic strategies for patients with suspected DVT. One such strategy allows a diagnosis of DVT to be excluded in certain patients after a single duplex ultrasound scan rather than serial scanning.[51] Many centres, however, now utilise strategies incorporating D-dimer testing

Table 14.3 • Clinical model predicting the pretest probability of DVT*

Clinical characteristic	Score
Active cancer (patient receiving treatment for cancer within previous 6 months or palliative)	1
Paralysis, paresis or recent plaster immobilisation of the lower extremeties	1
Recently bedridden for 3 days or more, or major surgery within 12 weeks	1
Localised tenderness along the distribution of the deep venous system	1
Entire leg swollen	1
Calf swelling at least 3 cm larger than that on asymptomatic leg (10 cm below tibial tuberosity)	1
Pitting oedema confined to symptomatic leg	1
Collateral superficial veins (non-varicose)	1
Previously documented DVT	1
Alternative diagnosis at least as likely as DVT	-2

* A score of 2 or higher indicates that the probability of DVT is likely; a score of less than 2 indicates that the probability of DVT is unlikely.

Reproduced from Wells PS et al. Evaluation of D-dimer in the diagnosis of suspected deep-vein thrombosis. N Engl J Med 2003; 349(13):1227–35. Copyright © 2003 Massachusetts Medical Society. All rights reserved.

which allow a diagnosis of DVT to be excluded in low-risk patients if D-dimers are not elevated without the need for further investigation.

D-dimer

D-dimers are the product of fibrinolysis of cross-linked fibrin, and are usually (but not always) increased in patients with active VTE (i.e. active thrombus formation). There are a number of different D-dimer assays (qualitative and quantitative) available, many of which have been evaluated to determine clinically meaningful cut-off values for the exclusion of VTE.[52] Patients with low D-dimers (below the cut-off value for that assay) with a low clinical pretest probability of DVT or PE do not generally need imaging performed to exclude a thrombosis, and can be said to have had VTE excluded (**Fig. 14.4**). It must be borne in mind, however, that D-dimers tend to be increased with increasing age, in pregnancy and in hospital inpatients (particularly those with malignancy, recent surgery or acute infection). The clinical utility of requesting a D-dimer assay in these patient groups is therefore limited, and most patients within these groups are likely to need imaging to exclude a thrombosis. D-dimer levels are reduced in patients on anticoagulant drugs (e.g. heparin or warfarin) and therefore should not be requested for the purpose of excluding a diagnosis of VTE in patients receiving anticoagulants; all such patients should have imaging performed.

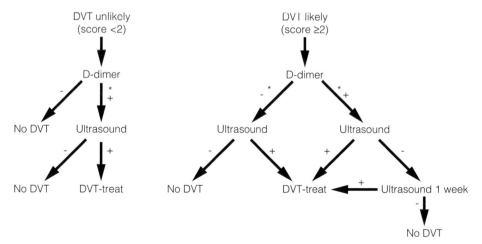

Figure 14.4 • Algorithms for the diagnosis of DVT incorporating clinical pretest probability scoring and D-dimer measurement. *LMWH if imaging delayed. Adapted from Wells PS. Integrated strategies for the diagnosis of venous thromboembolism. J Thromb Haemost 2007; 5(Suppl 1):41–50. With permission from Blackwell Publishing.

Imaging techniques for DVT

Venography

Venography is the 'gold standard' for a diagnosis of DVT; however, as it is painful and involves the use of contrast medium, its use today is limited to those patients in whom there is a high clinical suspicion yet negative imaging using other modalities. A diagnosis of DVT is made by venogram if filling defects are seen within the veins. Due to the (albeit small) risks of serious contrast reaction and venous thrombosis itself (due to endothelial damage by the contrast), venography has now been superseded by duplex ultrasound imaging.

Venous ultrasound

Venous ultrasound is now the investigation of choice for suspected DVT. It is non-invasive, relatively inexpensive and easily available. The lumen of a vein is anechoic, whether patent or occluded by thrombus, but the walls of a patent vein are easily opposed by pressure whereas those of a vein occluded by thrombus are not. The sensitivity of ultrasound for proximal DVT has been reported to be 97%, and for popliteal DVT 94%; the sensitivity is considerably less for calf DVT.[53] Many centres therefore only scan the proximal veins (down to the popliteal segment), repeating the investigation 1 week later if the initial scan was negative (in order to pick up the thrombi extending proximally). The development of clinical pretest probability tools and D-dimer testing has allowed the development of more streamlined diagnostic strategies (see below).

Particular attention should be applied to the interpretation of ultrasound scans when requested for the investigation of recurrent DVT. A scan report of echogenic or non-occlusive thrombus at the site of a previous clot could be due to chronic or 'old' DVT rather than a new event. Serial ultrasound (or venography) may be useful in such circumstances.

Impedance plethysmography (IP)

IP was extensively studied in the 1970s and 1980s and is currently still used to exclude DVT in a number of centres. A tourniquet is applied to the affected limb and changes in the volume of the limb measured after tourniquet removal. The sensitivity and specificity of IP for DVT (83% and 92% respectively) are lower than with ultrasound, hence the preference for ultrasound for the diagnosis of DVT by many hospitals.[53,54]

Computed tomography (CT)

CT has a 95% sensitivity for DVT (proximal and distal) and 97% specificity.[54] While it may not be routinely used for the diagnosis of peripheral venous occlusion, it is useful in the investigation of suspected proximal venous thrombosis (inferior and superior vena cava).

Magnetic resonance imaging (MRI) and angiography (MRA)

MRI and MRA can detect both peripheral and central venous thromboses, and are being studied for their role in the investigation of venous thrombosis. MRA is non-invasive, uses venous blood flow as the source of image contrast, but is not yet widely available. As with the other imaging modalities, MRA is sensitive and specific for proximal thrombosis, but has a lower sensitivity for distal thrombi. MRI is particularly useful for the investigation of suspected iliac thrombosis in pregnant women.

Summary of diagnostic methods in DVT

Ultrasonography by an experienced operator is now the investigation of choice for DVT. D-dimer results have now been widely incorporated into diagnostic algorithms, allowing the exclusion of DVT in patients at low risk with D-dimers below the cut-off for that assay (Fig. 14.3). Serial ultrasound scanning should be performed in those at moderate/high risk of DVT with an initial 'negative' ultrasound but D-dimers above the cut-off. More invasive investigations (e.g. CT, MRA, venography) should be reserved for those in whom there is thought to be iliac thrombosis not visualised by ultrasound, or if there is lack of concordance between clinical probability and the ultrasound scan result. Many centres will prefer to use CT or MRA rather than venography for the investigation of patients suspected of having an iliac thrombosis.

Diagnosis of pulmonary embolism

Clinical presentation and pretest probability

The symptoms and signs most commonly associated with a confirmed diagnosis of PE are (in order of descending frequency): dyspnoea, tachypnoea, pleuritic pain, apprehension, tachycardia, cough, haemoptysis, leg pain and clinical DVT. As those features with high specificity for PE (such as DVT) have a low sensitivity, and those with high sensitivity (e.g. dyspnoea) have a low specificity for PE, clinical history and examination are insufficient to exclude a diagnosis of PE.[55]

The diagnostic process has been improved considerably by the introduction of clinical decision rules (such as the Wells (Table 14.4) and Geneva scoring systems), which stratify patients with suspected PE into low-, moderate- or high-risk groups, in combination with D-dimer testing. In the original study by Wells et al.,[56] the prevalence of PE was 3.6%, 20.5% and 66.7% in low-, moderate- and high-risk patient groups respectively. Studies have shown that a diagnosis of PE can be safely excluded in low-risk patients who do not have increased D-dimers, thus avoiding further unnecessary investigations.

More recently, studies have demonstrated that the clinical utility of the Wells scoring system for PE can be improved by using only two categories of clinical probability (PE unlikely and PE likely) rather than three.

The Christopher study[57] demonstrated that 32% of patients with clinically suspected acute PE can have PE safely excluded by a combination of pretest clinical probability 'PE unlikely' and normal D-dimers, without the need for further investigation (**Fig. 14.5**).

Investigation for PE

Chest X-ray (CXR)

Radiographic findings in PE are usually non-specific on a CXR. Atelectasis and parenchymal abnormalities are most commonly seen (68%), whereas the Westermark sign of reduced pulmonary vascularity is rarely seen (6%). The CXR is, however, essential to exclude other diagnoses which may present in a similar fashion (such as infection or pulmonary oedema) and is necessary for the interpretation of a ventilation/perfusion scan (V/Q scan).

Electrocardiogram (ECG)

Many patients with PE will be tachycardic and have non-specific ECG changes, with fewer than 10% having the classical S1, Q3, T3 ECG changes at presentation. As with the CXR, however, it is useful in the exclusion of other conditions which can present with similar symptoms.

Pulmonary arteriography

Angiography involves the cannulation of a central vein, catheterisation of the pulmonary arteries and injection of contrast media under fluoroscopic control. It is expensive, requires both a trained radiologist and a cooperative patient, and therefore is now primarily reserved for cases where non-invasive tests remain indeterminate. It must be remembered as well that a negative result does not unequivocally exclude PE. The PIOPED investigators found that 1.5% of patients with a negative pulmonary angiogram presented with a PE in the year after the procedure, the majority within the next 30 days.[58] Therefore, although angiography is still considered to be the 'gold standard' for the diagnosis of PE, it is now rarely performed (only 15% of British radiography departments had the ability to undertake pulmonary angiography in 2003).[55]

Ventilation/perfusion (V/Q) scanning

Until recently, V/Q scanning was the imaging investigation of choice for those suspected of having had a PE. It is relatively easily performed and is less invasive and cheaper than pulmonary angiography. A scan showing one or more segmental, or two or more subsegmental, perfusion defects with normal ventilation is considered to be 'high probability' for PE, and has an 85–90% predictive value for PE.[58] A normal V/Q scan excludes the diagnosis of PE (1% VTE in

Table 14.4 • Variables used to determine patient pretest probability for pulmonary embolism*

Clinical variable	Score
Clinical signs and symptoms of DVT (minimum of leg swelling and pain with palpation of deep veins)	3
PE as or more likely than an alternative diagnosis	3
Heart rate >100	1.5
Immobilisation or surgery in the previous 4 weeks	1.5
Previous DVT/PE	1.5
Haemoptysis	1
Malignancy (on treatment, treated in the last 6 months or palliative)	1

* Score >4, probability of PE is 'likely'; 4, probability for PE is 'unlikely'. Alternatively, <2 is low probability, 2–6 moderate and >6 high.
Adapted from Wells PS. Integrated strategies for the diagnosis of venous thromboembolism. J Thromb Haemost 2007; 5(Suppl 1): 41–50.[50] With permission from Blackwell Publishing.

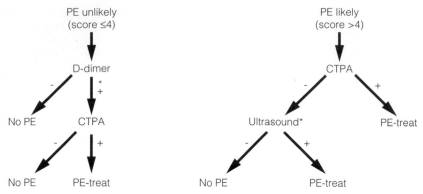

Figure 14.5 • Algorithms for the diagnosis of PE incorporating clinical pretest probability scoring and D-dimer measurement. *If multidetector CTPA is used, PE can be excluded in most cases without the need for ultrasound, but consider ultrasound if the patient has clinical symptoms or clinical probability is high. Adapted from Wells PS. Integrated strategies for the diagnosis of venous thromboembolism. J Thromb Haemost 2007; 5(Suppl 1):41–50. With permission from Blackwell Publishing.

follow-up); however, 35–40% of patients have 'non-diagnostic' scans of 'intermediate probability' and require further investigation. As a result, computed tomography pulmonary angiography (CTPA) is now increasingly used in place of V/Q scanning.

CTPA

Early single-slice CT scanners did not reliably visualise the subsegmental pulmonary arteries (sensitivity 53–100%); however, many centres now have access to multislice scanners which have increased sensitivity for clots involving the segmental and subsegmental vessels. Multislice CTPA scanners allow the entire pulmonary arterial tree to be visualised in less than 10 seconds, and in addition to demonstrating the presence or absence of a PE, an alternative cause for the patient's symptoms may be detected (not possible with V/Q scanning). It is now accepted that CTPA is not inferior to V/Q scanning in the exclusion of PE, and that anticoagulation can safely be withheld in patients with negative scans.[59]

Echocardiography

Echocardiography can be particularly useful in unstable patients for whom transport to the radiology department is unfeasible. Right ventricular free-wall hypokinesis and increased pulmonary pressures are highly suggestive of PE, and considered pathognomonic if ultrasound evidence of DVT is also seen. It may also allow differentiation between other clinical conditions which can present in a similar fashion, such as aortic dissection, myocardial infarction or pericardial tamponade.[60]

MRI

Currently, the clinical utility of MRI in the diagnosis of PE is low when compared with CTPA. Contrast-enhanced magnetic resonance angiography (ce-MRA) has been most widely adopted, with blood pool and fibrin-specific contrast agents under investigation. Although preliminary studies suggest ce-MRA has a similar sensitivity and specificity to other imaging techniques,[61] there is less access to patients (who may be clinically unstable) whilst in the magnet, the duration of scanning is longer and MRI scanning is generally less easily available. However, MRI scanning has some advantages: it does not require ionising radiation (beneficial for women of childbearing age and/or who are pregnant), MRI contrast agents are considered to have fewer side-effects than the iodinated media required for CT, and it is possible to carry out a comprehensive protocol of magnetic resonance venography and pulmonary angiography (taking less than 20 minutes in total). As a result consideration could be given to using MRI in patients with contraindications to contrast media, young women with a low clinical probability of PE, and pregnancy. However, the other imaging modalities discussed above remain the mainstay of investigation at the present time.

Investigation in pregnancy

VTE disease remains the leading cause of maternal mortality in the UK. Pregnancy is associated with a 10-fold increased risk of VTE; the risk begins early in the first trimester, with the puerperium being the time of greatest risk. Clinical assessment of DVT and PE is especially unreliable in pregnancy, and the minority of pregnant women undergoing objective investigation for VTE will have that diagnosis confirmed. It is important, therefore, that the risks of imaging (both to the mother and the fetus) are minimised. The Royal College of Obstetricians advises that pregnant women suspected of having a PE have a duplex ultrasound performed, with V/Q scanning or CTPA reserved for those with negative ultrasound scans.[62] CTPA has the disadvantage of a high radiation dose to the woman's breasts and an increased lifetime risk of developing breast cancer. Some centres therefore perform perfusion scans in those with negative leg duplex ultrasound scans, reserving CTPA scanning for those with abnormal perfusion scans.

Summary of diagnostic methods for PE

Patients presenting with symptoms suggestive of PE should have a clinical assessment and the pre-test probability determined. Those at low risk with D-dimers below the laboratory 'cut-off' for the exclusion of VTE do not usually need further investigation. For those with suspected PE in whom the diagnosis is 'PE likely' or 'PE unlikely but with positive D-dimers', CTPA has now superseded V/Q scanning as the imaging investigation of choice in many centres, and a negative multislice scan can safely exclude the presence of a PE. Pregnant women should have duplex ultrasound of the leg veins performed as the initial investigation.

Management of venous thromboembolic disease

Aims of treatment

The primary aims of the treatment of VTE are to relieve symptoms and to prevent thrombus extension and recurrent thrombotic events, thereby reducing the risks of the long-term complications of VTE (the post-thrombotic syndrome and chronic thromboembolic pulmonary hypertension). Anticoagulation is the mainstay of treatment of VTE for both DVT and PE.

 The first study of anticoagulation in PE was undertaken in 1960, in which patients were randomised to UFH infusion or placebo. The study was halted early due to the high mortality rate in patients receiving placebo; PE at autopsy was found to be the cause of death in the majority of these.[63]

Anticoagulation should be started as soon as an objective diagnosis has been made and should there be any delays in investigation, patients at moderate or high risk of VTE should have treatment started pending results of investigation. For most patients, this will mean immediate anticoagulation with an injectable anticoagulant (UFH, LMWH or fondaparinux), followed by oral anticoagulation with a vitamin K antagonist. Some patients (such as those with PE with haemodynamic compromise

or phlegmasia caerulea dolens) may benefit from thrombolytic therapy or surgical intervention. Studies are currently under way investigating the efficacy of new oral anticoagulant therapies (dabigatran etexilate, rivaroxaban, apixaban) for the treatment of VTE.

Anticoagulation

Unfractionated heparin

UFH is bound non-specifically to plasma and cellular proteins, is renally excreted, has an unpredictable dose response and a narrow therapeutic window; it therefore needs monitoring. It is usually administered by a continuous intravenous infusion after an initial loading dose (loading dose 80 U/kg followed by an infusion of 18 U/kg per hour) with subsequent dose adjustments made to maintain an APTT ratio of 1.5–2.5. Randomised clinical trials have shown that treatment with i.v. UFH for 5–7 days followed by more prolonged treatment with an oral anticoagulant is as efficacious as longer treatment with i.v. UFH.[64] Haemorrhage occurs in up to 5% of individuals receiving UFH infusions, the risk being greater in the elderly and those receiving antiplatelet therapies. Care should be taken to monitor for HIT (see above). Long-term treatment with UFH is associated with osteoporosis, and it is now rarely used in this fashion. Oral anticoagulation (see below) should be started concurrently with UFH, and the UFH stopped when the INR is therapeutic on two consecutive days.[64]

Low-molecular-weight heparins

LMWHs are made by depolymerisation of UFH, either by chemical or enzymatic means. Their predominant mode of action is to inhibit anti-Xa activity, although all have variable anti-IIa activity. In comparison to UFH, they have more reliable pharmacokinetics and a greater bioavailability, can be given by once or twice daily weight-adjusted subcutaneous administration and do not, routinely, require monitoring. In certain circumstances, however (e.g. in renal impairment or elderly patients with low body weight), monitoring may be of benefit. Peak anti-Xa levels should be measured 3–4 hours after LMWH injection, the therapeutic range being 1.0–2.0 IU/mL with once-daily injection and 0.5–1.0 IU/mL with twice-daily injections. The risk of bleeding is less with LMWH compared with UFH, as is the risk of HIT (platelet count monitoring should still be undertaken; see above).

 Studies have shown that for the treatment of DVT, outpatient LMWH administration at therapeutic licensed dosages is as safe and efficacious as UFH infusion.[64]

LMWHs have been shown to be as safe and effective as UFH in treating non-massive haemodynamically stable PE, but the optimal dosing schedule (once or twice daily) remains controversial. Studies are under way investigating the safety of outpatient PE management with LMWH.

LMWHs are the treatment of choice for VTE in pregnancy, as warfarin is teratogenic. As the half-life of LMWH in pregnancy is shorter, twice-daily regimens should be utilised for pregnant patients. Furthermore these patients should be managed in consultation with an obstetrician and a haematologist with an interest in obstetric haematology.[62]

Cancer patients deserve a specific mention. Studies comparing LMWH to standard warfarin anticoagulation in patients with acute VTE and malignancy demonstrated a significant reduction in the occurrence of recurrent VTE without an increase in bleeding in those receiving LMWH.[46] Although there was no reduction in mortality, LMWH was well tolerated and avoided the necessity of frequent INR checks; it therefore should be considered for patients with malignancy and VTE, especially whilst undergoing chemotherapy, which can cause unstable INRs.

Fondaparinux

Fondaparinux is a pentasaccharide which exerts a selective anti-Xa anticoagulant effect via antithrombin. Once-daily, subcutaneous, fixed-dose fondaparinux (7.5 mg subcutaneously once daily for patients 50–100 kg in weight) has been shown to be as effective and safe as UFH and LMWH for the management of acute symptomatic DVT and PE, and has a licence for these indications. Whilst it is more expensive than UFH and LMWH, it does not need monitoring, nor has it been associated with the development of HIT.[65]

Oral anticoagulation

Warfarin (or other coumarins) remains the treatment of choice for the majority of patients with VTE as, despite its obvious shortcomings, it is currently the only oral anticoagulant available. It has a narrow therapeutic window, there is considerable variability in dose response between subjects, it has numerous drug and food interactions and requires regular monitoring. All too frequently, there are dosing problems due to patient non-adherence or miscommunication between patient and health professional. Warfarin inhibits the metabolism of vitamin K, which is required for the essential post-translational modification (carboxylation) of the vitamin K-dependent coagulation factors (factors II, VII, IX and X). The rate of inhibition of these coagulation factors is dependent on their rate of synthesis; factor VII (with a half-life of 6 h) is rapidly inhibited, whereas it takes considerably longer for the activity of factor II (with a half-life of 72 h)

to fall. It usually takes 4–7 days for the activities of these vitamin K-dependent coagulation factors to fall to a level at which the patient is therapeutically anticoagulated.

Warfarin is monitored by the INR (derived from the prothrombin time). The early increase in the INR is due to the rapid fall in the activity of factor VII; therefore 'bridging' anticoagulation with UFH, LMWH or fondaparinux should be continued until the INR is >2 on two consecutive days. The target INR for a patient with DVT or PE (unless the thrombosis occurred on warfarin) is 2.5. Not surprisingly the most serious adverse complication of oral anticoagulation is bleeding. The risk is directly related to the intensity of anticoagulation and the length of therapy, and is greatest in the elderly, those with unstable anticoagulation and those with significant concomitant illnesses (including past history of gastrointestinal bleeding, renal or liver failure, anaemia, uncontrolled hypertension). The risk of major bleeding with coumarin anticoagulation is reported to be 0.5–6.5% per year, and fatal bleeding 0.1–1.0% per year.[66] For patients newly starting warfarin anticoagulation it is not (yet) possible to predict their dose, and induction algorithms (such as the modified Fennerty algorithm) should be used to guide dosing. Induction algorithms utilising a number of different variables (sex, age, weight, drug information, presence or absence of genetic polymorphisms in the CYP 2C9 and VKORC1 genes) are under investigation.

Duration of anticoagulation

There remains uncertainty about the optimal duration of anticoagulation following a VTE.

At least 3 months of anticoagulant therapy is required after a proximal DVT or PE; 3 months is probably sufficient if associated with a transient risk factor, whereas at least 6 months of anticoagulation should be advised for an idiopathic event. Calf vein thromboses, if diagnosed, should be treated with anticoagulation for 6–12 weeks.[67]

There is a very high risk of recurrence if 3 months of anticoagulation is given for a proximal idiopathic DVT.

Two recent studies have been performed with the aim of investigating whether low-intensity anticoagulation (target INR 1.5–2.0) is effective at preventing recurrent VTE.

The PREVENT study demonstrated a significant reduction in recurrent VTE without an increased risk of bleeding when low-intensity anticoagulation was compared with placebo.[68] The ELATE study showed that low-intensity anticoagulation was less effective at preventing recurrent VTE than those anticoagulated with a target INR of 2.5, with no difference in bleeding risk between the two groups.[69] When comparing these studies, there is clearly a dose–response effect. Combining the data from these two studies, the cumulative thrombosis rate at a target INR of 2.5 was 2.5%, 7.5% with a target INR of 1.5–1.9/2.0, and 20% without warfarin after 4 years. Therefore a target INR of 2.5 is most effective for prevention of VTE, and as there was no difference in bleeding between the targets of 1.75 and 2.5, a target INR of 2.5 should be the target for patients requiring long-term anticoagulation for VTE prevention.

As active cancer and anticancer treatment both increase the risk of VTE, consideration should be given to continuing anticoagulation until active malignancy has resolved and anticancer treatment finished.

Thrombophilic patients with VTE

Whilst it is now clear that the mode of presentation of the thrombotic event (idiopathic or precipitated) influences the likelihood of recurrence,[12] the presence or absence of an inherited thrombophilia is not as helpful in predicting the likelihood of recurrence. When decisions are being made regarding duration of anticoagulation, clinical features of the thrombotic event, such as site and severity of thrombosis (e.g. massive PE), presence or absence of ongoing risk factors (e.g. cancer), thrombophilia (e.g. antithrombin deficiency) and family history should all be taken into account. Decisions regarding duration of anticoagulation will generally be the same irrespective of the presence of an inherited thrombophilia.[66]

Novel anticoagulants

There are a number of new anticoagulants under investigation for the treatment of VTE. These are predominantly direct thrombin (factor IIa) or factor Xa inhibitors. They do not require monitoring of their anticoagulant effect and do not have the dietary and drug interactions that warfarin does; therefore there are obvious advantages when compared to warfarin. Ximelagatran, a direct thrombin inhibitor, underwent phase III trials for the successful treatment of VTE in 2002/03;[70] unfortunately, significantly abnormal liver function tests occurred in up to 10% of patients taking ximelagatran, so it did not come to market.

Currently, dabigatran etexilate (another direct thrombin inhibitor), rivaroxaban and apixaban (both direct Xa inhibitors) are undergoing phase III trials in VTE treatment and results appear promising.

Other treatments

Inferior vena caval (IVC) filters

There is only one randomised trial of the use of vena caval filters in the management of VTE.

 Four hundred patients with proximal DVT considered to be at high risk of PE were randomised to filter placement or not. At day 12 there were fewer new PEs in the filter group but no significant difference in symptomatic PE. By 2 years, symptomatic DVT was significantly more frequent in the filter group, that finding persisting at 8 years. The incidence of PE was significantly reduced in the group that had IVC filters in situ at 8 years (6.2% vs. 15.1%). These results suggest that IVC filters provide protection against PE, but are associated with a greater risk of DVT and provide no reduction in mortality.[71]

The remainder of the evidence for IVC filter use comes predominantly from descriptive case series; therefore there is little robust evidence to guide the clinician on their use. Both permanent and retrievable filters are available (some may be retrieved up to a few months after insertion). It is recommended that insertion of an IVC filter be considered to prevent PE in patients with VTE and a contraindication to anticoagulation; this includes patients with recent VTE who require cessation of anticoagulation for surgery. Anticoagulation should be commenced if the contraindication to its use resolves, and should be considered for all patients with IVC filters in situ (dependent on perceived risks of thrombosis from disease and bleeding associated with anticoagulant therapy). It is also reasonable to consider IVC filter insertion in patients who have PE despite therapeutic anticoagulation. If the indication for the filter is temporary, retrievable filters should be used (and then removed) if possible.

Thrombolysis

Thrombolysis has been used for the treatment of DVT, initially given systemically and more recently by local catheter. The major argument for the use of thrombolytic therapy in the treatment of DVT is to prevent the development of the post-thrombotic syndrome (PTS). It remains uncertain, however, whether the risk of PTS developing is reduced with thrombolytic therapy of the initial DVT.[63]

Nevertheless, thrombolytic therapy should be considered for patients with recent-onset massive ileofemoral DVT who remain at risk of limb gangrene secondary to venous occlusion despite anticoagulant therapy.

Thrombolysis is used for the treatment of massive (life-threatening, causing cardiogenic shock) PE. Thrombolysis achieves clot lysis more rapidly than anticoagulation alone, accelerates the reduction in pulmonary vascular obstruction, potentially increasing pulmonary perfusion and gas exchange.

It is now generally agreed that patients with PE resulting in cardiogenic shock are best treated with thrombolysis plus anticoagulation.[63] Although others have suggested that patients with right ventricular dysfunction should receive thrombolysis, due to the bleeding risk associated with thrombolytic therapy this has not been widely adopted.[60]

Prevention of venous thromboembolic disease: thromboprophylaxis

There is good evidence that most hospital patients have at least one risk factor for VTE (see above). Most studies of the prevention of VTE have used angiography or more recently ultrasonography to confirm the presence of a thrombotic event, with the majority of these being subclinical below-knee DVTs. Nevertheless, as there is a strong association between asymptomatic DVT and the development of symptomatic VTE (proximal DVT or PE),[8] it is necessary to institute strategies to reduce the risk to patients of developing a thrombosis. It is possible to identify groups at high risk of VTE, but not the specific patient who will go on to develop a thrombosis. Nor is it possible to identify the patient who might develop a sudden massive PE. In 70–80% of patients dying of a PE in hospital, a diagnosis of VTE was not considered prior to autopsy, and most patients with PE have had no symptoms suggestive of DVT. The prevalence of postoperative PE is now considerably lower than it was some years ago due to the use of improved surgical and anaesthetic techniques, early mobilisation of patients and the systematic introduction of chemical thromboprophylaxis. It is now well recognised that hospitalised medical patients (especially those with heart or respiratory failure, cancer, inflammatory disease or acute infection) are also at risk of VTE, and a number of well-conducted trials (MEDENOX, PREVENT, ARTEMIS)[72-74] have demonstrated the benefit of chemical thromboprophylaxis in this patient group. However, despite these trial findings, thromboprophylaxis remains poorly utilised in medical patients.

There are now many guidelines making recommendations for the reduction in the risk of VTE in surgical patients (and in other patient groups). These include the 2007 NICE (National Institute for Clinical Excellence) guideline 46 'Reducing the risk of VTE in inpatients undergoing surgery', the 2002 SIGN (Scottish Intercollegiate Guideline Network) publication Number 62 'Prophylaxis of venous thromboembolism' and the 2004 ACCP guideline 'Prevention of venous thromboembolism'.[8] What these guidelines have in common is the recommendation that patients be assessed for their risk of developing a venous thromboembolic event, based on both their individual predisposing factors and the risk associated with their illness or proposed surgical procedure (Table 14.5). Patients assessed as being at high risk of VTE should be given thromboprophylaxis. Major surgery is generally defined as surgery of >30 minutes duration.

Methods of thromboprophylaxis

Mechanical

Mechanical methods of prophylaxis include graduated elastic compression hosiery (GECS), intermittent pneumatic compression (IPC) devices, and venous foot-pumps. These methods are designed to reduce venous stasis and improve venous flow in the leg veins.

GECS devices have a compression profile of 18 mmHg at the ankle, 14 mmHg mid-calf and 8 mmHg at the knee. They are simple, safe when applied correctly (care should be taken not to apply in those with severe peripheral vascular disease) and moderately efficacious at preventing VTE without any increased risk of bleeding.

In 1994, a comprehensive meta-analysis concluded that graduated compression stockings produced a highly significant risk reduction in postoperative venous thomboembolic disease of 68% in moderate-risk patients.[75] A recent review of stockings in both surgical and medical patients confirmed their effectiveness in reducing risk of venous thromboembolic disease, particularly when used on a background of other methods of prophylaxis.[76]

There are a number of different manufacturers of IPC devices, which supply intermittent low pressure (typically 40 mmHg) for 1 minute with a 90-second period of decompression. This increases the velocity of venous return and blood flow and may also enhance fibrinolysis[77] and inhibition of the tissue factor

Table 14.5 • Levels of thromboembolism risk in surgical patients without prophylaxis

Level of risk	DVT (%)		PE (%)		Successful prevention strategies
	Calf	Proximal	Clinical	Fatal	
Low risk Minor surgery in patients <40 years with no additional risk factors	2	0.4	0.2	<0.001	No specific prophylaxis Early and 'aggressive' mobilisation
Moderate risk Minor surgery in patients with additional risk factors Major surgery in patients 40–60 years without additional risk factors	10–20	2–4	1–2	0.1–0.3	Prophylactic UFH (b.d.) or LMWH (3400 U daily), mechanical prophylaxis
High risk Major surgery in patients >60 years, or 40–60 years with additional risk factors	20–40	4–8	2–4	0.4–1.0	Prophylactic UFH (t.d.s.), LMWH (>3400 U daily), intermittent pneumatic compression
Highest risk Surgery in patients with multiple risk factors Hip or knee arthroplasty, hip fracture surgery Major trauma Spinal cord injury	40–80	10–20	4–10	0.2–5	LMWH (>3400 U daily), fondaparinux, oral coumarin (INR 2–3), or mechanical methods plus UFH/LMWH

Adapted from Geerts WH et al. Prevention of venous thromboembolism: the Seventh ACCP Conference on Antithrombotic and Thrombolytic Therapy. Chest 2004; 126(3, Suppl):338S–400S.[8] With permission from the American College of Chest Physicians.

pathway.[78] The two meta-analyses mentioned above[75,76] of the use of mechanical methods for thromboprophylaxis reported DVT rates of 9.9% and 17.6% for IPC versus 20.3% and 27% for placebo.

There is a newer high-pressure, rapid-inflation pneumatic compression device which can be used either as a foot pump alone, or a combination of foot and calf compression.

A Cochrane review in 2003 of the efficacy of mechanical pumping devices in hip fracture found that their use may protect against DVT and PE (7% with pumps vs. 22% without).[79] A randomised comparison of IPC and LMWH in 442 trauma patients showed similarly low rates of thromboembolic and bleeding complications, with the authors recommending use of IPC for thromboprophylaxis on the grounds of cost-effectiveness.[80]

A major limitation in the studies of mechanical thromboprophylaxis is the relatively small numbers of patients included. When used alone in high-risk procedures they appear to lack efficacy, and further assessment of their role is required.

Pharmacological methods

Many drugs have now been used in the prophylaxis of DVT. It has been known since 1959 that warfarin anticoagulation reduces significantly the incidence of thromboembolic disease when it is used as prophylaxis.[81] This method is not routinely used by surgeons, however, mainly because of the considerable risk of haemorrhage, either spontaneous or related to the surgery.

Aspirin

The Medical Research Council sponsored a double-blind, placebo-controlled study of 303 surgical patients which showed no reduction in postoperative

DVT with 600 mg aspirin taken immediately before and for 5 days after surgery.[82] A meta-analysis of thromboprophylaxis following total hip replacement including data from 56 randomised trials showed no benefit for aspirin in preventing DVT.[83] In the meta-analysis of the Antiplatelets Trialists' Collaboration,[84] aspirin was found to reduce DVT significantly, although the poor quality of some studies included has led to many doubts regarding this finding. However, aspirin may have a role in prophylaxis of low-risk groups.[84]

The largest randomised study comparing aspirin with placebo was carried out between 1992 and 1998 in surgical patients who required surgery for hip fracture or elective hip arthroplasty.[85] Aspirin (160 mg per day) or placebo were administered, but other thromboprophylaxis as was thought necessary could be given. Heparin was given in 26% of cases and GECS in 30%. The benefits of aspirin were confined to the hip fracture patients where 1.6 % of those who received aspirin had an objective VTE, compared with 2.5% receiving placebo. The data showed a trend towards a greater reduction after the first postoperative week, suggesting a benefit for extended prophylaxis. There was an excess of gastrointestinal bleeding in the aspirin group.

From the results of these studies,[82–85] aspirin appears to have some efficacy in the prevention of VTE, but as yet there is no evidence that it is the drug of choice as there are no studies directly comparing it with other pharmacological agents which are of proven efficacy, and the ACCP 2004 guidelines[8] advised against its use for thromboprophylaxis.

Heparins

The use of low-dose UFH for thromboprophylaxis has now largely been superseded by LWMH due to the latter's superior bioavailability, once-daily dosing and the reduced incidence of HIT.

A meta-analysis of UFH prophylaxis in surgery showed a reduction in DVT and PE by two-thirds when compared to placebo, with a 2% increase in minor bleeding events.[86] Studies have consistently shown reductions in DVT and PE by two-thirds with both UFH and LMWH, with a slightly reduced risk of bleeding with LMWH compared with UFH. Two meta-analyses have shown superior results with LMWH after total hip replacement with regard to postoperative DVT (risk reduction of 17–32%) and PE (risk reduction

of 50%).[87,88] Higher doses of LMWH should be given to high-risk general surgical patients as these provide greater protection than lower doses. In cancer patients, prophylaxis with dalteparin 5000 U daily was shown to be significantly more effective than 2500 U daily, without an increased risk of bleeding.[89]

As mentioned earlier, monitoring for HIT should be undertaken in all surgical patients receiving thromboprophylactic doses of UFH or LMWH.

Other agents

Fondaparinux is more effective than LMWH in preventing VTE following orthopaedic surgery (incidence of VTE with enoxaparin 13.7% compared with 6.8% with fondaparinux).[90] Fondaparinux does, however, have a longer half-life and is more expensive than the LMWHs. It is for these reasons that LMWHs remain the most frequently used drugs for thromboprophylaxis in orthopaedic surgery.

Dabigatran etexilate, an oral direct thrombin inhibitor has just been granted a licence for thromboprophylaxis in hip and knee replacement surgery.

In hip replacement surgery, 6.0% of patients receiving dabigatran 220 mg once daily had thromboses, compared to 6.7% in the enoxaparin 40 mg once-daily group.[91] After total hip replacement surgery, 36.4% of patients receiving dabigatran were shown to have venous thromboses, compared to 37.7% of those receiving enoxaparin. There was no increase in bleeding in those receiving dabigatran.[92]

Other oral anticoagulants (including rivaroxaban and apixaban, both anti-Xa agents) are undergoing studies for thromboprophylaxis and treatment of VTE.

Duration of thromboprophylaxis

Patients remain at increased risk of VTE once discharged after a surgical procedure. Clinical trials of extended prophylaxis (4 weeks of LMWH vs. 1 week LMWH) after general surgery showed a significant reduction in venographically detected thromboses in those with cancer.[8,93] Similarly, studies in patients undergoing hip replacement surgery have shown reductions in venographically detectable VTE with extended prophylaxis with LMWH.[94]

NICE guideline 46 recommended that all surgical patients receive mechanical thromboprophylaxis (thigh-length elastic compression hosiery), that all patients undergoing hip fracture, hip replacement or knee replacement surgery receive LMWH or fondaparinux, and that other patients undergoing major surgery receive LMWH if any other patient-related risk factors for VTE are present. The guideline also recommended that chemical thromboprophylaxis continue for 4 weeks for those having hip replacement or hip fracture surgery.[94,95]

Summary of methods of prophylaxis

The clinical evidence available shows effective prevention of DVT with LMWH and low-dose UFH, but at the cost of a small risk of potentially clinically significant bleeding. Mechanical methods have no associated risks but are probably less effective in prevention. Combinations of LMWH and mechanical methods, particularly GECS, have shown superior efficacy in DVT prevention in several studies. There is little evidence to support the use of aspirin for thromboprophylaxis. Newer agents such as dabigatran will become available in the next few years and will increase the available options for prophylaxis. Pending the results of ongoing trials, the following recommendations are generally applicable. In low-risk patients chemical thromboprophylaxis is unnecessary as the risk of thrombosis does not warrant the risk of bleeding associated with such therapies.[96] Moderate-risk patients should be given LMWH (unless there are major risks of haemorrhage), and lower doses may be sufficient. High-risk patients should be given higher-dose prophylactic LMWH (or fondaparinux or dabigatran etexilate) and should also receive mechanical thromboprophylaxis.

Key points

- Thromboembolic disease predominantly affects the elderly, being vanishingly rare in children. The risk is increased in young and middle-aged adults with the presence of inherited and acquired risk factors.
- Thromboembolism is common, developing in up to 25% of general surgical and over 40% of orthopaedic patients in the absence of thromboprophylaxis. PE is a well-recognised complication of surgery, and a significant cause of perioperative morbidity and death. There are frequently no signs of DVT prior to the onset of PE.
- Patients can be identified to be at risk of VTE both by surgical (i.e. procedure) and patient (i.e. thrombophilia or cancer) related factors. Undertaking a risk assessment and using appropriate thromboprophylaxis will reduce the risk of VTE.
- HIT is a relatively common complication of UFH and LMWH therapy, whether used for prophylaxis or treatment of VTE. Regular monitoring of the platelet count should be undertaken for the first 14 days of treatment, and HIT considered if the platelet count falls or the patient develops a thrombosis.
- If VTE is suspected, appropriate diagnostic strategies should be undertaken utilising clinical pretest probability, D-dimer assays and, where appropriate, imaging investigations. If there is a delay in investigation, if moderate or high risk, then therapeutic anticoagulation should be commenced.
- Anticoagulation for 5 days with UFH or LMWH is the mainstay of treatment for DVT and PE. If anticoagulation is contraindicated, IVC filter insertion should be considered.
- Thromboprophylaxis with a combination of mechanical and pharmacological agents (LMWH, fondaparinux or dabigatran etexilate) is effective in high-risk surgical patients. Further studies to evaluate the efficacy of newer mechanical methods are needed.

References

1. White RH. The epidemiology of venous thromboembolism. Circulation 2003; 107(23, Suppl):I4–8.

2. Naess IA, Christiansen SC, Romundstad P et al. Incidence and mortality of venous thrombosis: a population-based study. J Thromb Haemost 2007; 5:692–9.

3. Chalmers EA. Epidemiology of venous thromboembolism in children and neonates. Thromb Res 2006; 118:3–12.

4. Cohen AT, Agnelli G, Anderson FA et al. Venous thromboembolism in Europe. Thromb Haemost 2007; 98:756–64.

5. Buller HR, Sohne M, Middeldorp S. Treatment of venous thromboembolism. J Thromb Haemost 2005; 3:1554–60.

6. Spencer FA, Lessard D, Emery C et al. Venous thromboembolism in the outpatient setting. Arch Intern Med 2007; 167(14):1471–5.

7. Kearon C. Natural history of venous thromboembolism. Circulation 2003; 107(23):I22–30.

8. Geerts WH et al. Prevention of venous thromboembolism: the Seventh ACCP Conference on Antithrombotic and Thrombolytic Therapy. Chest 2004; 126(3, Suppl):338S–400S.

9. Pineda LA, Hatahwar VS, Grant BJ. Clinical suspicion of fatal pulmonary embolism. Chest 2001; 120(3):791–5.

10. Hansson PO, Sorbo J, Eriksson H. Recurrent venous thromboembolism after deep vein thrombosis: incidence and risk factors. Arch Intern Med 2000; 160(6):769–74.

11. Heit JA, Mohr DN, Silverstein MD et al. Predictors of recurrence after deep vein thrombosis and pulmonary embolism: a population-based cohort study. Arch Intern Med 2000; 106(6):761–8.

12. Baglin T, Luddington R, Brown K et al. Incidence of recurrent venous thromboembolism in relation to clinical and thrombophilic risk factors: prospective cohort study. Lancet 2003; 362:523–6.

13. Warlow C et al. Deep venous thrombosis of the legs after strokes. Part I: Incidence and predisposing factors. Br Med J 1976; 1:1178–83.

14. Comerota AJ et al. Operative venodilation: a previously unsuspected factor in the cause of postoperative deep vein thrombosis. Surgery 1989; 106:301–9.

15. Flynn PD et al. Thrombin generation by apoptotic vascular smooth muscle cells. Blood 1997; 89:4378–84.

16. Juhan-Vague I, Valadier J, Alessi MC et al. Deficient t-PA release and elevated PA inhibitor levels in patients with spontaneous or recurrent deep venous thrombosis. Thromb Haemost 1987; 57:67–72.

17. Thomas DP. Pathogenesis of venous thrombosis. In: Bloom AL, Forbes CD, Tuddenham EGD (eds) Haemostasis and thrombosis, 3rd edn. Edinburgh: Churchill Livingstone, 1994; pp. 1327–33.

18. Hamilton G, Platt SA. Deep vein thrombosis. In: Beard JD, Gaines PA (eds) Vascular and endovascular surgery. London: WB Saunders, 1998; pp. 351–96.

19. Gillet JL, Perrin MR, Allaert FA. Short-term and mid-term outcome of isolated symptomatic muscular calf vein thrombosis. J Vasc Surg 2007; 46(3):513–19.

20. Egeberg O. Inherited antithrombin deficiency causing thrombophilia. Thromb Diath Haemorrh 1965; 13:516–30.

21. Rosendaal FR. Risk factors for venous thrombotic disease. Thromb Haemost 1999; 82(2):610–19.

22. Lane DA et al. Inherited thrombophilia: part 1. Thromb Haemost 1996; 76:651–62.

23. Tait RC, Walker ID, Reitsma PH et al. Prevalence of protein C deficiency in the healthy population. Thromb Haemost 1995; 73(1):87–93.

24. Dahlback B et al. Familial thrombophilia due to a previously unrecognized mechanism characterized by poor anticoagulant reponse to activated protein C: prediction of a cofactor to activated protein C. Proc Natl Acad Sci USA 1993; 90:1004–8.

25. Lijfering WM, Coppens M, Veeger NJ et al. Hyperhomocysteinemia is not a risk factor for venous and arterial thrombosis, and is associated with elevated factor VIII levels. Thromb Res 2008 (Epub ahead of print).

26. Cristina L et al. High plasma levels of factor VIII and risk of recurrence of venous thromboembolism. Br J Haematol 2004; 124(4):504–10.

27. Ohira T, Cushman M, Tsai MY et al. ABO blood group, other risk factors and incidence of venous thrombembolism: the Longitudinal Investigation of Thromboembolism Etiology (LITE). J Thromb Haemost 2007; 5:1455–61.

28. Bolton-Maggs PH et al. The rare coagulation disorders review with guidelines for management from the United Kingdom Haemophilia Centre Doctors' Organisation. Haemophilia 2004; 10:593–628.

29. Zwicker J, Bauer KA. Thrombophilia. In: Kitchens CS, Alving BA, Kessler CM (eds) Consultative hemostasis and thrombosis. Elsevier Science, 2002; pp. 181–96.

30. Rand JH. The antiphospholipid syndrome. Hematology Am Soc Hematol Educ Program 2007; 136–42.

31. Galli M et al. Lupus anticoagulants are stronger risk factors for thrombosis than anticardiolipin antibodies in the antiphospholipid syndrome: a systematic review of the literature. Blood 2003; 101:1827–32.

32. Warkentin TE et al. Heparin-induced thrombocytopenia: recognition, treatment and prevention: the

Seventh ACCP Conference on Antithrombotic and Thrombolytic Therapy. Chest 2004; 126:311–37.

33. Keeling D, Davidson S, Watson H. The management of heparin-induced thrombocytopenia. Br J Haematol 2006; 133:259–69.

34. Wu O et al. Oral contraceptives, hormone replacement therapy, thrombophilias and risk of venous thromboembolism: a systematic review. The Thrombosis: Risk and Economic Assessment of Thrombophilia Screening (TREATS) Study. Thromb Haemost 2005; 94(1):17–25.

35. Rosendaal FR, Van Hylckama Vlieg A, Tanis BC et al. Estrogens, progestogens and thrombosis. J Thromb Haemost 2003; 1:1371–80.

36. Jick S et al. Further results on the risk of non-fatal venous thrombembolism in users of the contraceptive transdermal patch compared to users of oral contraceptives containing norgestimate and 35 μg of ethinyl estradiol. Contraception 2007; 76(1):4–7.

37. Daly E, Vessey MP, Hawkins MM et al. Risk of venous thromboembolism in users of hormone replacement therapy. Lancet 1996; 348:977–80.

A systematic review of the literature on VTE and thrombophilia in women using oral estrogen preparations that confirmed the increased risk of VTE with third-generation oral contraceptives.

38. Jick H, Derby LE, Myers MW et al. Risk of hospital admission for idiopathic venous thromboembolism among users of postmenopausal oestrogens. Lancet 1996; 348:981–3.

A case control study that confirmed a threefold increased risk of venous thromboembolic disease in current HRT users.

39. Grodstein F, Stampfer MJ, Goldhaber SZ et al. Prospective study of exogenous hormones and risk of pulmonary embolism in women. Lancet 1996; 348:983–7.

A prospective population-based study of the influence of HRT and the cOCP which confirmed the increased risk of PE with these preparations.

40. Wu O. Postmenopausal hormone replacement therapy and venous thromboembolism. Gend Med 2005; 2(Suppl A):S18–27.

41. Symington IS, Stack BH. Pulmonary thromboembolism after travel. Br J Dis Chest 1977; 71:138–40.

42. Chee YL, Watson H. Air travel and thrombosis. Br J Haematol 2005; 130:671–80.

43. Kuipers S et al. The absolute risk of venous thrombosis after air travel: a cohort study of 8755 employees of international organizations. PLoS Med 2007; 4(9):e290.

44. Cannegieter SC et al. Travel-related venous thrombosis: results from a large population-based case control study (MEGA study). PLoS Med 2006; 3(8):e307.

45. Prandoni P et al. Risk stratification and venous thromboprophylaxis in hospitalized medical and cancer patients. Br J Haematol 2008; 141:587–97.

46. Lee AY et al. Low-molecular-weight heparin versus a coumarin for the prevention of recurrent venous thromboembolism in patients with cancer. N Engl J Med 2003; 349(2):146–53.

The first study of extended LMWH anticoagulation for VTE. It demonstrated a clear reduction in recurrent thromboses in patients with VTE and cancer compared to adjusted-dose coumarin with no increase in bleeding.

47. White RH et al. Incidence of symptomatic venous thromboembolism after different elective or urgent surgical procedures. Thromb Haemost 2003; 90:446–55.

48. Thromboembolic Risk Factors (THRIFT) Consensus Group. Risk of, and prophylaxis for, venous thromboembolism in hospital patients. Br Med J 1992; 305:567–74.

Seminal consensus on risk stratification for venous thromboembolic disease in hospital populations.

49. Arumilli BR, Lenin Babu V, Paul AS. Painful swollen leg think beyond deep vein thrombosis or Baker's cyst. World J Surg Oncol 2008; 6:6.

50. Wells PS. Integrated strategies for the diagnosis of venous thromboembolism. J Thromb Haemost 2007; 5(Suppl 1):41–50.

51. Wells PS, Anderson DR, Bormanis J et al. Value of assessment of pretest probability of deep vein thrombosis in clinical management. Lancet 1997; 350:1795–8.

52. Keeling D et al. The Haemostasis and Thrombosis Task Force of the British Committee for Standards in Haematology. The diagnosis of deep vein thrombosis in symptomatic outpatients and the potential for clinical assessment and D-dimer assays to reduce the need for diagnostic imaging. Br J Haematol 2004; 124(1):15–25.

53. Kearon C, Julian AJ, Newman TE et al. Noninvasive diagnosis of deep vein thrombosis. Ann Intern Med 1998; 128:663–77.

54. Goodacre S, Sampson F et al. Measurement of the clinical and cost-effectiveness of non-invasive diagnostic testing strategies for deep vein thrombosis. Health Technol Assess 2006; 10(15):1–168, iii–iv.

55. The British Thoracic Society Standards of Care Committee, Pulmonary Embolism Guideline Development Group. BTS Guidelines for the Management of Suspected Acute Pulmonary Embolism, 2003. Thorax 2003; 48:470–84.

56. Wells PS, Anderson DR, Rodger M et al. Derivation of a simple clinical model to categorize patients probability of pulmonary embolism: increasing the models utility with the SimpliRED d-dimer. Thromb Haemost 2000; 83:416–20.

57. Writing group for the Christopher Study Investigators. Effectiveness of managing suspected

pulmonary embolism using an algorithm combining clinical probability, D-dimer testing, and computed tomography. JAMA 2006; 295:172–9.

58. The PIOPED Investigators. Value of the ventilation/perfusion scan in acute pulmonary embolism. Results of the prospective investigation of pulmonary embolism diagnosis (PIOPED). JAMA 1990; 263:2753–9.

59. Anderson DR, Kahn SR, Rodger MA et al. Computed tomographic pulmonary angiography vs ventilation perfusion lung scanning in patients with suspected pulmonary embolism. JAMA 2007; 298(23):2743–53.

60. Garcia D et al. Update on the diagnosis and management of pulmonary embolism. Br J Haematol 2005; 131:301–12.

61. Clemens S, Leeper KV. Newer modalities for detection of pulmonary emboli. Am J Med 2007; 120(10, Suppl 2):S2–12.

62. Royal College of Obstetricians and Gynaecologists Green Top Guideline No. 28. Thromboembolic disease in pregnancy and the puerperium: acute management.

63. Barritt DW, Jordan SC. Anticoagulant drugs in the treatment of pulmonary embolism. A controlled trial. Lancet 1960; 1:627S–644S.

   The initial, seminal study which demonstrated the effectiveness of anticoagulation for the management of PE.

64. Buller H et al. Antithrombotic therapy for venous thromboembolic disease: the Seventh ACCP Conference on Antithrombotic and Thrombolytic Therapy. Chest 2004; 126:401–28.

   Evidence-based guideline for the use of anticoagulants for the treatment of VTE recommending that outpatient LMWH is as safe as UFH for the management of DVT (grade I recommendation).

65. Shorr AF et al. Minimizing costs for treating deep vein thrombosis: the role for fondaparinux. J Thromb Thrombolysis 2007; 23(3):229–36.

66. Makris M et al. The management of coumarin-induced over-anticoagulation. Br J Haematol 2001; 114(2):271–80.

67. Baglin TP et al. Guidelines on oral anticoagulation (warfarin): third edition 2005 update. Br J Haematol 2006; 132:277–85.

68. Ridker PM, Goldhaber SZ, Danielson E et al. Long-term, low-intensity warfarin therapy for the prevention of recurrent venous thromboembolism. N Engl J Med 2003; 348:1425–34.

   This randomised placebo-controlled trial of low-intensity warfarin versus placebo for the prevention of recurrent VTE confirmed that VTE was reduced by warfarin anticoagulation.

69. Kearon C, Ginsberg JS, Kovacs MJ et al. (2003) Comparison of low-intensity warfarin therapy with conventional intensity warfarin therapy for long-term prevention of recurrent venous thromboembolism. N Engl J Med 2003; 349:631–9.

   A randomised double-blind study comparing warfarin target INR 2.5 to warfarin target INR 1.9 in the long-term prevention of VTE. It demonstrated that conventional-dose anticoagulation is superior to low-dose anticoagulation in the prevention of recurrent events.

70. Schulman S et al. Secondary prevention of venous thromboembolism with the oral direct thrombin inhibitor Ximelagatran. N Engl J Med 2003; 349:1713–21.

71. The PREPIC Study Group. Eight-year follow-up of patients with permanent vena cava filters in the prevention of pulmonary embolism: the PREPIC (Prevention du Risque d'Embolie Pulmonaire par Interruption Cave) randomized study. Circulation 2005; 112:416–22.

72. Samama MM et al. A comparison of enoxaparin with placebo for the prevention of venous thromboembolism in acutely ill medical patients. Prophylaxis in medical patients with enoxaparin study group. N Engl J Med 1999; 341:793–800.

73. Leizorovicz A et al. A randomized placebo controlled trial of dalteparin for the prevention of venous thromboembolism in 3706 acutely ill medical patients: the PREVENT medical thromboprophylaxis study trial. Circulation 2004; 110:874–9.

74. Cohen AT, Alikhan R, Arcelus JI et al. Assessment of venous thromboembolism risk and the benefits of thromboprophylaxis in medical patients. Thromb Haemost 2005; 94:750–9.

75. Wells PS, Lensing AW, Hirsh J. Graduated compression stockings in the prevention of postoperative venous thromboembolism. A meta-analysis. Arch Intern Med 1994; 154:67–72.

   Graduated compression stockings significantly reduce venous thromboembolic disease in moderate-risk patients (insufficient evidence in high-risk orthopaedic surgery).

76. Amaragiri SV, Lees TA. Elastic compression stocking for the prevention of deep vein thrombosis (Cochrane review). Cochrane Library, 2004; issue 1.

   A review of randomised controlled trials that confirms the efficacy of stockings in prevention of venous thromboembolic disease in hospitalised patients.

77. Comerota AJ, Chouhan V, Harada RN et al. The fibrinolytic effects of intermittent pneumatic compression: mechanism of enhanced fibrinolysis. Ann Surg 1997; 226:306–13.

78. Chouhan VD, Comerota AJ, Sun L et al. Inhibition of tissue factor pathway during intermittent pneumatic compression: a possible mechanism for antithrombotic effect. Arterioscler Thromb Vasc Biol 1999; 19:2812–17.

79. Handoll HHG, Farrar MJ, McBirnie J et al. Heparin, low molecular weight heparin and physical methods for preventing deep vein thrombosis and pulmonary embolism following surgery for hip fractures (Cochrane review). Cochrane Library, 2003; issue 4.

This updated Cochrane review confirms the efficacy of both LMWH and UFH in DVT prevention but finds insufficient evidence for pulmonary embolism; calf and foot pumps appear to prevent DVT.

80. Ginzburg E, Cohn SM, Lopez J et al. Randomized clinical trial of intermittent pneumatic compression and low molecular weight heparin in trauma. Br J Surg 2003; 90:1338–44.

Calf compression is as effective as LMWH in trauma patients.

81. Browse NL, Burnand KG, Irvine AT et al. Deep vein thrombosis: prevention. In: Browse NL, Burnand KG, Irvine AT. (eds) Diseases of the veins, 2nd edn. London: Arnold, 1999; pp. 359–83.

82. Watson H et al. Aspirin and other antiplatelet drugs in the prevention of venous thromboembolism. Blood Rev 2008; 22:107–16.

83. Imperiale TF et al. A meta-analysis of methods to prevent venous thromboembolism following total hip replacement. JAMA 1994; 271:1780–5.

84. Antiplatelet Trialists' Collaboration. Collaborative overview of randomized trials of antiplatelet therapy – III: Reduction in venous thrombosis and pulmonary embolism by antiplatelet prophylaxis among surgical and medical patients. Br Med J 1994; 308:235–46.

85. Pulmonary Embolism Prevention (PEP) Trial. Prevention of pulmonary embolism and deep vein thrombosis with low dose aspirin. Lancet 2000; 355:1295–302.

86. Collins R et al. Reduction in fatal pulmonary embolism and venous thrombosis by perioperative administration of subcutaneous heparin. Overview of results of randomized trials in general, orthopaedic and urological surgery. N Engl J Med 1988; 318:1162–73.

87. Leizorovicz A, Haugh MC, Chapuis FR et al. Low molecular weight heparin in prevention of perioperative thrombosis. Br Med J 1992; 305:913–20.

88. Nurmohamed MT, Rosendaal FR, Buller HR et al. Low-molecular weight heparin versus standard heparin in general and orthopaedic surgery: a meta-analysis. Lancet 1992; 340:152–6.

89. Bergqvist D, Burmark US, Flordal PA et al. Low molecular weight heparin started before surgery as prophylaxis against deep vein thrombosis: 2.500 versus 5000 Xai units in 2070 patients. Br J Surg 1995; 82:496–501.

This prospective, randomised, double-blind multicentre study confirmed the superior efficacy of higher doses of LMWH for thromboprophylaxis in cancer patients undergoing surgery.

90. Turpie AG et al. Superiority of fondaparinux over enoxaparin in preventing venous thromboembolism in major orthopedic surgery using different efficacy end points. Chest 2004; 126(2):501–8.

91. Eriksson BI et al. Dabigatran etexilate versus enoxaparin for prevention of venous thromboembolism after total hip replacement: a randomized, double-blind, non-inferiority trial. Lancet 2007; 370:949–56.

92. Eriksson BI et al. Oral dabigatran etexilate versus subcutaneous enoxaparin for the prevention of venous thromboembolism after total knee replacement: the REMODEL randomized trial. J Thromb Haemost 2007; 5:2178–85.

The above two studies were randomised, double-blind, comparative studies of dabigatran etexilate versus enoxaparin, which confirmed the effectiveness of dabigatran in the prevention of VTE with no increase in bleeding.

93. Bergqvist D, Lowe GD, Berstad A et al. Prevention of venous thromboembolism after surgery: a review of enoxaparin. Br J Surg 1992; 79:495–8.

94. Comp PC, Spiro TE, Friedman RJ et al. Prolonged enoxaparin therapy to prevent venous thromboembolism after primary hip or knee replacement. Enoxaparin Clinical Trial Group. J Bone Joint Surg Am 2001; 83A(3):336–45.

95. Eriksson BI, Lassen MR et al. Duration of prophylaxis against venous thromboembolism with fondaparinux after hip fracture surgery: a multicenter, randomized, placebo-controlled, double-blind study. PENTasaccharide in HIp-FRActure Surgery Plus Investigators. Arch Intern Med 2003; 163(11):1337–42.

96. Bounameaux H. Integrating pharmacologic and mechanical prophylaxis of venous thromboembolism. Thromb Haemost 1999; 82:931–7.

15

Patient assessment and surgical risk

Euan J. Dickson
Peter S. Chong

Introduction

Risk can be defined as a *concept* denoting a potential negative outcome that may arise from a future *event*. In the healthcare model it can be applied to three entities: patients, staff and system. **Patient assessment** is a means of attempting to quantify this negative impact in order to reduce risk to these entities, to enable informed discussion and decision-making with patients and relatives, and to ensure adequate infrastructure and resources prior to undertaking a given procedure.

Surgical risk from the patient's perspective broadly encompasses two factors: morbidity and mortality. It may also apply to staff, for example in exposure-prone procedures, and to the medical organisation in terms of efficiency and litigation. The principle aim of this chapter is to focus on surgical risk to the patient. Surgical risk can be further subdivided into **procedural risk**, e.g. anastomotic leak, and **patient-centred risk**, e.g. perioperative myocardial infarction. These constitute morbidity, and clearly either or both can lead to patient mortality.

The General Medical Council (GMC) has issued guidance on this matter[1] and defines the risk of proposed investigation or treatment using four criteria (Box 15.1).

Box 15.1 • GMC definition of risk of investigation/treatment

1. Side-effects
2. Complications
3. Failure of an intervention to achieve the desired aim
4. The potential outcome of taking no action

Why assess surgical risk?

Surgical risk assessment is a vital part of modern practice and has two major components. Firstly, what do we aim to achieve by investigating or treating the *patient*? Secondly, what can we expect of the patient's *physiology*? Answering these questions preoperatively helps to quantify risk for the individual patient and enhances *surgical decision-making*. This in turn facilitates the informed consent process and *patient decision-making*. It allows the anaesthetic and surgical team to make preprocedural preparation with respect to skill mix, equipment and logistical capabilities required during the perioperative phase. A further positive effect of this process is to aid *case mix adjustment*. There is increasing public release of activity/outcome figures, or 'league tables', in surgery which may be crude mortality or complication rates. Case mix adjustment allows units with a greater proportion of *high-risk patients* to compensate for any differences in their figures with respect to national outcomes. The overall aims of this complex process are summarised in Box 15.2.

Box 15.2 • Why assess surgical risk?

1. Allow informed consent
2. Facilitate surgical decision-making
3. To anticipate adverse events
4. To minimise risk to patients, staff and healthcare system

How can we assess surgical risk?

Broadly speaking we can assess surgical risk either *subjectively* or *objectively*, but the reality is that risk prediction is often a combination of both. **Subjective risk assessment** includes patient history, clinical examination, pattern recognition, accumulated clinical experience and, perhaps above all, 'the end of the bed test'. There are in fact data to support the concept that 'gut instinct' or surgical intuition can be more effective than formal risk prediction models in identifying the patient with a poor prognosis in the context of a particular procedure,[2] especially in the elective setting.[3] **Objective risk assessment** includes formal laboratory results, assessment of comorbidity and physiological function and an ever-increasing number of **risk prediction models and scoring systems**. Of these objective assessments, this chapter will focus predominantly on measuring surgical risk with the various models and scoring systems available.

Risk prediction models and scoring systems

Surgical risk prediction tools have been developed to objectively estimate morbidity and mortality rates for individual patients prior to the proposed intervention. It should be noted that there is no perfect tool, that the models available must not be used to guide decision-making in isolation and that there is probably no substitute for the combination of objective markers with surgical experience and intuition. Furthermore, the models available pertain to populations rather than individual patients, and therefore have limitations which need to be recognised before using them to inform surgical risk assessment. For example, the mortality rate for a surgical intervention in a particular population may be 5%, but for the individual patient it can only be 0% or 100%.

The scoring systems available usually incorporate physiological and comorbid data that have been selected using logistical regression techniques in a large database of patients, which may not be similar to the local population. A *coefficient* may be assigned in order to weight the variables and the resulting equation provides a *numerical indication of risk* for the patient, although it is frequently more meaningful to the operating surgeon. There are a variety of different systems available to the clinician and many are situation specific, although they are increasingly applied outwith the original setting in which they were validated. Examples of situation-specific models are given in Table 15.1.

Ideally the patients in the database on which the scoring system is developed and validated should be similar to the individual patient in question.

Table 15.1 • Examples of situation-specific risk prediction models

Facility	Intensive care unit	APACHE
Surgical procedure	Oesophagectomy	O-POSSUM
Pathology	Acute pancreatitis	Imrie Score
Physiological warning signs	Critically ill patient	MEWS

However, publication bias may mean that only the best data are published. While this has inherent flaws, it may also be viewed as an opportunity to benchmark one's own results against those from a centre of excellence.

Scoring systems

APACHE

The Acute Physiology and Chronic Health Evaluation (APACHE) system was developed between 1979 and 1981 to measure severity of illness in the intensive care unit patient. The original system consisted of two parts: an acute physiology score (weights 1–4), which indicated the extent of 34 potential acute physiological abnormalities, and a chronic health evaluation measured using a questionnaire which classified patients (A–D) according to their pre-existing health status. The score correlated well with hospital mortality, but the system was cumbersome, not validated and did not include probability calculations.

APACHE II

Introduced in 1985, APACHE II incorporated several important changes to the original system.[4] The number of physiological values was reduced from 34 to 12 by eliminating variables that were infrequently measured, redundant or of low clinical priority. The method for chronic health evaluation was also altered, abandoning the health status questionnaire and awarding points to reflect diminished physiological reserve due to ageing, immune deficiency and chronic cardiac, pulmonary, renal or liver disease.

APACHE II scores have a range of 0–71 and are based on three components (Table 15.2):

- the degree of abnormality of 12 physiological measures (acute physiology score);
- increasing age;
- chronic health abnormalities.

APACHE II physiology scoring is performed using worst values obtained in the first 24 hours in the intensive care unit (ICU), and reflects severity of

Table 15.2 ● -APACHE II

	Acute physiology score								
	+4	+3	+2	+1	0	+1	+2	+3	+4
Core temperature (°C)	≥41	39–40.9		38.2–38.9	36–38.4	34–35.9	32–33.9	30–31.9	≤29.9
Mean blood pressure (mmHg)	≥160	130–159	110–129		70–109		50–69		≤49
Heart rate (beats/min)	≥180	140–179	110–139		70–109		55–69	40–54	≤39
Respiratory rate (breaths/min)	≥50	35–49	25–34		12–24	10–11	6–9		≤5
If $F_iO_2 ≥ 0.5$: $A – aDO_2$ (mmHg)	≥500	350–499	200–349						
If $F_iO_2 < 0.5$: PO_2 (mmHg)		>70		<200	61–70		55–60	≤55	
Arterial pH	≥7.7	7.6–7.69		7.5–7.59	7.33–7.49		7.25–7.32	7.15–7.24	≤7.15
Serum Na⁺ (mmol/L)	≥180	160–179	155–159	150–154	130–149		120–129	111–119	≤110
Serum K⁺ (mmol/L)	≥7	6–6.9		5.5–5.9	3.5–5.4	3–3.4	2.5–2.9		<2.5
Serum creatinine (µmol/L)	≥300	171–299	121–170		50–120		<50		
N.B. double points score if acute renal failure									
Haematocrit (%)	≥60		50–59.9	46–49.9	30–45.9		20–29.9		<20
Leucocytes (per mm³)	≥40		20–39.9	15–19.9	3–14.9		1–2.9		<1
Neurological points = 15 – Glasgow Coma Score									

Age points

Years	≤44	45–54	55–64	65–74	≥75
Points	0	2	3	5	6

Chronic health evaluation points

2 points for elective postoperative admission or 5 points if emergency operation or non-operative admission, if patient has either:

- Biopsy-proven cirrhosis, portal hypertension or previous hepatic failure
- Chronic heart failure (NYHA grade 4)
- Chronic hypoxia, hypercapnia, severe exercise limitation, secondary polycythaemia or pulmonary hypertension
- Dialysis-dependent renal disease
- Immunosuppression by disease or drugs

illness and an escalating risk of hospital death. A weighting to reflect the prognostic impact of emergency surgery is added to reflect its independent effect on mortality. In addition the principal diagnosis leading to ICU admission is added as a category weight, with a choice of 40 disease and eight organ system categories. The APACHE II mortality prediction equation uses these scores and additional weightings to give a risk of death.

Problems with APACHE II

- It is outdated – one of the major limitations of APACHE II is that its risk predictions are based on the outcomes measured over 20 years ago and much has changed in intensive care therapy since then.
- The system was never designed to predict mortality for individual patients, and decisions about a patient's care need to take into consideration many aspects not covered by scoring systems.
- Selection bias refers to errors in prediction caused by differences in how patients, for whom outcomes are to be predicted, are actually selected compared with the criteria that were used in creating the reference database, i.e. it only works for the type of patients it was developed on. It does not work for burns or cardiothoracic patients, performs poorly in trauma patients and is not useful for children (under 15 years old).
- Lead-time bias refers to errors in prediction due to variations in the timing of intensive care admission. Scoring time starts after admission to ICU so a patient who has been aggressively resuscitated prior to admission will have a lower score than one treated in a similar way after admission.
- Some elements of the score are highly weighted (e.g. reduced Glasgow Coma Scale (GCS)), which is reasonable if the GCS is reduced due to brain injury, but not so if it is reduced due to something reversible, such as drugs or metabolic coma.
- Variation in data collection (there are some very subjective elements) will introduce variations in the predicted scores.

Despite these limitations, APACHE II has been validated in many countries and is widely used for a number of purposes. It has been used as a tool in clinical research as the score allows risk stratification of patients entered into research studies.

This capability has been used in outcome studies among patients with a broad range of diagnoses and in therapeutic trials, where the score measured at study entry ensures that treatment and control groups have an equivalent severity of illness.

A second major use of APACHE II has been to examine and compare the quality of intensive care as reflected by patient outcome. Many units collect APACHE II data to follow their own activity over time and compare against other units. The standardised mortality ratio (SMR) is often used to assess outcome, with an observed and predicted (by APACHE II) mortality being compared; an SMR >1 suggests outcomes worse than expected, while an SMR <1 implies the opposite. There are, however, many criticisms levelled against the use of SMR.

In North American and European studies, risk factors for disease have been combined with APACHE II scores to estimate group death rates which are compared with actual deaths as a measure of performance across ICUs.[5, 6] Observations of variation in ICU performance may then allow the identification of factors that are associated with improved outcome.

Finally, APACHE II has been used in studies aimed at optimising the allocation of intensive care resources, as patients with higher scores are at greater risk of requiring organ support.

APACHE III

APACHE III was developed in 1991 to expand and improve the prognostic estimates provided by APACHE II. The APACHE III database was collected between 1988 and 1990 and included data on patient and institutional characteristics of 17 440 intensive care admissions in the USA.[7]

Using equations constructed from the APACHE III database, the system can predict outcome. An APACHE III equation predicts hospital mortality for groups of intensive care admissions by linking first-day patient characteristics to the reference database. Although these predictions are based on patient outcomes between 1988 and 1990, they have been updated based on outcomes between 1993 and 1996 for over 37 000 intensive care admissions in the USA. Prognostic estimates use the APACHE III score and additional variables to reflect disease and selection for intensive care.

Patient selection is accounted for by weights reflecting whether ICU readmission or emergency surgery occurred, and hospital length of stay and location prior to ICU admission. These variables are included to control, at least in part, for differences in patient selection and response (or lack of response) to previous therapy, i.e. for selection and lead-time bias. When individual prognostic estimates are aggregated to the unit level, comparisons of actual and predicted outcomes provide a method for assessing ICU performance.[8]

In addition to hospital mortality, equations incorporating similar but not identical variables are used to predict outcomes which reflect intensive care resource use. These first-day capabilities include predictions of subsequent intensive care and hospital stay, therapeutic intervention score, risk for active life-supporting therapy, frequency of laboratory testing, and duration of mechanical ventilation.

The ability to predict an individual patient's probability of survival depends on assessment of response to therapy over time. The APACHE III prognostic system uses daily assessment of acute physiology scores to achieve this prediction. An individual's probability of hospital mortality is updated daily using a series of equations based on the patient's status on ICU day 1, on physiological status during the current day, and on physiological trends over the last 24 hours. These daily prognostic estimates can then be used to assist in making decisions about individual patients.[9]

As with any clinical measurement or investigation, those using the information from any of the APACHE scoring systems must consider their limitations. Missing values and data entry are potential sources of error and the confidence interval for each estimate widens for each successive day. Trends are more important than absolute values, and some indicators of response to therapy are not measured by the physiological variables. APACHE is now in its fourth revision but the latest versions have not been used as extensively as the more user-friendly APACHE II.

POSSUM

The Physiological and Operative Severity Score for the enUmeration of Mortality and morbidity (POSSUM) was first described in 1991.[10] It was designed as a scoring system to estimate morbidity and mortality following a surgical procedure and, by including data on the patient's physiological condition, it provides a *risk-adjusted prediction* of outcome. This facilitates more accurate comparison of hospital or surgeon performance. It can be used as an audit and clinical governance tool, and to provide information for individual patients as part of the consent process. POSSUM is the most widely applied, validated, surgical risk scoring system in the UK and has been modified by several authors to provide specialty-specific information. It may also need to be adjusted in the elderly as both POSSUM and P-POSSUM (see below) over-predict mortality in the group of patients undergoing major elective

Box 15.3 • POSSUM formula

$$\text{Ln } R/1 - R = -7.04 + (0.13 \times \text{physiological score}) + (0.16 \times \text{operative severity score})$$

gastrointestinal surgery. This may be corrected if an individual unit adjusts the calculations based on its own patient series.[11]

The original POSSUM score was developed after initially subjecting 62 parameters to multivariate analysis in order to determine the most powerful outcome predictors. Twelve physiological and six operative parameters were identified, and each of these factors were weighted to a value of 1, 2, 4 or 8 to simplify the calculation (Box 15.3).

P-POSSUM (Portsmouth)

The original POSSUM equation was derived using exponential analysis. It was re-evaluated in 1998 in Portsmouth by Whiteley et al., who reported concerns that it overestimated mortality in their patients, particularly in the lowest risk group, in which death was over-predicted by a factor of six.[12] They modified the POSSUM formula and, by subjecting the original 18 variables to linear analysis, they constructed the Portsmouth predictor equation for mortality (P-POSSUM). The modified formula (Box 15.4) returns a minimum predicted risk of mortality of 0.2% rather than 1.08% for the lowest risk group, and fitted well with the observed mortality rate. The P-POSSUM model, however, still overestimates mortality in low-risk groups and in certain surgical subspecialties. The latter finding has prompted the development of specialty-specific POSSUM for major elective surgery.

CR-POSSUM (Colorectal)

The value of POSSUM and P-POSSUM in predicting in-hospital mortality was examined in patients undergoing colorectal surgery in France. They were also compared to the AFC index (French Association for Surgery: Association Française de Chirurgie). P-POSSUM performed well but overestimated postoperative death in elective surgery twofold. POSSUM, however, overestimated postoperative death in all cases and the authors concluded that it had not been validated in France in the field of colorectal surgery. The predictive value of the AFC index was also good. It had the same sensitivity and specificity as P-POSSUM but required simpler calculations.[13]

Box 15.4 • P-POSSUM formula

$$\text{Ln } R/1 - R = -9.065 + (0.1692 \times \text{physiological score}) + (0.1550 \times \text{operative severity score})$$

The original POSSUM score and P-POSSUM were derived from a heterogeneous population of general surgical patients. They were analysed further with respect to high-risk colorectal surgery and found to under-predict death in the emergency patients.[14] There was also a lack of calibration of POSSUM and P-POSSUM at the extremes of age in both emergency and elective work. The authors concluded that remodelling the original scores may facilitate their application in colorectal surgery.

In 2004 the same group then reported a dedicated POSSUM system for patients undergoing colorectal surgery. This Colorectal-POSSUM model (CR-POSSUM) was developed by subjecting prospectively collected data to stepwise logistic regression analysis. After exclusions, the final study cohort included 4632 elective patients and 2107 emergency patients undergoing colorectal surgery in 15 UK hospitals between 1993 and 2001. An age-adjusted POSSUM model was also developed. The CR-POSSUM model was superior to both the age-adjusted model and P-POSSUM in predicting operative mortality.[15]

External validation of CR-POSSUM was provided in a review of predictive models for estimating postoperative mortality in patients undergoing colorectal surgery. Data were derived from three multicentre, UK studies involving a total of 16 006 patients: the original CR-POSSUM study population ($n = 6883$), the Association of Coloproctology of Great Britain and Ireland (ACPGBI) Colorectal Cancer (CRC) Database ($n = 8077$) and the ACPGBI Malignant Bowel Obstruction (MBO) Study ($n = 1046$). Of the models tested, CR-POSSUM was superior in predicting postoperative death.[16]

This conflicted to a certain extent with a later study in New Zealand involving 308 patients undergoing major colorectal surgery. In this cohort POSSUM, P-POSSUM and CR-POSSUM were all satisfactory predictive tools for postoperative mortality but the latter tended to be relatively less accurate. However, the authors noted that CR-POSSUM requires fewer individual patient parameters to be calculated and is therefore simpler to use.[17]

CR-POSSUM is not an accurate predictor of disease-specific colorectal mortality. A study from the Netherlands on patients undergoing elective sigmoid resection for either carcinoma or diverticular disease demonstrated that CR-POSSUM over-predicted mortality in the patients with malignant disease and under-predicted it in patients with benign disease. However, in the whole group CR-POSSUM predicted postoperative mortality accurately.[18]

A possible modification to the CR-POSSUM system was suggested following a single-centre UK study in 304 patients. CR-POSSUM proved to be a more accurate predictive model than POSSUM and P-POSSUM, and interestingly logistic regression demonstrated a significant correlation between albumin and mortality. It may be possible to improve the accuracy of CR-POSSUM further by modifying the equation to include serum albumin.[19]

O-POSSUM (Oesophagogastric)

A UK study of 204 patients demonstrated that POSSUM did not accurately predict morbidity and mortality in patients undergoing oesophagectomy.[20] A dedicated oesophagogastric model developed in a study population of 1042 patients was described in 2004. The O-POSSUM model used the following independent factors: age, physiological status, mode of surgery, type of surgery and histological stage. It provided a more accurate risk-adjusted prediction of death from oesophageal and gastric surgery for individual patients than P-POSSUM.[21] To date there have been several conflicting studies examining the predictive value and accuracy of O-POSSUM. A Dutch study of 663 patients undergoing potentially curative oesophagectomy in a tertiary referral centre (in-hospital mortality 3.6%) demonstrated that O-POSSUM over-predicted in-hospital mortality threefold and could not identify those patients with an increased risk of death.[22] This was confirmed in a smaller study in the UK ($n = 313$, in-hospital mortality 10.2%), which found that neither P-POSSUM nor O-POSSUM accurately predicted the risk of postoperative death. Again, O-POSSUM over-predicted total mortality whilst P-POSSUM had superior discriminatory power.[23] The most recent study evaluating the POSSUM models for predicting mortality in patients undergoing elective oesophagectomy was reported by a group in Hong Kong. The observed in-hospital mortality rate in 545 patients undergoing thoracic oesophagectomy for squamous cell carcinoma was 5.5%. In contrast, the rates predicted by POSSUM, P-POSSUM and O-POSSUM were 15.0%, 4.7% and 10.9% respectively. POSSUM over-predicted mortality across nearly all risk groups, whereas O-POSSUM over-predicted mortality in patients with low physiological scores and in older patients. The authors concluded that P-POSSUM provided the most accurate prediction of in-hospital mortality in patients undergoing oesophagectomy.[24] In summary, the data reported in the original study to construct O-POSSUM have not been validated in other centres. It may be that individual units have to modify the O-POSSUM model to take account of local factors.

V-POSSUM (Vascular)

A modification of the original POSSUM score – V-POSSUM – was devised for use specifically in patients undergoing arterial surgery. One study examined the records of 1313 patients and added 'extra items' to the original POSSUM dataset, although this did not appear to significantly improve the accuracy of prediction.[25] The model has, however, been used in further studies and has been modified further to only take account of the physiology component of the score (V-POSSUM physiology only). Before these modifications, the original POSSUM score was used for comparative audit in different vascular units.[26] Although P-POSSUM has been shown to be a better model for predicting death in both elective and emergency patients undergoing major arterial surgery in a single surgeon study, the data are conflicting.[27] For example, POSSUM is a reasonable model following elective abdominal aortic aneurysm (AAA) repair,[28] though one study suggests that neither P-POSSUM nor V-POSSUM is accurate in predicting mortality in the context of ruptured aortic aneurysms.[25] This finding that V-POSSUM may be of limited value in the context of emergency arterial surgery was confirmed by a larger and more recent evaluation of the appropriate POSSUM models in the context of ruptured abdominal aortic aneurysms (RAAAs).[29] When the P-POSSUM, RAAA-POSSUM, RAAA-POSSUM (physiology only), V-POSSUM and V-POSSUM (physiology only) models were all compared in 223 patients with RAAA (in-hospital mortality was 32.4%), all except V-POSSUM and P-POSSUM (physiology only) demonstrated no significant lack of fit.

As one may expect, the various POSSUM models are not accurate predictive tools in the context of elective carotid surgery. Both POSSUM and V-POSSUM over-predicted mortality in a large single-centre study (*n* = 499) of patients undergoing carotid endarterectomy.[30] This is not surprising given the nature of the surgery, and the reduced surgical insult compared to body cavity procedures.

A recent evaluation of V-POSSUM in New Zealand has indicated that it is a useful tool not only in the assessment of outcome, but of longitudinal surgical performance in major vascular surgery. Major vascular procedures (*n* = 454) were prospectively scored for V-POSSUM over a 10-year period. There was a trend towards improved surgical performance over time, with a drop in the observed to predicted ratios of deaths. This novel role has not yet been tested in the other POSSUM models, but given these data there may be the potential to use them to evaluate surgical training and performance in other surgical subspecialties.[31]

The original POSSUM equation has undergone several modifications in an effort to increase its overall accuracy as a risk prediction tool for in-hospital surgical mortality. Of these, P-POSSUM is the most widely used and validated general modification. Specialty-specific POSSUM has also been developed for use in colorectal, oesophagogastric and vascular patients with some improvement in risk stratification. The available data, however, suggest that the various POSSUM models may have to be recalibrated and modified based on data from the local population before their introduction as an adjunct to surgical risk assessment.

ASA

In 1963 the American Society of Anesthesiologists (ASA) adopted a five-point classification system for assessing the physical status of a patient prior to elective surgery. A sixth category was added later (Box 15.5).

The ASA grade is essentially a combination of the subjective opinion of the anaesthetist taken in conjunction with a more objective assessment of the patient's general fitness for surgery, and is used routinely in most centres in the UK. There are a number of studies assessing the utility and accuracy of the ASA grade in determining surgical risk and, as anticipated given the nature of this scoring system, the literature is conflicting.

One study of 113 anaesthetists in the UK demonstrated such marked variation in the inter-individual assessment of 10 hypothetical patients that the authors concluded that the ASA grade should not be used on its own to predict surgical risk.[32] A further study of 97 anaesthetists demonstrated that the agreement for the assessment of each hypothetical patient varied from 31% to 85%. The overall correlation was only *fair*, and the inter-observer inconsistency was similar to that in a study from 20 years previously.[33]

However, that largest study to date is more encouraging.[34] Of 16 227 patients undergoing elective surgery over a 5-year period, 215 died within 4 weeks

Box 15.5 • ASA classification

1. A normal healthy patient
2. A patient with mild systemic disease
3. A patient with severe systemic disease
4. A patient with severe systemic disease that is a constant threat to life
5. A moribund patient who is not expected to survive without the operation
6. A declared brain-dead patient whose organs are being removed for donor purposes

Note: If the surgery is an emergency, the ASA grade is followed by 'E' (for emergency) for example '3E'. Category 5 is always an emergency so should not be written without 'E'. The category 6E probably does not exist.

of operation. There was a significant correlation between perioperative mortality and the ASA grade. The mortality was lowest (0.4%) when the ASA grade was less than or equal to 2 and increased up to 7.3% in ASA grade 4 patients. The authors concluded that perioperative mortality can be predicted using the ASA grade.

 The ASA classification remains a quick, simple, widely used and reasonably accurate assessment of surgical risk in both the elective and emergency settings.

Other disease-specific scoring systems

There are several other disease-specific scoring systems (e.g. for acute pancreatitis and trauma) and the reader is referred to Chapters 8 and 13 for further information.

Scoring systems – organ failure

Organ failure has in the past been considered to be a dichotomous state, being either present or absent as determined by arbitrary and variable criteria. The term 'multiple organ dysfunction syndrome'[35] evolved as a result of the need to recognise this clinical entity as a continuum of physiological dysfunction rather than as an all-or-nothing event. It is now clear that outcome is a function of the number of failing organ systems and of the severity of derangement within each system. This has generated interest in the development of objective scoring systems for quantifying organ dysfunction. Several systems have emerged,[36–38] but there is still no universally accepted method for judging severity of organ dysfunction, and new systems continue to evolve. Scores such as APACHE and SAPS (Simplified Acute Physiology Score, discussed later) describe the risk of death at the time of admission, and incorporate elements of the acute physiological problem and the patient's underlying physiological reserve (usually age and comorbidity). Organ dysfunction scores, on the other hand, aim to evaluate how a patient progresses after resuscitation and how organ system dysfunction evolves over time, thereby assessing morbidity.[39]

Assessment of organ failure

The measurement of organ dysfunction is dependent on the availability of a reliable variable that reflects physiological disturbance of the relevant organ system. On the whole, it is dysfunction that is measured rather than the therapeutic interventions that are employed as part of organ support.

In most scores the following six organ systems are included:

1. **Respiratory** – based on the P_aO_2/F_iO_2 ratio or the need for mechanical ventilation.
2. **Renal** – scored by blood urea and creatinine levels and presence of oliguria.
3. **Haematological** – assessed by platelet count, prothrombin time and activated partial thromboplastin time. A low haematocrit or an abnormal white cell count may be included.
4. **Hepatic** – the degree of hyperbilirubinaemia is most useful. Levels of the liver enzymes may give additional information.
5. **Cardiovascular** – hypotension is the most useful parameter. Inotropic support may be included, though this is clearly a therapeutic measure.
6. **Neurological** – the Glasgow Coma Scale (GCS) is used to assess neurological dysfunction. In sedated patients a normal GCS is usually assumed for the purposes of scoring organ dysfunction.

Gastrointestinal function is generally omitted in organ failure scores as an accurate assessment of gastrointestinal function is currently not possible.

MODS

The Multiple Organ Dysfunction Score (MODS) was structured using a methodologically rigorous approach which recognises the dynamic nature of organ dysfunction and provides a quantitative measure of organ dysfunction. The score was developed through a systematic review of the literature to identify which systems, and what abnormalities in those systems, defined organ dysfunction and was developed from data taken from 692 surgical ICU patients. The score variables reflect physiological disturbance rather than the therapeutic intervention employed to maintain a clinical end-point. MODS employs an equation for 'pressure-adjusted heart rate' as the main determinant of cardiovascular function, as no single and readily available parameter was viewed to reflect it (Table 15.3).

The standard MODS is calculated by summing the worst scores for each of the individual systems over the ICU stay. **Figure 15.1** demonstrates the increasing ICU and hospital mortality and increasing ICU length of stay seen with increasing MODS.

MODS can be used in a number of additional ways, such as the baseline score at admission, for

Table 15.3 • MODS

Organ system	0	1	2	3	4
Respiratory* PO_2/F_iO_2	>300	226–300	151–225	76–150	≤75
Renal† Serum creatinine (µmol/L)	≤100	101–200	201–350	351–500	>500
Hepatic Serum bilirubin (µmol/L)	≤20	21–60	61–120	121–240	>240
Cardiovascular‡ PAR	≤10.0	10.1–15.0	15.1–20.0	20.1–30.0	>30.0
Haematological Plalelet count (platelets/mL)	>120	81–120	51–80	21–50	≤20
Neurological§ GCS	15	13–14	10–12	7–9	≤6

Selected values are those obtained at a standard time of day (preferably morning) rather than the worst values during the day: missing data receive a score of zero.
* The PO_2/FO_2 ratio is calculated without reference to the use of mode of mechanical ventilation, and without reference to the use or level of positive end-expiratory pressure.
† The serum creatinine level is measured without reference to the use of dialysis.
‡ PAR, pressure-adjusted heart rate.
§ Glasgow Coma Score is preferably calculated by the patient's nurse, and is scored conservatively (for the patient receiving sedation or muscle relaxants, normal function is assumed unless there is evidence of intrinsically altered mentation).
Reproduced from Marshall JC, Cook DJ, Christou NV et al. Multiple organ dysfunction score: a reliable descriptor of a complex clinical outcome. Crit Care Med 1995; 23(10):1638–52. With permission from the Society of Critical Care Medicine/Lippincott, Williams & Wilkins.

serial scores on a daily basis, for new organ dysfunction developing after admission (ΔMODS) and in combination with mortality for combined outcome.

SOFA

The European Society of Intensive Care Medicine developed the Sepsis-related Organ Failure Assessment (SOFA) score as a measure of the degree of individual organ dysfunction in all critically ill patients. The elements of the score were developed at a consensus conference of intensivists and validated on 1449 general ICU patients in 40 European centres. Unlike MODS it incorporates aspects of treatment (mechanical ventilation and inotrope use), and different utilisation of these therapies by different units might alter SOFA scoring locally. It aims to assess morbidity and therefore complements other scales which focus on mortality (Table 15.4).

As with MODS, increasing SOFA scores correlate with increasing mortality (**Fig. 15.2**). A number of versions of the SOFA score are used, including initial SOFA score (0–24 hours), Delta-SOFA score (differences between subsequent scores), and the highest and mean SOFA scores obtained during the ICU stay.

Reasons for measurement of organ dysfunction

Prognosis
The degree of organ dysfunction early during the ICU stay is an important determinant of the ultimate risk of mortality. Organ dysfunction scores calculated within the first 24 hours of ICU admission correlate strongly with ultimate risk of mortality, ranging from 2% for patients with a score of 0, to 100% for patients with a score of greater than 12.[40]

Clinical trials
An objective measure of organ failure provides a means of stratifying patients in clinical trials and the trend in MODS over time provides an evaluation of net clinical improvement or deterioration

Figure 15.1 • Performance of the Multiple Organ Dysfunction Score in the entire study population. Increasing values of the score demonstrated a strong correlation with the intensive care unit (ICU) mortality rate **(a)** (stippled bars, development set; solid bars, validation set), with hospital mortality rate **(b)** and with the ICU stay in surviving patients **(c)**. Reproduced from Marshall JC, Cook DJ, Christou NV et al. Multiple organ dysfunction score: a reliable descriptor of a complex clinical outcome. Crit Care Med 1995; 23(10):1638–52. With permission from the Society of Critical Care Medicine/Lippincott, Williams & Wilkins.

to a given therapy. These measurements are more sensitive than mortality to clinically important effects of therapy, and can enhance studies by permitting smaller sample sizes.

ICU morbidity

The time course and magnitude of deteriorating organ function can give an indication of ICU morbidity. A quantitative measure of the degree of morbidity that develops following ICU admission can be obtained by calculating a ΔMODS, or a measurement of organ dysfunction over time. The ΔMODS provides a measure of ICU morbidity that can provide an important quality control measure. Mortality also increases incrementally with increasing values of the ΔMODS, an observation that is independent of admission organ failure score.[41]

It is easy to appreciate that organ dysfunction scores can influence discussions of prognosis with medical teams and families, but the greatest potential use of these scores is as an objective measure of clinical outcome that can be used in clinical trials, and systems for describing organ dysfunction are a requirement in studies of the pathophysiology of this complex condition.

Lastly, it must be remembered that all scoring systems are developed and validated on large patient populations and cannot be applied directly to decisions on individual patients. Scores that provide an estimate of predicted mortality should not be used to determine whether aggressive treatment should be withdrawn or escalated.

Scoring systems – critical care

SAPS

The Simplified Acute Physiology Score (SAPS) was published in 1984 and was based upon 14 biological and clinical variables which were measured during the first 24 hours of ICU admission.[42] It was designed to predict the risk of mortality in the intensive care patient and was evaluated in 679 consecutive patients (40% surgical) admitted to eight ICUs in France. SAPS replaced the Acute Physiology Score, which was a more complex and time-consuming method for predicting risk of death in this patient population.

The revised version of this score, SAPS II, was reported in 1993 and was based on a large, international multicentre study.[43] SAPS II was developed using patient data from 137 ICUs and included 13 152 patients in total. The new score comprised 17 variables: 12 physiology variables, age, type of admission (scheduled surgical, unscheduled surgical or medical) and three underlying disease variables (acquired immunodeficiency syndrome, metastatic cancer and haematological malignancy). SAPS II

Table 15.4 • SOFA score

	SOFA score			
	1	**2**	**3**	**4**
Respiration				
P_aO_2/F_iO_2 (mmHg)	<400	<300	<200	<100
(kPa)	(<53.3)	(<40)	(<26.7)	(<13.3)
			← with respiratory support →	
Coagulation				
Platelets (× 10^9/L)	<150	<100	<50	<20
Liver				
Bilirubin (mg/dL (μmol/L))	1.2–1.9	2.0–5.9	6.0–11.9	>12.0
	(20–32)	(33–101)	(102–204)	(>204)
Cardiovascular				
Hypotension*	MAP <70 mmHg	Dopamine < 5 or dobutamine (any dose)	Dopamine >5 or epinephrine ≤0.1 or norepinephrine ≤0.1	Dopamine >15 or epinephrine >0.1 or norepinephrine >0.1
Central nervous system				
Glasgow Coma Scale	13–14	10–12	6–9	<6
Renal				
Creatinine (mg/dL (μmol/L))	1.2–1.9	2.0–3.4	3.5–4.9	>5.0
or	(110–170)	(171–299)	(300–440)	(>440)
Urine output (mL/day)			<500	<200

* Adrenergic agents administered for at least 1 h (doses are in μg/kg per min). MAP, mean arterial pressure.

provided an accurate prediction of risk of death in the intensive care patient in this study.

There have been numerous studies over the past two decades examining the utility and accuracy of SAPS and SAPS II in risk prediction in different patient populations and also comparative research with other models. The remainder of this section focuses on SAPS II, which has essentially replaced the original scoring system. Although this model can be used to predict prognosis, compare ICU performance and to stratify patients for clinical research, it appears to share the same problems inherent in many of the other scoring systems in that it is population specific.[44] It may therefore require customisation,[45,46] recalibration[47] or validation in the target population[48] before use. One suggested method for improving the overall accuracy of this model, and to increase its utility as a comparative tool, is to combine regional data and then recalibrate as a national reference system to allow more meaningful comparison of quality of care and performance amongst units.[49] Perhaps the most effective method of recalibration in this context is to calculate new logistic regression coefficients and then validate the modified score within the target population as demonstrated in a large study of 22 Scottish ICUs (n = 10393 patients).[50]

SAPS II compared favourably to other models of risk prediction, including APACHE II, when analysed in the context of a large international ICU database (n = 14745 patients); both of these systems were superior to their older counterparts in this study.[5]

The application of SAPS II has been extended to include the initial set of variables in the patient presenting to the emergency department.[51] Although superior to the other models tested in this study, SAPS II only demonstrated moderate accuracy in predicting actual in-hospital death (area under the receiver operating characteristic curve 0.72, 95% CI 0.57–0.87). This serves as an important reminder that this scoring system has been designed and validated in the ICU setting and derived from variables collected during the initial 24 hours, rather than simply a general risk prediction model for the acutely unwell patient.

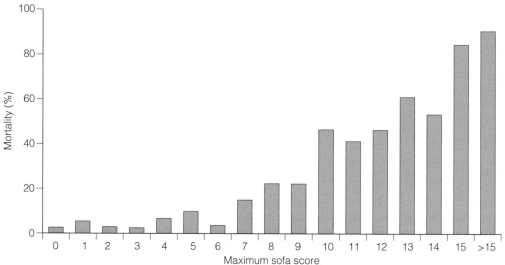

Figure 15.2 • Maximum Sequential Organ Failure Assessment (SOFA) score and mortality. Maximum SOFA score is defined as the highest score achieved by each patient during his/her ICU stay. Top: distribution of survivors (hatched bars) and non-survivors (solid bars) by maximum SOFA score; bottom: mortality rate associated with maximum SOFA score. The mortality rate was >90% in patients whose maximum SOFA score was >15. A cut-off value of a maximum SOFA score of 15 had a sensitivity of 30.7%, a specificity of 98.9% and a correct classification of 84.2%. Reproduced from Vincent JL et al. Use of the SOFA score to assess the incidence of organ dysfunction/failure in intensive care units: results of a multicenter, prospective study. Crit Care Med 1998; 16(11):1793–800. With permission from the Society of Critical Care Medicine/Lippincott, Williams & Wilkins.

Communicating risk

The use of risk prediction models and scoring systems as an adjunct to decision-making is an increasingly important part of surgical practice. This information must then be communicated effectively to the patient to allow fully informed choice. Recent guidance from the GMC states that:

"Clear, accurate information about the risks of any proposed investigation or treatment, presented in a way patients can understand, can help them make informed decisions. The amount of information about risk that the clinician should share with patients will depend on the individual patient and what they want,

or need, to know. Discussions with patients should therefore focus on their individual situation and the risk to them."[1]

Further recommendations by the GMC on the communication of risk to a patient are shown in Box 15.6.

Numbers or words?

In communicating risk there are several techniques to impart the concept of how likely it is that the patient will have a complication of the procedure, or die as a result of it. These broadly fall into using numerical data or descriptive details of risk. As always, this communication must be tailored to the needs and expectations of the individual patient and it is likely that a combination of these techniques will be most appropriate.

Percentages alone are often not well understood, and as they apply to a population rather than an individual patient, they may be misleading. Odds, relative risk and absolute risk may be too complex, but quoting for example 'a 1 in 10 or 1 in 100 chance' may be helpful. Using relativity (comparison with a concept the patient understands) or examples ('of the last 50 patients this has happened to …') may also clarify the concept of surgical risk to the patient.

Finally, it is worth remembering that the perceived surgical risk that concerns the surgeon is not necessarily what the patient is worried about. Assessing, discussing and communicating risk has the primary aim of allowing patients to understand what may happen to them, and to help them make an informed choice about investigation or therapeutic options. However, as a consequence of this, coupled with careful documentation, it affords the surgeon some protection against litigation.

Box 15.6 • GMC recommendations on the communication of risk to a patient

As well as all the elements of 'good medical practice', in the process of obtaining consent you should:

- Be patient tailored – involve the patient and make decisions together
- Identify potential adverse outcomes of the proposed action, and of no action
- Understand the patient's views and preferences
- Always tell of risks if they are very serious or very common
- Be balanced (benefits and risks)
- Be simple and clear
- Be consistent
- Be accurate
- Check the patient's understanding
- Allow the patient to ask questions
- Back up with other sources of information
- Document discussions clearly and accurately
- Know procedure if the patient refuses to hear the risks
- Keep up to date in your field so your information is likewise
- Give the patient time to reflect – a 'cooling off period'

Key points

- Surgical risk from the patient's perspective broadly encompasses two factors: morbidity and mortality. It can be further subdivided into procedural risk and patient-centred risk.
- Surgical risk includes side-effects, complications, failure of an intervention to achieve the desired aim, and the potential outcome of taking no action.
- Risk assessment is vital to quantify morbidity and mortality for the individual patient, to facilitate the informed consent process and to enhance surgical decision-making.
- Patient assessment includes subjective and objective tools. Of these, 'the end of the bed test' and risk prediction models/scoring systems are probably the most valuable.
- Surgical risk prediction tools have been developed to objectively estimate morbidity and mortality rates for individual patients prior to the proposed procedure, but **there is no perfect model**.
- The most widely used risk prediction tools for mortality include APACHE II, SAPS II and the various POSSUM models. These are an adjunct to, rather than a replacement for, surgical decision-making. They have been validated in specific populations which may not have similar characteristics to the individual patient in question.
- MODS and SOFA are probably the most useful systems for documenting organ failure and predicting the risk of mortality in the critically ill patient.
- In communicating surgical risk there are several techniques to impart the concept of how likely it is that the patient will have a complication of the procedure, or die as a result of it. This should be tailored to the individual patient and may include numerical data or descriptive details of risk.

References

1. GMC. Consent: patients and doctors making decisions together. General Medical Council, 2008.

2. Hartley MN, Sagar PM. The surgeon's 'gut feeling' as a predictor of post-operative outcome. Ann R Coll Surg Engl 1994; 76(6 Suppl):277–8.

3. Markus PM, Martell J, Leister I et al. Predicting postoperative morbidity by clinical assessment. Br J Surg 2005; 92(1):101–6.

4. Knaus WA, Draper EA, Wagner DP et al. APACHE II: a severity of disease classification system. Crit Care Med 1985; 13(10):818–29.

5. Castella X, Artigas A, Bion J et al. A comparison of severity of illness scoring systems for intensive care unit patients: results of a multicenter, multinational study. The European/North American Severity Study Group. Crit Care Med 1995; 23(8):1327–35.

6. Rowan KM, Kerr JH, Major E et al. Intensive Care Society's Acute Physiology and Chronic Health Evaluation (APACHE II) study in Britain and Ireland: a prospective, multicenter, cohort study comparing two methods for predicting outcome for adult intensive care patients. Crit Care Med 1994; 22(9):1392–401.

7. Knaus WA, Wagner DP, Draper EA et al. The APACHE III prognostic system. Risk prediction of hospital mortality for critically ill hospitalized adults. Chest 1991; 100(6):1619–36.

8. Zimmerman JE, Shortell SM, Knaus WA et al. Value and cost of teaching hospitals: a prospective, multicenter, inception cohort study. Crit Care Med 1993; 21(10):1432–42.

9. Wagner DP, Knaus WA, Harrell FE et al. Daily prognostic estimates for critically ill adults in intensive care units: results from a prospective, multicenter, inception cohort analysis. Crit Care Med 1994; 22(9):1359–72.

10. Copeland GP, Jones D, Walters M. POSSUM: a scoring system for surgical audit. Br J Surg 1991; 78(3):355–60.

11. Wakabayashi H, Sano T, Yachida S et al. Validation of risk assessment scoring systems for an audit of elective surgery for gastrointestinal cancer in elderly patients: an audit. Int J Surg 2007; 5(5):323–7.

12. Whiteley MS, Prytherch DR, Higgins B et al. An evaluation of the POSSUM surgical scoring system. Br J Surg 1996; 83(6):812–15.

13. Slim K, Panis Y, Alves A et al. Predicting postoperative mortality in patients undergoing colorectal surgery. World J Surg 2006; 30(1):100–6.

14. Tekkis PP, Kessaris N, Kocher HM et al. Evaluation of POSSUM and P-POSSUM scoring systems in patients undergoing colorectal surgery. Br J Surg 2003; 90(3):340–5.

15. Tekkis PP, Prytherch DR, Kocher HM et al. Development of a dedicated risk-adjustment scoring system for colorectal surgery (colorectal POSSUM). Br J Surg 2004; 91(9):1174–82.

16. Al-Homoud S, Purkayastha S, Aziz O et al. Evaluating operative risk in colorectal cancer surgery: ASA and POSSUM-based predictive models. Surg Oncol 2004; 13(2–3):83–92.

17. Vather R, Zargar-Shoshtari K, Adegbola S et al. Comparison of the POSSUM, P-POSSUM and Cr-POSSUM scoring systems as predictors of postoperative mortality in patients undergoing major colorectal surgery. Aust NZ J Surg 2006; 76(9):812–16.

18. Oomen JL, Cuesta MA, Engel AF. Comparison of outcome of POSSUM, p-POSSUM, and cr-POSSUM scoring after elective resection of the sigmoid colon for carcinoma or complicated diverticular disease. Scand J Gastroenterol 2007; 42(7):841–7.

19. Bromage SJ, Cunliffe WJ. Validation of the CR-POSSUM risk-adjusted scoring system for major colorectal cancer surgery in a single center. Dis Colon Rectum 2007; 50(2):192–6.

20. Zafirellis KD, Fountoulakis A, Dolan K et al. Evaluation of POSSUM in patients with oesophageal cancer undergoing resection. Br J Surg 2002; 89(9):1150–5.

21. Tekkis PP, McCulloch P, Poloniecki JD et al. Risk-adjusted prediction of operative mortality in oesophagogastric surgery with O-POSSUM. Br J Surg 2004; 91(3):288–95.

22. Lagarde SM, Maris AK, de Castro SM et al. Evaluation of O-POSSUM in predicting in-hospital mortality after resection for oesophageal cancer. Br J Surg 2007; 94(12):1521–6.

23. Nagabhushan JS, Srinath S, Weir F et al. Comparison of P-POSSUM and O-POSSUM in predicting mortality after oesophagogastric resections. Postgrad Med J 2007; 83(979):355–8.

24. Lai F, Kwan TL, Yuen WC et al. Evaluation of various POSSUM models for predicting mortality in patients undergoing elective oesophagectomy for carcinoma. Br J Surg 2007; 94(9):1172–8.

25. Prytherch DR, Sutton GL, Boyle JR. Portsmouth POSSUM models for abdominal aortic aneurysm surgery. Br J Surg 2001; 88(7):958–63.

26. Copeland GP, Jones D, Wilcox A et al. Comparative vascular audit using the POSSUM scoring system. Ann R Coll Surg Engl 1993; 75(3):175–7.

27. Midwinter MJ, Tytherleigh M, Ashley S. Estimation of mortality and morbidity risk in vascular surgery using POSSUM and the Portsmouth predictor equation. Br J Surg 1999; 86(4):471–4.

28. Irvine CD, Shaw E, Poskitt KR et al. A comparison of the mortality rate after elective repair of aortic aneurysms detected either by screening or incidentally. Eur J Vasc Endovasc Surg 2000; 20(4):374–8.

29. Bown MJ, Cooper NJ, Sutton AJ et al. The postoperative mortality of ruptured abdominal aortic aneurysm repair. Eur J Vasc Endovasc Surg 2004; 27(1):65–74.

30. Kuhan G, Abidia AF, Wijesinghe LD et al. POSSUM and P-POSSUM overpredict mortality for carotid endarterectomy. Eur J Vasc Endovasc Surg 2002; 23(3):209–11.

31. Mosquera D, Chiang N, Gibberd R. Evaluation of surgical performance using V-POSSUM risk-adjusted mortality rates. Aust NZ J Surg 2008; 78(7):535–9.

32. Haynes SR, Lawler PG. An assessment of the consistency of ASA physical status classification allocation. Anaesthesia 1995; 50(3):195–9.

33. Mak PH, Campbell RC, Irwin MG. The ASA Physical Status Classification: inter-observer consistency. American Society of Anesthesiologists. Anaesth Intensive Care 2002; 30(5):633–40.

34. Prause G, Ratzenhofer-Comenda B, Pierer G et al. Can ASA grade or Goldman's cardiac risk index predict peri-operative mortality? A study of 16,227 patients. Anaesthesia 1997; 52(3):203–6.

35. Bone RC, Balk RA, Cerra FB et al. Definitions for sepsis and organ failure and guidelines for the use of innovative therapies in sepsis. The ACCP/SCCM Consensus Conference Committee. American College of Chest Physicians/Society of Critical Care Medicine. Chest 1992; 101(6):1644–55.

36. Marshall JC, Cook DJ, Christou NV et al. Multiple organ dysfunction score: a reliable descriptor of a complex clinical outcome. Crit Care Med 1995; 23(10):1638–52.

37. Le G Jr, Klar J, Lemeshow S et al. The Logistic Organ Dysfunction system. A new way to assess organ dysfunction in the intensive care unit. ICU Scoring Group. JAMA 1996; 276(10):802–10.

38. Vincent JL, Moreno R, Takala J et al. The SOFA (Sepsis-related Organ Failure Assessment) score to describe organ dysfunction/failure. On behalf of the Working Group on Sepsis-related Problems of the European Society of Intensive Care Medicine. Intensive Care Med 1996; 22(7):707–10.

39. Marshall JC. Measuring organ dysfunction in the intensive care unit: why and how? Can J Anaesth 2005; 52(3):224–30.

40. Marshall JC. Multiple organ dysfunction syndrome (MODS). In: Sibbald WJ, Vincent JL (eds) Clinical trials for the treatment of sepsis. Berlin: Springer-Verlag, 1995; pp. 122–38.

41. Bernard GR et al. Quantification of organ failure for clinical trials and clinical practice. Am J Respir Crit Care Med 1995; 151:A323 (abstract).

42. Le G Jr, Loirat P, Alperovitch A et al. A simplified acute physiology score for ICU patients. Crit Care Med 1984; 12(11):975–7.

43. Le G Jr, Lemeshow S, Saulnier F. A new Simplified Acute Physiology Score (SAPS II) based on a European/North American multicenter study. JAMA 1993; 270(24):2957–63.

44. Lemeshow S, Le G Jr. Modeling the severity of illness of ICU patients. A systems update. JAMA 1994; 272(13):1049–55.

45. Le G Jr, Lemeshow S, Leleu G et al. Customized probability models for early severe sepsis in adult intensive care patients. Intensive Care Unit Scoring Group. JAMA 1995; 273(8):644–50.

46. Glance LG, Osler TM, Dick AW. Identifying quality outliers in a large, multiple-institution database by using customized versions of the Simplified Acute Physiology Score II and the Mortality Probability Model II0. Crit Care Med 2002; 30(9):1995–2002.

47. Harrison DA, Brady AR, Parry GJ et al. Recalibration of risk prediction models in a large multicenter cohort of admissions to adult, general critical care units in the United Kingdom. Crit Care Med 2006; 34(5):1378–88.

48. Moreno R, Miranda DR, Fidler V et al. Evaluation of two outcome prediction models on an independent database. Crit Care Med 1998; 26(1): 50–61.

49. Beck DH, Smith GB, Pappachan JV. The effects of two methods for customising the original SAPS II model for intensive care patients from South England. Anaesthesia 2002; 57(8):785–93.

50. Livingston BM, MacKirdy FN, Howie JC et al. Assessment of the performance of five intensive care scoring models within a large Scottish database. Crit Care Med 2000; 28(6):1820–7.

51. Jones AE, Fitch MT, Kline JA. Operational performance of validated physiologic scoring systems for predicting in-hospital mortality among critically ill emergency department patients. Crit Care Med 2005; 33(5):974–8.

16

Perioperative and intensive care management of the surgical patient

Michael Grounds
Andrew Rhodes

Introduction

Over the last 50 years the incidence of death directly attributable to anaesthesia has decreased. In the 1950s a number of studies demonstrated that the postoperative mortality solely associated with anaesthesia was approximately 1 in 2500[1–3] and by 1987, in the *Report of a confidential enquiry into perioperative deaths (CEPOD)*,[4] this cause of death had fallen to 1 in 185 000. This chapter deals with the perioperative and intensive care management of these patients with a specific focus on how ensuring that each patient has adequate cardiovascular performance for their needs during the perioperative period can reduce their risk of complications and death.

Postoperative critical care is a key factor to the improvement of outcome in surgical patients, particularly to those patients who are at high risk of postoperative morbidity and mortality. Thus postoperative critical care admission should always be considered when the preoperative physiological condition of the patient suggests that there is a reasonable probability or risk of postoperative complications and organ dysfunction. In order to provide this postoperative critical care it is obviously necessary to be able to identify these high-risk patients preoperatively.

How big is the problem?

In a recent analysis of over four million surgical procedures in the UK, a subgroup of high-risk patients was identified.[5] The mortality in this group of 513 924 patients was 12.3%. The overall mortality rates were 0.44% for elective and 5.4% for emergency surgery. This high-risk group of patients accounted for 83.8% of all deaths but only 12.5% of procedures. For the 31 633 patients admitted to an intensive care unit (ICU) electively there was a mortality rate of 10.1% and the 24 764 emergency surgical cases carried a mortality of 28.6%. Despite the high mortality rates, fewer than 15% of these patients were admitted to the ICU and the highest mortality rate (39%) was found in patients who required ICU admission following initial care in a ward environment.

Repeated publications by the National Confidential Enquiry into Postoperative Deaths (NCEPOD) have cited inadequate preoperative preparation, inappropriate intraoperative monitoring and poor postoperative care as contributing causes of perioperative mortality. The Department of Health issued guidelines as to which patients should be admitted to critical care units in 1996.[6] In particular, they suggested that postoperative patients who needed close monitoring for more than a few hours after surgery should be admitted. However, the great variation in underlying pathology and premorbid physiology of these patients makes it very difficult to provide hard and fast rules as to which patients will benefit from perioperative admission to either ICUs or high dependency units (HDUs). What is clear from a number of studies is that at present the care of patients before admission to ICU is often suboptimal.[7,8] This situation is partly exacerbated by the paucity of both ICU and HDU beds in the UK[9–11] and the fact that patients were often admitted later and with a worse severity of illness.

Why do patients die after surgery?

Major surgery is associated with a significant stress response[12] that is vital for the body to recover and heal from the surgical trauma. This reponse manifests in many different ways; however, a common delineating pattern is one of a hyperdynamic circulation with increased oxygen requirements from $110\,mL/min$ per m^2 at rest to $170\,mL/min$ per m^2 postoperatively.[13] If the body is unable to increase the cardiac output in response to the surgical stress, then the increased need for oxygen cannot be met and the patient develops tissue dysoxia and cellular dysfunction. This has been described by some authors as an acquired oxygen debt.[14] If left, this will result in organ failure and death. The important point to recognise is that the normal response to surgery is to increase the cardiac output and the delivery of oxygen to the tissues. Any patient who for whatever reason is unable to develop this response is at higher risk of subsequent complications.

What is a high-risk surgical patient?

The early identification of patients who are at high risk of postoperative complications and death is vital in order to ensure that correct care and therapy is initiated at an optimal time in order to reduce the associated morbidity and mortality. On the whole this patient group is characterised by undergoing major surgery whilst having concurrent medical illnesses that limit their physiological reserve to compensate for the stressful situation (Box 16.1). More sophisticated analyses of these relationships have been described. In particular, elective surgical patients can be assessed by cardiopulmonary exercise testing,[13,15] in which a strong correlation has been demonstrated between anaerobic threshold and perioperative mortality. The anaerobic threshold is the point where aerobic metabolism fails to provide adequate adenosine triphosphate and anaerobic metabolism starts to reduce the resultant deficit. The threshold is determined by monitoring inhaled and exhaled levels of oxygen and carbon dioxide during escalating levels of exercise. This provideds an objective measure of physiological reserve.

Box 16.1 • Criteria for identifying high-risk surgical patients developed by Shoemaker[14]

> Previous severe cardiorespiratory illness, including myocardial infarction, stroke, chronic obstructive pulmonary disease, etc., including admission to critical care unit for cardiorespiratory illness
>
> Late-stage vascular disease
>
> Age >70 years with limited physiological reserve, particularly limited cardiorespiratory reserve
>
> Extensive surgery for carcinoma: oesophagectomy, gastrectomy, cystectomy in patient with limited physiological reserve
>
> Acute abdominal catastrophe with haemodynamic instability: peritonitis, perforated viscus, pancreatitis
>
> Acute massive blood loss >8 units at time of surgery
>
> Proven septicaemia: positive blood culture or septic focus
>
> Acute respiratory failure: P_aO_2 <8.0 kPa or F_iO_2 >0.4 or mechanical ventilation >48 hours
>
> Acute renal failure: urea >20 mmol/L or creatinine >260 mmol/L

Variables associated with postoperative complications and death

Several authors[16,17] have examined the prognostic ability or power of many variables that can be monitored in the postoperative setting. One group[5] found that none of the routinely measured variables such as heart rate, blood pressure, central venous pressure, urine output or any marker of acid–base status was able to predict subsequent postoperative complications. The variables independently associated with subsequent significant complications were the central venous oxygen saturation and the cardiac index. This association between oxygen flux in the perioperative period and subsequent complications is not new and is essentially the same as work published by Shoemaker et al.[14] some 30 years previously, who identified the key variables as being cardiac index, oxygen delivery and oxygen consumption. It was from this body of work that the theories surrounding the targeting of oxygen delivery to values of over $600\,mL/min$ per m^2 in the perioperative period to improve patient outcome originated.

The role of the splanchnic circulation

There is some evidence of the role of the splanchnic circulation in the pathogenesis of postoperative morbidity and mortality. It has been shown that increasing global tissue oxygen delivery will increase splanchnic oxygen delivery.[18–20] It would appear that in the early stages of shock any inadequacy of tissue oxygen delivery predominantly effects the splanchnic circulation.[21] The splanchnic circulation is particularly sensitive to hypoperfusion states, and the reduction in flow to the splanchnic bed is out of proportion to the overall reduction in cardiac output and is usually the last major system blood flow to recover when the hypoperfusion state improves.[22–34] It is thought that this splanchnic hypoperfusion leads to disruption of the enteric mucosal barrier with translocation of endotoxins and micro-organisms into the systemic circulation.[25–28] This translocation initiates a cytokine pathway, increasing the risk of sepsis and organ failure. This risk of splanchnic hypoperfusion and translocation increases with age, the urgency of the surgery and the preoperative presence of bowel obstruction. The translocation of bacteria and endotoxins induces cytokine release by tissue macrophages, activates the complement and coagulation systems, and produces a proinflammatory state. These cytokines themselves can impair oxygen delivery to the splanchnic circulation, further increasing translocation.

Strategies to improve outcomes

The concept of augmenting cardiac output in the perioperative period to improve the outcome of surgical patients has been described by many authors as 'optimisation' or 'goal-directed therapy'. The main aim of all optimisation strategies for high-risk surgical patients has been to ensure that the circulatory status of the patients is adequate for their needs in the perioperative period. This has been achieved with a number of differing protocols utilising different time periods, resuscitation end-points and pharmacological agents. There are little to no data describing the relative efficacy of the different protocols when compared with each other as they have nearly all been compared against 'standard' care. Almost all studies where this approach has been used have led to an improved outcome.

Oxygen delivery

In order to understand the rationale behind many of the protocols that have been utilised in the perioperative setting, it is vital to appreciate the important variables that determine oxygen delivery. These variables can be summarised according to the following equations:

Oxygen content $= ([1.34 \times Hb \times (S_aO_2/100)] + (0.023 \times P_aO_2))$

Oxygen delivery = Cardiac output × Oxygen content

It therefore becomes clear that in order to ensure that an adequate volume of oxygen is delivered to the body's vital organs the haemoglobin concentration (Hb), the arterial saturation of haemoglobin with oxygen (S_aO_2) and the cardiac index must all be at a satisfactory level. Maximising all three of these variables to clinically acceptable levels is the aim of resuscitation in any given patient, although not always achievable. The haemoglobin level is governed by the clinical situation as well as the underlying pathophysiological process, but many experts aim to keep the haemoglobin level above 9 g/dL in a stable perioperative setting. The S_aO_2 is usually targeted to be over 95% with increased inspired oxygen and/or continuous positive airways pressure (CPAP) if necessary, so the main variable that can be manipulated is the cardiac output. There is a growing understanding that atelectasis in the postoperative period is not just associated with hypoxaemia but also with a proinflammatory response that potentiates tissue injury. As a result the use of CPAP or other non-invasive positive pressure ventilation (NIPPV) therapy has the potential to improve many physiological parameters without serious side-effects in certain high-risk groups of patients, but whether this leads to improved outcome or reduced hospital stay is not yet clear and requires further investigation.

Cardiac output can be increased with several easy-to-use protocols. The targeting of cardiac index does necessitate the measurement and monitoring of this variable, which nowadays can be done relatively non-invasively. Once measured, if the cardiac output is perceived to be too low, then it is increased with intravenous volume therapy and then, if it has still not improved sufficiently, pharmacologically using appropriate cardiovascular pharmaceutical agents which will improve cardiac output.

Measurement and monitoring of cardiac output

There are a variety of technologies available to monitor cardiac output. Traditionally a pulmonary artery catheter has been used which enables a thermodilution curve to be constructed across the right ventricle, thus enabling cardiac output to be calculated from the Stewart–Hamilton equation. In recent times this tool has become highly controversial due to a lack of evidence demonstrating a beneficial effect on outcome and the perceived invasiveness of its approach, but its use in this situation for improvent of outcome for patients at high risk of complications and death after major surgery is not in dispute. Many new devices and techniques are now available which can provide the same information in a less invasive fashion. Oesophageal Doppler analysis of the descending aorta has been widely described in the perioperative period, while titrating therapy with pulse power analysis has recently been shown to reduce length of stay and postoperative complications.

Protocol-driven therapy to augment oxygen delivery

Inappropriately low values of cardiac index, oxygen delivery and oxygen consumption result in abnormal microcirculatory blood flow as a result of vasoconstriction in the capillary beds. Unfortunately it is not possible to detect these tissue hypoxic states with traditional monitored variables; therefore it is necessary to monitor and titrate therapy to cardiac index and oxygen delivery. Shoemaker et al.[30] utilised targets of cardiac index, oxygen delivery and consumption (4.5 L/min per m^2, DO_2 >600 mL/min per m^2 and VO_2 >170 mL/min per m^2) that had been previously demonstrated to be the median values for survivors following major surgery, in order to show that the repayment of an incurred oxygen debt within 8 hours resulted in an improved outcome. It has been consistently shown[30–36] that reductions in mortality and morbidity are obtained when these levels of oxygen delivery are achieved and that in conjunction with the decreased complications there is a reduced length of stay. It is worth noting that many patients are unable to achieve adequate levels of oxygen delivery without assistance in this setting. Not all patients will achieve these targets even with

assistance. For these patients an increase in oxygen delivery may still be beneficial, although it is unclear exactly how hard to drive them so that the complications do not override any benefit accrued. Most successful trials have targeted an oxygen delivery of 600 mL/min per m^2. This therefore seems a sensible target to use in this setting. This does not mean, however, that this is the best target as others that may be better may be available but simply have yet to be studied. Other goals or targets are available, for instance maximal stroke volume or central venous saturations and serum lactate. Until they have been proven to be beneficial, however, it would be prudent to continue with the published data.

Reductions in mortality, morbidity and hospital stay have consistently been shown to occur with improved tissue levels of oxygen delivery.[29–35]

Fluid resuscitation

It is important to recognise that protocol-driven therapy of this nature is not about giving more intravenous fluid to the patients; it is about giving the right amount at the right time. There is evidence that excessive fluid administration is detrimental in critically ill and postoperative patients (**Fig. 16.1**). It is likely that inappropriate volume overload has just as many detrimental effects as inadequate volume resuscitation. This mandates the need to monitor

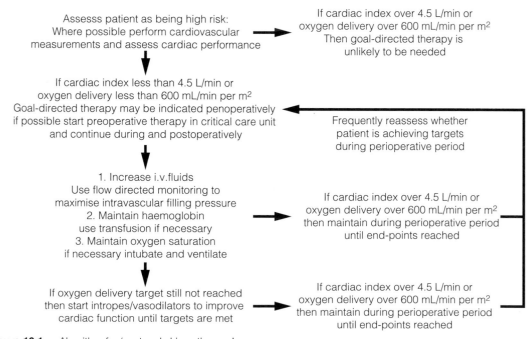

Figure 16.1 • Algorithm for 'protocol-driven therapy'.

very carefully fluid administration in critically ill or high-risk patients where simple measures or markers of preload status are often inadequate. Defining the end-point at which filling is optimal and the need for inotropic therapy begins is difficult. Plateauing of the stroke volume, flow correction time as determined by oesophageal Doppler and stroke volume variation (with the pulse pressure analysis) can all be used to define the end-point. It seems intuitive and important that the end-points of resuscitation are reached with the minimal amount of volume and inotropic therapy possible.

Timing of protocol-driven therapy

The timing of goal-directed therapy (GDT) is vitally important in order to achieve the benefits demonstrated in the published studies. Most of the studies that have had significant impact on mortality have been started before surgery and then continued on throughout the perioperative period. Due to resource constraints this is difficult to implement, so many authors have since studied the effects of GDT either only during surgery or during the postoperative period. Although nearly all of these studies have also demonstrated benefit, the effects are not as dramatic as when therapy is started in the preoperative period. Whether this is a real effect or whether it is an artefact of study design is difficult to ascertain. A pragmatic response is to intiate therapy as soon as is practically possible – either during or immediately after surgery. It makes no sense to wait until after problems have developed. In practice this means that the GDT should be started as early as possible and continued until the patient is stable in the postoperative period (Box 16.2). The duration, timing and setting of therapy will mandate the type of monitoring technology used – for instance, awake patients do not readily tolerate the oesophageal Doppler probe.

 Goal-directed therapy to optimise the patient's circulation and therefore tissue oxygenation should be commenced as soon as possible and continued into the postoperative period.

Box 16.2 • Clinical guidelines for the implementation of goal-directed therapy in high-risk surgical patients

Identify the high-risk patient

See Box 16.1 for Shoemaker criteria

Particularly identify elderly patients with poor cardiorespiratory reserve, ischaemic heart disease with evidence of heart failure

Identify the operation

Operations likely to last longer than 1.5 hours

Lack of postoperative critical care facilities

Emergency surgery, particularly abdominal surgery

Perioperative goal-directed therapy

1. Assess the patient preoperatively: where possible perform cardiovascular measurements to assess cardiac performance. Measure cardiac output and oxygen delivery

2. If cardiac index >4.5 L/min per m^2 and/or oxygen delivery >600 mL/min per m^2 (body surface area), then no further goal-directed therapy will be necessary. Patient can proceed to anaesthesia and surgery

3. If cardiac index <4.5 L/min per m^2 and/or oxygen delivery <600 mL/min per m^2 (body surface area), then further goal-directed therapy may be indicated either prior to surgery or, if this is not possible, then immediately following surgery in a dedicated critical care area

4. If cardiac index <4.5 L/min per m^2 and/or oxygen delivery <600 mL/min per m^2 (body surface area):
   (a) Increase intravenous fluids: direct therapy using flow-directed monitoring equipment to maximise intravascular filling pressure
   (b) Maintain adequate haemoglobin concentration with blood transfusion if necessary
   (c) Maintain blood oxygen saturation at 95% or greater with supplemental oxygenation or artificial ventilation

5. If despite these measures cardiac index is <4.5 L/min per m^2 and/or oxygen delivery <600 mL/min per m^2 (body surface area), then consider the use of cardiovascular performance-enhancing therapy. Although a number of different inotropic and vasodilator therapies have been used (including adrenaline and dobutamine), the best results seem to have been achieved using dopexamine, which acts mainly as a vasodilator with some positive inotropic effects. Start dopexamine at 0.5 μg/kg per min and increase the rate of infusion incrementally every 10–15 minutes until either the target oxygen delivery has been achieved or there is an increase in heart rate 20% greater than the patient's resting rate or there are signs of ischaemia on the ECG. (If the patient is very tachycardic prior to starting inotropes, it is important to recognise this and not try to increase cardiac output at the expense of increasing the already raised heart rate.) Maintain intravascular filling pressure during this period of inotrope therapy

Maintain this goal-directed therapy into the postoperative period until there is evidence that the intraoperative oxygen debt is repaid (return of base deficit to normal, blood lactate concentration within normal range)

Chapter 16

Conclusions

This overview of the literature relating to the high-risk surgical patient and current improvements associated with goal-directed therapy leads to some inevitable conclusions:

1. There is good evidence to suggest that patients with poor cardiorespiratory reserve have a higher mortality and complication rate when undergoing major surgery. Most of these patients can be identified by simple clinical methods before surgery.
2. It is likely that there are significant numbers of patients undergoing different types of surgery who may be at substantial risk of developing major complications or death.
3. A number of randomised controlled clinical studies have consistently demonstrated the improvement in outcome that can be achieved in these patients by the use of goal-directed therapy aimed at temporarily improving the cardiovascular performance of high-risk patients so that non-survivors have the same cardiorespiratory performance as survivors.
4. Studies have shown that benefit may be obtained in a wide range of surgery, including vascular surgery, colorectal surgery, trauma, orthopaedics, major cancer surgery and cardiac surgery.
5. From the work by Shoemaker and colleagues it would seem that about 8% of the surgical population would fulfil this definition of being at high risk of complications or death following major surgery. It would appear that these patients have a postoperative 30-day mortality of 20–30%, representing 90–95% of all surgical deaths. This number is likely to increase with an ageing population on whom increasingly complex surgery is being performed.
6. Although optimising the circulation produces significant reductions in mortality and postoperative complications in the higher-risk patient, it is now clear that important reductions in complications can be achieved in patients who have a lower mortality but for whom a significant complication risk exists.
7. It is also apparent that optimising the circulation can be carried out using several different techniques and at different times (i.e. preoperatively, intraoperatively and postoperatively).

Key points

- Patients with poor cardiorespiratory reserve undergoing major operations have a high postoperative complication and mortality rate. The mortality rate is much higher if these patients have emergency operations.
- These patients can be identified preoperatively by simple clinical history and examination.
- This high postoperative complication and mortality rate can be significantly reduced by goal-directed therapy aimed at enhancing the cardiorespiratory performance of these patients with poor physiological reserve during the perioperative period.
- Goal-directed therapy aims to ensure that tissue oxygen delivery is enhanced to levels shown to confer survival without postoperative complications.

References

1. Beecher HK, Todd DP. A study of the deaths associated with anaesthesia and surgery. Ann Surg 1954; 140:2–5.
2. Edwards G, Morton HJV, Pask EA et al. Deaths associated with anaesthesia. Anaesthesia 1956; 11:194–220.
3. Dornette WHL, Orth OS. Death in the operating room. Anesth Analg 1956; 3:545–69.
4. Buck N, Devlin HB, Lunn JN. The report of a confidential enquiry into perioperative deaths. London: Nuffield Provincial Hospitals Trust and the King Edward's Hospital Fund for London, 1987.
5. Pearse RM, Harrison DA, James P et al. Identification and characterisation of the high-risk surgical population in the United Kingdom. Crit Care 2006; 10(3):R81.

6. Department of Health. Guidelines on admission to and discharge from intensive care and high dependency units. London: NHS Executive, 1996.

7. McQuillan P, Pilkington S, Allan A et al. Confidential enquiry into quality of care before admission to intensive care. BMJ 1998; 316(7148):1853–8.

8. Garrard C, Young D. Suboptimal care of patients before admission to intensive care is caused by a failure to appreciate or apply the ABCs of life support. BMJ 1998; 316(7148):1841–2.

9. Purdie JA, Ridley SA, Wallace PG. Effective use of regional intensive therapy units. BMJ 1990; 300(6717):79–81.

10. Henao FJ, Daes JE, Dennis RJ. Risk factors for multi-organ failure: a case control study. J Trauma 1991; 31:74–80.

11. Bion J. Rationing intensive care. BMJ 1995; 310(6981):682–3.

12. Desborough JP. The stress response to trauma and surgery. Br J Anaesth 2000; 85:109–17.

13. Older P, Hall A, Hader R. Cardiopulmonary exercise testing as a screening test for perioperative management of major surgery in the elderly. Chest 1999; 116:355–62.

14. Shoemaker WC, Appel PL, Kram HB. Role of oxygen debt in the development of organ failure, sepsis and death in high-risk surgical patients. Chest 1992; 102:208–15.

15. Gibbons RJ, Balady GJ, Timothy Bricker J et al. ACC/AHA 2002 guideline update for exercise testing: summary article. A report of the American College of Cardiology/American Heart Association Task Force on Practice Guidelines (Committee to Update the 1997 Exercise Testing Guidelines). J Am Coll Cardiol 2002; 40:1531–40.

16. Shoemaker WC. Cardiorespiratory patterns of surviving and non-surviving postoperative patients. Surg Gynecol Obstet 1972; 134:810–14.

17. Shoemaker WC, Montgomery ES, Kaplan E et al. Physiologic patterns in surviving and nonsurviving shock patients. Use of sequential cardiorespiratory variables in defining criteria for therapeutic goals and early warning of death. Arch Surg 1973; 106:630–6.

18. Ruokonen E, Takala J, Kari A. Regional blood flow and oxygen transport in patients with the low cardiac output syndrome after cardiac surgery. Crit Care Med 1993; 21:1304–11.

19. Ruokonen E, Takala J, Kari A et al. Regional blood flow and oxygen transport in septic shock. Crit Care Med 1993; 21:1296–303.

20. Uusaro A, Ruokonen E, Takal J. Splanchnic oxygen transport after cardiac surgery: evidence for inadequate tissue perfusion after stabilization of hemodynamics. Intensive Care Med 1996; 22:26–33.

21. Gutierrez G, Bismar H, Dantzker DR et al. Comparison of gastric intramucosal pH with measures of oxygen transport and consumption in critically ill patients. Crit Care Med 1992; 20: 451–7.

22. Adar R, Franklin A, Spark RF et al. Effect of dehydration and cardiac tamponade on superior mesenteric artery flow: role of vasoactive substances. Surgery 1976; 79:534–43.

23. Bailey RW, Bulkley GB, Hamilton SR et al. Protection of the small intestine from nonocclusive mesenteric ischemic injury due to cardiogenic shock. Am J Surg 1987; 153:108–16.

24. McNeill JR, Stark RD, Greenway CV. Mortality and morbidity in gastro-oesophageal cancer surgery: initial results of ASCOT multi-centre prospective cohort study. BMJ 2003; 327:1192–7.

25. Ohri SK, Somasundaram S, Koak Y et al. The effect of intestinal hypoperfusion on intestinal absorption and permeability during cardiopulmonary bypass. Gastroenterology 1994; 106:318–23.

26. Brooks SG, May J, Sedman P et al. Translocation of enteric bacteria in humans. Br J Surg 1993; 80:901–2.

27. O'Boyle CJ, MacFie J, Mitchell CJ et al. Microbiology of bacterial translocation in humans. Gut 1998; 42:29–35.

28. Deitch EA. Multiple organ failure. Pathophysiology and potential future therapy. Ann Surg 1992; 216:117–34.

29. Shoemaker WC, Appel PC, Cram HB et al. Prospective trial of supranormal values of survivors as therapeutic goals in high risk surgical patients. Chest 1988; 94:1176–86.

30. Boyd O, Grounds RM, Bennett ED. A randomized clinical trial of the effect of deliberate perioperative increase of oxygen delivery on mortality in high risk surgical patients. JAMA 1993; 270:2699–708.

This was the first full well-conducted, randomised controlled study of goal-directed therapy for perioperative enhancement of the cardiovascular systems of these high-risk surgical patients. It was stopped before it was completed by the local hospital research ethics committee because the surgeons felt that it was obvious which group their patients were in and felt it was unethical to continue when the benefits were so obvious.

31. Wilson J, Woods I, Fawcett J et al. Reducing the risk of major elective surgery: randomised controlled trial of preoperative optimization of oxygen delivery. BMJ 1999; 318:1099–103.

This study is important because not only did it have a control group where clinicians not involved with the study were able to decide on the postoperative treatment and send patients back to the ward postoperatively (which is common practice in many hospitals in the UK due to lack of critical care facilities), but it also divided the group admitted to intensive care into two groups for therapeutic intervention and thus showed that there could be a difference in outcome if different drugs were used for goal-directed therapy.

32. Lobo SM, Salgado PF, Castillo VG et al. Effects of maximizing oxygen delivery on morbidity and mortality in high-risk surgical patients. Crit Care Med 2000; 28:3396–404.

33. Bishop MH, Shoemaker WC, Appel PL et al. Prospective, randomized trial of survivor values of cardiac index, oxygen delivery, and oxygen consumption as resuscitation end points in severe trauma. J Trauma 1995; 38:780–7.

34. Polonen P, Rukonen E, Hippelainen M et al. A prospective, randomized study of goal-orientated hemodynamic therapy in cardiac surgical patients. Anesth Analg 2000; 90:1052–9.

35. Pearse R, Dawson D, Fawcett J et al. Early goal-directed therapy after major surgery reduces complications and duration of hospital stay. A randomized controlled study. Crit Care 2005; 9:R687–93.

17

Surgical nutrition

Steven D. Heys
William G. Simpson

Introduction

The importance of nutrition in all fields of clinical practice has become well recognised and none more so than in the management of patients who are undergoing surgery and/or are faced with critical illness. Despite this increasing understanding of the importance of nutrition in health, up to 40% of hospitalised patients can be classified as being malnourished and many of these patients are not recognised clinically as having this problem. In patients undergoing gastrointestinal surgery, for example, the prevalence of 'mild' and 'moderate' malnutrition has been estimated to be approximately 50% and 30% respectively.

The clinical significance of this is vitally important because when patients have malnutrition the disturbances in function at the organ and cellular level can manifest as the following:

- altered partitioning and impairment of normal homeostatic mechanisms;
- muscle wasting and impairment of skeletal muscle function;
- impaired respiratory muscle function;
- impaired cardiac muscle function;
- atrophy of smooth muscle in the gastrointestinal tract;
- impaired immune function;
- impaired healing of wounds and anastomoses.

The key point, therefore, is that as a result of these malnutrition-induced changes, patients have an increased risk of postoperative morbidity and mortality. To further complicate the situation with respect to nutrition, patients undergoing surgery will also be fasted for varying periods of time (preoperatively and/or postoperatively). Moreover, if patients then experience postoperative complications (e.g. sepsis), these effects may be further potentiated and the disturbances of cellular and organ function occurring in malnutrition then made even more complex.

In this chapter the following areas, which are important for surgical practice, will be outlined:

- the principles of the metabolic responses to trauma and sepsis;
- nutritional requirements for surgical patients;
- identification of patients who are malnourished or are at risk;
- nutritional support principles for surgical practice and modifications in defined common clinical situations;
- modulation of nutritional support with key nutrients – application to clinical practice.

Metabolic response to trauma and sepsis

Trauma

Whilst a detailed knowledge of complex biochemical pathways is not necessary, it is important to understand the principles of the metabolic changes which occur following trauma. Therefore, the first thing to consider is the principles of these metabolic and biochemical changes, the metabolic response to trauma and when a patient undergoes surgery or develops sepsis. This forms the basis for understanding nutritional support in critically ill patients.

A major advance in understanding occurred more than 50 years ago when Sir David Cuthbertson described the loss of nitrogen from skeletal muscle that occurred following trauma.[1] Cuthbertson concluded that the response to injury could be considered as occurring in two phases (**Fig. 17.1**):

1. the 'ebb' phase, which is a short-lived response associated with hypovolaemic shock, increased sympathetic nervous system activity and reduced metabolic rate;
2. the 'flow' phase, which is associated with a loss of body nitrogen and resultant negative nitrogen balance.

These changes result in the following:

Ebb phase

- decreased resting energy expenditure;
- decreased gluconeogenesis;
- increased glycogenolysis.

Flow phase

- increased resting energy expenditure;
- increased heat production, pyrexia;
- increased muscle catabolism and wasting and loss of body nitrogen;
- increased breakdown of fat and reduced fat synthesis;
- increased gluconeogenesis and glucose intolerance.

If the changes of the 'ebb phase' are not replaced by the 'flow phase', then despite any advances in surgery, anaesthesia and intensive care support, death of the patient is the inevitable outcome.

The central nervous system and the neurohypophyseal axis play key roles in mediating these metabolic changes following trauma, with a range of hormones and cytokines being key regulators. Afferent nerve impulses also stimulate the hypothalamus to secrete hypothalamic releasing factors that, in turn, stimulate the pituitary gland to release prolactin, arginine vasopressin (also known as antidiuretic hormone), growth hormone and adrenocorticotrophic hormone (ACTH). The changes in hormone levels in plasma following trauma are outlined in Box 17.1, with the stress hormones (adrenaline, cortisol, glucagon) playing pivotal roles.

Changes in protein metabolism

The increased loss of nitrogen following trauma is due to protein breakdown occurring at a rate in excess of synthesis.[2] This occurs whether the patient is fed or fasted. The magnitude of the nitrogen loss is proportional to degree of operative trauma and a major site of protein breakdown is skeletal muscle (contains 80% of the body's amino acid pool with 60% being glutamine).[3] The amino acids released can be used for:

- hepatic production of glucose from alanine (the latter being produced by transamination reactions from other amino acids);
- energy substrates for gut, lymphocytes and other rapidly proliferating tissues;
- maintenance of renal acid–base balance (arginine);
- synthesis of proteins necessary for structural repair;
- hepatic production of proteins with immunological or tissue repair functions;
- as fuel in muscle.

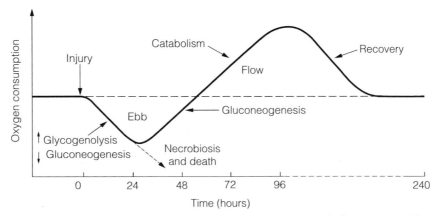

Figure 17.1 • Diagrammatic representation of the ebb and flow phases in the metabolic response to injury. Reproduced from Broom J. Sepsis and trauma. In: Garrow JS, James WPT (eds) Human nutrition and dietetics, 9th edn. Edinburgh: Churchill Livingstone, 1993; pp. 456–64. With permission from Churchill Livingstone.

Box 17.1 • Changes in hormone levels in plasma following trauma

Catecholamines

Rapid increases in concentrations of adrenaline and noradrenaline within a few minutes of injury due to increased activity of sympathetic nervous system. Levels return to normal within 24 hours

Glucagon

Rises within a few hours; maximal levels 12–48 hours post-trauma

Insulin

Initially plasma levels are low following trauma, but rise to above normal levels and reach a maximum several days after the injury

Cortisol

Rapid increase in cortisol (due to stimulation by ACTH), returning to normal 24–48 hours later; may remain elevated for up to several days. Has 'permissive' effects with other hormones such as catecholamines

Growth hormone

Levels increased following trauma; usually return to normal levels within 24 hours

Thyroid hormones

Following trauma, the biochemical features of 'sick euthyroid syndrome' may be present: thyroid-stimulating hormone (TSH) levels normal or low, levels of free thyroxine (T4) and tri-iodothyronine (T3) normal, whereas the total levels are altered because of changes in binding protein concentration. In addition, reverse T3 is generally high. These effects may be prolonged for some weeks

Other disturbances of thyroid function may, however, be present, including 'transient hyperthyrotropinaemia of illness' – a transiently raised TSH, not to be confused with hypothyroidism

Renin, aldosterone

Aldosterone levels increased after trauma, returning to normal within 12 hours. Its secretion is stimulated by renin, which in turn is produced in response to reduced renal perfusion

Testosterone

Plasma levels fall after trauma and may remain low for up to 7 days

Vasopressin/antidiuretic hormone

Plasma levels rise following trauma and may remain elevated for several days

Prolactin

Secretion increased following trauma but function in trauma is unknown

Cytokines

Increased secretion of interleukin (IL)-2, IL-6, tumour necrosis factor, etc.; interrelationship between these changes leads to differential responses seen in trauma and sepsis

Changes in carbohydrate metabolism

Glucose is the main fuel used by many different tissues being essential for some. When it is not available for absorption from the gastrointestinal tract, it is endogenously produced from glycogen (glycogenolysis) or other precursors (gluconeogenesis), e.g. amino acids. Glucose can be utilised for energy or converted into glycogen or fat. Following trauma, there is an increase in hepatic glycogen breakdown (caused by increased sympathetic activity),[4] with these stores being substantially depleted within 24 hours.[5] There is also an associated reduction in peripheral utilisation of glucose. Insulin antagonists are also involved in this metabolic response (see Box 17.1).

Resistance to insulin occurs in patients who have been injured. The circulating concentrations of glucose and insulin are elevated following injury, but there is a more marked rise in insulin concentration. The circulating insulin level usually reaches a maximum several days after the injury, before returning towards normal levels.

In general, the carbohydrate response is to produce hyperglycaemia both in the immediate 'shock' ('ebb' phase) and later 'flow' phase of the metabolic response. The origin of the increased glucose differs between these two phases – whilst reduced peripheral utilisation of glucose is common to both phases, the glycogenolysis of the ebb phase must be replaced by gluconeogenesis in the flow phase. In the critically ill patient the advent of hypoglycaemia is an indication of major problems – glycogenolysis has slowed with depletion of glycogen stores, but gluconeogenesis is not yet adequate.

Changes in fat metabolism

After trauma, there is an increase in the turnover of fatty acids and glycerol. Lipolysis of triacylglycerols is increased, with the production of free fatty acids and glycerol (although raised levels of lactate, for example in hypovolaemic shock, induce re-esterification leading to raised plasma triglyceride levels). The glycerol can be used by the liver for gluconeogenesis and the fatty acids can also be used as a fuel source.[6] Fatty acids are also metabolised in the liver to form ketone bodies, which are used as a preferential fuel source by many tissues (remember that the human liver cannot use fatty acids for gluconeogenesis).

Sepsis

The metabolic response to sepsis is characterised by alterations in protein, carbohydrate and fat metabolism. The changes occurring in patients with sepsis have definite and increasingly well-defined differences from those with trauma.[7] In patients with sepsis, the following are the key changes:

- There is breakdown of skeletal muscle and nitrogen losses can be substantial (more than 15–20 g per day). Amino acids released from muscle are utilised by the liver for production of acute-phase and visceral proteins, and as substrates for the increase in gluconeogenesis.
- There is increased production of glucose by the liver (e.g. by both gluconeogenesis and glycogenolysis), resulting in an elevated plasma glucose.
- In contrast to the situation following trauma, there is an increased rate of glucose uptake and oxidation by peripheral tissues.
- Circulating levels of free fatty acids may increase or decrease in patients with sepsis.[8] The reasons for these differences may be explained by the differing times during the septic episode at which concentrations were measured.
- There is an increase in breakdown of fat stores in adipose tissue by lipolysis and hypertriglyceridaemia.
- Decrease in the peripheral uptake of these triacylglycerols and defective ketogenesis in the presence of sepsis (in contrast to the situation occurring after trauma) are observed.

A significant abnormality in the patient with sepsis is the disruption of the microstructure of the hepatocyte mitochondria, particularly of the inner membrane. There is a block in energy transduction pathways, with consequent reduction in the aerobic metabolism of both glucose and fatty acids. The body therefore depends on the *anaerobic* metabolism of glucose, which also results in lactate production. It is essential therefore that there is an adequate supply of glucose from gluconeogenic pathways. If this is impaired or inadequate, then hypoglycaemia (and death) may ensue. The development of hypoglycaemia during sepsis is an indicator of an extremely poor prognosis and is usually associated with inevitable mortality.

Nutritional requirements

Proteins and amino acids

Protein is required for the maintenance of normal health and cellular function. Proteins have many functions, including being essential components of cellular structure. They are required for the synthesis of a variety of secretory proteins produced by many organs. The average daily intake of protein is approximately 80 g in the UK, with a recommended daily intake of 0.8 g/kg body weight and with nitrogen comprising approximately 16% of its weight. However, more than 50% of the world's population exist on less!

Conventionally, amino acids have been classified as either 'essential' or 'non-essential'. The 'essential' amino acids cannot be synthesised endogenously and are required in the diet, whereas the 'non-essential' amino acids are so necessary that humans have retained the ability to synthesise them. Both groups of amino acids are necessary for normal tissue growth and metabolism.

Dietary intake and endogenous synthesis of amino acids in the body maintain the relevant pool of amino acids, replacing those that have been lost by excretion in the urine, losses from the skin and gastrointestinal tract, utilisation as precursors for non-protein synthetic pathways, irreversible modification and irreducible oxidation.

Under certain circumstances (e.g. sepsis, trauma, growth) endogenous synthesis of some amino acids normally considered to be 'non-essential' is inadequate; therefore, these amino acids are described as 'conditionally essential'. It seems likely that only three amino acids are actually non-essential: L-alanine, L-glutamate and L-aspartate, which are produced by a simple transamination reaction. These are the three most important amino acids in times of starvation:

- alanine for hepatic gluconeogenesis;
- glutamate as a hepatic fuel source;
- aspartate for maintaining renal acid–base balance.

Energy requirements

Energy transduction is accomplished by the breakdown of carbohydrate, fat and proteins. The energy available from various common nutrients is:

- fat 9.3 kcal/g (38.9 kJ/g);
- glucose 4.1 kcal/g (17.1 kJ/g);
- protein 4.1 kcal/g (17.1 kJ/g);
- alcohol 7.1 kcal/g (29.7 kJ/g).

The principal carbohydrates in the diet are polysaccharides (starch and dietary fibre), dextrins and free sugars (monosaccharides), disaccharides, oligosaccharides and sugar alcohols. Dietary fat includes triacylglycerol, containing long-chain fatty acids (C_{16}–C_{18} triacylglycerols) and medium-chain fatty acids (C_6–C_{12} triacylglycerols) and cholesterol.

If the energy intake of an individual is greater than energy expenditure, extra carbohydrate intake, on reaching the liver via the portal vein, will be channelled into glycogen synthesis until hepatic glycogen stores are replete; thereafter, glucose is metabolised to fatty acids and fat synthesis occurs. Additional fat intake will be stored in adipose tissue as triacylglycerol. In contrast, if there is a negative energy balance, then glycogen, followed by fat and protein, will be broken down to provide energy.

Total daily energy expenditure comprises the following:

- resting metabolic expenditure (RME), which is energy required for cardiorespiratory function and synthesis and maintenance of electrochemical gradients across cell membranes;
- activity energy expenditure (depends on type of physical work undertaken);
- diet induced energy expenditure.

Normally, approximately 25–30 kcal/kg (105–125 kJ/g) are required daily; the magnitude of changes in requirements in some common conditions are given in Box 17.2.

Micronutrients

Vitamins

Vitamins are organic compounds essential for normal growth and maintenance of body functions,
playing key roles in many metabolic processes in health and disease. In general, vitamins are classified into:

- fat soluble (A, D, E and K);
- water soluble (C and the B vitamins – folic acid, B_{12}, B_1, B_2, B_3, pantothenic acid, biotin and B_6).

The exact requirement for vitamins during trauma and sepsis is unclear and may alter depending on the type of metabolic support provided. Details of individual vitamins are beyond the scope of this chapter and can be found elsewhere, but examples are given in Box 17.3.

Trace elements

Trace elements are inorganic elements that are important in regulation of metabolic processes.[5] For example, zinc is necessary for wound healing as is a cofactor in enzymes involved in protein and nucleic acid synthesis. Others of importance to surgical patients include iron (involved in energy transfer, hence vital for repair), copper (collagen synthesis) and selenium (synthesis of antioxidant enzyme systems, protecting against peroxidation processes occurring in tissue damage and repair, and necessary for combating sepsis). A detailed description of other trace elements, their requirements and structure can be found in standard texts.[9]

It should be remembered that micronutrients, if given at high doses, could have toxic effects on tissues. In particular, toxicity can be a problem with excesses of vitamins A and D, iron, selenium, zinc

Box 17.2 • Additional energy requirements in disease states

Trauma: 0.3 × RME
Elective surgery: 0.1 × RME
Sepsis: up to 0.5 × RME
Severe sepsis: up to 0.6 × RME
Massive burns: 1 × RME

Box 17.3 • Functions of some vitamins important in surgical practice

Vitamin A

Stabilises epithelial cell membranes; necessary for fibroblast differentiation and collagen secretion

Vitamin D

Role in calcium and phosphate regulation

Vitamin E

Immunostimulant and free radical scavenger

Vitamin K

Required for liver synthesis of clotting factors

Vitamin B_{12}

Important in synthesis of proteins and nucleic acids

Ascorbic acid

Important in hydroxylation (e.g. collagen synthesis) and energy transduction

Thiamine

Necessary for carbohydrate metabolism and ATP synthesis

and copper. Care must be taken when these micro-nutrients are provided for a prolonged period to ensure that toxicity does not occur.

Identification of patients who are malnourished

It is important to determine the nutritional status in all patients undergoing surgery and identify those who are malnourished, or who are at risk of becoming so. Assessments used previously in clinical practice are:

- anthropometric measures;
- biochemical assessments and body composition measurements;
- evaluation of body function (skeletal and respiratory muscle function, immune responses).

Anthropometric measures

Height and weight

Height and weight are two commonly used indices of nutritional status. A body weight value for a particular patient can be compared with a series of standard values to assess degree of leanness or adiposity.[10] These tables take no account of frame size and body mass index (BMI; weight divided by the square of the height) is a good anthropometric indicator of total body fat in adults.

Loss of body weight has been used as an indicator of nutritional status. This is determined by subtracting current weight from recall weight when the patient was 'well' or from the 'ideal' weight, obtained from published tables. The loss of more than 10% of body weight, or more than 4.5 kg of recall weight, is associated with a significant increase in postoperative mortality. The shorter the period of weight loss, the more significant this is in predicting increased postoperative complications. By combining weight loss and rate of weight loss, malnutrition can be defined as a BMI of less than the 10th percentile with a weight loss of 5% or more.[11]

Subcutaneous fat thickness

Other anthropometric measurements have been used. The most commonly used index of total body fat is skinfold thickness (50% of total body fat is subcutaneous, depending on age, sex and fat pad). Triceps skinfold thickness is most commonly measured but assessment of skinfolds at multiple sites is better and correlates with total body fat. Regression equations for the estimation of total body fat from these measurements are available.[12] However, skinfold thickness measurements are susceptible to intra-observer and inter-observer variability, which limits clinical use.

Biochemical measures

Serum proteins

Albumin is the major protein in serum and the relationship between serum proteins and malnutrition was recognised over 150 years ago.[13] Low serum albumin levels are associated with increased risk of complications in patients undergoing surgery.[14] In experimental starvation, however, serum albumin levels may not fall for several weeks[15] because, although synthesis decreases, only 30% of the total exchangeable albumin is in the intravascular space, with the remainder being extravascular. In addition, albumin has a relatively long half-life of approximately 21 days. It has been estimated that the flux of albumin between the intravascular and extravascular compartments is about 10 times the rate of albumin synthesis.[16]

Previous studies have shown that a 30% loss of body weight with long periods of semi-starvation was associated with an increase in serum albumin concentration, confirming that serum albumin concentration bears no relationship to nutritional status. Furthermore, serum albumin acts as a negative marker of the acute-phase response, and so is lowered in malignancy, trauma and sepsis, even in the presence of an adequate intake. Serum albumin should therefore *not* be used as an assessment of nutritional state, although low levels point to the increased nutritional risk associated with underlying disease.

Alternatives to using albumin as a marker of nutritional status by measuring other serum protein concentrations, including transferrin (half-life 7 days), retinol-binding protein (half-life 1–2 hours) and pre-albumin (half-life 2 days) have been suggested. Changes in their serum concentrations might theoretically reflect acute changes in nutritional state more accurately than albumin. The serum levels of these proteins are, however, also altered in stress, sepsis and cancer, and so, as for albumin, they are not useful for assessing nutritional status in routine clinical practice.

Nitrogen balance

Most of the nitrogen lost from the body is excreted in urine, mainly as urea (approximately 80% of total urinary nitrogen). Urea alone may be measured as an approximate indicator of losses, or total urinary nitrogen may be measured, although this latter technique is not widely available. In addition, there are also losses of nitrogen from the skin and in stool of approximately 2–4 g per day. One equation used for balance studies is:

$$\text{Nitrogen balance(g)} = (\text{dietary protein(g)} \times 0.16) - (\text{urine urea nitrogen(g)} + 2\text{g stool} + 2\text{g skin})$$

where urine urea nitrogen (g) = urine urea (mmol) × 28.

Although nitrogen balance has not been shown to be a prognostic indicator, it is an important way of assessing a patient's nutritional requirements and the response to provision of nutritional support.

Body composition

More complicated techniques for assessing the body's different compartments (e.g. fat, fat-free mass, total body nitrogen and total body mineral contents) have become available but these require specialised equipment and may not be readily applicable to clinical practice. Relatively simple techniques, such as bio-electrical impedance, can be used clinically.

Bioelectrical impedance

This entails the passage of an alternating electrical current between electrodes attached to the hand and foot. The current passes through the water and electrolyte compartment of lean tissues and the drop in voltage between the electrodes is measured.[17] This change in voltage gives an estimation of total body resistance, which depends principally on total body water and electrolyte content (i.e. lean body mass). Bioelectrical impedance is an accurate measure of body composition in stable subjects; it becomes less reliable in patients with oedema and electrolyte shifts, and its value in critically ill patients is unclear.[13]

Tests of function

Immune competence

In malnutrition there is a reduction in total circulating lymphocyte count and impairment in immune functions, e.g. decreased skin reactivity to mumps, *Candida* and tuberculin (these should be antigens to which the individual has been previously exposed) and reduced lymphocyte responsiveness to mitogens in vitro.[18, 19]

A correlation between depressed immune function and postoperative morbidity and mortality has been demonstrated, and depression of total circulating lymphocyte count is associated with a poorer prognosis in surgical patients.[20] However, these alterations in immune function are non-specific and affected by trauma, surgery, anaesthetic and sedative drugs, pain and psychological stress,[21] and are not generally applicable to clinical practice.

Muscle function

Skeletal muscle

Various aspects of skeletal muscle structure and function are deranged in malnutrition. In patients undergoing surgery, handgrip strength (cheap and easy to perform) may predict patients who develop postoperative complications (sensitivity >90%). However, grip strength is influenced by factors such as patients' motivation and cooperation. Furthermore, such tests may be difficult to apply to critically ill patients. Alternatively, stimulation of the ulnar nerve at the wrist with a variable electrical stimulus results in contraction of the adductor pollicis muscle, the force of which reflects nutritional intake.[22]

Respiratory muscle

The function of the respiratory muscles is impaired by malnutrition and can be detected by deterioration in respiratory function tests, in particular vital capacity.[23] Measurements of inspiratory muscle strength have the advantage that they can be performed in patients who are intubated and are affected by intercurrent illnesses.

Nutrition risk index

A nutrition risk index is an index of nutritional status based on combinations of variables. Although several indices exist, one that is commonly used depends on serum albumin, current weight and the patient's usual weight:

$$\text{Nutrition risk index} = 1.519 \times \text{serum albumin (g/L)} \\ + 0.417 \times (\text{current weight}/ \\ \text{usual weight}) \times 100$$

The score obtained is used to categorise nutritional state: <83.5, 'severely' malnourished; 83.5–97.5, 'mildly' malnourished; 97.5–100, 'borderline' malnourished. However, such an index bears no relationship to the patient's nutritional status but is a prognostic index.

How should nutritional status be assessed in clinical practice?

Although the various techniques outlined above can help to predict the risks of complications, there is at present no reliable technique for assessing nutritional status. There is, however, increasing support for using the following techniques, which are applicable to clinical practice.

The Malnutrition Universal Screening Tool (MUST)

This is a simple, yet effective, tool developed by the British Association for Parenteral and Enteral Nutrition (BAPEN). Details are available from the website, which we recommend you read carefully (www.BAPEN.org.uk). This tool has been endorsed by external organisations and its routine use is recommended for all hospital admissions in the UK. As a minimum standard in clinical practice, the MUST tool should be used to assess nutritional risk.

Essentially, MUST consists of a series of five steps:

1. Measure height and weight to obtain BMI (in kg/m^2) – this is then given a numerical score (>20 = 0; 18.5–20 = 1; >18.5 = 2).
2. Note percentage unplanned weight loss in the previous 3–6 months – then give this a numerical score (<5% = 0; 5–10% = 1; >10% = 2).

3. Establish the 'acute disease effect' and also give this a numerical score (if patient is acutely ill and there is or will be no nutritional intake for more than 5 days = 2).
4. Add scores from steps 1, 2 and 3 together to obtain the 'overall risk of malnutrition'.
5. A decision is taken as to what to do depending on the resultant score.

Significance of the resultant score and clinical management

- **Score 0 (low risk)** – repeat the screening process at a future time.
- **Score 1 (medium risk)** – observe by noting the patient's dietary intake for the next 3 days. If this improves then there is little concern. However, if there is no improvement, this is of clinical concern and one should follow the local policies for what to do next, e.g. referral to nutrition support team/dietician.
- **Score 2 or more (high risk)** – these patients should be referred to the nutrition support team/dietician to try to increase their nutritional intake and there should be policies in place for the nutritional support given to these patients.

 The MUST tool should be used routinely to assess nutritional risk for all hospital admissions (www.BAPEN.org.uk).

Subjective global assessment
Useful indicators for bedside assessment of nutritional status applicable to clinical practice have been identified,[24] and include estimation of protein and energy balance, assessment of body composition and evaluation of physiological function.

Assessment of protein and energy balance
Protein and energy balance can be assessed either by a dietician or by a clinician, who determines the frequency and size of meals eaten. This information is compared with the patient's rate of loss of body weight and BMI.

Assessment of body composition
Loss of body fat can be determined by observing the physical appearance of the patient (loss of body contours) and feeling the patient's skinfolds between finger and thumb. In particular, if the dermis can be felt on pinching the biceps and triceps skinfolds, then considerable weight loss has occurred.

The stores of protein in the body can be assessed from various muscle groups including temporalis, deltoid, suprascapular, infrascapular, biceps and tri-

ceps, and the interossei of the hands. When tendons of the muscles are prominent and bony protruberances of the scapula are obvious, greater than 30% of the total body protein stores have been lost.

Assessment of physiological function
Assessments of function are made by observing the patient's activities. Grip strength is determined by asking patients to squeeze the clinician's index and middle fingers for at least 10 seconds, and respiratory function by asking them to blow hard on a strip of paper held 10 cm from the patient's lips. The measurement of metabolic expenditure requires specialised equipment, but additional metabolic stresses on the patient can be determined from clinical examination. Extra metabolic stresses will occur if trauma or surgery has taken place or there is evidence of significant sepsis (elevated temperature and/or white blood cell counts, tachycardia, tachypnoea, positive blood cultures) or active inflammatory bowel disease. In addition, patients should be asked about their ability to heal wounds, changes in exercise tolerance and their 'tiredness'.

Re-feeding syndrome
Once a patient's need for nutritional support has been identified, it is important to consider whether the patient is at risk of re-feeding syndrome. This is described in detail elsewhere, but in essence it is the inability of a patient's metabolism to handle macronutrients. After approximately 10 days without nutritional intake, the metabolism adapts to the state of starvation. Re-feeding with full 'normal' required amounts of macronutrients will induce a sudden reversal of this adaptation, with an anabolic drive which may result in catastrophic depletion of available potassium, phosphate and magnesium. Before re-feeding, the serum biochemistry may appear 'normal', and so the possibility of re-feeding must be anticipated on history alone. The other essential nutrient liable to become depleted in this situation is thiamine. This must be replenished before feeding is commenced in the starved patient to prevent development of Wernicke–Korsakoff syndrome. The potential for this is considerably higher in patients with a history of chronic excessive ethanol intake, and so even greater caution is required.

 Thiamine deficiency must always be considered in patients who have had no nutritional intake for more than 1 week, who have a history of excessive alcohol intake, or in the presence of an unexplained metabolic acidosis.

Nutritional support in surgical practice

Route of nutritional support

The route of administration of nutritional support may be through either the gastrointestinal tract (enteral) or the intravenous (parenteral) route. The enteral route is the preferred method of nutrient delivery whenever possible and the parenteral route is used for patients with primary intestinal failure.

Enteral nutritional support

If there is an intact and functioning gastrointestinal tract, enteral feeding should be used if oral intake is insufficient. Enteral feeding is contraindicated to various degrees in patients with intestinal obstruction, paralytic ileus, vomiting and diarrhoea, high-output intestinal fistulas or in the presence of major intra-abdominal sepsis.

Why enteral nutrition is important

Studies in animals have shown that in the absence of nutrients into the intestinal lumen, changes occur in the intestinal mucosa. There is loss of height of villi, reduction in cellular proliferation and the mucosa becomes atrophic.[25,26] Activities of enzymes found in association with the mucosa are reduced and permeability of the mucosa to macromolecules increased.[27] Stimulation of the intestinal tract by nutrients is important for release of many gut-related hormones, including those responsible for gut motility and stimulation of secretions necessary for normal maintenance of the mucosa. The gut acts as a barrier to bacteria, both physically and by release of chemical and immunological substances. There is evidence to suggest that atrophy of the intestinal mucosa is associated with loss of intercellular adhesion and opening of intercellular channels. This predisposes to increased translocation of bacteria and endotoxin from the gut lumen into portal venous and lymphatic systems.[28] Loss of gut integrity may account for a substantial proportion of septicaemic events in severely ill patients. However, the extent to which it contributes to sepsis in patients is not fully understood.

Routes of access for enteral nutritional support

Nasoenteric tubes

Nasogastric feeding via fine-bore tubes (polyvinyl chloride or polyurethane) may be used in patients who require nutritional support for a short period of time. There has been considerable debate as to whether positioning the feeding tube beyond the pylorus into the duodenum will result in reduction in the risks of regurgitation of gastric contents and pulmonary aspiration (occurs in up to 30% of patients fed this way). This is most likely in patients with impaired gastric motility. In the latter patients, the fine-bore tube can be manipulated through the pylorus into the duodenum, reducing the risk of gastric aspiration. Other complications associated with the use of nasoenteric tubes include:

- pulmonary atelectasis;
- oesophageal necrosis, stricture formation;
- tracheo-oesophageal fistulas;
- sinusitis, postcricoid ulceration.

More recently, double lumen tubes have been used – one lumen resides in the stomach and is used to aspirate gastric contents, the other longer lumen is placed in the jejunum for feeding, thus reducing risks of aspiration. This can be successful even in patients with relatively high gastric aspirates, previously thought to be a contraindication for feeding via the enteral route.

Gastrostomy tubes

A gastrostomy tube can be placed into the stomach at laparotomy, although percutaneous endoscopic or percutaneous fluoroscopic techniques are preferred. Details of how these are performed can be found in standard texts.

The establishment and use of a gastrostomy has certain disadvantages and there is a recognised morbidity:

- infection of the skin at the puncture site;
- necrotising fasciitis or deeper-sited sepsis;
- damage to adjacent intra-abdominal viscera;
- leakage of gastric contents into the peritoneal cavity;
- haemorrhage from the stomach;
- persistent gastrocutaneous fistula following removal of the feeding tube.

The overall mortality rate for a gastrostomy is 1–2%, with major and minor complications occurring in up to 15% of patients. Mechanical complications associated with the tube include blockage, fracture and displacement. Furthermore, 'dumping' and diarrhoea are more common when the tip of the tube lies in the duodenum or jejunum.[29]

Jejunostomy tubes

A feeding jejunostomy is usually carried out at the time of laparotomy if it is envisaged that a patient will need nutritional support for a longer period. Details of the operative technique are also in standard operative texts and the smaller needle-catheter tubes are to be preferred. Advantages of a feeding jejunostomy compared with a gastrostomy are:

- less stomal leakage;
- gastric and pancreatic secretions are reduced because the stomach is bypassed;
- less nausea, vomiting or bloating;
- reduced risk of pulmonary aspiration.

Nutrient solutions available for enteral nutrition

A range of nutrient solutions are available for use in enteral nutritional support and examples can be found in specialised texts. However, there are four main categories of enteral diet.

Polymeric diets

Polymeric diets are 'nutritionally complete' diets and provided to patients whose gastrointestinal function is good. They contain whole protein as the source of nitrogen, and energy is provided as complex carbohydrates and fat. They also contain vitamins, trace elements and electrolytes in standard amounts.

Elemental diets

Elemental diets are required if the patient is unable to produce an adequate amount of digestive enzymes or has a reduced area for absorption (e.g. severe pancreatic insufficiency or short-bowel syndrome). Elemental diets contain nitrogen as oligopeptides. Free amino acids are not as easily absorbed as dipeptide and tripeptide mixtures. The energy source is provided as glucose polymers and medium-chain triacylglycerols. Each oligopeptide molecule contributes as much to the osmolarity of the solution as one molecule of intact protein, and it can be difficult to provide complete requirements without producing side-effects associated with an osmotic load, e.g. 'dumping' and diarrhoea.

Special formulations

Special formulations have been developed for patients with particular diseases. Examples of such diets include: (i) those with increased concentrations of branched-chain amino acids and low in aromatic amino acids for patients with hepatic encephalopathy; (ii) those with a higher fat but lower glucose energy content for patients who are artificially ventilated; and (iii) diets containing key nutrients that modulate the immune response (see later).

Modular diets

Modular diets are not commonly used but allow provision of a diet rich in a particular nutrient for specific patients. For example, the diet may be enriched in protein if the patient is protein deficient or in sodium if sodium deficient. These modular diets can be used to supplement other enteral regimens or oral intake.

Enteral nutrition delivery and complications

Previously, when starting an enteral nutrition feeding regimen, patients received either a reduced rate of infusion or a lower strength formula for the first 2 or 3 days to reduce gastrointestinal complications. Recent studies have demonstrated this is not required and nutritional support can commence using full-strength feeds at the desired rate in those not at risk of developing 're-feeding syndrome'. Cyclical feeding (e.g. 16 hours feeding with a post-absorptive period of 8 hours) is optimal and more closely mimics the natural feeding cycle than other types of feeding regimens.[30]

Enteral nutrition should be administered through a volumetric pump. If not available, then it is possible to use a gravity drip flow but care should be taken to reduce the risk of a large bolus being administered. In patients whose conscious level is impaired or confined to bed, the head of the bed should be elevated by 25° to reduce risks of pulmonary aspiration. Some clinicians prefer patients to be sitting upright when receiving enteral nutrition. The stomach contents should be aspirated every 4 hours during feeding and if a residual volume of more than 100 mL is found, enteral nutrition is temporarily discontinued.

The aspirate is checked again after 2 hours, and when satisfactory volumes are aspirated (<100 mL) feeding is re-instituted. If more than 400 mL per 24 hours is aspirated, then feeding is discontinued. Gastric emptying may be improved by the administration of cisapride or erythromycin, which may allow feeding to be continued.

Metabolic disturbances are less likely with enteral feeding. The other complications of enteral nutrition are those associated with the route of access to the gastrointestinal tract (Box 17.4).

Parenteral nutritional support

Patients who require nutritional support but with enteral feeding contraindicated will require parenteral nutrition. These include:

- patients with a non-functioning or inaccessible gastrointestinal tract;
- those with high-output enteric fistulas (enteral nutrition may stimulate gastrointestinal secretion – discussed further later);
- those for whom it is not possible to provide sufficient intake of nutrients enterally (e.g. because of a short segment of residual bowel or malabsorption, severe burns, major trauma).

Detailed guidance for total parenteral nutrition (TPN) in patients has been published by the American Society of Parenteral and Enteral

Box 17.4 • Complications of enteral nutrition

Gastrointestinal

Diarrhoea, nausea, vomiting, abdominal discomfort and bloating, regurgitation and aspiration of feed/stomach contents

Mechanical

Dislodgement of the feeding tube, blockage of the tube, leakage of stomach/small intestine contents onto the skin with the use of jejunostomies or gastrostomies

Metabolic

Excess or deficiency of glucose, electrolytes, minerals or trace elements, Some of these will be noted through routine testing protocols, e.g hyperkalaemia, but others such as hypophosphataemia may be missed if not specifically anticipated

Infective

Local effects (e.g. diarrhoea, vomiting) or systemic effects (e.g. pyrexia, malaise)

Nutrition (ASPEN).[31] Current ASPEN guidelines are also available on their website (www.nutrition-care.org) and should be studied.

Parenteral routes of access

Central venous access

Central venous access is obtained by positioning a catheter into the superior vena cava through sub-clavian or internal jugular veins. The catheter either emerges through the skin (usually after being tun-nelled in the subcutaneous fat) or is connected to a port placed in the subcutaneous fat of the anterior chest wall. A variety of techniques for insertion of central venous lines are used. For example, cathe-ters may be introduced into the internal jugular or subclavian or vein directly by 'blind' percutaneous puncture, using small hand-held ultrasound imaging or by 'cut-down' techniques utilising the cephalic vein to access the subclavian vein. Radiologists can also be asked to insert lines under fluoroscopic con-trol. Details of these techniques, their advantages and disadvantages can be found elsewhere.[32–34] However, it is important that whoever inserts a cen-tral venous line is expert, well practised and carries out the procedure under full aseptic techniques.

Technical aspects of feeding lines

Central lines are manufactured from polyurethane or silicone. Both of these materials are tolerated well with low thrombogenic potential. However, polyurethane does have advantages:

- it is stiffer than silicone at room temperature, but at body temperature is pliable;

- it has a higher tensile strength than silicone and is less likely to fracture;
- polyurethane catheters have smaller outside diameters making cannulation easier, as well as a greater resistance to thrombus development on their surfaces.

Catheter manufacturers have attempted to reduce risks of bacterial colonisation of the line by bonding antiseptics (e.g. chlorhexidene) and antibiotics (e.g. silver sulphadiazine) into the catheter's fabric. Some catheters have an antimicrobial cuff, usually made of Dacron, around their external surface. This acts as a barrier to microorganisms, which may migrate from subcutaneous tissues along the external aspect of the catheter to its tip. Although studies have suggested that risks of septicaemia are reduced by using a cuff around the catheter, this makes positioning of the catheter more difficult technically. Complications of central venous catheters are shown in Box 17.5.

Catheter care

Appropriate dressings of the catheter are essential. The dressing should be changed weekly and the skin exit site cleaned weekly with chlorhexidine. A variety of dressings have been used at the skin exit, but sterile gauze and a transparent adherent type of dressing are satisfactory.

Infection of the catheter tip is the most serious type of infection. The patient usually is pyrexial and may have systemic signs of sepsis. This may be diagnosed by blood (at least three cultures 1 hour apart) and catheter cultures.[35] Antibiotic therapy may result in recovery, but in some the feeding line has to be removed to eradicate the infection. However, less serious infection may occur in the skin at the exit site of the catheter. This is recognised by skin erythema, possibly associated with fluid exudate and pus.

Peripheral venous access

Peripheral venous cannulation, using a sterile technique, may be used to supply nutrients intra-venously avoiding complications associated with

Box 17.5 • Complications of central venous catheter placement and incidence of occurrence

Catheter-related sepsis: variable, but reported in up to 40% of catheters

Thrombosis of central vein: variable, but reported in up to 20% of catheters

Pleural space damage: pneumothorax (5–10%), haemothorax (2%)

Major arterial damage: subclavian artery (1–2%)

Catheter problems: thrombosis (1–2%), embolism (<1%), air embolism (<1%)

Miscellaneous problems: brachial plexus (<1%), thoracic duct damage (<1%)

central venous catheters. Peripheral intravenous nutrition is likely to be used in patients who do not require nutritional support for long enough to justify risks of central vein cannulation or in whom central vein cannulation is contraindicated (e.g. central line insertion sites are traumatised, increased risks of infective complications, thrombosis of the central veins or significant clotting defects).

Problems associated with the delivery of intravenous nutrition using the peripheral route include:

- a limit to nutrient quantity deliverable – this is not the route of choice in those with high requirements for protein or energy;
- a high incidence of complications, particularly phlebitis (occurs in up to 45% of patients), and it is essential to ensure good peripheral venous access.

The lifespan of a peripheral intravenous cannula can be prolonged by treating it as if it is a central line with regard to aseptic care, and by using a narrow-gauge cannula giving better mixing and flow characteristics of the nutrient solution. Risks of phlebitis can be reduced by frequent changes of infusion site, ultrafine-bore catheters or using a vasodilator patch over the cannulation site (e.g. transdermal glyceryl trinitrate). Furthermore, peripheral intravenous nutrition can only be used where fat emulsion is part of the single-phase administration of nutrients to avoid thrombophlebitis.

Nutrients used in parenteral feeding solutions

Various nutrient solutions (amino acids, glucose and fat) are available and a complete list is given in the *British National Formulary* (http://www. bnf.org/bnf/). There are also available a variety of pre-mixed bags containing various concentrations of amino acids and glucose, with or without fat, which are suitable for different clinical situations. These mixtures do not usually contain vitamins or trace elements, which must be given in addition to avoid development of metabolic complications. Care should be taken that patients receive sufficient electrolytes and minerals to satisfy requirements.

Nitrogen sources

Nitrogen sources are solutions of crystalline L-amino acids containing all essential and a balanced mixture of the non-essential amino acids required. Amino acids that are relatively insoluble (e.g. L-glutamine, L-arginine, L-taurine, L-tyrosine, L-methionine) may be absent or present in inadequate amounts.

Attention has focused on the provision of L-glutamine because of its key roles in metabolism. It can be supplied as *N*-acetylglutamine (hydrolysed in the renal tubule to free L-glutamine) or as L-glutamine dipeptides such as alanylglutamine (broken down to release free L-glutamine).[36] An alternative approach has been to supplement parenteral nutrition with ornithine α-ketoglutarate. This is promising but further investigation is necessary to clarify their roles before introduction into practice.

Energy sources

Energy is supplied as a balanced combination of dextrose and fat. Glucose is the primary carbohydrate source and the main form of energy supply to the majority of tissues. During critical illness the body's preferred calorie source is fat (fasted or fed states).[37,38] There are controversies as to the utilisation of fat in sepsis because of defects in energy substrate metabolism at the oxidative level.

Glucose utilisation may be impaired in certain patients and glucose is then metabolised through other pathways. This results in increased production of fatty acids and increased oxidation of fatty acids, resulting in increased carbon dioxide (excreted through the lungs). In addition, if glucose is the only energy source, patients may develop essential fatty acid (linolenic, linoleic) deficiency.

Fat (e.g. soyabean oil emulsions) is also given as an energy source. Usually, approximately 30–50% of the total calories are given as fat with non-protein calorie to nitrogen ratio varying from 150:1 to 200:1 (lower in hypercatabolic conditions). The provision of exogenous lipids has also been associated with problems. Intravenous fat emulsions can impair lung function, inhibit the reticuloendothelial system and modulate neutrophil function.[39, 40]

Other nutrients

Commercially available preparations of trace elements (e.g. Additrace®) and vitamins, water soluble (e.g. Solivito®) and fat soluble (e.g. Vitlipid®), supply daily requirements. Larger amounts, particularly of the water-soluble vitamins, may be required initially if recent nutritional intake has been inadequate. Additionally, total fluid volume and amounts of electrolytes can be modified daily to meet particular requirements.

Delivery and administration of TPN

In practice, commercially available solutions for parenteral infusion are mixed under sterile conditions in laminar flow facilities. The feeding regimen is made up in an inert 3- to 4-L bag (ethyl vinyl acetate), comprising all nutrients and stored for up to 1 week, although compatibility between different constituents must be ensured. No additions of drugs should be made as this could make the emulsion unstable, affect the bioavailability of the drug or compromise sterility. Advantages of pre-mixed bags include:

- cost-effectiveness;
- reduced infective risks;
- more uniform administration of a balanced solution over a prolonged period;
- decreased lipid toxicity as a result of the greater dilution of the lipid emulsion and longer duration of infusion;
- ease of delivery and storage and reduced long-term accumulation of triacylglycerols (occurs with glucose-based TPN).

Recently, prepared bags are available where the fat emulsion is stored separately from the aqueous solution and is mixed by bag rupture immediately prior to administration. Such bags should be used for short-term support only, because overall nutrient composition may not be appropriate.

Complications of parenteral nutritional support

Instant availability of nutrients provided by the intravenous route can lead to metabolic complications if the composition or flow rate is inappropriate. Rapid infusion of high concentrations of glucose can precipitate hyperglycaemia, which may be further complicated by lactic acidosis. Electrolyte disturbances may present problems, not least because the intravenous feeding regimen is usually prescribed in advance for 24 hours. Prediction of the patient's nutrient requirements must be complemented by frequent monitoring. The provision of nutrients may lead to further electrolyte abnormalities when potassium, magnesium and phosphate enter the intracellular compartment. This is particularly noticeable in patients whose previous nutrient intake was especially poor, as highlighted previously. Others complications of TPN are shown in Box 17.6.

Monitoring patients receiving nutritional support

Enteral nutrition

Patients receiving nutritional support should be monitored by accurate recording of fluid balance and daily weighing. Daily intake of calories and nitrogen should be documented. Biochemical assessments include twice-weekly measurements of renal and liver function, regular checks of phosphate, calcium, magnesium, albumin and protein levels and haematological indices, until the patient is stabilised. Then, weekly or fortnightly measurements are necessary.

Box 17.6 • Metabolic complications of parenteral nutrition

Glucose disturbances

Hyperglycaemia: excessive administration of glucose inadequate insulin, sepsis

Hypoglycaemia: rebound hypoglycaemia occurs if glucose is stopped abruptly but insulin levels remain high

Lipid disturbances

Hyperlipidaemia: directly through excess administration of lipid, or indirectly, through excess calories which will be converted to fat or reduced metabolism (e.g. renal failure, liver failure)

Fatty acid deficiency: essential fatty acid deficiency leads to hair loss, dry skin, impaired wound healing

Nitrogen disturbances

Hyperammonaemia: occurs if deficiency of L-arginine, L-ornithine, L-aspartate or L-glutamate in infusion. Also occurs in liver diseases

Metabolic acidosis: caused by excessive amounts of chloride and monochloride amino acids

Electrolyte disturbances

Hyperkalaemia: excessive potassium administration or reduced losses

Hypokalaemia: inadequate potassium administration or excessive loss

Hypocalcaemia: inadequate calcium replacement, losses in pancreatitis, hypoalbuminaemia

Hypophosphataemia: inadequate phosphorus supplementation, also tissue compartment fluxes

Liver disturbances

Elevations in aspartate aminotransferase, alkaline phosphatase and γ-glutamyl transferase may occur because of enzyme induction secondary to amino acid imbalances or deposition of fat and/or glycogen in liver

Ventilatory problems

If excessive amounts of glucose are given, the increased production of CO_2 may precipitate ventilatory failure in nonventilated patients

Other methods of assessment may be used at regular intervals to ascertain patient progress (see nutritional assessment section above). Routes of access should be regularly examined to ensure that the catheter is correctly positioned and mechanically satisfactory.

Parenteral nutrition

The patient's clinical condition and fluid balance should be evaluated daily (weight, signs of fluid depletion or overload). Biochemical indices are monitored; serum electrolytes, urea, creatinine and glucose are checked daily, serum albumin, protein, calcium, magnesium, phosphate and liver function are checked twice per week. Haematological indices (haemoglobin, white blood cell count, haematocrit) are checked twice weekly. Urinalysis is performed four times daily initially in case glycosuria occurs, as this induces further fluid and electrolyte losses. If glycosuria occurs, it may be necessary to commence intravenous insulin on a sliding scale with hourly blood glucose monitoring. It is important to note that if the TPN fluid is stopped, insulin requirements will reduce immediately; it is safest to discontinue the insulin at the same time as the TPN, reviewing the sliding scale.

Other assessments, e.g. muscle function, nitrogen balance, measurement of trace elements and vitamins, may be performed. The catheter, site of access and equipment infusing the feeding solution must all be carefully examined for possible complications or dysfunction.

Nutritional support teams

It is clear that for optimal provision of nutritional support, a multidisciplinary nutritional support team is required. This may comprise a clinician with a special interest in nutritional support and understanding of metabolic pathways, a biochemist, a pharmacist, a dietician and a nursing specialist. The provision of nutritional support by such a team results in the most cost-effective use of nutritional support and the least risk of infective, metabolic and feeding line complications.[41]

Nutritional support in defined clinical situations

Nutritional support in the perioperative period

Parenteral nutrition

There is debate as to which patients require preoperative and/or postoperative nutritional support. Many studies have evaluated the effects of nutritional support in the perioperative period; clinical benefit with supplemental nutrition has not been a consistent finding. This may be because the studies were small, with many different end-points (e.g. morbidity, mortality), frequently without proper randomisation or allowance for malnutrition prior to the study commencing.

A meta-analysis has examined 27 randomised controlled trials (almost 3000 patients) of nutritional support in the perioperative period.[42] The results are important and provide a basis for the rational use of nutritional support in this situation. The key findings are detailed in Table 17.1. When TPN was given in the preoperative period there was a reduction in complication rates (relative risk 0.52, 95% CI 0.30–0.91) in malnourished patients but not when nutritional state was adequate. However, there was no difference in mortality. Analysis of patients in the postoperative period indicated no reduction in complications (relative risk 1.08, 95% CI 0.81–1.43) or mortality in patients receiving TPN. Subgroup analyses indicated that nutritional support in the preoperative period be considered for:

- those with a serum albumin <30–32 g/L;
- patients with a weight loss of 15% or more, associated with impairment of physiological function;
- patients with a nutrition (prognostic) risk index <83.5.

Table 17.1 • Effect of perioperative nutritional support on morbidity and mortality in surgical patients

	Complications (RR and 95% CI)	Mortality (RR and 95% CI)
Malnourished patients	0.53 (0.30–1.91)	1.13 (0.78–71)
Adequate nutrition	0.95 (0.75–1.21)	0.90 (0.66–1.2)
Preoperative TPN	0.70 (0.52–0.95)	0.85 (0.6–1.20)
Postoperative TPN	1.01 (0.70–1.96)	1.08 (0.73–1.58)
Overall effects	0.81 (0.65–1.01)	0.97 (0.76–1.24)

CI, confidence interval; RR, relative risk; TPN, total parenteral nutrition.

Nutritional support should be given to malnourished patients for at least 7–10 days preoperatively to reduce postoperative morbidity.[42] Nutritional support in the postoperative period should be considered for:

- patients in whom it is anticipated that normal oral intake is unlikely for 7 days or more after surgery;
- those with severe sepsis or burns;
- those with enterocutaneous fistulas (particularly if high output);
- patients who have lost 15% or more of their usual weight prior to surgery being undertaken.

Enteral nutrition

As discussed, the enteral route is the preferred route except in specific circumstances where not possible (e.g. intestinal obstruction, ileus, intestinal ischaemia, etc.) or used in combination with TPN if the nutritional requirements cannot be provided by the enteral route alone. A recent analysis of studies of enteral nutrition given to patients in the perioperative period has been carried out and published as European Society of Parenteral and Enteral Nutrition (ESPEN) guidelines[43] (http://www.espen.org/Education/documents/ENSurgery.pdf).

The ESPEN guidance is summarised as follows.[43] Patients who should receive perioperative nutritional support:

- Those expected not to eat for >7 days perioperatively.
- Those unable to have an oral intake >60% of their recommended intake for >10 days.

Patients who should receive preoperative enteral nutritional support:

- Preoperative nutritional support should be given for 10–14 days to those with 'severe' nutritional risk, which is defined as either a BMI <18.5 kg/m^2, recent weight loss of 10–15% in the previous 6 months or serum albumin <30 g/L (with no evidence of renal or hepatic failure). For such patients it is recommended that surgery should be delayed if possible to allow nutritional support.

Patients who should receive postoperative nutritional support:

- Early enteral nutritional feeding (i.e. <24 h after surgery) is recommended for patients who have undergone upper gastrointestinal anastomosis with the tip of a feeding tube placed distal to the anastomosis.

Nutritional support in patients with acute pancreatitis

Severe pancreatitis produces a major catabolic stress with rapid loss of muscle proteins. The daily nitrogen requirements of such patients are high, reaching 1.2–2.0 g/kg of protein (0.2–0.3 g/kg of nitrogen). Daily energy requirements also increase with disease severity to be 28–35 kcal/kg. Previously, patients with pancreatitis were fasted in order to avoid pancreatic stimulation. However, views have now changed[44,45] and a recent systematic review[46] has shown that patients with acute severe pancreatitis should commence enteral support early (within 5 days). This resulted in better outcomes with reduced infectious complications and hospital stay, but without effect on mortality.[44–46]

Patients with severe acute pancreatitis should commence early enteral nutritional support as this is associated with a better outcome.[46]

Nutritional supplementation in inflammatory bowel disease

A significant number of patients with Crohn's disease and ulcerative colitis become malnourished. The reasons for this include decreased nutrient intake, malabsorption by the small intestine (decreased length, bacterial overgrowth, protein-losing enteropathy) and increased calorie/nitrogen requirements in those with coexistent sepsis. There may be deficiencies of specific vitamins and trace elements.

Nutritional support, therefore, may have different roles: (i) to provide nutritional requirements and correct nutritional deficiencies the patient may have; (ii) the possibility that provision of TPN with bowel rest in Crohn's disease may be therapeutically beneficial. The results of studies addressing this latter point are inconclusive,[47,48] suggesting that parenteral nutrition itself does not have a therapeutic effect in inflammatory bowel disease. Furthermore, there is evidence showing that enteral nutrition is as effective as TPN in these patients.[49] This has the added benefits of maintaining gut mucosa integrity in addition to stimulating production of gut hormones necessary for function.

While systematic reviews have shown some potential for enteral nutrition in this regard, further studies are required to clarify the use of nutrition in this way.[50,51]

Nutritional support in enterocutaneous fistulas

Nutritional support has an important role to play in management of patients with enterocutaneous fistulas as up to 50% are malnourished. The importance of adequate nutritional support was demonstrated by Chapman et al.,[52] who found that if patients with fistulas received nutritional support with TPN and enteral feeding (>3000 kcal (12.6 MJ) daily), spontaneous fistula healing with a reduced mortality occurred compared with patients with fistulas receiving less than 1000 kcal (4.1 MJ) daily. The management of such patients commences with correction of fluid and electrolyte deficits and elimination of septic foci. Nutritional support is required to correct any nutritional deficits and provides maintenance requirements when the patient is stabilised. Whether TPN or enteral nutrition is more effective is unknown. Other techniques for providing nutritional support have included collecting the intestinal output from the proximal end of the fistula and re-infusing it into the distal part of the small intestine or by giving enteral nutrition via the fistula. If the fistula output is low, enteral nutritional support should be considered because of the benefits.[53]

 Enteral nutrition has theoretical benefits due to its effects on gut mucosa and case series have suggested that healing rates with enteral nutrition are comparable to those of parenteral nutrition.[53]

Nutritional support in patients with burns

Major burns induce severe hypermetabolic and hypercatabolic states. There is increased skeletal muscle breakdown, nitrogen losses of 15 g daily or more, and up to a doubling of metabolic rate. In patients with burns of greater than 20% of their body surface area, nutritional support is required, orally or by nasoenteric feeding. There may be clinical benefits by introducing feeding early, and with glutamine supplementation.[54,55] This appears to be associated with reduced infectious complications and better wound healing and is recommended by the ESPEN guidelines.[56]

 Glutamine supplementation should be given to patients with substantial burns to reduce their complications and improve healing. If enteral nutritional support is not possible, e.g. with gastric stasis, ileus or other coexistent injuries, parenteral nutrition is required.

Several formulae exist for calculating the protein and calorie requirements.[57] However, up to 20–25 g of nitrogen per day may be required initially, with a non-protein calorie to nitrogen ratio of 100–200. Energy is provided as carbohydrate and lipids, with the calorie requirement being 35–50% as lipid.

Nutritional supplementation with key nutrients: application to clinical practice

Certain nutrients can have effects on cellular and tissue function. Some of these nutrients modulate immune and inflammatory responses if given in excess of normal intake or requirements. The use of nutrients ('nutriceuticals') in this way has been termed 'nutritional pharmacology'. Examples and specific effects include:

- L-arginine – stimulates aspects of immune function, improves nitrogen retention after surgery, enhances wound healing;[58, 59]
- L-glutamine – stimulates immune function, reduces nitrogen loss postoperatively, may be important in maintaining gut-barrier function;[60]
- branched-chain amino acids – may control protein synthesis in muscle and stimulate whole-body protein synthesis, especially in severely traumatised patients;[61]
- essential fatty acids – stimulation or inhibition of immune function, anti-inflammatory effects;[62, 63]
- polyribonucleotides and ribonucleic acid – stimulate immune function;
- vitamins, trace elements – stimulation of immune function, antioxidant effects, wound healing;
- selenium – stimulation of immune function, prevention of tissue damage, anti-inflammatory effects.[64]

The clinical benefits of supplementation with key nutrients have been difficult to demonstrate but special interest has focused on the role of L-glutamine supplementation (e.g. 30 g daily).

 Individual studies have found some benefits for patients treated with glutamine supplementation, and systemic reviews have identified trends to suggest that parenteral or enteral glutamine supplementation reduces mortality, the development of infection and organ failure in patients with critical illness. Parenteral nutrition containing glutamine given to patients undergoing elective surgery may also reduce postoperative infections. However, it is still not possible to draw definitive conclusions for general clinical practice.[65]

Combinations of these nutrients and their place in practice

Several studies have evaluated the use of combina tions of key nutrients in clinical practice in patients with critical illnesses (trauma, surgery for malignant disease, burns), but particularly in upper gastrointestinal cancer. A combination of L-arginine, *n*-3 essential fatty acids and ribonucleic acid is commercially available (Impact; Sandoz Nutrition, Minneapolis, MN, USA) and has been used in many trials. The supplemented nutrition has been given in the postoperative period (nasoenteric tube or feeding jejunostomy), starting within 12–48 hours of the critical events and continued for several days.

The first meta-analysis of the studies that have compared supplemented nutritional versus standard nutritional diets (**Figs 17.2** and **17.3**) showed that supplemented nutrition had clinical benefits:[66]

- reduction in infectious complications (wound infections, intra-abdominal abscesses, septicaemia), with an odds ratio of 0.47 (95% CI 0.32–0.70);

- reduction in length of hospital stay, with a weighted mean difference of –2.4 days (95% CI –4 to –1).

However, there was no significant difference in mortality. A subsequent meta-analysis of 17 trials has confirmed this benefit.[67]

Many of these studies had methodological limitations but, nevertheless, the role of immunonutrition in critically ill patients was further investigated by ESPEN[56] (http://www.espen.org/Education/documents/ENICU.pdf). The conclusions drawn from the consensus based on the available evidence was that an immune-modulating nutrition (enriched with arginine, nucleotides and omega-3 fatty acids) was beneficial and recommended for the following:

- patients with mild sepsis (APACHE II score <15);
- patients undergoing elective major intra-abdominal surgery for cancer to receive 5–7 days of immune-enhancing nutrition (arginine, omega-3 fatty acids and polyribonucleotides);
- patients with acute respiratory distress syndrome (ARDS) should receive enteral

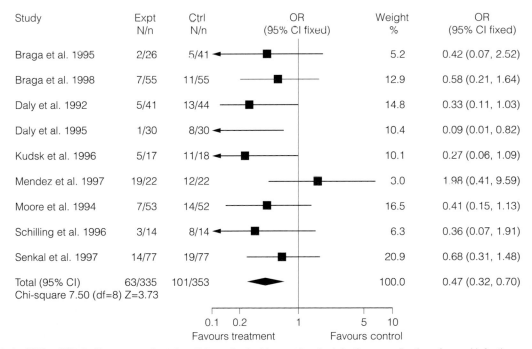

Figure 17.2 • Effect of immuno-enhancing diets on the incidence of major infective complications (wound infections, intra-abdominal abscesses, pneumonia, septicaemia). Expt, patients receiving immuno-enhancing diets; Ctrl, patients receiving standard nutrition; n, number of events; N, number of patients in each group on an intention-to-treat basis; OR, odds ratio; CI, confidence interval. (Study sources are given in Heys et al.[60]) Reproduced from Heys SD, Walker LG, Smith IC et al. Enteral nutritional supplementation with key nutrients in patients with critical illness and cancer. A meta-analysis of randomised controlled clinical trials. Ann Surg 1999; 229:467–77. With permission from Lippincott, Williams & Wilkins.

Study	Expt N	Expt mean (sd)	Ctrl N	WMD (95% CI fixed)	Weight %	WMD (95% CI fixed)
Braga et al. 1995	26	13.50(4.89)	26		16.5	-1.70 (-5.574, -2.174)
Braga et al. 1998	55	13.70(4.80)	55		61.4	-2.40 (-4.410, -0.390)
Daly et al. 1992	41	18.80(10.90)	45		13.1	-1.60 (-5.959, 2.759)
Daly et al. 1995	30	16.00(5.48)	30		6.9	-6.00 (-12.018, 0.018)
Schilling et al. 1996	14	14.50(7.90)	14		2.1	0.50 (-10,279, 11.279)
Total (95% CI)	164		170		100.0	-2.365 (-3.94, -1.171)

Chi-square 1.91 (df=4) Z=2.94

-10   -5   0   5   10

Favours treatment   Favours control

Figure 17.3 • Effect of immuno-enhancing diets on the length of hospital stay. WMD, weighted mean difference; CI, confidence interval. (Study sources are given in Heys et al.[66]) Reproduced from Heys SD, Walker LG, Smith IC et al. Enteral nutritional supplementation with key nutrients in patients with critical illness and cancer. A meta-analysis of randomised controlled clinical trials. Ann Surg 1999; 229:467–77. With permission from Lippincott, Williams & Wilkins.

nutrition supplemented with omega-3 fatty acids and antioxidants.

In addition, there were situations identified where immunonutrition should not be given due to potentially adverse effects:

- patients with severe sepsis;
- patients unable to tolerate more than 700 mL/day of immunonutrition.

Immune-modulating nutrition is associated with a reduction in septic complications and a reduced hospital stay. It should be considered in patients with mild sepsis (APACHE II score <15), patients undergoing elective major intra-abdominal surgery for cancer and in patients with ARDS.[56,66,67]

Key points

- Malnutrition is associated with loss of body weight and impairments in organ function.
- The metabolic changes that occur in patients undergoing surgery or in those who have experienced trauma and sepsis can be compounded by inadequate nutritional support.
- Nutritional requirements must take into consideration the underlying pathophysiological changes.
- An assessment of nutritional status should be made in all patients.
- If nutritional support is considered necessary, the route and composition of this support should be considered carefully.
- Remember re-feeding syndrome and possible thiamine deficiency.
- The role of certain key nutrients and their effects, either individually or in combination, on aspects of organ and immune function should be taken into consideration when planning nutritional interventions.
- There is now emerging evidence to indicate that manipulating the composition of nutritional support can affect patient outcome.
- Careful monitoring of patients receiving nutritional support and the role of the multidisciplinary team is essential for all patients.

References

1. Cuthbertson DP. Observations on the disturbances of metabolism produced by injury to the limbs. Q J Med 1932; 1:233–46.

2. O'Keefe SJD, Sender PM, James WPT. Catabolic loss of body nitrogen in response to surgery. Lancet 1974; ii:1035–8.

3. Bergstrom J, Furst P, Noree L-O et al. Intracellular free amino acid concentration in human muscle tissue. J Appl Physiol 1973; 36:693–8.

4. Stoner HB. Studies on the mechanism of shock. The quantitative aspects of glycogen metabolism after limb ischaemia in the rat. Br J Exp Pathol 1958; 39:635–51.

5. Allsop JR, Wolfe RR, Burke JF. Glucose kinetics and responsiveness to insulin in the rat injured by burn. Surg Gynecol Obstet 1978; 147:565–73.

6. Nordenstrom J, Carpentier YA, Askanazi J et al. Free fatty acid mobilisation and oxidation during total parenteral nutrition in trauma and infection. Ann Surg 1983; 198:725–35.

7. Broom J. Sepsis and trauma. In: Garrow JS, James WPT (eds) Human nutrition and dietetics, 9th edn. Edinburgh: Churchill Livingstone, 1993; pp. 456–64.

8. Rich AJ, Wright PD. Ketosis and nitrogen excretion in undernourished surgical patients. J Parenteral Enteral Nutr 1979; 3:350–4.

9. Demling RH, DeBiasse MA. Micronutrients in critical illness. Crit Care Clin 1995; 11:651–73.

10. Metropolitan Life Assurance Company. Statist Bull 1959; 40:1.

11. Pettigrew RA. Assessment of malnourished patients. In: Burns HG (ed.) Clinical gastroenterology. London: Baillière Tindall, 1988; pp. 729–49.

12. Durnin JVGA, Womersley J. Body-fat assessed from total body density and its estimation from skin-fold thickness: measurements on 481 men and women aged from 16 to 72 years. Br J Nutr 1987; 32:77–97.

13. Kushner RE, Kunigk A, Alspaugh M et al. Validation of bioelectrical-impedance analysis as a measurement of change in body composition in obesity. Am J Clin Nutr 1990; 52:219–23.

14. Ryan JA, Taft DA. Preoperative nutritional assessment does not predict morbidity and mortality in abdominal operations. Surg Forum 1980; 31:96–8.

15. Rothschild MA, Oratz M, Schreiber SS. Albumin metabolism. Gastroenterology 1973; 64:324–37.

16. Fleck A, Raines G, Hawker F et al. Increased vascular permeability: a major cause of hypoalbuminaemia in disease and injury. Lancet 1985; i:781–4.

17. Lukaski HC. Methods for the assessment of human body composition. Am J Clin Nutr 1987; 46:537–56.

18. Eremin O, Broom J. Nutrition and the immune response. In: Eremin O, Sewell HF (eds) The immunological basis of surgical science and practice. Oxford: Oxford University Press, 1992; pp. 133–44.

19. Bistrian BR, Blackburn GL, Scrimshaw NJ et al. Cellular immunity in semistarved hospitalized adults. Am J Clin Nutr 1975; 28:1148–55.

20. Seltzer MH, Bastidas JA, Cooper DM et al. Instant nutritional assessment. J Parenteral Enteral Nutr 1979; 3:157–9.

21. Heys SD, Khan AL, Eremin O. Immune suppression in surgery. Postgrad Surg 1995; 5:62–7.

22. Lopes J, Russke DM, Whitwell J et al. Skeletal muscle function in malnutrition. Am J Clin Nutr 1982; 36:602–10.

23. Daley BJ, Bistrian BR. Nutritional assessment. In: Zaloga GP (ed.) Nutrition in critical care. St Louis: Mosby Year Book, 1994; p. 28.

24. Hill G, Windsor JA. Nutritional assessment in clinical practice. Nutrition 1995; 11(Suppl):198–201.

25. Johnson LR, Copeland EM, Dudrick SJ et al. Structural and hormonal alterations in the gastrointestinal tract of parenterally fed rats. Gastroenterology 1975; 68:1177–83.

26. Levine GM, Deren JJ, Steiger E et al. Role of oral intake in maintenance of gut mass and disaccharide activity. Gastroenterology 1974; 67:975–82.

27. Wilmore D, Smith R, O'Dwyer S et al. The gut: a central organ after sepsis. Surgery 1988; 104:917–23.

28. Fong Y, Marano MA, Barber A et al. Total parenteral nutrition and bowel rest modify the metabolic response to endotoxin in humans. Ann Surg 1989; 210:449–56.

29. Grimble GK, Payne-James JJ, Rees RGP et al. Nutrition support. London: Medical Tribune UK, 1989; pp. 32–51.

30. Gayle D, Pinchcofsky-Devlin RD, Kaminski MV. Visceral protein increase associated with interrupted versus continuous enteral hyperalimentation. J Parenteral Enteral Nutr 1985; 9:474–6.

31. ASPEN Board of Directors and The Clinical Guidelines Task Force. Guidelines for the use of parenteral and enteral nutrition in adult and pediatric patients. J Parenter Enteral Nutr 2002; 26S:1SA–138SA.

32. Adam A. Insertion of long term central venous catheters: time for a new look. Br Med J 1995; 311:341–2.

33. Robertson LJ, Mauro MA, Jaques PF. Radiologic placement of Hickman catheters. Radiology 1989; 170:1007.

34. Lameris JS, Post PJM, Zonderland HM et al. Percutaneous placement of Hickman catheters: comparison of sonographically guided and blinded techniques. Am J Roentgenol 1990; 155:1097–9.

35. Maki DG, Ringer M. Evaluation of dressing regimens for prevention of infection with peripheral intravenous catheters. JAMA 1987; 258:2396–403.

36. Furst P, Albers D, Stehle P. Stress-induced intracellular glutamine depletion. The potential use of glutamine containing peptides in parenteral nutrition. In: Adibi SA, Fekl W, Oehmke M (eds) Dipeptides as new substrates in nutrition therapy. Munich: Karger, 1987; pp. 117–36.

37. Levinson MR, Groeger JS, Jeevanandam M et al. Free fatty acid turnover and lipolysis in septic mechanically ventilated cancer-bearing humans. Metabolism 1988; 37:618–25.

38. Shaw JHF, Woolfe RR. Energy and protein metabolism in sepsis and trauma. Aust NZ J Surg 1987; 57:41–7.

39. Venus B, Patel CB, Mathru M et al. Pulmonary effects of lipid infusion in patients with acute respiratory failure (abstract). Crit Care Med 1984; 12:293.

40. Seidner DL, Mascioli EA, Istfan NW et al. Effects of long chain triacylglycerol emulsions on reticuloendothelial system function in humans. J Parenteral Enteral Nutr 1989; 13:614–19.

41 http://www.nice.org.uk/guidance/index.jsp?action=download&co=29980. Accessed 1 January 2008. Guidelines for the role and function of multidisciplinary nutritional support teams.

42. Heyland DK, Montalvo M, MacDonald S et al. Total parenteral nutrition in the surgical patient: a meta-analysis. Can J Surg 2001; 44:102–11.

A meta-analysis of randomised controlled trials of parenteral nutritional support which attempts to draw together the evidence as to which patients benefit from TPN.

43. Weimann A, Braga M, Harsanyi L et al. ESPEN guidelines on enteral nutrition: surgery including organ transplantation. Clin Nutr 2006; 25:224–44.

Evidence-based guidelines summarising the current evidence and making recommendations for clinical practice in patients during the perioperative period.

44. Croad NR. The management of acute severe pancreatitis. Br J Intensive Care 1999; 2:38–45.

45. Kanwar A, Windsor ACJ, Li A et al. Benefits of early enteral nutrition in acute pancreatitis. Br J Surg 1997; 84:875.

46. McClave SA, Chang WK, Dhaliwal R et al. Nutrition support in acute pancreatitis: a systematic review of the literature. J Parenter Enteral Nutr 2006; 30:143–56.

Current updated position evaluating evidence for clinical nutritional support in patients with acute pancreatitis.

47. Dickinson RJ, Ashton MG, Axon ATR et al. Controlled trial of intravenous hyperalimentation as an adjunct to the routine therapy of acute colitis. Gastroenterology 1980; 79:1199–204.

48. Muller JM, Keller HW, Erasmi H et al. Total parenteral nutrition as sole therapy in Crohn's disease: a prospective study. Br J Surg 1983; 70:40–3.

49. Jones VA. Comparison of total parenteral nutrition and enteral diet in induction of remission in Crohn's disease: long term maintenance of remission by personalised food exclusion. Dig Dis Sci 1987; 32(Suppl):1005–75.

50 Zachos M, Tondeur M, Griffiths AM. Enteral nutrition therapy for induction of remission in Crohn's disease. Cochrane Database Syst Rev 2001; CD000542.

51 Akobeng AK, Thomas AG. Enteral nutrition for maintenance of remission in Crohn's disease. Cochrane Database Syst Rev 2007; CD005984.

52. Chapman R, Foran R, Dunphey JE. Management of intestinal fistulas. Am J Surg 1964; 108:157–64.

53. Lloyd DA, Gabe SM, Windsor AC. Nutrition and management of enterocutaneous fistula. Br J Surg 2006; 93:1045–55.

54. Windle EM. Glutamine supplementation in critical illness: evidence, recommendations, and implications for clinical practice in burns care. J Burn Care Res 2006; 27:764–72.

55. Wasiak J, Cleland H, Jeffery R. Early versus late enteral nutrition in adults with burn injury: a systematic review. J Hum Nutr Rev 2007; 20:75–83.

56. Kreymann KG, Berger MM, Deutz NEP et al. ESPEN guidelines on enteral nutrition:intensive care. Clin Nutr 2006; 25:210–23.

Evidence-based guidelines summarising the current evidence and making recommendations for clinical practice.

57. Chiarelli A, Siliprandi L. Burns. In: Zagola GP (ed.) Nutrition in critical care. St Louis: Mosby Year Book, 1994; pp. 587–97.

58. Brittenden J, Park KGM, Heys SD et al. l-Arginine stimulates host defences in patients with breast cancer. Surgery 1994; 115:205–12.

59. Brittenden J, Heys SD, Ross JA et al. Nutritional pharmacology: effects of l-arginine on host defences, responses to trauma and tumour growth. Clin Sci 1994; 86:123–32.

60. Heys SD, Park KGM, Garlick PJ et al. Nutrition and malignancy: implications for surgical practice. Br J Surg 1992; 79:614–23.

61. Heys SD, Gough DB, Kahn AL et al. Nutritional pharmacology and malignant disease: a therapeutic modality in patients with cancer? Br J Surg 1996; 83:608–19.

62. Purasiri P, Murray A, Richardson S et al. Modulation of cytokine production in vivo by dietary essential fatty acids in patients with colorectal cancer. Clin Sci 1994; 87:711–17.

63. Purasiri P, McKechnie A, Heys SD et al. Modulation in vitro of human natural cytotoxicity, lymphocyte proliferative response to mitogens and cytokine production by essential fatty acids. Immunology 1997; 92:166–72.

64. Avenell A, Noble DW, Barr J et al. Selenium supplementation for critically ill adults. Cochrane Database Syst Rev 2004; 4:CD003703.

65. Avenell A. Glutamine in critical care: current evidence from systematic reviews. Proc Nutr Soc 2006; 65:236–41.

66. Heys SD, Walker LG, Smith IC et al. Enteral nutritional supplementation with key nutrients in patients with critical illness and cancer. A meta-analysis of randomised controlled clinical trials. Ann Surg 1999; 229:467–77.

This is the first meta-analysis which indicated that immunonutrition could result in clinically important benefits for patients in terms of reduction in infectious complications postoperatively.

67. Heyland DK, Novak F, Drover JW et al. Should immunonutrition become routine in critically ill patients? JAMA 2001; 286:944–53.

This is an updated meta-analysis of randomised controlled trials that confirms the previous meta-analysis and extends it further by examining different subgroups of patients in an attempt to try to understand further which patients are the most likely to benefit from immunonutrition.

18

Abdominal sepsis and abdominal compartment syndrome

Iain D. Anderson

Introduction

Abdominal sepsis accounts for many of the serious and all too often fatal emergency conditions which the general surgeon is called upon to treat. It may arise primarily from conditions as seemingly simple and routine as appendicitis, to more complicated and serious conditions such as diverticulitis and perforated peptic ulcer disease. Alternatively it may arise as a consequence of complications of surgery, particularly intestinal anastomotic leakage. While, with experience and a few basic principles, even complex cases of abdominal sepsis can be relatively straightforward to manage, not infrequently the diagnosis is obscured and delayed and, as a consequence, treatment is complicated and prolonged. Some 90% of general surgical deaths follow emergency admission,[1] and much of this morbidity and mortality expresses itself through the processes of abdominal sepsis. Delay to operation is the single most common reason for adverse outcome and anastomotic leak the single commonest cited complication in fatal cases. These will be recurring themes in this chapter as even with optimal treatment of abdominal sepsis, multiple organ failure (MOF) may ensue and MOF is more likely and often fatal when treatment is slow or suboptimal. In the intensive care unit (ICU), abdominal sepsis constitutes a substantial proportion of the patients with MOF. Severe sepsis has become increasingly common in recent decades but with little overall improvement in mortality.[2] Given its frequency and severity, a sound understanding of abdominal sepsis

must be integral to every general surgeon's professional armamentarium.

This chapter will address the diagnosis and management of abdominal sepsis, including the complex patient in the ICU, where sequelae such as compartment syndrome, management of the open abdomen and intestinal fistulation can create particular difficulty. The reader is referred to Chapter 16 for a description of the intensive care management of the surgical patient, Chapters 6, 8, 9, 10 and 13 for more detail on specific causal conditions, and to Chapter 17 for surgical nutrition.

The slippery slope of sepsis

The mechanism behind the systemic inflammatory response syndrome (SIRS), sepsis, organ dysfunction and later MOF in relation to the intensive care management of the surgical patient has been discussed in Chapter 16. It can be tempting to see these phenomena as being solely of interest to the intensivist but, in reality, they are also useful and important concepts for the general surgeon. SIRS is common enough amongst surgical patients on the ward, although it is usually resolved by appropriate treatment of the underlying problem. Sometimes it persists and particularly when it does so beyond 48 hours, outcome is worsened as progression to organ dysfunction is much more likely. The next step beyond this is organ failure, which still typically carries a mortality of the order of 40%. Mortality, in general, increases with the number of organ systems affected and with the severity of physiological disturbance at onset.[3] While the onset of SIRS does not accurately predict development of sepsis or the multiple organ dysfunction syndrome (MODS), the progression from SIRS to severe sepsis is associated with increasing risk of organ failure.[4] Approximately 30% of septic patients develop at least one organ dysfunction.[5] Therefore, timely recognition of SIRS, particularly if persistent, alerts the clinician to a potentially deteriorating situation at a time when prompt intervention may yet avert catastrophe. By the time the patient with abdominal sepsis has developed shock, the mortality increases from less than 10% to greater than 50%.[6,7]

The identification and active management of SIRS and early organ dysfunction is therefore an important first step as, once organ dysfunction is under way, the patient is on a slippery slope which can lead them rapidly downwards despite the best treatment. It is essential that the surgeon appreciates that these processes often start insidiously on the ward and that early detection is vital as management is most successful at this stage. While there are objective criteria which define organ dysfunction, clinical findings are useful pointers. Hypoxia, oliguria, hypotension, deranged liver function tests or clotting, thrombocytopenia, acidosis and confusion are some of the plethora of signs that indicate that a severe systemic derangement is in process or not far away. All these are seen commonly amongst surgical patients outwith the ICU environment. Almost any organ system can be involved in abdominal sepsis and thus the presenting features are numerous, although the site of the original insult and any comorbid processes will often be an influence.

 The importance of detecting the often subtle signs of abdominal sepsis at the earliest stage cannot be overemphasised and while the rate with which organ dysfunction develops in individual patients will vary, the requirement for rapid identification and treatment remains key.[4]

Metabolic changes and their surgical implications

Sepsis is associated with a range of profound hormonal and metabolic disturbances, including hypermetabolism, protein catabolism and insulin resistance, amongst other systemic effects. Many have direct impact on the success of surgery in these patients and are only reversed once sepsis is dealt with. There is inevitable muscle breakdown with loss of respiratory muscles as well as large limb muscles. Tissues can become oedematous, delicate and easily damaged during surgery, and thrombocytopenia and coagulopathy make operative bleeding more likely. Wound healing may be impaired, glucose levels

raised, immune function is suppressed and secondary infection more common. Hypoalbuminaemia is common in sepsis, reflecting plasma volume and capillary leakage more than impaired nutritional status. It is also an indicator of adverse outcome.[8] Measurement of plasma albumin and C-reactive protein may provide valuable information with regard to the progress of the septic patient.

Systematic assessment

Although effective management of patients with severe sepsis may entail complex investigations and procedures, the results of these manoeuvres are often suboptimal or even lethal, without adequate prior resuscitation. A systematic approach such as that described in the *Care of the Critically Ill Surgical Patient* (CCrISP) course[9] has much to recommend it as it provides a common management structure for problems of any type or severity. Having a structured approach in times of crisis may also be important in reducing the likelihood of management errors. It certainly provides a common language and transparency which lets other health professionals understand interventions more easily. With complex abdominal sepsis, a team approach is required: firstly, because help will often be needed from radiology, anaesthesia and intensive care; secondly, because the illness will often run a prolonged time course of days or weeks and hence many doctors will be involved. A common approach and clear communication will be fundamental to success.

Patients with abdominal sepsis will present with some degree of instability and CCrISP advocates rapid **immediate management** following ABC principles of assessment with simultaneous correction of life-threatening conditions and initiation of high-flow oxygen therapy, fluid resuscitation and basic monitoring as needed. Although some patients will deteriorate catastrophically and require immediate intensive care support, simple resuscitation will more commonly buy sufficient time for a more thorough **full assessment** to be carried out. This aims to determine the cause and severity of any problem and to exclude other conditions that would prove deleterious if untreated. It includes a thorough appraisal of the patient's notes and charts.

As the clinical manifestations of abdominal sepsis can be subtle and varied (Box 18.1), a high index of suspicion, combined with anticipation of potential complications, is essential. This holds true when dealing with the critically ill patient but also for the patient recovering after major surgery and for the emergency admission. Complications can usually be anticipated from the surgical condition in question, any operation recently carried out and knowledge of comorbid conditions from which the patient suffers. Frequently,

Box 18.1 • General manifestations of abdominal sepsis in the ward or HDU patient

Pyrexia or hypothermia
Tachycardia
Tachypnoea
Confusion
Oedema
Metabolic acidosis
Hypoalbuminaemia
Thrombocytopenia
Ileus
Poor peripheral perfusion
Hypotension
Hypoxia
Lethargy
Oliguria
Raised lactate
Hyponatraemia
Leucocytosis or neutropenia

the range of possible diagnoses is large (Box 18.2) and, in order to capture these adequately, the initial diagnostic net must be cast wide before drawing it in rapidly with the assistance of selective investigations. Reaching a provisional diagnosis and management plan rapidly is important as outcome worsens with delay and deterioration, as indicated above.

Patients should improve after clinical interventions. Failure to progress, or deterioration, suggests a new problem or an unresolved one. The same systematic CCrISP approach forms the basis of ongoing assessment of the critically ill, or at-risk, patient on the critical care unit or ward. As repeated complications and setbacks are likely in complex cases, the surgeon must be prepared for a long campaign not a single battle, and be prepared to take a leading role in ongoing management.

Antimicrobial therapy in abdominal sepsis

Definitive management of sepsis requires identification of the source of infection and its treatment. In abdominal sepsis, this will usually entail surgery

Box 18.2 • Some possible differential diagnoses in patients presenting with abdominal sepsis on the ward (this depends on presenting features)

Sepsis of other origin (urine, line, chest, etc.)
Cardiac (ischaemia, infarction, dysrhythmias, failure)
Cerebral (toxic confusion, ischaemia)
Pulmonary (atelectasis, collapse, infection, pulmonary embolism)
Fluid imbalance
Other non-septic abdominal complications (e.g. ileus, bleeding)

or radiological intervention. That said, the role of antimicrobial therapy is also vital.[10] When sepsis is suspected, blood cultures, urine, wound swabs and sputum should be submitted for urgent Gram staining and culture, with all sources of sepsis considered. Cultures from the main source of sepsis are several times more likely to be positive (75% vs. 18%)[11] than blood cultures, but both are important in the critically ill patient. Once cultures are taken, best-guess antibiotic therapy should begin immediately as delay may influence outcome. The role of cultures is to enable the antibiotics to be changed successfully if the patient fails to respond. The choice of antibiotic will be influenced by the clinical circumstances to cover the expected range of infecting organisms. The route of administration must ensure adequate plasma levels and the drugs should penetrate adequately into the tissues. Intravenous infusion is usually necessary. In most instances, pathogens will be bacteria, but antifungal agents may be required. Whenever there is doubt concerning the optimal choice of antibiotics, the advice of a medical microbiologist should be urgently sought. For most abdominal sepsis, coverage of Gram-negative and anaerobic bacteria will be necessary. With biliary sepsis, approximately 15% of cases will involve streptococci species which are resistant to cephalosporins, so the addition of a modern penicillin is a common approach. With postoperative hospital acquired infection, cover against a broader and more resistant spectrum of organisms will be needed.[10] Fungal infection (usually *Candida* species) is not uncommon in complex abdominal sepsis requiring ICU care and so antifungal therapy will be needed in addition to usual methods to control the source of sepsis.

Imaging in abdominal sepsis

Various imaging techniques may be employed to localise an infective focus (see also Chapter 5). Computed tomography (CT), usually with gastrointestinal and/or intravenous contrast enhancement, can provide excellent information in thoracic, abdominal and pelvic sepsis, provided that the patient can be transferred safely to the scanner and imaged without too much interference from infusions, drains and metallic prostheses. CT is excellent at primary diagnosis and at least as useful in the complex or postoperative case where clinical examination is more difficult.[12] Contrast can be usefully inserted up drains or down stomas when needed. Comparison with previous scans is important and the input of a senior, specialist radiologist will increase the accuracy of the report. In emergency cases, the surgeon should ideally be present at the scan so that decisions about any interventional radiological procedure can be made jointly.

It should not be considered that CT or any other diagnostic test is perfect. Even in expert hands, there is a small but significant rate of missed diagnoses and when emergency scans are interpreted by trainees, the rate is probably higher.

The chest radiograph remains an integral part of patient assessment and ultrasound has the advantages of being portable, harmless and repeatable. However, the greatest utility of ultrasound probably lies with the assessment of biliary and renal pathology and the monitoring of identified collections. It is limited by operator dependency and a negative scan will offer little reassurance when the clinical picture is concerning. When a focus of subacute sepsis cannot be identified radiologically, isotopic methods such as labelled white cell scanning using indium-111 may help.

The role of diagnostic laparotomy is now limited. Occasional patients are too unstable to undergo CT safely and occasionally the index of suspicion remains too strong to ignore after an apparently normal scan. On the other hand, when faced with an unstable patient with a clear indication for laparotomy, delaying surgery for CT would usually be inappropriate. Most commonly, however, the surgical patient can be stabilised sufficiently for safe scanning to take place and the assistance which CT gives in terms of accurate diagnosis and selective therapeutic intervention should not be underestimated.

Aims of treatment in abdominal sepsis

The management of abdominal sepsis in the emergency surgical admission is that of the underlying disease, as covered elsewhere in this book. The aim is to deal not only with the sepsis, but also to deal definitively with the underlying disease process or cause. In all patients, pus must be drained and dead tissue removed with specimens submitted for urgent microbiology. While loculated sepsis can be drained percutaneously, generalised peritonitis remains an indication for laparotomy. Exceptions to this rule include primary spontaneous bacterial peritonitis and acute pancreatitis.

Whether treatment is radiological or surgical, adequate preparation is essential (see also Chapter 16). Coagulopathy must be excluded or corrected beforehand and blood for transfusion should be available. Although drainage may be an essential prerequisite to resolution of sepsis, it is not infrequent for bacteraemia, as a consequence of the intervention, to cause a temporary deterioration in the patient's condition. Indeed, a bacteraemia may represent the 'second hit' that precipitates MODS. Such circumstances should be anticipated, and an appropriate level of postprocedure care arranged beforehand. The importance of adequate systemic support for the patient having imaging or image-guided intervention should nowadays be self-evident. Surgeons have a role to play in this, which may involve delivery of that care or the coordination of it with the assistance of anaesthetists. Percutaneous procedures may be less invasive than open surgery but will only be effective if good drainage is achieved. Many percutaneous drains are narrow and inadequate when infected fluid is viscous or contains necrotic tissue. Larger or multiple drains may be more effective and daily flushing can help. When radiological drains are placed for abdominal sepsis, the responsibility lies with the surgical team to ensure that the patient's condition improves as expected. Failure to respond to radiological intervention is another indication for laparotomy. The urgency of treatment should be re-emphasised as it influences outcome significantly. In a complex system such as a hospital, it is all too easy for multiple small delays to add up. Managing the multidisciplinary hospital team to achieve prompt and timely intervention is a considerable skill which requires active and continued leadership from the surgeon.

With more complex cases and with older and sicker patients, treatment may need to be tempered in order to be survivable. However, there is a balance to be struck as inadequate treatment will condemn the patient to recurrent sepsis and likely death, and the opinion of senior colleagues and specialist centres can sometimes be invaluable. When open surgery is performed for sepsis, the procedure will vary according to the underlying pathology. Nonetheless, general principles apply and one principle is that the most straightforward adequate procedure is often preferable to a complex and time-consuming operation. The aim is to improve the patient's condition without risking further complication. For example, there is a current trend towards primary bowel resection and anastomosis in acute settings, but this should be avoided in unstable patients, the presence of significant comorbidity or heavy contamination. This traditional approach still remains the norm among UK surgeons, typified by the persisting preference for Hartmann's procedure for severe complicated diverticulitis in the emergency setting.[13] Generous saline lavage is recommended on completion of the procedure but there is nothing to be gained either by removing fibrinous debris piecemeal or by postoperative lavage.[10] Delayed skin wound closure may be preferable to primary suture, or wounds may be left to close by secondary intention if sepsis is substantial.

Obtaining informed consent for treatment will involve both patient and relatives. The potential severity of the situation should not be underestimated and the possibility of death, stoma creation, the need for intensive care treatment and further surgery will usually need to be discussed explicitly.

Box 18.3 • Surgeon's role on the ICU

Daily surgical input to:
Wound and stoma care
Tubes and drains
Nutrition
Ongoing management of sepsis
Further operations
Compartment syndrome
Postoperative bleeding
Preparation for HDU/ward
Treatment/advice regarding the underlying surgical disease

The majority of patients presenting acutely with abdominal sepsis will undergo successful treatment and recover. To maximise success, the systematic approach indicated above is again needed, with attention to the many facets of systemic care during the postoperative period. Identifying problems as early as possible and dealing with them effectively is essential. Often the early phase of care will be delivered on the surgical high dependency unit (HDU) or ICU. Although we, as surgeons, may feel uncomfortable on ICU, there are a range of skills which we are usually best placed to deliver (Box 18.3).

Abdominal sepsis on the ICU

Not infrequently, the surgeon is also involved with the assessment and management of patients already on the ICU who develop recurrent abdominal sepsis. These patients pose considerable difficulties and many of the considerations also apply to patients well enough not to be on the ICU but who develop complications (typically a leaking anastomosis) or recurrent sepsis. The outcome of patients with abdominal sepsis who require ICU treatment is dependent upon the factors shown in Box 18.4, with successful control or eradication of the source of sepsis being essential for survival among patients with MOF.[14] When sepsis is eradicated successfully from these patients by surgery over 60% survive, whereas survival is close to zero if significant

Box 18.4 • Factors associated with survival in patients with abdominal sepsis on the ICU

Age
Severity of acute illness (APACHE II score on admission)
Eradication of source of sepsis
Source of sepsis
Speed of treatment (absence of septic shock)

abdominal sepsis continues. Survival also falls in a manner closely related to advancing age.

While recent years have seen the introduction of successful novel therapies for sepsis, particularly activated protein C, its impact is still much less than adequate and timely surgical or radiological intervention when needed and this remains the foremost priority. However, the surgeon should be aware of the coagulopathic effect of activated protein C.[15]

Assessment on the ICU

Assessing patients on the ICU is difficult for several reasons. Firstly, the patients are often complex yet unfamiliar, perhaps having been treated previously by other surgeons. Secondly, sedated, postoperative patients in organ failure show their abdominal sepsis in different ways to a new emergency admission with peritonitis. Abdominal signs are unlikely to be evident unless gross (e.g. flank cellulitis, bowel contents in a drain, necrotic stoma), and the diagnosis of recurrent abdominal sepsis is often made from deterioration in vital organ function (see Chapter 16) and suspicion based on previous treatment and imaging. Again, contrast-enhanced CT is the gold-standard investigation and of great value, but occasional patients will be too unwell to travel to the scanner. For them, exploratory laparotomy may still occasionally be necessary. Interpreting CT images in the recently operated abdomen is not easy. With expert help, the CT will not only confirm the diagnosis but can also potentially identify areas where there is no evidence of inflammation. In a difficult re-operative procedure with adhesions, that knowledge can save time and reduce the risk of surgical damage to other organs. Percutaneous drainage has a similar role here as in primary inflammation and similar caveats apply.

The importance of the surgeon making their own thorough assessment cannot be overestimated as the stakes are high. The surgeon should be satisfied that the diagnosis is secure and that surgery is the best course of action. Part of that process will be engaging in detailed discussion with the intensivist to weigh up alternative diagnoses and sources of sepsis, and the risks and benefits of intervention at this point in time. Often this is not clear-cut as patients may have multiple potential sources (e.g. simultaneous pneumonia and abdominal sepsis) or other complicating factors, usually revolving around comorbid diseases or other ICU treatments. That said, any significant abdominal sepsis will require treatment.

In some patients it will be clear that there is no realistic prospect of survival, either of the required operation or, more commonly, of the inevitably prolonged ICU course thereafter. Once the need and appropriateness of intervention is decided upon, plans are made and discussed with the family. Further delay, other than to correct specific abnormalities such as clotting factors, is usually then counter-productive. While the risks of surgery are often self-evident to all, these patients can sometimes be described as being 'too sick **not** to have an operation'. As before, clear indications for life-saving surgery include generalised peritonitis, multiple collections and presence of dead tissue. Those who fail to respond to percutaneous drainage also need a laparotomy if they are to survive. Patients with deteriorating organ function and a strong suspicion of abdominal pathology also remain a significant group in whom laparotomy may be necessary.

Causes of abdominal sepsis in the ICU

The principal causes of recurrent abdominal sepsis in the ICU are shown in Box 18.5. Leaking anastomosis remains the commonest single cause and should be actively suspected in all at-risk patients who are critically ill or deteriorating. Enterotomy during difficult surgery is also not uncommon, occurring in approximately 20% of patients,[16] and these can also leak. Gastrostomy or other tubes inserted into the gut occasionally leak: this is more likely when tissue healing is poor.

The management of most conditions follows standard specialty lines but certain causes are more specific to the ICU. Acute acalculous cholecystitis may lead to biliary peritonitis. Non-specific derangement of liver biochemistry is common but not universal. Ultrasound may reveal gallbladder thickening, and demonstration of intramural gas is particularly concerning. The treatment is either urgent cholecystostomy or occasionally cholecystectomy (see also Chapter 8).[17]

Small-bowel ischaemia can occur secondary to low cardiac output, embolisation or venous sludging. Vasopressors can precipitate non-occlusive ischaemia, which has a high mortality.[18] Early diagnosis is notoriously difficult but bloody diarrhoea is ominous. In the severely ill, the treatment is resection with exteriorisation. Large-bowel ischaemia is usually left-sided and is associated with low cardiac

output and aortic surgery. Often only the mucosa is affected and treatment can be non-operative,[19] but systemic upset or peritonitis are indications for resection with exteriorisation. In pseudomembranous colitis, secondary to infection with *Clostridium difficile*, mucosal sloughing is not universally seen on sigmoidoscopy. Most patients settle with treatment with enteral metronidazole or vancomycin. However, subtotal colectomy with exteriorisation may be necessary in severe disease. Neutropenic colitis is associated with chemotherapy for haematological malignancy. The right colon is usually affected, and plain radiography may show dilatation and oedema. Initial supportive management with broad-spectrum antibiotics is recommended. Resection is reserved for peritonitis or failure to progress.[20]

Intestinal obstruction is not usually seen as an indication for re-operation unless there is suggestion of strangulation or another indication for surgery such as a concomitant abscess. Most patients will settle eventually and the risk of operative damage or recurrent obstruction outweighs the benefit.[21]

Re-operating in abdominal sepsis

Re-operating in abdominal sepsis is always difficult: the timing of the most recent operation will influence the degree of difficulty and hence the risk of future complications. Beyond 72 hours adhesions will make surgery increasingly difficult and the risk of bowel damage increases: often the adhesions are stronger than the bowel. Entry to the abdomen can be difficult and an extension of the previous midline incision may help. Adhesions are generally most dense around any site of inflammation, as well as a recent incision. Here, having a preoperative CT scan comes into its own, guiding the surgeon as to the relative necessity to dissect in any difficult area. While a full laparotomy is ideal, prolonged dissection of adhesions in an area not thought from CT to contain inflammation or a collection may not be merited.

The surgeon must deal with the sepsis as thoroughly as possible but also simply and quickly. Prolonged and complex procedures will likely lead to a systemic deterioration in the patient and the prospects of bowel anastomoses healing under these adverse circumstances is not as high as one would like. The ability of the patient to withstand further surgery for further complications is very much lower next time around[14] and the surgeon should see the present operation as the best opportunity for salvaging the patient. Intestinal reconstruction can be attempted when the patient is well and recovered, some months later.

Hence, in general terms the simplest and safest procedure will be best. This holds true especially in

Box 18.5 • The principal causes of recurrent abdominal sepsis in the ICU

Leaked anastomosis or enterotomy
Leaking gastrostomies and other tubes
Abscesses or collections
Dead or ischaemic gut
Acalculous cholecystitis
Antibiotic-associated colitis
Continuing sepsis from 'common' peritonitis
(perforation, diverticular, etc.)

the patient who already has incipient or established organ failure: drain sepsis, debride any necrotic tissue and exteriorise any leaking bowel or anastomoses as stomas. Most controversy relates to the management of enteric and colorectal anastomotic leaks. While in a well patient, with a small leak and minimal contamination, preservation of a repaired anastomosis with proximal defunctioning and local drainage may be appropriate, it is all too often foolhardy in the critically ill. Preserving the anastomosis might work but there is a significant risk of further peritonitis and likely death as further acute surgery will seldom be successful. A first salvage operation in an ICU patient will successfully eradicate sepsis over 40% of the time but a second operation carries a success rate of only 25% and a third operation only 7%.[14] This is reflected in the rate of survival.

In difficult cases, the surgeon must be ready to employ alternative strategies, although it remains essential to drain significant collections of pus or enteric content and to debride any necrotic tissue. In the multiply operated septic abdomen, it may not be possible to take down and exteriorise the prime source of sepsis because of dense adhesions or the anatomical location (oesophagus, duodenum). For inaccessible pelvic sepsis arising from distal small bowel or colon, it may be possible to identify and exteriorise a proximal loop of jejunum without entering and damaging the matted pelvic loops other than to achieve necessary drainage. This will usually relieve the sepsis but at the price of a high-output stoma and prolonged intravenous feeding. For oesophagogastric or duodenal sepsis, all that may be possible is to drain collections and leave large tube or sump drains beside the leaking anastomosis or other septic focus. Placing a second tube in the hole to create a controlled fistula is also of merit. Proximal intestinal contents or secretions can sometimes be diverted away by tube gastrostomy or other techniques although each has its complications. A further option in difficult situations or resistant cases is to gain entry to locules of pus or enteric content, then to leave the abdomen open as a laparostomy (**Fig. 18.1**). Further pus or enteric content will usually find its way to the surface, assisted by subsequent manual lavage on the ICU or in theatre as necessary.

In addition to their role in draining proximal gut secretions, gastrostomy and enterostomy tubes can be usefully placed to facilitate future, and often prolonged, enteral feeding. The same tube can serve both roles: drainage initially, then feeding as intestinal function returns, provided there is no persisting distal bowel leak. These laparotomies are often oozy and contaminated, and many surgeons would leave large drains (24Ch tube or sump) in

Figure 18.1 • Laparostomy with polyglactin mesh, gastrostomy, jejunostomy, cholecystostomy and drains.

the subphrenic spaces and pelvis at the end of the procedure. This is particularly so for certain deep cavities (e.g. psoas abscess) or when further leakage is likely or inevitable. Large Foley catheters can be used to intubate inaccessible bowel to create a controlled fistula (typically the duodenum) and it is often advisable to place an additional large drain just outside the bowel. There is a particular role for local lavage in pancreatic necrosis (see Chapter 8) but, otherwise, continuing lavage down abdominal drains in the postoperative period is of no proven benefit.

Outcome from surgery for abdominal sepsis in the ICU patient depends on many factors which vary between patients as the patient group is heterogeneous. Age and eradication of sepsis have been discussed but numbers of failed organs, comorbid conditions and the underlying surgical disease are also important. Overall, 30–40% will survive[14] but a further factor which is associated with survival is the early response to the first operation in the ICU. If the patient has improved clinically within 48 hours then survival is much better (80%) than if the patient does not improve in this time frame (10%). Given the cost of intensive care, attempts have been made using a variety of scoring systems to define numerically those patients with no chance of survival. There exist general scores such as Acute Physiology and Chronic Health Evaluation (APACHE) and specific scoring systems for peritonitis such as the Mannheim Peritonitis Index. However, to date, the heterogeneity of the patient group and the nature of scoring systems in general (see also Chapter 15) has not made it possible to use them for decision-making in individual patients. Clinical experience and judgement remain important and the scoring systems remain primarily useful tools for audit and research.

Damage control laparotomy

Damage control laparotomy (DCL) is a concept which has expanded from its initial role in trauma surgery (see also Chapter 13). Trauma patients become hypothermic, acidotic and coagulopathic, and surgery becomes unsurvivable. Rapid, immediately life-saving surgery ('staple, pack and go') is carried out and the patient returned to ICU for warming and resuscitation, with more definitive surgery deferred for 24–48 hours once coagulopathy has been corrected and homeostasis returned towards normal. In abdominal sepsis, similar considerations can be applied to severely unstable patients where it can be better to make an active decision to quickly drain pus, remove dead tissue, stop bleeding by packing and close overtly leaking bowel with staples (without resection) before terminating the operation.[22]

Packing areas, usually the pelvis, to obtain haemostasis is a lesser form of the same concept. This is sometimes required when prolonged attempts at haemostasis seem increasingly futile on account of coagulopathy. Packs should generally be removed as early as possible once clotting is restored and usually the next day. The small bowel becomes adherent remarkably quickly and can be damaged as packs are removed. Packs should be removed cautiously under direct vision with saline irrigation and gentle finger separation.

Second-look or planned re-laparotomy

This term refers to the planned re-exploration of the abdomen, planned at the previous procedure in order to re-operate before any clinical deterioration occurs. The term distinguishes it from 'laparotomy on demand', which is now the more common approach and where the abdomen is only explored when a new problem is diagnosed. After DCL, a second look is obviously required to complete the necessary definitive procedures, but the term is more commonly applied to 'looking again' after laparotomy for intestinal ischaemia. The extent of intestinal ischaemia may not be fully evident at the first operation and, particularly if the bowel has been re-anastomosed, looking again at 48–72 hours, depending on progress, can identify further ischaemia before the patient deteriorates. In some cases of intestinal ischaemia where they may be doubt as to the extent, it may be preferable to resect and staple off the bowel ends, forcing the surgeon to re-explore 48 hours or so later, rather than gamble on anastomsing bowel which might be subclinically ischaemic and subsequently break down.

Repeated planned re-laparotomies have been used aggressively for abdominal sepsis with MOF in both Europe and North America for some years. In this method of treatment, the abdomen is typically re-operated upon every 24–48 hours for several days to wash out the peritoneal cavity and remove any ongoing sepsis. However, a recent randomised trial has shown that this approach is associated with a worse outcome compared to the 're-laparotomy on demand' approach.[23] In this randomised trial of 232 patients with severe secondary peritonitis, two possible surgical treatment strategies following an initial emergency laparotomy were compared: planned re-laparotomy and re-laparotomy only when the patient's condition demands it ('on demand'). Patients had severe secondary peritonitis and an APACHE II score of 11 or greater. There was no significant difference in mortality (29% on demand vs. 36% planned; $P = 0.22$) or morbidity (40% on demand ($n = 32$) vs. 44% planned ($n = 32$); $P = 0.58$). A total of 31% of first re-laparotomies were negative in the on-demand group versus 66% in the planned group ($P < 0.001$). Patients in the on-demand group had shorter median ICU stays (7 vs. 11 days; $P = 0.001$) and shorter median hospital stays (27 vs. 35 days; $P = 0.008$). Direct medical costs per patient were reduced by 23% using the on-demand strategy. Although on occasions there may be a case for a single second-look laparotomy in patients with severe faecal peritonitis, even this is debatable. However, the inability of planned second-look laparotomy to alter outcome should not divert the surgeon from maintaining a low threshold for early laparotomy on demand when indicated, as delaying necessary surgery worsens outcome.[14]

 In patients undergoing surgery for severe secondary peritonitis, re-laparotomy on demand is preferable to 'planned re-laparotomy'.[23]

Leaving the abdomen open (laparostomy)

In adverse circumstances, the abdomen is occasionally left open as a last resort in allowing pus and enteric contents to drain. More often it is left open in preference to closing it with undue tension. Abdominal compartment syndrome (see below) may also lead to an open abdomen. Leaving the abdomen open in appropriate circumstances can avoid or reduce septic, enteric and wound complications. It also allows improved systemic function, faster weaning from the ventilator and can facilitate early enteral nutrition. However, it is deforming, increases evaporative losses and exposes the bowel to risk of damage and fistulation. Prolonged healing is usually required with a risk of late herniation. These deleterious effects are significant enough to make one caution against unnecessary use of laparostomy.[10] It is undoubtedly a valuable and life-saving technique when needed but it is also a significant future burden to the patient in its own right.

In closing the abdomen during laparotomy for abdominal sepsis, the surgeon should close the fascia conventionally but avoid tension. Tension sutures have little to recommend them and their continued use is not supported. If bowel distension, oedema, haemorrhage (or packing) combine to make closure impossible, then there are several options open to the surgeon, depending on a number of factors, including the likely time course of recovery. In general, each end of the wound is closed conventionally to the point of reasonable tension and the central defect left open. For short-lived oedema (e.g. after aortic aneurysm repair or traumatic haemorrhage) the defect can be covered with abdominal packing, which is changed daily until such time as the defect can be closed or a longer-term solution implemented (see below). Alternatively a version of the Bogota bag can be used (**Fig. 18.2**). In this technique, a sterile 3-litre intravenous fluid bag is slit open and sutured to the fascia, covering and protecting the bowel and providing it with a clean, moist environment. There are various commercial plastic sheets which can also be used. Again, as the oedema subsides, usually within 72 hours or so, this can be removed and the abdomen either closed or a longer-term technique instituted. In recurrent sepsis, where recovery is likely to be slow, some form of mesh can be used to restrain the viscera. Absorbable polyglactin meshes have become popular recently and are preferred to non-absorbable meshes, as there is less likelihood of fistulation to underlying bowel. Furthermore, with non-absorbable meshes, as the wound gradually granulates over and re-epithelialisation takes place, redundant and protruding parts of mesh may require subsequent 'trimming'. Whichever technique is employed, the later development of an incisional hernia is almost inevitable, but might be less so with the non-absorbable mesh. If the contamination is particularly severe such that a further laparotomy and lavage is planned in 24–48 hours, then mesh placement can be deferred until then. Likewise if oozing requires gauze packing then mesh placement can be effected when the gauze is removed. The mesh and bowels must still be kept moist and protected, and a double-sandwich dressing of semipermeable adhesive dressing with moist gauze between the layers of dressing achieves this admirably. Early dressing changes should be carried out by the surgical team. If there is a lot of effluent or tissue fluid, then use of low-grade suction can help provide control. As the wound shrinks, these bulky dressings can be changed to a large fistula bag, even if there is no fistula. Use of the commercial vacuum dressings is popular as they provide a ready-made technique for the non-expert unit, but may be associated with an increased rate of fistulation from the exposed bowel.[24]

Abdominal compartment syndrome

Normally, intra-abdominal pressure is low (<10 mmHg), but it is increasingly recognised that it can be raised in abdominal sepsis (and other acute abdominal conditions, particularly trauma) to the significant detriment of the patient. The condition is recognised with increasing frequency and is probably not as uncommon in our practice as thought.[25] As abdominal pressure rises, venous return is impaired and with it cardiac output. The tense abdomen can cause pulmonary compromise, oliguria and mesenteric ischaemia, and in some patients even raised intracranial pressure. These features constitute the abdominal compartment syndrome (ACS) – similar in some ways to a tension pneumothorax, within the abdomen.[26]

ACS is most commonly caused by multiple factors which mutually exist after certain emergency operations, typically those for peritonitis, abdominal aneurysm repair and abdominal trauma. Tissue oedema results from the combined effects of tissue injury, surgery, intravenous fluid infusion and leaky capillaries, while bowel distension and haematomas also contribute. Not surprisingly, ACS is seen most commonly after fascial closure but it can also occur in the abdomen which has been left open and packed, especially if there is ongoing haemorrhage. Operations likely to cause ACS include those involving significant haemorrhage, retroperitoneal or intestinal oedema, bowel distension, aortic clamping, hypothermia, massive transfusion or prolonged surgery, and these circumstances should heighten the surgeon's awareness of ACS as a potential complication. ACS is not restricted to emergency surgery and

Figure 18.2 • Bogota bag.

prolonged elective surgery with a scarred and rigid abdominal wall may also lead to this condition. The anaesthetist may signal an unacceptable rise in the ventilatory pressure as the abdomen is closed but more commonly ACS develops on the critical care unit, some 12–30 hours after surgery. Oligoanuria and raised ventilatory pressures are the usual presenting features.

ACS can be detected simply by measuring the intravesical pressure. The bladder is filled with 50 mL of normal saline, after which the pressure is measured through the aspiration port of the catheter tubing using a transducer. With modest increases in abdominal pressure (20–25 mmHg) intravenous fluid therapy can offset lesser effects, but once a pressure of approximately 25–35 mmHg is reached, the abdomen will need to be decompressed and left open by the techniques discussed above. The presence of worsening organ failure is a further pointer towards surgery and any ongoing surgical issues will need to be managed appropriately when the abdomen is decompressed. If packs need to be removed then it will be necessary to ensure that clotting is corrected and that appropriate support for any specialist procedure (e.g. vascular, hepatobiliary) is available.

Intestinal fistulas

Intestinal fistulas pose their own particular problems and can greatly complicate patient management. They contribute to sepsis, malnutrition, fluid and electrolyte imbalances, difficulties in wound care, as well as posing an enormous psychological challenge to the patient.

A fistula is defined as an abnormal communication between two epithelial lined surfaces. There are many types and exhaustive description is beyond the remit of this chapter. The great majority of those seen within the context of severe abdominal sepsis follow surgery and result from anastomotic leakage or an inadvertent enterotomy, either overlooked or unsuccessfully repaired.

An intestinal fistula, from somewhere in the intestinal tract to the laparotomy wound, will occur occasionally in every gastrointestinal surgeon's practice, arising most commonly as a result of anastomotic leakage or bowel damage. While a few will show signs of severe sepsis, more often than not there is a period of apparent ileus, wound infection and clinical stagnation. When the wound ruptures or is opened to treat the infection, the enteric or faecal nature of the contents will become apparent. This may not be convincing to begin with as the enteric flow is usually preceded by a volume of pus and blood, as with most postoperative wound infections. Postoperative fistulas may also occur through

drains or along recent drain sites, to the vaginal vault (especially in those who have undergone previous hysterectomy) and occasionally to the rectum or other parts of the gut.

However, fistulas are more likely to occur after emergency surgery, usually carried out for another postoperative complication, commonly sepsis, obstruction or bleeding. In these operations, the inherent difficulty of the procedure, brought about by adhesions, bowel distension and softened tissues, makes further bowel damage a real possibility. If that damage is not, or cannot, be repaired effectively, if there is persisting obstruction of the intestine postoperatively, a postoperative phlegmon or an open abdomen, then the likelihood of fistulation escalates considerably. Postoperatively, the combination of small-bowel obstruction and an undrained abscess is also likely to result in a fistula as the obstructed bowel eventually softens and gives way at or into the collection. Thus it will be evident that repairing a leaking anastomosis once the patient is septic and local tissues oedematous and friable is all too often doomed to failure. Bowel exposed in an open abdomen will also invariably be subject to some degree of trauma unless the dressings or appliances are handled and changed expertly. Again, if there is distal obstruction, a local and exposed suture line or local trauma, a fistula will often occur. Perhaps 10–20% of 'laparostomies' will fistulate and this sometimes happens even with expert care.

A significant number of intestinal fistulas heal spontaneously, although they will cause misery and morbidity while they do so. The factors which contribute to persistence of a fistula are shown in Box 18.6.

The best-known approach to fistula care is that described at the specialist fistula unit in Salford,

Box 18.6 • Factors contributing to the occurrence and persistence of postoperative fistulas

Occurrence

Repaired anastomosis
Inadvertent enterotomy (repaired or missed)
New anastomosis in unfavourable circumstances
Persisting abscess or phlegmon causing obstruction
Fistulating disease
Open abdomen

Persistence

Distal obstruction (including constipation)
Open abdomen
Disconnected bowel ends
Local abscess
High output from fistula
Complex fistula
Mucocutaneous continuity

and known by the acronym SNAP (Sepsis, Nutrition, Anatomy, Procedure). The most pressing effects of a fistula relate to intra-abdominal sepsis. There can also be wound sepsis, usually in the form of cellulitis, although occasionally local necrosis can occur. Once the necessary resuscitation is in hand, an early priority is CT of the abdomen, preferably with both gut and intravenous contrast. The frequency of intra-abdominal abscess formation is high, in the region of 66%,[27] and often these are not evident clinically. Without diagnosis and control of the sepsis, the prognosis is bleak. Management strategies follow the principles outlined above.

Almost as urgent, and an integral part of early management, is wound care and control of the fistula effluent. When there is a small fistula orifice in a drain site or through part of a wound, the effluent can be controlled with a stoma bag. At the other extreme, when bowel contents are leaking into a laparostomy, management may be very difficult. Large fistula bags are available but even these may not be large enough for a new laparostomy. The author's unit often uses a sandwich dressing initially, as described above, with low-grade suction attached to soft rubber catheters placed near the fistula site. The same suction technique can be placed inside a fistula bag when appropriate in order to reduce the frequency of bag leakage. Commercially available vacuum dressings can also be of great assistance.

Important ancillary techniques include reducing fistula output by avoiding enteral feeding and reducing gastric acid output with proton-pump inhibitors. Codeine and loperamide can subsequently be used to contribute to this control of gut secretions. Octreotide will also significantly reduce gut secretion in some patients but, in the author's experience, its effect is inferior to the steps already described. It is perhaps most useful in pancreatic fistulas and upper small-bowel fistulas.

Immediate fluid management will have been considered as the patient was resuscitated but attention will have to turn rapidly to the optimal means of nutrition. The deleterious effect which enteral nutrition often has on output and wound care, particularly in the early stages, has been noted above. Additionally, enteral feeding may also 'feed' the abdominal sepsis, if there is complexity to the fistula with a further unrecognised proximal hole in the bowel. There is often partial obstruction associated with the sepsis and with most fistulas it is often better and more reliable to resort to parenteral nutrition while the patient stabilises and the situation with regard to sepsis, wound care and fistula anatomy each become clearer. Indeed, it is often better to see parenteral nutrition as the ongoing mainstay of nutritional support in intestinal fistulation with abdominal sepsis. In some circumstances, enteral nutrition can take over some, or even all, of the role, but this will usually take time and is only possible in selected patients.

Fistulas can be categorised as high or low output (high >500 mL per 24 hours). This cut-off represents a level above which the fistula is likely to have a significant effect on fluid balance and nutrition. Some proximal fistulas have outputs of one or more litres per day and fluid balance will be challenging in its own right. Senior surgical staff will need to commit to adequate supervision of the recording of the various inputs and outputs, particularly in the initial unstable and complicated phase of care. Fistula output will often reduce with time and, when possible, some healing begins to occur. A typical anastomotic wound fistula will be a side hole and if there is free distal flow, no sepsis, no bowel disease and no distal obstruction (or constipation), then healing may occur. It is unknown whether restricted oral intake helps, but it is intuitive to minimise the flow through the hole to encourage healing. As healing occurs, usually after 2–4 weeks, oral intake can be increased. If there is no healing by 6 weeks and no apparently reversible factor (e.g. abscess, constipation), then many would assume the fistula will not heal and allow more liberal oral intake.

In the ICU setting, once sepsis is excluded or controlled and the open abdomen, if present, is starting to granulate, oral or enteral feeding can begin cautiously, maintaining a careful watch for recurrent sepsis. The nutritional effect of this will depend on the length and condition of gut available for absorption and it will often take time for enteral feeding to be tolerated. During this phase, combined enteral and parenteral feeding is used.

It will be clear from the above that further surgery is usually only advocated to deal with abdominal sepsis. Further operations at this stage to try and correct the fistula often cause more harm than good through loss of bowel (risking short-bowel syndrome) or the creation of yet more fistulas. If surgery is undertaken then the approach follows that described above for abdominal sepsis. Surgery for fistulas is best deferred until the patient is well physically, nutritionally and emotionally, and only after the anatomy has been defined radiologically. This is often some months later and in complex cases is a highly specialist undertaking.

Chronic abdominal sepsis

Intestinal fistulas often settle down and can run a course of chronic abdominal sepsis where there is low-grade inflammation but no organ failure. This can be punctuated with further acute episodes and it may be difficult to be certain if the sepsis comes from the feeding line, urinary catheter, chest, wounds or abdomen. Unusual bacteria or fungi can be involved and occasionally less common sites become infected (e.g. myocardium or heart valves secondary to feeding lines). During this period there is a continuing requirement for close daily monitoring with senior surgical input, often for several months, if the patient is to recover. Ongoing parenteral nutrition is often integral to this and, again, the help of a specialist unit can be invaluable. In these units, the support of specialist nursing staff in maintaining sepsis-free nutrition and providing expert fistula care is fundamental to success. The overall recovery or otherwise of the patient will be indicated by the clinical and biochemical picture combined. A falling white count and C-reactive protein with a steady rise in the serum albumin, together with increasing general well-being, are all good signs. Further surgery should probably be deferred for at least 6 months after the last laparotomy in order to allow the abdomen to become less hostile, and prolapse of stomas or fistulas is a useful indicator that re-peritonealisation has occurred. Restorative surgery is still usually prolonged and difficult, and reconstructing the abdominal wall after laparostomy has its own difficulties.

The gastrointestinal tract in critical illness

Gastrointestinal diseases frequently cause abdominal sepsis and MODS. However, the gut may contribute to the deterioration of a patient with MODS or MOF even when their primary pathology involves other systems. Additionally, only 50% of patients with abdominal sepsis and MOF survive even when the septic focus has been eradicated successfully.[7] The gut may play a part in these phenomena: it may be the source of the 'second hit' that precipitates progression to MOF and some have labelled it the 'motor of multiple organ failure'.[28] Exposure to endotoxin or splanchnic reperfusion injury may increase mucosal permeability[29] and bacterial translocation[30] to reticuloendothelial tissue, where previously primed macrophages and Kupffer cells are activated. This hypothesis may explain why enteric bacteraemia is observed in MODS even when there is no obvious septic focus within the abdomen,[31] and why enteral nutrition may be protective.

Abdominal conditions that may complicate critical illness

Abdominal problems may complicate, as well as cause, serious illness. Signs may be subtle, particularly in ventilated patients, and a high index of clinical suspicion is necessary.

Acute massive gastric dilatation predisposes to aspiration and can limit diaphragmatic excursion and impair ventilation. If untreated, massive dilatation may progress to emphysematous gastric necrosis. Immediate treatment comprises support of breathing and nasogastric intubation.

Delayed gastric emptying is associated with diabetic autonomic neuropathy, subtotal gastrectomy, or gastroenterostomy performed for obstruction. Distal intestinal motility is usually normal but nasogastric intubation is required to prevent aspiration and facilitate fluid and electrolyte management. Intravenous metoclopramide (10 mg three times daily) or erythromycin (1 mg/kg four times daily) may hasten resolution, but recovery often takes several weeks, during which nutritional support will be required.

Postoperative small-bowel ileus usually resolves within days, regardless of the extent of bowel handling.[32] Drugs, especially opiates, or electrolyte abnormalities (hypokalaemia, uraemia) may delay resolution, but failure to progress may also indicate ongoing retroperitoneal or abdominal pathology. Ileus may be difficult to distinguish from adhesive obstruction, and contrast studies may clarify the situation (see also Chapter 5). Adhesive obstruction frequently resolves but refractory cases occasionally require laparotomy. However, in a hostile abdomen, such as found in abdominal sepsis, considerable caution should be exercised in subjecting the patient to further surgery.[21] Whereas a 5- to 7-day period of non-operative treatment might be acceptable in the presence of straightforward adhesion obstruction (and on occasions perhaps even longer if nutrition is supported), one should be prepared to wait for considerably longer when faced with a hostile abdomen, provided specific indications for surgery are not present. These indications include a known point of unrelieved obstruction or where there is a septic focus.

Colonic pseudo-obstruction (see also Chapter 10) is associated with chronic cardiorespiratory disease, a well as immobility, electrolyte abnormalities and fractures of the spine, pelvis and lower limbs. Distension may be dramatic but tenderness is uncommon. If massive colonic dilatation or peritonism develops, urgent exclusion of organic obstruction by contrast enema or endoscopy is necessary. Decompression may be achieved by rigid sigmoidoscopy or colonoscopy.

Severe illness, mechanical ventilation and coagulopathy predispose to peptic ulceration, and liberal prophylaxis with proton-pump inhibitor therapy is essential.

Sepsis and intravenous nutrition can produce non-specific derangements of liver biochemistry. Abnormal liver tests may also reflect infective hepatitis, liver abscesses, or drug or transfusion reactions. Imaging is indicated to exclude biliary obstruction and may also reveal occult collections, which might contribute to hepatic dysfunction. Urgent biliary decompression is required for extra-hepatic obstruction, particularly in the presence of cholangitis. In most other circumstances, treatment of liver dysfunction is supportive until resolution occurs. Cholestatic medication should be stopped, but intravenous nutrition can be continued unless liver function deteriorates. Encephalopathy, hypo-glycaemia, acidosis or coagulopathy may indicate hepatic decompensation and the need for special-ist hepatology care. Chronic liver disease or recent hepatic resection predispose to liver failure, and the link between hepatic and renal failure must not be ignored. Adequate hydration is essential and sodium overload must be avoided.

Nutrition in critical illness

Nutritional support will be required in the major-ity of critically ill patients (see Chapter 17). Enteral feeding is preferred because it is relatively safe, effi-cacious and economical; furthermore, it may pre-serve the gut mucosal barrier. Enteral nutrition is contraindicated in the presence of small-bowel ileus or when there is inadequate bowel available for absorption. In such circumstances parenteral nutri-tion is required. Jejunostomy catheters or nasojeju-nal tubes may allow enteral feeding, even when there is a proximal anastomosis or delayed gastric empty-ing, providing distal motility is adequate. Studies indicate that enteral feeding is safe not only imme-diately after surgery but also in acute pancreatitis, and neither ventilation nor absent bowel sounds are contraindications to enteral feeding providing gastric emptying is normal.

Nutrition as therapy

Starvation and parenteral nutrition are associated with compromised gut mucosal barrier function and bacterial translocation in animals. Whether or not similar events occur in humans, nutritional therapy has been proposed as a means to reduce the incidence of sepsis and there is now good evi-dence to support this. Early enteral nutrition has been shown to be associated with a reduction in infective complications (chest, urinary, abdominal) after blunt trauma,[33] and these findings have been supported by a meta-analysis of eight randomised prospective studies.[34]

The importance of early enteral feeding is now generally accepted, especially after injury, and many surgeons now place a feeding jejunostomy as part of appropriate trauma laparotomies.[33,34]

Several nutrients have been ascribed specific phar-macological properties in addition to their role as energy or nitrogen sources. Enteral feeds contain-ing arginine, omega-3 polyunsaturated fatty acids and ribonucleic acids may be beneficial for sep-tic patients. In animals, glutamine appears essen-tial to maintain mucosal integrity, and intravenous replacement reverses changes associated with star-vation or parenteral nutrition. However, evidence that glutamine-supplemented parenteral nutrition alters clinical outcome is still accumulating (see Chapter 17).

Key points

- Abdominal sepsis is a leading cause of death in acute surgical practice and cases still carry a high mortality.
- A systematic approach, based on a sound understanding of pathophysiology, is essential to successful sepsis management. Adequate resuscitation, safe, timely diagnosis, rapid definitive treatment, and accurate and ongoing reassessment are important parts of this system.
- Identifying and treating adequately the underlying cause of sepsis ('the septic focus') is fundamental to a successful outcome.
- Radiological intervention for localised sepsis is growing in importance.
- Indications for laparotomy include generalised peritonitis, necrotic tissue, multifocal abscesses and failure of radiological intervention.
- Re-laparotomy is often difficult and advanced techniques may be required.
- Abdominal sepsis often runs a prolonged course in which the surgeon will have to play an ongoing role.

References

1. Scottish Audit of Surgical Mortality 2005. http://www.sasm.org.uk/Reports/2005Report/ScottishAuditofSurgicalMortality2005_data.pdf

2. Friedman G, Silva E, Vincent JL. Has the mortality of septic shock changed with time. Crit Care Med 1998; 26:2078–86.

3. Zimmerman JE, Knauss WA, Wagner DP et al. A comparison of risks and outcomes for patients with organ system failure: 1982–90. Crit Care Med 1996; 24:1633–41.

4. Rangel-Frausto MS, Pittet D, Costigan M et al. The natural history of the systemic inflammatory response syndrome (SIRS). A prospective study. JAMA 1995; 273:117–23.

5. Pinskey MR, Vincent JL, Deviere J et al. Serum cytokine levels in human septic shock. Relation to multiple-system organ failure and mortality. Chest 1993; 103:565–75.

6. American College of Chest Physicians/Society of Critical Care Medicine Consensus Conference. Definitions for sepsis and organ failure and guidelines for the use of innovative therapies in sepsis. Crit Care Med 1992; 20:864–74.

7. McLauchlan GJ, Anderson, ID, Grant IS et al. Outcome of patients with abdominal sepsis treated in an intensive care unit. Br J Surg 1995; 82:524–9.

8. McCluskey A, Thomas AN, Bowles BJ et al. The prognostic value of serial measurements of serum albumin concentration in patients admitted to an intensive care unit. Anaesthesia 1996; 51:724–7.

9. Anderson ID. Assessing the critically ill surgical patient. In: Anderson ID (ed.) Care of the critically ill surgical patient. London: Arnold, 1999; pp. 7–15.

10. Boermeester MA. Surgical approaches to peritonitis. Br J Surg 2007; 94:1317–18.

11. Goldie AS, Fearon KCH, Ross JA et al. Natural cytokine antagonists and endogenous anti-endotoxin core antibodies in sepsis syndrome. JAMA 1995; 274:172–7.

12. Go HL, Baarslag HJ, Vermeulen H et al. A comparative study to validate the use of ultrasonography and computed tomography in patients with post-operative intra-abdominal sepsis. Eur J Radiol 2005; 54:383–7.

13. Constantinides VA, Tekkis PP, Senapati A et al Prospective multicentre evaluation of adverse outcomes following treatment for complicated diverticular disease. Br J Surg 2006; 93:1503–13.

14. Anderson ID, Fearon KCH, Grant IS. Laparotomy for abdominal sepsis in the critically ill. Br J Surg 1996; 83:535–9.

15. Bernard GR, Vincent JL, Laterre PF et al. Efficacy and safety of recombinant human activated protein C for severe sepsis. N Engl J Med 2001; 344:699–709.

16. van Goor H. Consequences and complications of peritoneal adhesions. Colorectal Dis 2007; 9(Suppl 2):25–34.

17. Barie PS, Fisher E. Acute acalculous cholecystitis. J Am Coll Surg 1995; 180:232–4.

18. Bassiouny HS. Non occlusive mesenteric ischaemia. Surg Clin North Am 1997; 77:319–26.

19. Robert JH, Mentha G, Rohner A. Ischaemic colitis: two distinct patterns of severity. Gut 1993; 34:4–6.

20. Willams NS, Scott ADN. Neutropenic colitis. Br J Surg 1997; 84:1200–5.

21. Sajja SB, Schein M. Early postoperative small bowel obstruction. Br J Surg 2004; 91(6):683–91.

22. Jansen JO, Loudon MA. Damage control surgery in a non-trauma setting. Br J Surg 2007; 94:789–90.

23. van Ruler O, Mahler CW, Boer KR et al. Comparison of on-demand vs planned relaparotomy strategy in patients with severe peritonitis: a randomized trial. JAMA 2007; 298:865–72.

A randomised trial of 232 patients which demonstrated that better results were associated with the re-laparotomy on-demand group.

24. Teubner A, Anderson ID, Scott NA. Intra-abdominal hypertension and the abdominal compartment syndrome. Br J Surg 2004; 91:1527.

25. Moore AFK, Hargest R, Martin M. Intra-abdominal hypertension and the abdominal compartment syndrome. Br J Surg 2004; 91:1102–10.

26. Hong JJ, Cohn SM, Perez JM et al. Prospective study of the incidence and outcome of intra-abdominal hypertension and the abdominal compartment syndrome. Br J Surg 2002; 89:591–6.

27. Harris CA, Nicholson DA, Anderson ID. Computed tomography: a vital adjunct in the management of complex postoperative abdominal sepsis Br J Surg 1998; 85:861–2.

28. Meakins JL, Marshall JC. The gut: the 'motor' of MOF. Arch Surg 1986; 121:197–201.

29. O'Dwyer ST, Michie HR, Zeigler TR et al. A single dose of endotoxin increases intestinal permeability in healthy humans. Arch Surg 1988; 123:1459–64.

30. Deitch EA, Berg R, Specian R. Endotoxin promotes the translocation of bacteria from the gut. Arch Surg 1987; 122:185–90.

31. Border JR, Hasset JM, LaDuca J et al. Gut origin in septic states in blunt multiple trauma (ISS-40) in the ICU. Ann Surg 1987; 206:427–48.

32. Condon RE, Cowles VE, Schulte WJ et al. Resolution of post-operative ileus in humans. Ann Surg 1986; 203:574–81.

33. Moore FA, Moore EE, Jones TN et al. TEN versus TPN following major torso trauma: reduced septic morbidity. J Trauma 1989; 29:916–23.

34. Moore FA, Feliciano DV, Andrassy RJ et al. Early enteral feeding compared with parenteral reduces postoperative septic complications: the results of a meta-analysis. Ann Surg 1992; 216:172–83.

Early enteral nutrition is associated with improved outcome after blunt abdominal trauma.

Index

M

S